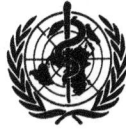

WORLD HEALTH ORGANIZATION

INTERNATIONAL AGENCY FOR RESEARCH ON CANCER

# IARC MONOGRAPHS

## ON THE

# EVALUATION OF CARCINOGENIC

# RISKS TO HUMANS

*Chromium, Nickel and Welding*

## VOLUME 49

This publication represents the views and expert opinions
of an IARC Working Group on the
Evaluation of Carcinogenic Risks to Humans,
which met in Lyon,

5–13 June 1989

1990

# IARC MONOGRAPHS

In 1969, the International Agency for Research on Cancer (IARC) initiated a programme on the evaluation of the carcinogenic risk of chemicals to humans involving the production of critically evaluated monographs on individual chemicals. In 1980 and 1986, the programme was expanded to include the evaluation of the carcinogenic risk associated with exposures to complex mixtures and other agents.

The objective of the programme is to elaborate and publish in the form of monographs critical reviews of data on carcinogenicity for agents to which humans are known to be exposed, and on specific exposure situations; to evaluate these data in terms of human risk with the help of international working groups of experts in chemical carcinogenesis and related fields; and to indicate where additional research efforts are needed.

This project is supported by PHS Grant No. 5 UO1 CA33193–07 awarded by the US National Cancer Institute, Department of Health and Human Services. Additional support has been provided since 1986 by the Commission of the European Communities.

ISBN 92 832 1249 5

ISSN 0250–9555

Distributed for the International Agency for Research on Cancer
by the Secretariat of the World Health Organization

PRINTED IN THE UK

# CONTENTS

# CONTENTS

# CONTENTS

# CONTENTS

# CONTENTS

# CONTENTS

## CONTENTS

# NOTE TO THE READER

The term 'carcinogenic risk' in the *IARC Monographs* series is taken to mean the probability that exposure to an agent will lead to cancer in humans.

Inclusion of an agent in the *Monographs* does not imply that it is a carcinogen, only that the published data have been examined. Equally, the fact that an agent has not yet been evaluated in a monograph does not mean that it is not carcinogenic.

The evaluations of carcinogenic risk are made by international working groups of independent scientists and are qualitative in nature. No recommendation is given for regulation or legislation.

Anyone who is aware of published data that may alter the evaluation of the carcinogenic risk of an agent to humans is encouraged to make this information available to the Unit of Carcinogen Identification and Evaluation, International Agency for Research on Cancer, 150 cours Albert Thomas, 69372 Lyon Cedex 08, France, in order that the agent may be considered for re-evaluation by a future Working Group.

Although every effort is made to prepare the monographs as accurately as possible, mistakes may occur. Readers are requested to communicate any errors to the Unit of Carcinogen Identification and Evaluation, so that corrections can be reported in future volumes.

# IARC WORKING GROUP ON THE EVALUATION OF CARCINOGENIC RISKS TO HUMANS: CHROMIUM, NICKEL AND WELDING

## Lyon, 5–13 June 1989

## LIST OF PARTICIPANTS

### Members[1]

A. Andersen, The Cancer Registry of Norway, Montebello, Oslo 3, Norway

D. Baker, Division of Environmental and Occupational Epidemiology, Department of Community Medicine, Mount Sinai School of Medicine, 1 Gustave L. Levy Place, Box 1057, New York, NY 10029, USA

D. Beyersmann, Division 2, Biochemistry, University of Bremen, 2800 Bremen 33, Federal Republic of Germany

M. Costa, Department of Environmental Medicine, New York University Medical Center, 550 First Avenue, New York, NY 10016, USA

S. de Flora, Institute of Hygiene and Preventive Medicine, University of Genoa, via Pastore 1, 16132 Genoa, Italy

J.P.W. Gilman, Biomedical Sciences Department, University of Guelph, Guelph, Ontario, Canada

P. Grandjean, Odense University, Institute of Community Health, Department of Environmental Medicine, J.B. Winsløws Vej 19, 5000 Odense C, Denmark

C.N. Gray, Institute of Occupational Health, University Road West, PO Box 363, Birmingham B15 2TT, UK

---

[1]Unable to attend: C.G. Elinder, Huddinge Hospital, Department of Renal Medicine, 141 86 Huddinge, Sweden; S. Langård, Telemark Central Hospital, Department of Occupational Medicine, Olavsgt 26, 39000 Porsgrunn, Norway

K.S. Kasprzak, Laboratory of Comparative Carcinogenesis, Division of Cancer Etiology, National Cancer Institute, NCI-FCRF Building 538, Room 205, Frederick, MD 21701, USA

L.S. Levy, Industrial Toxicology Unit, Institute of Occupational Health, University Road West, PO Box 363, Birmingham B15 2TT, UK

O. Møller Jensen, The Danish Cancer Registry, Rosenvaengets Hovedvej 35, 2100 Copenhagen Ø, Denmark (*Chairman*)

N.K. Mottet, Department of Pathology, SM-30, University of Washington, School of Medicine, Seattle, WA 98195, USA

T. Norseth, National Institute of Occupational Health, Gydas Vei No. 8, PO Box 8149 Dep, Oslo 1, Norway (*Vice-Chairman*)

J. Peto, Institute of Cancer Research, Division of Epidemiology, Clifton Avenue, Sutton, Surrey SM2 5PX, UK

K.-H. Schaller, University Institute for Occupational and Social Medicine, Schillerstrasse 25, 8520 Erlangen, FRG

L. Simonato, Centre of Environmental Carcinogenesis, University of Padua, via Facciolati 71, 35100 Padua, Italy

R. Stern, Occupational Health, World Health Organization, 8 Scherfigsvej, 2100 Copenhagen Ø, Denmark

F.W. Sunderman, Jr, Department of Laboratory Medicine, University of Connecticut School of Medicine, 263 Farmington Avenue, Farmington, CT 06032, USA

S. Swierenga, Genetic Toxicology Section, Bureau of Drug Research, Health Protection Branch, Health and Welfare Canada, Tunney's Pasture, Ottawa, Ontario K1A OL2, Canada

A. Tossavainen, Institute of Occupational Health, Topeliuksenkatu 41 a A, 00250 Helsinki, Finland

**Representatives and observers**

*Representative of the National Cancer Institute*

R.B. Hayes, Division of Cancer Etiology, National Cancer Institute, Executive Plaza North, Room 418, 6130 Executive Blvd, North Bethesda, MD 20892, USA

*Representative of Tracor Technology Resources Inc.*

S. Olin, Tracor Technology Resources Inc., 1601 Research Boulevard, Rockville, MD 20850, USA

*Representative of the Commission of the European Communities*

M. Draper/E. Krug, Commission of the European Communities, Health and Safety Directorate, Bâtiment Jean Monnet, BP 1907, 2920 Luxembourg

*Representative of the Chemical Manufacturers' Association*

M. Kennebeck, American Welding Society, 550 NW LeJeune Road, PO Box 351040, Miami, FL 33135, USA

*Representative of the Chromium Association*

M. Huvinen, Outokumpu Ltd, 00100 Helsinki, Finland

*Representative of the Institut de Soudure* (Welding Institute)

C. Bozec, ERAMET-SLN (Entreprise de Recherche et d'Activités — Métaux — Société Le Nickel), 33, avenue du Maine, 75755 Paris Cédex 15, France

*Representative of the Nickel Producers' Environmental Research Association*

J.S. Warner, Inco Limited, PO Box 44, Royal Trust Tower, Suite 220, Toronto-Dominion Centre, Toronto, Ontario M5K 1N4, Canada

## Secretariat

A. Aitio, Unit of Carcinogen Identification and Evaluation

E. Cardis, Unit of Biostatistics Research and Informatics

M.-J. Ghess, Unit of Carcinogen Identification and Evaluation

E. Heseltine, Lajarthe, Montignac, France

T. Kauppinen, Institute of Occupational Health, Topeliuksenkatu 41 a A, 00250 Helsinki, Finland

M. Kogevinas, Unit of Analytical Epidemiology

K. L'Abbé[1], Unit of Analytical Epidemiology

D. McGregor[2], 50 Standish Road, New Milford, CT 06776, USA

D. Mietton, Unit of Carcinogen Identification and Evaluation

R. Montesano, Unit of Mechanisms of Carcinogenesis

I. O'Neill, Unit of Environmental Carcinogenesis and Host Factors

C. Partensky, Unit of Carcinogen Identification and Evaluation

I. Peterschmitt, Unit of Carcinogen Identification and Evaluation, Geneva, Switzerland

T. Shirai, Unit of Mechanisms of Carcinogenesis

D. Shuker, Unit of Environmental Carcinogenesis and Host Factors

---

[1]Present address: Industrial Diseases Standard Panel, Ontario Ministry of Labour, 10 King Street East, 7th floor, Toronto, Ontario M5C 1C3, Canada

[2]Present address: International Agency for Research on Cancer, Unit of Carcinogen Identification and Evaluation

L. Shuker, Unit of Carcinogen Identification and Evaluation

E. Smith, International Programme on Chemical Safety, World Health Organization, 1211 Geneva 27, Switzerland

L. Tomatis, Director

V.S. Turusov, Cancer Research Centre, USSR Academy of Medical Sciences, Kashirskoye Shosse 24, 115478 Moscow, USSR

J.D. Wilbourn, Unit of Carcinogen Identification and Evaluation

H. Yamasaki, Unit of Mechanisms of Carcinogenesis

*Secretarial assistance*

J. Cazeaux

M. Lézère

M. Mainaud

S. Reynaud

# PREAMBLE

# IARC MONOGRAPHS PROGRAMME ON THE EVALUATION OF CARCINOGENIC RISKS TO HUMANS[1]

## PREAMBLE

### 1. BACKGROUND

In 1969, the International Agency for Research on Cancer (IARC) initiated a programme to evaluate the carcinogenic risk of chemicals to humans and to produce monographs on individual chemicals. The *Monographs* programme has since been expanded to include consideration of exposures to complex mixtures of chemicals (which occur, for example, in some occupations and as a result of human habits) and of exposures to other agents, such as radiation and viruses. With Supplement 6(1), the title of the series was modified from *IARC Monographs on the Evaluation of the Carcinogenic Risk of Chemicals to Humans* to *IARC Monographs on the Evaluation of Carcinogenic Risks to Humans*, in order to reflect the widened scope of the programme.

The criteria established in 1971 to evaluate carcinogenic risk to humans were adopted by the working groups whose deliberations resulted in the first 16 volumes of the *IARC Monographs* series. Those criteria were subsequently re-evaluated by working groups which met in 1977(2), 1978(3), 1979(4), 1982(5) and 1983(6). The present preamble was prepared by two working groups which met in September 1986 and January 1987, prior to the preparation of Supplement 7(7) to the *Monographs* and was modified by a working group which met in November 1988(8).

### 2. OBJECTIVE AND SCOPE

The objective of the programme is to prepare, with the help of international working groups of experts, and to publish in the form of monographs, critical

[1]This project is supported by PHS Grant No. 5 UO1 CA33193–07 awarded by the US National Cancer Institute, Department of Health and Human Services, and with a subcontract to Tracor Technology Resources, Inc. Since 1986, this programme has also been supported by the Commission of the European Communities.

reviews and evaluations of evidence on the carcinogenicity of a wide range of human exposures. The *Monographs* may also indicate where additional research efforts are needed.

The *Monographs* represent the first step in carcinogenic risk assessment, which involves examination of all relevant information in order to assess the strength of the available evidence that certain exposures could alter the incidence of cancer in humans. The second step is quantitative risk estimation, which is not usually attempted in the *Monographs*. Detailed, quantitative evaluations of epidemiological data may be made in the *Monographs*, but without extrapolation beyond the range of the data available. Quantitative extrapolation from experimental data to the human situation is not undertaken.

These monographs may assist national and international authorities in making risk assessments and in formulating decisions concerning any necessary preventive measures. The evaluations of IARC working groups are scientific, qualitative judgements about the degree of evidence for carcinogenicity provided by the available data on an agent. These evaluations represent only one part of the body of information on which regulatory measures may be based. Other components of regulatory decisions may vary from one situation to another and from country to country, responding to different socioeconomic and national priorities. *Therefore, no recommendation is given with regard to regulation or legislation, which are the responsibility of individual governments and/or other international organizations.*

The *IARC Monographs* are recognized as an authoritative source of information on the carcinogenicity of chemicals and complex exposures. A users' survey, made in 1988, indicated that the *Monographs* are consulted by various agencies in 57 countries. Each volume is generally printed in 4000 copies for distribution to governments, regulatory bodies and interested scientists. The *Monographs* are also available *via* the Distribution and Sales Service of the World Health Organization.

## 3.   SELECTION OF TOPICS FOR MONOGRAPHS

Topics are selected on the basis of two main criteria: (a) that they concern agents and complex exposures for which there is evidence of human exposure, and (b) that there is some evidence or suspicion of carcinogenicity. The term agent is used to include individual chemical compounds, groups of chemical compounds, physical agents (such as radiation) and biological factors (such as viruses) and mixtures of agents such as occur in occupational exposures and as a result of personal and cultural habits (like smoking and dietary practices). Chemical analogues and compounds with biological or physical characteristics similar to those of suspected carcinogens may also be considered, even in the absence of data on carcinogenicity.

The scientific literature is surveyed for published data relevant to an assessment of carcinogenicity; the IARC surveys of chemicals being tested for carcinogenicity(9) and directories of on-going research in cancer epidemiology(10) often indicate those exposures that may be scheduled for future meetings. Ad-hoc working groups convened by IARC in 1984 and 1989 gave recommendations as to which chemicals and exposures to complex mixtures should be evaluated in the *IARC Monographs* series(11,12).

As significant new data on subjects on which monographs have already been prepared become available, re-evaluations are made at subsequent meetings, and revised monographs are published.

## 4.   DATA FOR MONOGRAPHS

The *Monographs* do not necessarily cite all the literature concerning the subject of an evaluation. Only those data considered by the Working Group to be relevant to making the evaluation are included.

With regard to biological and epidemiological data, only reports that have been published or accepted for publication in the openly available scientific literature are reviewed by the working groups. In certain instances, government agency reports that have undergone peer review and are widely available are considered. Exceptions may be made on an ad-hoc basis to include unpublished reports that are in their final form and publicly available, if their inclusion is considered pertinent to making a final evaluation (see pp. 33 *et seq.*). In the sections on chemical and physical properties and on production, use, occurrence and analysis, unpublished sources of information may be used.

## 5.   THE WORKING GROUP

Reviews and evaluations are formulated by a working group of experts. The tasks of this group are five-fold: (i) to ascertain that all appropriate data have been collected; (ii) to select the data relevant for the evaluation on the basis of scientific merit; (iii) to prepare accurate summaries of the data to enable the reader to follow the reasoning of the Working Group; (iv) to evaluate the results of experimental and epidemiological studies; and (v) to make an overall evaluation of the carcinogenicity of the exposure to humans.

Working Group participants who contributed to the considerations and evaluations within a particular volume are listed, with their addresses, at the beginning of each publication. Each participant who is a member of a working group serves as an individual scientist and not as a representative of any organization, government or industry. In addition, representatives from national and international agencies and industrial associations are invited as observers.

## 6.   WORKING PROCEDURES

Approximately one year in advance of a meeting of a working group, the topics of the monographs are announced and participants are selected by IARC staff in consultation with other experts. Subsequently, relevant biological and epidemiological data are collected by IARC from recognized sources of information on carcinogenesis, including data storage and retrieval systems such as Chemical Abstracts, Medline and Toxline — including EMIC and ETIC for data on genetic and related effects and teratogenicity, respectively.

The major collection of data and the preparation of first drafts of the sections on chemical and physical properties, on production and use, on occurrence, and on analysis are carried out under a separate contract funded by the US National Cancer Institute. Efforts are made to supplement this information with data from other national and international sources. Representatives from industrial associations may assist in the preparation of sections on production and use.

Production and trade data are obtained from governmental and trade publications and, in some cases, by direct contact with industries. Separate production data on some agents may not be available because their publication could disclose confidential information. Information on uses is usually obtained from published sources but is often complemented by direct contact with manufacturers.

Six months before the meeting, reference material is sent to experts, or is used by IARC staff, to prepare sections for the first drafts of monographs. The complete first drafts are compiled by IARC staff and sent, prior to the meeting, to all participants of the Working Group for review.

The Working Group meets in Lyon for seven to eight days to discuss and finalize the texts of the monographs and to formulate the evaluations. After the meeting, the master copy of each monograph is verified by consulting the original literature, edited and prepared for publication. The aim is to publish monographs within nine months of the Working Group meeting.

## 7.   EXPOSURE DATA

Sections that indicate the extent of past and present human exposure, the sources of exposure, the persons most likely to be exposed and the factors that contribute to exposure to the agent, mixture or exposure circumstance are included at the beginning of each monograph.

Most monographs on individual chemicals or complex mixtures include sections on chemical and physical data, and production, use, occurrence and analysis. In other monographs, for example on physical agents, biological factors, occupational exposures and cultural habits, other sections may be included, such as: historical perspectives, description of an industry or habit, exposures in the work place or chemistry of the complex mixture.

The Chemical Abstracts Services Registry Number, the latest Chemical Abstracts Primary Name and the IUPAC Systematic Name are recorded. Other synonyms and trade names are given, but the list is not necessarily comprehensive.

Some of the trade names may be those of mixtures in which the agent being evaluated is only one of the ingredients.

Information on chemical and physical properties and, in particular, data relevant to identification, occurrence and biological activity are included. A separate description of technical products gives relevant specifications and includes available information on composition and impurities.

The dates of first synthesis and of first commercial production of an agent or mixture are provided; for agents which do not occur naturally, this information may allow a reasonable estimate to be made of the date before which no human exposure to the agent could have occurred. The dates of first reported occurrence of an exposure are also provided. In addition, methods of synthesis used in past and present commercial production and different methods of production which may give rise to different impurities are described.

Data on production, foreign trade and uses are obtained for representative regions, which usually include Europe, Japan and the USA. It should not, however, be inferred that those areas or nations are necessarily the sole or major sources or users of the agent being evaluated.

Some identified uses may not be current or major applications, and the coverage is not necessarily comprehensive. In the case of drugs, mention of their therapeutic uses does not necessarily represent current practice nor does it imply judgement as to their clinical efficacy.

Information on the occurrence of an agent or mixture in the environment is obtained from data derived from the monitoring and surveillance of levels in occupational environments, air, water, soil, foods and animal and human tissues. When available, data on the generation, persistence and bioaccumulation are also included. In the case of mixtures, industries, occupations or processes, information is given about all agents present. For processes, industries and occupations, a historical description is also given, noting variations in chemical composition, physical properties or levels of occupational exposure with time.

Statements concerning regulations and guidelines (e.g., pesticide registrations, maximal levels permitted in foods, occupational exposure limits) are included for some countries as indications of potential exposures, but they may not reflect the most recent situation, since such limits are continuously reviewed and modified. The absence of information on regulatory status for a country should not be taken to imply that that country does not have regulations with regard to the exposure.

The purpose of the section on analysis is to give the reader an overview of current methods cited in the literature, with emphasis on those widely used for regulatory purposes. No critical evaluation or recommendation of any of the methods is meant or implied. Methods for monitoring human exposure are also given, when available. The IARC publishes a series of volumes, *Environmental Carcinogens: Methods of Analysis and Exposure Measurement(13)*, that describe validated methods for analysing a wide variety of agents and mixtures.

## 8. BIOLOGICAL DATA RELEVANT TO THE EVALUATION OF CARCINOGENICITY TO HUMANS

The term 'carcinogen' is used in these monographs to denote an agent or mixture that is capable of increasing the incidence of malignant neoplasms; the induction of benign neoplasms may in some circumstances (see p. 26) contribute to the judgement that the exposure is carcinogenic. The terms 'neoplasm' and 'tumour' are used interchangeably.

Some epidemiological and experimental studies indicate that different agents may act at different stages in the carcinogenic process, probably by fundamentally different mechanisms. In the present state of knowledge, the aim of the *Monographs* is to evaluate evidence of carcinogenicity at any stage in the carcinogenic process independently of the underlying mechanism involved. There is as yet insufficient information to implement classification according to mechanisms of action(6).

Definitive evidence of carcinogenicity in humans can be provided only by epidemiological studies. Evidence relevant to human carcinogenicity may also be provided by experimental studies of carcinogenicity in animals and by other biological data, particularly those relating to humans.

The available studies are summarized by the Working Group, with particular regard to the qualitative aspects discussed below. In general, numerical findings are indicated as they appear in the original report; units are converted when necessary for easier comparison. The Working Group may conduct additional analyses of the published data and use them in their assessment of the evidence and may include them in their summary of a study; the results of such supplementary analyses are given in square brackets. Any comments are also made in square brackets; however, these are kept to a minimum, being restricted to those instances in which it is felt that an important aspect of a study, directly impinging on its interpretation, should be brought to the attention of the reader.

For experimental studies with mixtures, consideration is given to the possibility of changes in the physicochemical properties of the test substance during collection, storage, extraction, concentration and delivery. Either chemical or toxicological interactions of the components of mixtures may result in nonlinear dose-response relationships.

An assessment is made as to the relevance to human exposure of samples tested in experimental systems, which may involve consideration of: (i) physical and chemical characteristics, (ii) constituent substances that indicate the presence of a class of substances, (iii) tests for genetic and related effects, including genetic activity profiles, (iv) DNA adduct profiles, (v) oncogene expression and mutation; suppressor gene inactivation.

## 9. EVIDENCE FOR CARCINOGENICITY IN EXPERIMENTAL ANIMALS

For several agents (e.g., 4-aminobiphenyl, bis(chloromethyl)ether, diethylstilboestrol, melphalan, 8-methoxypsoralen (methoxsalen) plus ultra-violet radiation, mustard gas and vinyl chloride), evidence of carcinogenicity in experimental animals preceded evidence obtained from epidemiological studies or case reports. Information compiled from the first 41 volumes of the *IARC Monographs*(14) shows that, of the 44 agents and mixtures for which there is *sufficient* or *limited evidence* of carcinogenicity to humans (see p. 34), all 37 that have been tested adequately experimentally produce cancer in at least one animal species. Although this association cannot establish that all agents and mixtures that cause cancer in experimental animals also cause cancer in humans, nevertheless, *in the absence of adequate data on humans, it is biologically plausible and prudent to regard agents and mixtures for which there is sufficient evidence of carcinogenicity in experimental animals (see pp. 34-35) as if they presented a carcinogenic risk to humans.*

The monographs are not intended to summarize all published studies. Those that are inadequate (e.g., too short a duration, too few animals, poor survival; see below) or are judged irrelevant to the evaluation are generally omitted. They may be mentioned briefly, particularly when the information is considered to be a useful supplement to that of other reports or when they provide the only data available. Their inclusion does not, however, imply acceptance of the adequacy of the experimental design or of the analysis and interpretation of their results. Guidelines for adequate long-term carcinogenicity experiments have been outlined (e.g., 15).

The nature and extent of impurities or contaminants present in the agent or mixture being evaluated are given when available. Mention is made of all routes of exposure that have been adequately studied and of all species in which relevant experiments have been performed. Animal strain, sex, numbers per group, age at start of treatment and survival are reported.

Experiments in which the agent or mixture was administered in conjunction with known carcinogens or factors that modify carcinogenic effects are also reported. Experiments on the carcinogenicity of known metabolites and derivatives may be included.

### (a) Qualitative aspects

An assessment of carcinogenicity involves several considerations of qualitative importance, including (i) the experimental conditions under which the test was performed, including route and schedule of exposure, species, strain, sex, age, duration of follow-up; (ii) the consistency of the results, for example, across species and target organ(s); (iii) the spectrum of neoplastic response, from benign tumours to malignant neoplasms; and (iv) the possible role of modifying factors.

Considerations of importance to the Working Group in the interpretation and evaluation of a particular study include: (i) how clearly the agent was defined and, in the case of mixtures, how adequately the sample characterization was reported; (ii) whether the dose was adequately monitored, particularly in inhalation experiments; (iii) whether the doses used were appropriate and whether the survival of treated animals was similar to that of controls; (iv) whether there were adequate numbers of animals per group; (v) whether animals of both sexes were used; (vi) whether animals were allocated randomly to groups; (vii) whether the duration of observation was adequate; and (viii) whether the data were adequately reported. If available, recent data on the incidence of specific tumours in historical controls, as well as in concurrent controls, should be taken into account in the evaluation of tumour response.

When benign tumours occur together with and originate from the same cell type in an organ or tissue as malignant tumours in a particular study and appear to represent a stage in the progression to malignancy, it may be valid to combine them in assessing tumour incidence. The occurrence of lesions presumed to be preneoplastic may in certain instances aid in assessing the biological plausibility of any neoplastic response observed.

Of the many agents and mixtures that have been studied extensively, few induced only benign neoplasms. Benign tumours in experimental animals frequently represent a stage in the evolution of a malignant neoplasm, but they may be 'endpoints' that do not readily undergo transition to malignancy. However, if an agent or mixture is found to induce only benign neoplasms, it should be suspected of being a carcinogen and it requires further investigation.

### (b)   Quantitative aspects

The probability that tumours will occur may depend on the species and strain, the dose of the carcinogen and the route and period of exposure. Evidence of an increased incidence of neoplasms with increased level of exposure strengthens the inference of a causal association between the exposure and the development of neoplasms.

The form of the dose-response relationship can vary widely, depending on the particular agent under study and the target organ. Since many chemicals require metabolic activation before being converted into their reactive intermediates, both metabolic and pharmacokinetic aspects are important in determining the dose-response pattern. Saturation of steps such as absorption, activation, inactivation and elimination of the carcinogen may produce nonlinearity in the dose-response relationship, as could saturation of processes such as DNA repair(16,17).

*(c)  Statistical analysis of long-term experiments in animals*

Factors considered by the Working Group include the adequacy of the information given for each treatment group: (i) the number of animals studied and the number examined histologically, (ii) the number of animals with a given tumour type and (iii) length of survival. The statistical methods used should be clearly stated and should be the generally accepted techniques refined for this purpose(17,18). When there is no difference in survival between control and treatment groups, the Working Group usually compares the proportions of animals developing each tumour type in each of the groups. Otherwise, consideration is given as to whether or not appropriate adjustments have been made for differences in survival. These adjustments can include: comparisons of the proportions of tumour-bearing animals among the 'effective number' of animals alive at the time the first tumour is discovered, in the case where most differences in survival occur before tumours appear; life-table methods, when tumours are visible or when they may be considered 'fatal' because mortality rapidly follows tumour development; and the Mantel-Haenszel test or logistic regression, when occult tumours do not affect the animals' risk of dying but are 'incidental' findings at autopsy.

In practice, classifying tumours as fatal or incidental may be difficult. Several survival-adjusted methods have been developed that do not require this distinction(17), although they have not been fully evaluated.

## 10.  OTHER RELEVANT DATA IN EXPERIMENTAL SYSTEMS AND IN HUMANS

*(a)  Structure-activity considerations*

This section describes structure-activity correlations that are relevant to an evaluation of the carcinogenicity of an agent.

*(b)  Absorption, distribution, excretion and metabolism*

Concise information is given on absorption, distribution (including placental transfer) and excretion. Kinetic factors that may affect the dose-reponse relationship, such as saturation of uptake, protein binding, metabolic activation, detoxification and DNA repair processes, are mentioned. Studies that indicate the metabolic fate of the agent in experimental animals and humans are summarized briefly, and comparisons of data from animals and humans are made when possible. Comparative information on the relationship between exposure and the dose that reaches the target site may be of particular importance for extrapolation between species.

*(c)  Toxicity*

Data are given on acute and chronic toxic effects (other than cancer), such as organ toxicity, immunotoxicity, endocrine effects and preneoplastic lesions. Effects on reproduction, teratogenicity, feto- and embryotoxicity are also summarized briefly.

### (d)  Genetic and related effects

Tests of genetic and related effects may indicate possible carcinogenic activity. They can also be used in detecting active metabolites of known carcinogens in human or animal body fluids, in detecting active components in complex mixtures and in the elucidation of possible mechanisms of carcinogenesis.

The adequacy of the reporting of sample characterization is considered and, where necessary, commented upon. The available data are interpreted critically by phylogenetic group according to the endpoints detected, which may include DNA damage, gene mutation, sister chromatid exchange, micronuclei, chromosomal aberrations, aneuploidy and cell transformation. The concentrations (doses) employed are given and mention is made of whether an exogenous metabolic system was required. When appropriate, these data may be represented by bar graphs (activity profiles), with corresponding summary tables and listings of test systems, data and references. Detailed information on the preparation of these profiles is given in an appendix to those volumes in which they are used.

Positive results in tests using prokaryotes, lower eukaryotes, plants, insects and cultured mammalian cells suggest that genetic and related effects (and therefore possibly carcinogenic effects) could occur in mammals. Results from such tests may also give information about the types of genetic effect produced and about the involvement of metabolic activation. Some endpoints described are clearly genetic in nature (e.g., gene mutations and chromosomal aberrations), others are to a greater or lesser degree associated with genetic effects (e.g., unscheduled DNA synthesis). In-vitro tests for tumour-promoting activity and for cell transformation may detect changes that are not necessarily the result of genetic alterations but that may have specific relevance to the process of carcinogenesis. A critical appraisal of these tests has been published(15).

Genetic or other activity detected in the systems mentioned above is not always manifest in whole mammals. Positive indications of genetic effects in experimental mammals and in humans are regarded as being of greater relevance than those in other organisms. The demonstration that an agent or mixture can induce gene and chromosomal mutations in whole mammals indicates that it may have the potential for carcinogenic activity, although this activity may not be detectably expressed in any or all species tested. Relative potency in tests for mutagenicity and related effects is not a reliable indicator of carcinogenic potency. Negative results in tests for mutagenicity in selected tissues from animals treated *in vivo* provide less weight, partly because they do not exclude the possibility of an effect in tissues other than those examined. Moreover, negative results in short-term tests with genetic endpoints cannot be considered to provide evidence to rule out carcinogenicity of agents or mixtures that act through other mechanisms. Factors may arise in many tests that could give misleading results; these have been discussed in detail elsewhere(15).

The adequacy of epidemiological studies of reproductive outcomes and genetic and related effects in humans is evaluated by the same criteria as are applied to epidemiological studies of cancer.

## 11. EVIDENCE FOR CARCINOGENICITY IN HUMANS

### (a) Types of studies considered

Three types of epidemiological studies of cancer contribute data to the assessment of carcinogenicity in humans — cohort studies, case-control studies and correlation studies. Rarely, results from randomized trials may be available. Case reports of cancer in humans are also reviewed.

Cohort and case-control studies relate individual exposures under study to the occurrence of cancer in individuals and provide an estimate of relative risk (ratio of incidence in those exposed to incidence in those not exposed) as the main measure of association.

In correlation studies, the units of investigation are usually whole populations (e.g., in particular geographical areas or at particular times), and cancer frequency is related to a summary measure of the exposure of the population to the agent, mixture or exposure circumstance under study. Because individual exposure is not documented, however, a causal relationship is less easy to infer from correlation studies than from cohort and case-control studies.

Case reports generally arise from a suspicion, based on clinical experience, that the concurrence of two events — that is, a particular exposure and occurrence of a cancer — has happened rather more frequently than would be expected by chance. Case reports usually lack complete ascertainment of cases in any population, definition or enumeration of the population at risk and estimation of the expected number of cases in the absence of exposure.

The uncertainties surrounding interpretation of case reports and correlation studies make them inadequate, except in rare instances, to form the sole basis for inferring a causal relationship. When taken together with case-control and cohort studies, however, relevant case reports or correlation studies may add materially to the judgement that a causal relationship is present.

Epidemiological studies of benign neoplasms and presumed preneoplastic lesions are also reviewed by working groups. They may, in some instances, strengthen inferences drawn from studies of cancer itself.

*(b)  Quality of studies considered*

It is necessary to take into account the possible roles of bias, confounding and chance in the interpretation of epidemiological studies. By 'bias' is meant the operation of factors in study design or execution that lead erroneously to a stronger or weaker association than in fact exists between disease and an agent, mixture or exposure circumstance. By 'confounding' is meant a situation in which the relationship with disease is made to appear stronger or to appear weaker than it truly is as a result of an association between the apparent causal factor and another factor that is associated with either an increase or decrease in the incidence of the disease. In evaluating the extent to which these factors have been minimized in an individual study, working groups consider a number of aspects of design and analysis as described in the report of the study. Most of these considerations apply equally to case-control, cohort and correlation studies. Lack of clarity of any of these aspects in the reporting of a study can decrease its credibility and its consequent weighting in the final evaluation of the exposure.

Firstly, the study population, disease (or diseases) and exposure should have been well defined by the authors. Cases in the study population should have been identified in a way that was independent of the exposure of interest, and exposure should have been assessed in a way that was not related to disease status.

Secondly, the authors should have taken account in the study design and analysis of other variables that can influence the risk of disease and may have been related to the exposure of interest. Potential confounding by such variables should have been dealt with either in the design of the study, such as by matching, or in the analysis, by statistical adjustment. In cohort studies, comparisons with local rates of disease may be more appropriate than those with national rates. Internal comparisons of disease frequency among individuals at different levels of exposure should also have been made in the study.

Thirdly, the authors should have reported the basic data on which the conclusions are founded, even if sophisticated statistical analyses were employed. At the very least, they should have given the numbers of exposed and unexposed cases and controls in a case-control study and the numbers of cases observed and expected in a cohort study. Further tabulations by time since exposure began and other temporal factors are also important. In a cohort study, data on all cancer sites and all causes of death should have been given, to avoid the possibility of reporting bias. In a case-control study, the effects of investigated factors other than the exposure of interest should have been reported.

Finally, the statistical methods used to obtain estimates of relative risk, absolute cancer rates, confidence intervals and significance tests, and to adjust for confounding should have been clearly stated by the authors. The methods used should preferably have been the generally accepted techniques that have been refined since the mid-1970s. These methods have been reviewed for case-control studies(19) and for cohort studies(20).

### (c)  Quantitative considerations

Detailed analyses of both relative and absolute risks in relation to age at first exposure and to temporal variables, such as time since first exposure, duration of exposure and time since exposure ceased, are reviewed and summarized when available. The analysis of temporal relationships can provide a useful guide in formulating models of carcinogenesis. In particular, such analyses may suggest whether a carcinogen acts early or late in the process of carcinogenesis(6), although such speculative inferences cannot be used to draw firm conclusions concerning the mechanism of action and hence the shape (linear or otherwise) of the dose-response relationship below the range of observation.

### (d)  Criteria for causality

After the quality of individual epidemiological studies has been summarized and assessed, a judgement is made concerning the strength of evidence that the agent, mixture or exposure circumstance in question is carcinogenic for humans. In making their judgement, the Working Group considers several criteria for causality. A strong association (i.e., a large relative risk) is more likely to indicate causality than a weak association, although it is recognized that relative risks of small magnitude do not imply lack of causality and may be important if the disease is common. Associations that are replicated in several studies of the same design or using different epidemiological approaches or under different circumstances of exposure are more likely to represent a causal relationship than isolated observations from single studies. If there are inconsistent results among investigations, possible reasons are sought (such as differences in amount of exposure), and results of studies judged to be of high quality are given more weight than those from studies judged to be methodologically less sound. When suspicion of carcinogenicity arises largely from a single study, these data are not combined with those from later studies in any subsequent reassessment of the strength of the evidence.

If the risk of the disease in question increases with the amount of exposure, this is considered to be a strong indication of causality, although absence of a graded response is not necessarily evidence against a causal relationship. Demonstration of a decline in risk after cessation of or reduction in exposure in individuals or in whole populations also supports a causal interpretation of the findings.

Although a carcinogen may act upon more than one target, the specificity of an association (i.e., an increased occurrence of cancer at one anatomical site or of one morphological type) adds plausibility to a causal relationship, particularly when excess cancer occurrence is limited to one morphological type within the same organ.

Although rarely available, results from randomized trials showing different rates among exposed and unexposed individuals provide particularly strong evidence for causality.

When several epidemiological studies show little or no indication of an association between an exposure and cancer, the judgement may be made that, in the aggregate, they show evidence of lack of carcinogenicity. Such a judgement requires first of all that the studies giving rise to it meet, to a sufficient degree, the standards of design and analysis described above. Specifically, the possibility that bias, confounding or misclassification of exposure or outcome could explain the observed results should be considered and excluded with reasonable certainty. In addition, all studies that are judged to be methodologically sound should be consistent with a relative risk of unity for any observed level of exposure and, when considered together, should provide a pooled estimate of relative risk which is at or near unity and has a narrow confidence interval, due to sufficient population size. Moreover, no individual study nor the pooled results of all the studies should show any consistent tendency for relative risk of cancer to increase with increasing level of exposure. It is important to note that evidence of lack of carcinogenicity obtained in this way from several epidemiological studies can apply only to the type(s) of cancer studied and to dose levels and intervals between first exposure and observation of disease that are the same as or less than those observed in all the studies. Experience with human cancer indicates that, in some cases, the period from first exposure to the development of clinical cancer is seldom less than 20 years; latent periods substantially shorter than 30 years cannot provide evidence for lack of carcinogenicity.

## 12. SUMMARY OF DATA REPORTED

In this section, the relevant experimental and epidemiological data are summarized. Only reports, other than in abstract form, that meet the criteria outlined on p. 21 are considered for evaluating carcinogenicity. Inadequate studies are generally not summarized: such studies are usually identified by a square-bracketed comment in the text.

### (a) Exposures

Human exposure is summarized on the basis of elements such as production, use, occurrence in the environment and determinations in human tissues and body fluids. Quantitative data are given when available.

### (b) Experimental carcinogenicity data

Data relevant to the evaluation of carcinogenicity in animals are summarized. For each animal species and route of administration, it is stated whether an increased incidence of neoplasms was observed, and the tumour sites are indicated. If the agent or mixture produced tumours after prenatal exposure or in single-dose experiments, this is also indicated. Dose-response and other quantitative data may be given when available. Negative findings are also summarized.

### (c) Human carcinogenicity data

Results of epidemiological studies that are considered to be pertinent to an assessment of human carcinogenicity are summarized. When relevant, case reports and correlation studies are also considered.

### (d) Other relevant data

Structure-activity correlations are mentioned when relevant.

Toxicological information and data on kinetics and metabolism in experimental animals are given when considered relevant. The results of tests for genetic and related effects are summarized for whole mammals, cultured mammalian cells and nonmammalian systems.

Data on other biological effects in humans of particular relevance are summarized. These may include kinetic and metabolic considerations and evidence of DNA binding, persistence of DNA lesions or genetic damage in exposed humans.

When available, comparisons of such data for humans and for animals, and particularly animals that have developed cancer, are described.

## 13. EVALUATION

Evaluations of the strength of the evidence for carcinogenicity arising from human and experimental animal data are made, using standard terms.

It is recognized that the criteria for these evaluations, described below, cannot encompass all of the factors that may be relevant to an evaluation of carcinogenicity. In considering all of the relevant data, the Working Group may assign the agent, mixture or exposure circumstance to a higher or lower category than a strict interpretation of these criteria would indicate.

### (a) Degrees of evidence for carcinogenicity in humans and in experimental animals and supporting evidence

It should be noted that these categories refer only to the strength of the evidence that an exposure is carcinogenic and not to the extent of its carcinogenic activity (potency) nor to the mechanism involved. A classification may change as new information becomes available.

An evaluation of degree of evidence, whether for a single substance or a mixture, is limited to the materials tested, and these are chemically and physically defined. When the materials evaluated are considered by the Working Group to be sufficiently closely related, they may be grouped for the purpose of a single evaluation of degree of evidence.

(i)   *Human carcinogenicity data*

The applicability of an evaluation of the carcinogenicity of a mixture, process, occupation or industry on the basis of evidence from epidemiological studies depends on the variability over time and place of the mixtures, processes, occupations and industries. The Working Group seeks to identify the specific exposure, process or activity which is considered most likely to be responsible for any excess risk. The evaluation is focused as narrowly as the available data on exposure and other aspects permit.

The evidence relevant to carcinogenicity from studies in humans is classified into one of the following categories:

*Sufficient evidence of carcinogenicity*: The Working Group considers that a causal relationship has been established between exposure to the agent, mixture or exposure circumstance and human cancer. That is, a positive relationship has been observed between the exposure and cancer in studies in which chance, bias and confounding could be ruled out with reasonable confidence.

*Limited evidence of carcinogenicity*: A positive association has been observed between exposure to the agent, mixture or exposure circumstance and cancer for which a causal interpretation is considered by the Working Group to be credible, but chance, bias or confounding could not be ruled out with reasonable confidence.

*Inadequate evidence of carcinogenicity*: The available studies are of insufficient quality, consistency or statistical power to permit a conclusion regarding the presence or absence of a causal association.

*Evidence suggesting lack of carcinogenicity*: There are several adequate studies covering the full range of levels of exposure that human beings are known to encounter, which are mutually consistent in not showing a positive association between exposure to the agent, mixture or exposure circumstance and any studied cancer at any observed level of exposure. A conclusion of 'evidence suggesting lack of carcinogenicity' is inevitably limited to the cancer sites, conditions and levels of exposure and length of observation covered by the available studies. In addition, the possibility of a very small risk at the levels of exposure studied can never be excluded.

In some instances, the above categories may be used to classify the degree of evidence for carcinogenicity for specific organs or tissues.

(ii)   *Experimental carcinogenicity data*

The evidence relevant to carcinogenicity in experimental animals is classified into one of the following categories:

*Sufficient evidence of carcinogenicity*: The Working Group considers that a causal relationship has been established between the agent or mixture and an increased incidence of malignant neoplasms or of an appropriate combination of benign and malignant neoplasms (as described on p. 26) in (a) two or more species of animals or (b) in two or more independent studies in one species carried out at different times or in different laboratories or under different protocols.

Exceptionally, a single study in one species might be considered to provide sufficient evidence of carcinogenicity when malignant neoplasms occur to an unusual degree with regard to incidence, site, type of tumour or age at onset.

In the absence of adequate data on humans, it is biologically plausible and prudent to regard agents and mixtures for which there is *sufficient evidence* of carcinogenicity in experimental animals as if they presented a carcinogenic risk to humans.

*Limited evidence of carcinogenicity.* The data suggest a carcinogenic effect but are limited for making a definitive evaluation because, e.g., (a) the evidence of carcinogenicity is restricted to a single experiment; or (b) there are unresolved questions regarding the adequacy of the design, conduct or interpretation of the study; or (c) the agent or mixture increases the incidence only of benign neoplasms or lesions of uncertain neoplastic potential, or of certain neoplasms which may occur spontaneously in high incidences in certain strains.

*Inadequate evidence of carcinogenicity.* The studies cannot be interpreted as showing either the presence or absence of a carcinogenic effect because of major qualitative or quantitative limitations.

*Evidence suggesting lack of carcinogenicity.* Adequate studies involving at least two species are available which show that, within the limits of the tests used, the agent or mixture is not carcinogenic. A conclusion of evidence suggesting lack of carcinogenicity is inevitably limited to the species, tumour sites and levels of exposure studied.

(iii)  *Supporting evidence of carcinogenicity*

Other evidence judged to be relevant to an evaluation of carcinogenicity and of sufficient importance to affect the overall evaluation is then described. This may include data on tumour pathology, genetic and related effects, structure-activity relationships, metabolism and pharmacokinetics, physicochemical parameters, chemical composition and possible mechanisms of action. For complex exposures, including occupational and industrial exposures, the potential contribution of carcinogens known to be present as well as the relevance of materials tested are considered by the Working Group in its overall evaluation of human carcinogenicity. The Working Group also determines to what extent the materials tested in experimental systems are relevant to those to which humans are exposed. The available experimental evidence may help to specify more precisely the causal factor(s).

*(b)  Overall evaluation*

Finally, the body of evidence is considered as a whole, in order to reach an overall evaluation of the carcinogenicity to humans of an agent, mixture or circumstance of exposure.

An evaluation may be made for a group of chemical compounds that have been evaluated by the Working Group. In addition, when supporting data indicate that other, related compounds for which there is no direct evidence of capacity to induce cancer in animals or in humans may also be carcinogenic, a statement describing the rationale for this conclusion is added to the evaluation narrative; an additional evaluation may be made for this broader group of compounds if the strength of the evidence warrants it.

The agent, mixture or exposure circumstance is described according to the wording of one of the following categories, and the designated group is given. The categorization of an agent, mixture or exposure circumstance is a matter of scientific judgement, reflecting the strength of the evidence derived from studies in humans and in experimental animals and from other relevant data.

### Group 1 — *The agent (mixture) is carcinogenic to humans.*
*The exposure circumstance entails exposures that are carcinogenic to humans.*

This category is used only when there is *sufficient evidence* of carcinogenicity in humans.

### Group 2

This category includes agents, mixtures and exposure circumstances for which, at one extreme, the degree of evidence of carcinogenicity in humans is almost sufficient, as well as those for which, at the other extreme, there are no human data but for which there is experimental evidence of carcinogenicity. Agents, mixtures and exposure circumstances are assigned to either 2A (probably carcinogenic) or 2B (possibly carcinogenic) on the basis of epidemiological, experimental and other relevant data.

### Group 2A — *The agent (mixture) is probably carcinogenic to humans.*
*The exposure circumstance entails exposures that are probably carcinogenic to humans.*

This category is used when there is *limited evidence* of carcinogenicity in humans and *sufficient evidence* of carcinogenicity in experimental animals. Exceptionally, an agent, mixture or exposure circumstance may be classified into this category solely on the basis of *limited evidence* of carcinogenicity in humans or of *sufficient evidence* of carcinogenicity in experimental animals strengthened by supporting evidence from other relevant data.

### Group 2B — *The agent (mixture) is possibly carcinogenic to humans.*
*The exposure circumstance entails exposures that are possibly carcinogenic to humans.*

This category is generally used for agents, mixtures and exposure circumstances for which there is *limited evidence* of carcinogenicity in humans in the absence of *sufficient evidence* of carcinogenicity in experimental animals. It may also be used when there is *inadequate evidence* of carcinogenicity in humans or when human data are nonexistent but there is *sufficient evidence* of carcinogenicity in experimental animals. In some instances, an agent, mixture or exposure circumstance for which there is *inadequate evidence* of or no data on carcinogenicity in humans but *limited evidence* of carcinogenicity in experimental animals together with supporting evidence from other relevant data may be placed in this group.

*Group 3 — The agent (mixture, exposure circumstance) is not classifiable as to its carcinogenicity to humans.*

Agents, mixtures and exposure circumstances are placed in this category when they do not fall into any other group.

*Group 4 — The agent (mixture, exposure circumstance) is probably not carcinogenic to humans.*

This category is used for agents, mixtures and exposure circumstances for which there is *evidence suggesting lack of carcinogenicity* in humans together with *evidence suggesting lack of carcinogenicity* in experimental animals. In some instances, agents, mixtures or exposure circumstances for which there is *inadequate evidence* of or no data on carcinogenicity in humans but *evidence suggesting lack of carcinogenicity* in experimental animals, consistently and strongly supported by a broad range of other relevant data, may be classified in this group.

## References

1. IARC (1987) *IARC Monographs on the Evaluation of Carcinogenic Risks to Humans*, Supplement 6, *Genetic and Related Effects: An Updating of Selected* IARC Monographs *from Volumes 1 to 42*, Lyon

2. IARC (1977) *IARC Monographs Programme on the Evaluation of the Carcinogenic Risk of Chemicals to Humans. Preamble* (IARC intern. tech. Rep. No. 77/002), Lyon

3. IARC (1978) *Chemicals with* Sufficient Evidence *of Carcinogenicity in Experimental Animals* — IARC Monographs *Volumes 1-17* (IARC intern. tech. Rep. No. 78/003), Lyon

4. IARC (1979) *Criteria to Select Chemicals for* IARC Monographs (IARC intern. tech. Rep. No. 79/003), Lyon

5. IARC (1982) *IARC Monographs on the Evaluation of the Carcinogenic Risk of Chemicals to Humans*, Supplement 4, *Chemicals, Industrial Processes and Industries Associated with Cancer in Humans. IARC Monographs, Volumes 1 to 29*, Lyon

6. IARC (1983) *Approaches to Classifying Chemical Carcinogens According to Mechanism of Action* (IARC intern. tech. Rep. No. 83/001), Lyon

7. IARC (1987) *IARC Monographs on the Evaluation of Carcinogenic Risks to Humans*, Supplement 7, *Overall Evaluations of Carcinogenicity: An Updating of* IARC Monographs *Volumes 1 to 42*, Lyon

8.  IARC (1988) *Report of an IARC Working Group to Review the Approaches and Processes Used to Evaluate the Carcinogenicity of Mixtures and Groups of Chemical* (IARC intern. tech. Rep. No. 88/002), Lyon

9.  IARC (1973-1988) *Information Bulletin on the Survey of Chemicals Being Tested for Carcinogenicity*, Numbers 1-13, Lyon

    Number 1 (1973)   52 pages
    Number 2 (1973)   77 pages
    Number 3 (1974)   67 pages
    Number 4 (1974)   97 pages
    Number 5 (1975)   88 pages
    Number 6 (1976)  360 pages
    Number 7 (1978)  460 pages
    Number 8 (1979)  604 pages
    Number 9 (1981)  294 pages
    Number 10 (1983) 326 pages
    Number 11 (1984) 370 pages
    Number 12 (1986) 385 pages
    Number 13 (1988) 404 pages

10. Coleman, M. & Wahrendorf, J., eds (1988) *Directory of On-going Studies in Cancer Epidemiology 1988* (IARC Scientific Publications No. 93), Lyon, IARC [and previous annual volumes]

11. IARC (1984) *Chemicals and Exposures to Complex Mixtures Recommended for Evaluation in* IARC Monographs *and Chemicals and Complex Mixtures Recommended for Long-term Carcinogenicity Testing* (IARC intern. tech. Rep. No. 84/002), Lyon

12. IARC (1989) *Chemicals, Groups of Chemicals, Mixtures and Exposure Circumstances to be Evaluated in Future IARC Monographs, Report of an ad hoc Working Group* (IARC intern. tech. Rep. No. 89/004), Lyon

13. *Environmental Carcinogens. Methods of Analysis and Exposure Measurement*:

    Vol. 1. *Analysis of Volatile Nitrosamines in Food* (IARC Scientific Publications No. 18). Edited by R. Preussmann, M. Castegnaro, E.A. Walker & A.E. Wasserman (1978)

    Vol. 2. *Methods for the Measurement of Vinyl Chloride in Poly(vinyl chloride), Air, Water and Foodstuffs* (IARC Scientific Publications No. 22). Edited by D.C.M. Squirrell & W. Thain (1978)

    Vol. 3. *Analysis of Polycyclic Aromatic Hydrocarbons in Environmental Samples* (IARC Scientific Publications No. 29). Edited by M. Castegnaro, P. Bogovski, H. Kunte & E.A. Walker (1979)

    Vol. 4. *Some Aromatic Amines and Azo Dyes in the General and Industrial Environment* (IARC Scientific Publications No. 40). Edited by L. Fishbein, M. Castegnaro, I.K. O'Neill & H. Bartsch (1981)

    Vol. 5. *Some Mycotoxins* (IARC Scientific Publications No. 44). Edited by L. Stoloff, M. Castegnaro, P. Scott, I.K. O'Neill & H. Bartsch (1983)

    Vol. 6. N-*Nitroso Compounds* (IARC Scientific Publications No. 45). Edited by R. Preussmann, I.K. O'Neill, G. Eisenbrand, B. Spiegelhalder & H. Bartsch (1983)

Vol. 7. *Some Volatile Halogenated Hydrocarbons* (IARC Scientific Publications No. 68). Edited by L. Fishbein & I.K. O'Neill (1985)

Vol. 8. *Some Metals: As, Be, Cd, Cr, Ni, Pb, Se, Zn* (IARC Scientific Publications No. 71). Edited by I.K. O'Neill, P. Schuller & L. Fishbein (1986)

Vol. 9. *Passive Smoking* (IARC Scientific Publications No. 81). Edited by I.K. O'Neill, K.D. Brunnemann, B. Dodet & D. Hoffmann (1987)

Vol. 10. *Benzene and Alkylated Benzenes* (IARC Scientific Publications No. 85). Edited by L. Fishbein & I.K. O'Neill (1988)

14. Wilbourn, J., Haroun, L., Heseltine, E., Kaldor, J., Partensky, C. & Vainio, H. (1986) Response of experimental animals to human carcinogens: an analysis based upon the IARC Monographs Programme. *Carcinogenesis, 7*, 1853-1863

15. Montesano, R., Bartsch, H., Vainio, H., Wilbourn, J. & Yamasaki, H., eds (1986) *Long-term and Short-term Assays for Carcinogenesis — A Critical Appraisal* (IARC Scientific Publications No. 83), Lyon, IARC

16. Hoel, D.G., Kaplan, N.L. & Anderson, M.W. (1983) Implication of nonlinear kinetics on risk estimation in carcinogenesis. *Science, 219*, 1032-1037

17. Gart, J.J., Krewski, D., Lee, P.N., Tarone, R.E. & Wahrendorf, J. (1986) *Statistical Methods in Cancer Research*, Vol. 3, *The Design and Analysis of Long-term Animal Experiments* (IARC Scientific Publications No. 79), Lyon, IARC

18. Peto, R., Pike, M.C., Day, N.E., Gray, R.G., Lee, P.N., Parish, S., Peto, J., Richards, S. & Wahrendorf, J. (1980) Guidelines for simple, sensitive significance tests for carcinogenic effects in long-term animal experiments. In: *IARC Monographs on the Evaluation of the Carcinogenic Risk of Chemicals to Humans*, Supplement 2, *Long-term and Short-term Screening Assays for Carcinogens: A Critical Appraisal*, Lyon, pp. 311-426

19. Breslow, N.E. & Day, N.E. (1980) *Statistical Methods in Cancer Research*, Vol. 1, *The Analysis of Case-control Studies* (IARC Scientific Publications No. 32), Lyon, IARC

20. Breslow, N.E. & Day, N.E. (1987) *Statistical Methods in Cancer Research*, Vol. 2, *The Design and Analysis of Cohort Studies* (IARC Scientific Publications No. 82), Lyon, IARC

# GENERAL REMARKS

This forty–ninth volume of *IARC Monographs* covers chromium and its compounds, nickel and its compounds and occupational exposures in welding. Chromium and nickel are widely used as components of stainless steel and other high alloy steels. Even though mild steel is the most common material welded, a considerable proportion of welders are regularly or occasionally exposed to fumes from stainless steel containing chromium and nickel compounds.

Chromium and its compounds have been evaluated previously in the *Monographs* (IARC, 1973, 1979, 1980, 1982, 1987). The monograph on chromium and chromium compounds is, for practical purposes, divided into subsections, on the basis of the oxidation state and solubility of the compounds. The principal oxidation states of chromium are 0, III and VI; in addition, oxidation states II, IV and V occur, and sometimes the agents tested were of mixed or unknown oxidation states. The latter are described under the title 'other chromium compounds'. The compounds tested for carcinogenicity are described in more detail than other compounds of the group in sections on chemical and physical properties, production, use and occurrence. Welding of stainless steel with exposure to chromium is described in detail in the monograph on welding and is cross-referenced in the monograph on chromium and chromium compounds.

In general, stainless-steel welders (mostly fabricators) are exposed primarily to fumes that differ from those in mild-steel welding mainly in their comparatively high content of chromium and nickel. Mild-steel welders work on a variety of materials in a range of situations (e.g., shipyards, construction work), which lead to exposure to a range of particulates such as fume, grinding dust and asbestos (see IARC, 1977) and to gaseous substances (e.g., from pyrolytic decomposition of antirust paint on construction plates and the oxides of nitrogen).

Nickel and its compounds have also been evaluated previously (IARC, 1973, 1976, 1979, 1982, 1987). As for chromium, the present monograph on nickel and nickel compounds has been divided into subsections. The purpose of this subdivision was prompted by the fact that since a wide variety of nickel compounds has been tested for carcinogenicity, a grouping of data on individual nickel compounds would be useful. The studies on stainless-steel welding and on welders exposed to nickel are described in the monograph on welding. These studies are, however, cross-referenced in the monograph on nickel and nickel compounds when they are considered to contribute to the evaluation of nickel and its compounds.

Welding and welding fumes have not been evaluated previously, although some of the studies on welders are reviewed in the monographs on chromium and nickel. The chemical composition of welding fumes and gases is determined by the material being welded (e.g., mild steel, stainless steel, aluminium) and the welding technique used (manual metal arc, metal inert gas, tungsten inert gas). When painted steel is welded, the basic components of welding fumes — the metals, metal oxides and metal salts — may be accompanied by a complex mixture of other compounds. In addition to welding fumes and gases, welders are also often exposed to ultraviolet light (see IARC, 1986), to electromagnetic fields and, in some cases, to other agents originating from their work (e.g., grinding dust) or from other work carried out at the same place (e.g., asbestos in shipyards).

The epidemiological studies summarized in the monograph on welding were selected on the basis that the majority of the population under study probably consisted of welders. For example, if the occupational group studied was specified as 'welders and solderers', the study was included because the number of solderers is usually much lower than that of welders. On the other hand, studies on 'metal workers' and 'sheet metal workers' were excluded, although in these wide occupational categories there is a minority of persons who are involved in welding operations. Similarly, it is probable that the studies on 'welders' as an unspecified occupation may have included a fair number of stainless-steel welders. It should be noted that laboratory experiments with samples of welding fume may not reflect, in terms of chemical composition, human exposures during the welding process.

*Solubility*

Chromium and nickel compounds are often classified as 'soluble' or 'insoluble'. Such a classification can be useful for describing the physical properties and industrial applications of the various compounds, but has sometimes also been used as a crude index of bioavailability in toxicological investigations. Some confusion has arisen because the terms 'soluble' and 'insoluble' have not always been defined adequately and because a variety of test methods has been used. In the preparation of the monographs in this volume, use was made of the accepted physical definition of 'solubility' in terms of the equilibrium concentration of a single chemical substance in saturated solution in a specified solvent at a given temperature. The 'soluble fraction' of a substance or mixture is usually measured by leaching the substance for a specified time under defined test conditions, and the results obtained are highly dependent upon the precise method used. It should be noted that different forms of nominally the same compound can have very different solubilities and rates of dissolution, and the dissolution rate is affected by particle size, purity and crystallinity.

The dissolution process can involve physical and chemical mechanisms, and the resulting compounds in solution might be chemically different from the source compound in the test material. For example, nickel subsulfide ($Ni_3S_2$) can be oxidized by dissolved oxygen, entering solution as nickel sulfate (Ciccarelli & Wetterhahn, 1984). Interpretation of the results of leaching measurements can be difficult: a low result, for example, might imply either a mixture with a small soluble fraction or a pure soluble material which dissolves relatively slowly. In few cases can the results of such tests, or data on solubility, for a substance in one solvent system be extrapolated reliably to other solvent systems.

*Bioavailability*

'Bioavailability' is a term used to denote the fraction of a substance that is absorbed, delivered to a target site and/or is responsible for a specific toxic or carcinogenic effect. Clearly, water solubility of an agent will often be an important factor in its availability within the body. It is, however, not the only relevant determinant of bioavailability. All dissolved chromium species, for example, may not pass equally through cell membranes: chromates in solution readily cross cell membranes, while Cr[III] does not. Chromates, moreover, have a range of solubilities in water and in body fluids, and agents such as lead chromate may release very few chromate ions for passage through cell membranes. Passage through cell membranes is only one route by which an agent may reach a target within a cell: particulate compounds of chromium and nickel may be phagocytized and thus become bioavailable.

The bioavailability of a potentially carcinogenic entity that is common to other members of its class of closely related compounds is an important factor in its carcinogenic potency, as demonstrated by differences in the levels of carcinogenic response observed in experimental and epidemiological studies. Not only is sufficient delivery of metal ion important, but in excess it can produce toxic effects (e.g., inhibitory phagocytosis), limiting uptake or survival of preneoplastic cells.

The classification scheme used in the *IARC Monographs* is qualitative and is based solely on the strength of evidence from the studies considered. Because of differences in observed levels of carcinogenic response, potency, and therefore dissolution and bioavailability as well, play a role in this qualitative evaluation. Alternatively, differences in the degree of evidence may merely reflect the fact that the entity has not been adequately tested over the range of compounds in which it occurs.

*Biological monitoring*

Biological monitoring of chromium, nickel and welding exposures shows that absorption into the human body has taken place. Such studies were considered, but several factors, such as sampling time, toxicokinetic factors and analytical validity, were taken into account, and the Working Group did not attempt to use such data to compare absorbed doses in different exposure situations.

*Availability and reporting of data*

There is a paucity of evidence for and against the possible carcinogenic hazards of oral exposures to chromium or nickel compounds in foods or potable water. There is also a lack of precision in characterizing the chemical species and physical properties of the tested compounds and welding processes described in these monographs, which hinders interpretation of the data.

*Adequacy of animal experiments*

Chromium and nickel are major world commodities, and these metals and their compounds constitute occupational exposures, principally by inhalation, for many millions of workers. Many long-term tests for carcinogenesis have been carried out by application to internal tissues (by injection or implantation); however, few bioassays of exposure by inhalation were available for evaluation. The paucity of data on the effects of inhalation of these compounds is partially offset by evidence from studies by intratracheal and intrabronchial exposure.

Carcinogenic effect is often strongly related to duration of exposure, in both humans and animals; thus, negative results for a single application of a soluble compound in an animal experiment cannot provide reasonable evidence that an agent will not be carcinogenic under conditions of prolonged or repeated application. This fact may provide a possible explanation for some of the negative results observed. In the absence of data from studies of soluble, acutely toxic substances by prolonged inhalation, some evidence may be obtained from repeated exposure of the same target cell population, as by repeated multiple injections of a toxic nickel-containing compound into the peritoneal cavity. The requirements for the carcinogenicity testing of metals need further elaboration.

*Genetic and related effects*

Most of the available short-term test results have been incorporated in the text. These include the results of anchorage-independent growth assays using Syrian hamster BHK21 fibroblasts. This assay in particular demonstrated that many metal compounds can induce changes in the normal growth pattern of the cells; however, neither this assay nor that for fetal mouse cell transformation was evaluated for the final summary (Section 4.4), because technical and interpretative difficulties are associated with both of them.

*Interpretation of moderately elevated lung cancer rates*

Apparently moderate elevations in lung cancer rates among occupationally exposed groups may occur as a result of confounding exposures to cigarette smoke and other carcinogens. Accurate smoking histories are rarely available in epidemiological studies of industrial workers, and, due to the differences in smoking prevalences, national or even regional lung cancer rates may not provide an appropriate basis for calculating expected numbers in industrial cohort studies. Furthermore, workers in a particular industry may also be exposed to carcinogens in other occupations during their working lives. For example, in several recent industrial studies, high lung cancer rates have been reported among short-term workers, which seem unlikely to be due to the specific period of employment. In the absence of an increasing trend with duration of exposure, a relative risk for lung cancer lower than about 1.5 should be interpreted with caution, although larger excesses are unlikely to be due entirely to smoking or to other exposures.

## References

Ciccarelli, R.B. & Wetterhahn, K.E. (1984) Molecular basis for the activity of nickel. In: Sunderman, F.W., Jr, ed., *Nickel in the Human Environment* (IARC Scientific Publications No. 53), Lyon, IARC, pp. 201-213

IARC (1973) *IARC Monographs on the Evaluation of Carcinogenic Risk of Chemicals to Man, Vol. 2, Some Inorganic and Organometallic Compounds*, Lyon, pp. 100-125, 126-149

IARC (1976) *IARC Monographs on the Evaluation of Carcinogenic Risk of Chemicals to Man, Vol. 11, Cadmium, Nickel, Some Epoxides, Miscellaneous Industrial Chemicals and General Considerations on Volatile Anaesthetics*, Lyon, pp. 75-112

IARC (1977) *IARC Monographs on the Evaluation of Carcinogenic Risk of Chemicals to Man, Vol. 14, Asbestos*, Lyon

IARC (1979) *IARC Monographs on the Evaluation of the Carcinogenic Risk of Chemicals to Humans*, Suppl. 1, *Chemicals and Industrial Processes Associated with Cancer in Humans. IARC Monographs, Volumes 1 to 20*, Lyon, pp. 29-30, 38

IARC (1980) *IARC Monographs on the Evaluation of the Carcinogenic Risk of Chemicals to Humans*, Vol. 23, *Some Metals and Metallic Compounds*, Lyon, pp. 205-323

IARC (1982) *IARC Monographs on the Evaluation of the Carcinogenic Risk of Chemicals to Humans*, Suppl. 4, *Chemicals, Industrial Processes and Industries Associated with Cancer in Humans. IARC Monographs, Volumes 1 to 29*, Lyon, pp. 91-93, 167-170

IARC (1986) *IARC Monographs on the Evaluation of the Carcinogenic Risk of Chemicals to Humans*, Vol. 40, *Some Naturally Occurring and Synthetic Food Components, Furocoumarins and Ultraviolet Radiation*, Lyon, pp. 379-415

IARC (1987) *IARC Monographs on the Evaluation of Carcinogenic Risks to Humans*, Suppl. 7, *Overall Evaluations of Carcinogenicity: An Updating of* IARC Monographs *Volumes 1-42*, Lyon, pp. 165-168, 264-269

# THE MONOGRAPHS

# CHROMIUM AND CHROMIUM COMPOUNDS

Chromium and chromium compounds were considered by previous IARC Working Groups, in 1972, 1979, 1982 and 1987 (IARC, 1973, 1979, 1980a, 1982, 1987a). Since that time, new data have become available, and these are included in the present monograph and have been taken into consideration in the evaluation.

# 1. Chemical and Physical Data

The list of chromium alloys and compounds given in Table 1 is not exhaustive, nor does it necessarily reflect the commercial importance of the various chromium-containing substances, but it is indicative of the range of chromium alloys and compounds available.

## 1.1 Synonyms, trade names and molecular formulae of chromium and selected chromium-containing compounds

**Table 1. Synonyms (Chemical Abstracts Service names are given in bold), trade names and atomic or molecular formulae of chromium and selected chromium compounds**

| Chemical name | Chem. Abstr. Services Reg. No.[a] | Synonyms and trade names | Formula[b] |
|---|---|---|---|
| **Metallic chromium [0] and chromium [0] alloys** | | | |
| Chromium | 7440-47-3 | **Chrome** | Cr |
| Cobalt-chromium alloy[c] | 11114-92-4 (91700-55-9) | **Chromium alloy (nonbase), Co, Cr; cobalt alloy (nonbase), Co, Cr** | - |
| Cobalt-chromium-molybdenum alloy[c] | 12629-02-6 (8064-15-1; 11068-92-1; 12618-69-8; 55345-18-1; | **Cobalt alloy (base), Co 56-68, Cr 25-29, Mo 5-6, Ni 1.8-3.8, Fe 0-3, Mn 0-1, Si 0-1, C 0.2-0.3 (ASTM A567-1)** | |

**Table 1 (contd)**

| Chemical name | Chem. Abstr. Services Reg. No.[a] | Synonyms and trade names | Formula[b] |
|---|---|---|---|
| | 60382-64-1; 83272-15-5; 85131-98-2; 94076-26-3) | Akrit CoMo35; AMS 5385D; Celsit 290; F 75; HS 21; Protasul-2; Stellite 21; Vinertia; Vitallium; X25CoCr-Mo62 28 5; Zimalloy | |
| Chromium-containing stainless steels[c] | 71631-40-8 (51204-69-4, 59601-19-3, 84723-14-8, 94197-89-4, 98286-69-2) | **Iron alloy (base), Fe 64-72, Cr 21-23, Ni 4.5-6.5, Mo 2.5-3.5, Mn 0-2, Si 0-1, N 0.1-0.2 (ASTM A276-S31803)** | - |
| | | AF 22; AF 22-130; AISI 318L; Alloy 2205; Arosta 4462; AST 2205; Avesta 2205; Avesta 223FAL; CR22; 22Cr; 22Cr5Ni; CrNiMoN22-5-3; DIN 1.4462; ES 2205; FAL 223; 744LN; Mann AF-22; Nirosta 4462; NKK-Cr22; Novonox FALC 223; NU 744 LN; NU stainless 744LN; Remanit 4462; SAF 2205; Sandvik SAF 2205; SS 2377; Stainless steel 2205; Uddeholm Nu744LN; UHB 744LN; UNS S31803; Uranus 45N; UR45N; Vallourec VS22; VEW A903; VLX 562; VS 22; X2CrNiMoN2253; Z2 CND 22.5 AZ | |
| Ferro-chrome[d] | 11114-46-8 (11133-75-8, 11143-43-4, 12604-52-3) | **Chromium alloy (base), Cr, C, Fe, N, Si; ferrochromium;** carbon ferrochromium; chrome ferroalloy; chromium ferroalloy | - |
| Iron-nickel-chromium alloy | 11121-96-3 | **Iron alloy (base), Fe 39-47, Ni 30-35, Cr 19-23, Mn 0-1.5, Si 0-1, Cu 0-0.8, Al 0-0.6, Ti 0-0.6, C 0-0.1 (ASTM B163-800)** | - |
| | | AFNOR ZFeNC45-36; AISI 332; Alloy 800; Alloy 800NG; Cr20Ni32TiAl; 20Cr32NiTiAl; DIN 1.4876; FeCr21Ni32TiAl; IN 800; Incoloy 800; JIS NCF800; N800; NCF800; NCF 800 HTB; NCF steel; Nickel 800; Nicrofer 3220; Ni33Cr21TiAl; POLDI AKR 17; Pyromet 800; Sanicro 31; Thermax 4876; TIG N800 | |
| Nickel-chromium alloy | 12605-70-8 | Nichrome; **Nickel alloy (base), Ni 57-62, Fe 22-28, Cr 14-18, Si 0.8-1.6, Mn 0-1, C 0-0.2 (ASTM B344-60 Ni, 16 Cr)** | - |
| | | Chromel C; Kh15N60N; NiCr6015; PNKh; Tophet C | |
| **Chromium [III] compounds** | | | |
| Basic chromic sulfate | 12336-95-7 (39380-78-4) | Basic chromium sulfate; **chromium hydroxide sulfate** ($Cr(OH)(SO_4)$); chromium sulfate; monobasic chromium sulfate; sulfuric acid, chromium salt, basic | $Cr(OH)SO_4$ |
| | | Chromedol; Chrometan; Chrome tan; Peachrome | |
| | 64093-79-4 | **Neochromium** | $Cr(OH)SO_4 \cdot Na_2SO_4 \cdot H_2O$ |

## Table 1 (contd)

| Chemical name | Chem. Abstr. Services Reg. No.[a] | Synonyms and trade names | Formula[b] |
|---|---|---|---|
| Chromic acetate | 1066-30-4 | **Acetic acid, chromium (3+) salt**; chromium acetate; chromium [III] acetate; chromium triacetate | $Cr(OCOCH_3)_3$ |
| Chromic chloride | 10025-73-7 | **Chromium chloride ($CrCl_3$)**; chromium [III] chloride; chromium trichloride; C.I. 77295; trichlorochromium | $CrCl_3$ |
| Chromic hydroxide | 1308-14-1 | Chromic acid ($H_3CrO_3$); **chromium hydroxide ($Cr(OH)_3$)**; chromium [III] hydroxide; chromium (3+) hydroxide; chromium trihydroxide | $Cr(OH)_3$ |
| Chromic nitrate | 13548-38-4 (20249-21-2) | Chromium nitrate; chromium [III] nitrate; chromium (3+) nitrate; chromium trinitrate; **nitric acid, chromium (3+) salt** | $Cr(NO_3)_3$ |
| Chromic oxide | 1308-38-9 | Chrome oxide; chromia; **chromium oxide ($Cr_2O_3$)**; chromium [III] oxide; chromium sesquioxide; chromium (3+) trioxide; C.I. 77288; C.I. Pigment Green 17; dichromium trioxide | $Cr_2O_3$ |
| | | Anadonis Green; Casalis Green; Chrome Green; Chrome Ochre; Chrome Oxide Green BX; Chrome Oxide Green GN-M; Chromium Oxide Pigment; Chromium 111 Oxide; Chromium Oxide Green; Chromium Oxide X1134; 11661 Green; Green Chrome Oxide; Green Chromic Oxide; Green Chromium Oxide; Green Cinnabar; Green Oxide of Chromium; Green Oxide of Chromium OC-31; Green Rouge; Guignet's Green; Leaf Green; Levanox Green GA (hydrated chromic oxide); Oil Green; Oxide of Chromium; P-106F10; Pure Chromium Oxide Green 59; Ultramarine Green | |
| Chromic perchlorate | 13537-21-8 | Chromium perchlorate; chromium triperchlorate; **perchloric acid, chromium (3+) salt** | $Cr(ClO_4)_3$ |
| Chromic phosphate | 7789-04-0 | Chromium monophosphate; chromium orthophosphate; chromium phosphate; **phosphoric acid, chromium (3+) salt (1:1)**; phosphoric acid, chromium [III] salt | $CrPO_4$ |
| | | Arnaudon's Green (hemiheptahydrate); Plessy's Green (hemiheptahydrate) | |
| Chromic sulfate | 10101-53-8 (39378-25-1) | Chromium sulfate (2:3); chromium [III] sulfate; dichromium sulfate; dichromium tris(sulfate); dichromium trisulfate; **sulfuric acid, chromium (3+) salt (3:2)**; C.I. 77305 | $Cr_2(SO_4)_3$ |
| | | Baychrom A; Baychrom F; Chromitan B; Chromitan MS; Chromitan NA; Cromitan B; Koreon | |
| Chromite ore | 1308-31-2 (61026-56-0) | Chrome ore; **chromite ($Cr_2FeO_4$)**; chromite mineral; iron chromite | $Cr_2O_3.FeO$ |
| Nickel chromate | 12018-18-7 | **Chromic acid ($H_2CrO_4$), nickel salt (1:1)** | $NiCrO_4$ |

## Table 1 (contd)

| Chemical name | Chem. Abstr. Services Reg. No.[a] | Synonyms and trade names | Formula[b] |
|---|---|---|---|
| Potassium chromic sulfate | 10141-00-1 (14766-82-6; 81827-72-7; 81827-73-8) | Chrome alum; chrome potash alum; chromic potassium sulfate; chromium potassium sulfate; potassium chromium alum; potassium chromium sulfate; potassium disulfatochromate [III]; **sulfuric acid, chromium (3 +) potassium salt (2:1:1)**<br><br>Chrome Alum 0% Basicity; Crystal Chrome Alum | $KCr(SO_4)_2$ |

### Chromium[VI] compounds

| | | | |
|---|---|---|---|
| Ammonium chromate | 7788-98-9 | Chromic acid, ammonium salt; **chromic acid ($H_2CrO_4$), diammonium salt**; diammonium chromate; neutral ammonium chromate | $(NH_4)_2CrO_4$ |
| Ammonium dichromate | 7789-09-5 | Ammonium bichromate; ammonium chromate; **chromic acid ($H_2Cr_2O_7$), diammonium salt**; diammonium dichromate; dichromic acid, diammonium salt | $(NH_4)_2Cr_2O_7$ |
| Barium chromate | 10294-40-3 (12000-34-9; 12231-18-4) | Barium chromate (VI); barium chromate (1:1); barium chromate oxide; **chromic acid ($H_2CrO_4$), barium salt (1:1)**; C.I. 77103; C.I. Pigment Yellow 31<br><br>Baryta Yellow; Lemon Chrome; Lemon Yellow; Permanent Yellow; Steinbuhl Yellow; Ultramarine Yellow | $BaCrO_4$ |
| Basic lead chromate | 1344-38-3 (54692-53-4) | C.I. 77601; **C.I. Pigment Orange 21**; C.I. Pigment Red; lead chromate oxide<br><br>Arancio Cromo; Austrian Cinnabar; Basic Lead Chromate Orange; Chinese Red; Chrome Orange; Chrome Orange 54; Chrome Orange 56; Chrome Orange 57; Chrome Orange 58; Chrome Orange Dark; Chrome Orange Extra Light; Chrome Orange G; Chrome Orange Medium; Chrome Orange NC-22; Chrome Orange R; Chrome Orange 5R; Chrome Orange RF; Chrome Orange XL; Chrome Red; C.P. Chrome Orange Dark 2030; C.P. Chrome Orange Extra Dark 2040; C.P. Chrome Orange Light 2010; C.P. Chrome Orange Medium 2020; Dainichi Chrome Orange R; Dainichi Chrome Orange 5R; Genuine Acetate Orange Chrome; Genuine Orange Chrome; Indian Red; International Orange 2221; Irgachrome Orange OS; Light Orange Chrome; No. 156 Orange Chrome; Orange Chrome; Orange Nitrate Chrome; Pale Orange Chrome; Persian Red; Pigment Orange 21; Pure Orange Chrome M; Pure Orange Chrome Y; Red Lead Chromate; Vynamon Orange CR | $PbO.PbCrO_4$ |
| Calcium chromate | 13765-19-0 | Calcium chromium oxide; calcium monochromate; **chromic acid ($H_2CrO_4$), calcium salt (1:1)**; C.I. 77223; C.I. Pigment Yellow 33<br><br>Calcium Chrome Yellow; Gelbin; Yellow Ultramarine | $CaCrO_4$ |

## Table 1 (contd)

| Chemical name | Chem. Abstr. Services Reg. No.[a] | Synonyms and trade names | Formula[b] |
|---|---|---|---|
| Chromium [VI] chloride | 14986-48-2 | Chromium hexachloride; (OC-6-11)-chromium chloride (CrCl₆) | $CrCl_6$ |
| Chromium trioxide | 1333-82-0 (12324-05-9; 12324-08-2) | Chromia; chromic acid; chromic [VI] acid; chromic acid, solid; chromic anhydride; chromic trioxide; **chromium oxide ($CrO_3$)**; chromium [VI] oxide; chromium (6+) trioxide; monochromium trioxide | $CrO_3$ |
| Chromyl chloride | 14977-61-8 | Chlorochromic anhydride; chromium chloride oxide; chromium dichloride dioxide; **chromium, dichlorodioxo-(T-4)**; chromium dioxide dichloride; chromium dioxychloride; chromium oxychloride; dichlorodioxochromium | $CrO_2Cl_2$ |
| Lead chromate | 7758-97-6 (8049-64-7) | **Chromic acid ($H_2CrO_4$), lead (2+) salt (1:1)**; C.I. 77600; C.I. Pigment Yellow 34; crocoite; lead chromium oxide; phoenicochroite; plumbous chromate<br><br>Canary Chrome Yellow 40-2250; Chrome Green; Chrome Green UC61; Chrome Green UC74; Chrome Green UC76; Chrome Lemon; Chrome Yellow; Chrome Yellow 5G; Chrome Yellow GF; Chrome Yellow LF; Chrome Yellow Light 1066; Chrome Yellow Light 1075; Chrome Yellow Medium 1074; Chrome Yellow Medium 1085; Chrome Yellow Medium 1295; Chrome Yellow Medium 1298; Chrome Yellow Primrose 1010; Chrome Yellow Primrose 1015; Cologne Yellow; Dainichi Chrome Yellow G; LD Chrome Yellow Supra 70 FS; Leipzig Yellow; Paris Yellow; Pigment Green 15; Primrose Chrome Yellow; Pure Lemon Chrome L3GS | $PbCrO_4$ |
| Molybdenum orange | 12656-85-8 | **C.I. Pigment Red 104**<br><br>Chrome Vermilion; Krolor Orange RKO 786D; Lead chromate molybdate sulfate red; Mineral Fire Red 5DDS; Mineral Fire Red 5GGS; Mineral Fire Red 5GS; Molybdate Orange; Molybdate Orange Y 786D; Molybdate Orange YE 421D; Molybdate Orange YE 698D; Molybdate Red; Molybdate Red AA 3; Molybden Red; Molybdenum Red; Renol Molybdate Red RGS; Vynamon Scarlet BY; Vynamon Scarlet Y | $PbMoO_4 \cdot PbCrO_4 \cdot PbSO_4$ |
| Potassium chromate | 7789-00-6 | Bipotassium chromate; **chromic acid ($H_2CrO_4$), dipotassium salt**; dipotassium chromate; dipotassium monochromate; neutral potassium chromate; potassium chromate [VI] | $K_2CrO_4$ |

## Table 1 (contd)

| Chemical name | Chem. Abstr. Services Reg. No.[a] | Synonyms and trade names | Formula[b] |
|---|---|---|---|
| Potassium dichromate | 7778-50-9 | **Chromic acid ($H_2Cr_2O_7$), dipotassium salt**; dichromic acid, dipotassium salt; dipotassium bichromate; dipotassium dichromate; potassium bichromate; potassium dichromate [VI] | $K_2Cr_2O_7$ |
| Sodium chromate | 7775-11-3 | **Chromic acid ($H_2CrO_4$), disodium salt**; chromium disodium oxide; chromium sodium oxide; disodium chromate; neutral sodium chromate; sodium chromium oxide | $Na_2CrO_4$ |
| Sodium dichromate | 10588-01-9 (12018-32-5) | Bichromate of soda; **chromic acid ($H_2Cr_2O_7$), disodium salt**; chromium sodium oxide; dichromic acid, disodium salt; disodium dichromate; sodium bichromate; sodium dichromate [VI] | $Na_2Cr_2O_7$ |
| Strontium chromate | 7789-06-2 (54322-60-0) | **Chromic acid ($H_2CrO_4$), strontium salt (1:1)**; C.I. Pigment Yellow 32; strontium chromate [VI]; strontium chromate (1:1) | $SrCrO_4$ |
| | | Deep Lemon Yellow; Strontium Chromate 12170; Strontium Chromate A; Strontium Chromate X-2396; Strontium Yellow; Sutokuro T | |
| Zinc chromate[e] | 13530-65-9 (1308-13-0; 1328-67-2; 14675-41-3) | **Chromic acid ($H_2CrO_4$), zinc salt (1:1)**; chromium zinc oxide; zinc chromium oxide; zinc tetraoxychromate; zinc tetroxychromate | $ZnCrO_4$ |
| | | Buttercup Yellow | |
| Zinc chromate hydroxides | 15930-94-6 (12206-12-1; 66516-58-3) | Basic zinc chromate; chromic acid ($H_6CrO_6$), zinc salt (1:2); chromic acid ($H_4CrO_5$), zinc salt (1:2), monohydrate; chromium zinc hydroxide oxide; zinc chromate hydroxide; zinc chromate [VI] hydroxide; **zinc chromate oxide ($Zn_2(CrO_4)O$), monohydrate**; zinc hydroxychromate; zinc tetrahydroxychromate; zinc yellow[f] | $Zn_2CrO_4(OH)_2$ and others |
| Zinc potassium chromates (hydroxides) | 11103-86-9 (12527-08-1; 37809-34-0) | Basic zinc potassium chromate; chromic acid ($H_6Cr_2O_9$), potassium zinc salt (1:1:2); **potassium hydroxyoctaoxodizincatedichromate(1-)**; potassium zinc chromate hydroxide; zinc yellow[f] | $KZn_2(CrO_4)_2(OH)$ and others |
| **Other chromium compounds** | | | |
| Chromium carbonyl | 13007-92-6 (13930-94-4) | **Chromium carbonyl ($Cr(CO)_6$)**; chromium hexacarbonyl; hexacarbonyl chromium | $Cr(CO)_6$ |
| Chromic chromate | 24613-89-6 | **Chromic acid ($H_2CrO_4$), chromium (3+) salt (3:2)**; chromium chromate | $Cr_2(CrO_4)_3$ |
| Chromium [II] chloride | 10049-05-5 | **Chromium chloride ($CrCl_2$)**; chromium dichloride; chromous chloride | $CrCl_2$ |

**Table 1 (contd)**

| Chemical name | Chem. Abstr. Services Reg. No.[a] | Synonyms and trade names | Formula[b] |
|---|---|---|---|
| Chromium [IV] dioxide | 12018-01-8 | Chromium dioxide; **chromium oxide (CrO₂)**; chromium [IV] oxide | $CrO_2$ |

[a] Replaced CAS Registry numbers are given in parentheses.

[b] Compounds with the same synonym or trade name can have different formulae.

[c] Thousands of alloys of chromium with other metals are listed by the Chemical Abstracts Registry Service; approximately 1300 contain cobalt, over 400 also contain molybdenum and nearly 100 are chromium-containing stainless steels. An example of each is listed here.

[d] Chemical Abstracts Registry Service lists several ferrochromium alloys; one example is given.

[e] The term 'zinc chromate' is also used to refer to a wide range of commercial zinc and zinc potassium chromates.

[f] 'Zinc yellow' can refer to several zinc chromate pigments; it has the CAS No. 37300-23-5.

## 1.2 Chemical and physical properties of pure substances

Known physical properties of some of the chromium compounds considered in this monograph are given in Table 2. Data on solubility refer to saturated solutions in water or other specified solvents. Hexavalent chromium compounds are customarily classed as soluble or insoluble in water; such a classification is useful in industry but might not be relevant to determining the biological properties of a compound. There is thus no general agreement on the definition of solubility: in practice, the aqueous solubility of Cr[VI] compounds has been classified as prompt (1 min) and short-term (30 min) (Van Bemst *et al.*, 1983). In laboratory studies, solubilization depends on, e.g., the medium used in in-vitro tests; for human exposures, solubility is related to the chemical environment in the respiratory tract. Examples of soluble hexavalent chromium compounds are sodium chromate (873 g/l at 30°C) and potassium chromate (629 g/l at 20°C). Hexavalent chromium compounds classed as insoluble include barium chromate (4.4 mg/l at 28°C) and lead chromate (0.58 mg/l at 25°C) (Windholz, 1983; Weast, 1985). Compounds with solubilities towards the middle of this range are not easily classified, and technical-grade compounds, such as the various zinc chromates, can have a wide range of solubilities.

## 1.3 Technical products and impurities

### (a) Chromite ore

Chromite ore consists of varying percentages of chromium, iron, aluminium and magnesium oxides as the major components. It has been classified into three

**Table 2. Physical properties of chromium and chromium compounds[a]**

| Chemical name | Atomic/ molecular weight | Melting– point (°C) | Boiling– point (°C) | Typical physical description | Solubility |
|---|---|---|---|---|---|
| **Metallic chromium [0]** | | | | | |
| Chromium | 51.996 | 1900 | 2642 | Steel–grey, lustrous metal or powder | Insoluble in water; soluble in dilute hydrochloric acid and sulfuric acid; insoluble in nitric acid or nitrohydrochloric acid |
| **Chromium[III] compounds** | | | | | |
| Basic chromic sulfate[b] | 165.06 | – | – | Green powder | Soluble in water (approximately 700 g/l at 35°C[b]) |
| Chromic acetate (hydrate) | 229.14 (247.15) | – | – | Grey–green powder (blue–violet needles) | Slightly soluble in water; insoluble in ethanol; soluble in cold water, acetone (2 g/l at 15°C) and methanol (45.4 g/l at 15°C) |
| Chromic chloride (hexahydrate) | 158.36 (266.45) | 1150 (83) | Sublimes at 1300 | Violet crystalline scales | Anhydrous form is insoluble in cold water, slightly soluble in hot water, but insoluble in ethanol, acetone, methanol and diethyl ether. The hydrated form is very soluble in water (585 g/l), soluble in ethanol, slightly soluble in acetone and insoluble in diethyl ether. |
| Chromic nitrate (7.5 hydrate) (nonahydrate) | 238.03 (373.13) (400.15) | – (100) (60) | Decomposes Decomposes at 100 | Pale–green powder (brown crystals) (deep–violet crystals) | Soluble in water. Both hydrated forms soluble in water; the nonahydrate is soluble in acids, alkali, ethanol and acetone |
| Chromic oxide | 151.99 | 2435 | 4000 | Light to dark–green, fine crystals | Insoluble in water, acids, alkali and ethanol |
| Chromic phosphate (dihydrate) | 147 (183.00) | >1800°C | – | Violet crystalline solid | Insoluble in water. Hydrated form is slightly soluble in cold water; soluble in most acids and alkali but not in acetic acid |

**Table 2 (contd)**

| Chemical name | Atomic/molecular weight | Melting-point (°C) | Boiling-point (°C) | Typical physical description | Solubility |
|---|---|---|---|---|---|
| Chromic sulfate | 392.16 | — | — | Violet or red powder | Insoluble in water; slightly soluble in ethanol; insoluble in acids |
| Potassium chromic sulfate (dodecahydrate) | 283.23 (499.39) | (89) | (400) | (Violet ruby-red to black crystals) | Hydrated form is soluble in water (243.9 g/l at 25°C; 500 g/l in hot water); slightly soluble in dilute acids; insoluble in ethanol |
| **Chromium[VI] compounds** | | | | | |
| Ammonium chromate | 152.07 | 180 | — | Yellow acicular crystals | Soluble in water (405 g/l); insoluble in ethanol, slightly soluble in ammonia, acetone and methanol |
| Ammonium dichromate | 252.06 | 170 (dec)^c | — | Orange-red crystals | Soluble in water (308 g/l at 15°C; 890 g/l at 30°C) and ethanol; insoluble in acetone |
| Barium chromate | 253.33 | — | — | Yellow crystals | Very slightly soluble in water (4.4 mg/l at 28°C); soluble in mineral acids |
| Basic lead chromate | 546.37 | — | — | Red crystalline powder | Insoluble in water; soluble in acids and alkali |
| Calcium chromate (dihydrate) | 156.09 (192.10) | (200) | — | Yellow crystalline powder | Slightly soluble in water and ethanol; soluble in acids. Hydrated form is soluble in water (163 g/l at 20°C; 182 g/l at 45°C), acids and ethanol |
| Chromium trioxide | 99.99 | 196 | Decomposes at 250^c | Dark-red crystals, flakes or granular powder | Soluble in water (625 g/l at 20°C; 674.5 g/l at 100°C), ethanol, diethyl ether and sulfuric and nitric acids |
| Chromyl chloride | 154.90 | -96.5 | 117 | Dark-red volatile liquid | Decomposes in water and ethanol; soluble in ether, acetic acid, carbon tetrachloride, carbon disulfide, benzene, nitrobenzene, chloroform and phosphorous oxychloride |

**Table 2 (contd)**

| Chemical name | Atomic/molecular weight | Melting-point (°C) | Boiling-point (°C) | Typical physical description | Solubility |
|---|---|---|---|---|---|
| Lead chromate | 323.18 | 844 | Decomposes | Yellow to orange-yellow crystalline powder | Very slightly soluble in water (0.58 mg/l at 25°C); soluble in most acids and alkali but not in acetic acid or ammonia |
| Nickel chromate | 174.71 | — | — | — | Insoluble in water; soluble in nitric acid and hydrogen peroxide |
| Potassium chromate | 194.20 | 968.3 | Decomposes[c] | Lemon-yellow crystals | Soluble in water (629 g/l at 20°C; 792 g/l at 100°C); insoluble in ethanol |
| Potassium dichromate | 294.19 | 398 | Decomposes at 500 | Bright orange-red crystals | Soluble in water (49 g/l at 0°C; 1020 g/l at 100°C); insoluble in ethanol |
| Sodium chromate | 161.97 | 792 | Decomposes[c] | Yellow crystals | Soluble in water (873 g/l at 30°C) and methanol (3.44 g/l at 25°C); slightly soluble in ethanol |
| Sodium dichromate (dihydrate) | 262.00 (298.00) | 356.7 | Decomposes at 400[c] | Reddish to bright-orange crystals | Soluble in water (2380 g/l at 0°C; 5080 g/l at 80°C; and methanol (513.2 g/l at 19.4°C); insoluble in ethanol |
| Strontium chromate | 203.61 | Decomposes[d] | — | Yellow crystalline powder | Slightly soluble in water (1.2 g/l at 15°C; 30 g/l at 100°C); soluble in hydrochloric, nitric and acetic acids and ammonium salts |
| Zinc chromate | 181.37 | — | — | Lemon-yellow crystals | Insoluble in cold water; decomposes in hot water; soluble in acids and liquid ammonia |
| Zinc chromate hydroxide | 280.74 | — | — | Fine yellow powder | Slightly soluble in water; soluble in dilute acids, including acetic acid |
| **Other chromium compounds** | | | | | |
| Chromium carbonyl | 220.06 | Decomposes at 110 | Explodes at 210 | Colourless crystals or white solid | Insoluble in water; slightly soluble in carbon tetrachloride and iodoform; insoluble in ethanol, diethyl ether and acetic acid |

**Table 2 (contd)**

| Chemical name | Atomic/ molecular weight | Melting– point (°C) | Boiling– point (°C) | Typical physical description | Solubility |
|---|---|---|---|---|---|
| Chromium [II] chloride | 122.90 | 824 | — | White lustrous needles or fused fibrous mass | Soluble in water; insoluble in ethanol and diethyl ether |
| Chromium dioxide | 83.99 | 300 | — | Brown–black crystalline powder | Insoluble in water; soluble in nitric acid |

[a]From Windholz (1983) and Weast (1985), unless otherwise specified
[b]From British Chrome & Chemical Ltd (1988)
[c]From Udy (1956)
[d]From Hartford (1979)

general grades associated with their use and chromic oxide content: metallurgical (greater than 46%), chemical (40-46%) and refractory (less than 40%) grades (Papp, 1985). During the past two decades, technological advances have allowed considerable interchangeability among the various grades, particularly the so-called chemical grade which can be utilized in all three industries. A more definitive classification is: (i) 'high-chromium' chromite (metallurgical-grade), containing a minimum of 46% chromic oxide and a chromium:iron ratio greater than 2:1; (ii) 'high-iron' chromite (chemical-grade), with 40-46% chromic oxide and a chromium:iron ratio of 1.5:1 to 2:1; and (iii) 'high-aluminium' chromite (refractory-grade), containing more than 20% aluminium oxide and more than 60% aluminium oxide plus chromic oxide (Papp, 1983).

Chromite from one US processor had the following typical analysis: chromium (as chromic oxide), 45.57%; iron (as ferric oxide), 29.80%; aluminium (as aluminium oxide), 13.80%; magnesium (as magnesium oxide), 9.28%; silicon (as silicon dioxide), 1.13%; and calcium (as calcium oxide), 0.40% (Cyprus Specialty Metals, 1988).

### (b)    Metallic chromium and chromium alloys

*Chromium (pure) metal* is a minor product of the metallurgical processing of chromium. It is available as electrolytic chromium (98.7-99.5% Cr; Elkem Metals Co., 1986), aluminothermic chromium (98.3% Cr (Morning, 1975) and 99.0-99.8% Cr (Delachaux, 1989)) and vacuum aluminothermic chromium (99.5-99.8% Cr; Delachaux, 1989). Electrolytic chromium and aluminothermic chromium typically contain traces of silicon, carbon, phosphorus, sulfur, iron, aluminium, nitrogen, oxygen and hydrogen (Elkem Metals Co., 1986; Belmont Metals, 1989). Chromium metal rapidly forms an oxide layer at the surface in air; such oxidation of finely divided chromium powder can result in the conversion of a large fraction of the metal to metal oxide upon prolonged storage (Sunderman et al., 1974).

*Ferrochromiums* are the main intermediates in the metallurgical processing of chromium. There are three categories: high-carbon, low-carbon and ferrochromium silicon. The compositions of typical ferrochromiums are given in Table 3 (Morning, 1975).

*Chromium-containing steels* are usually stainless steels and are iron-base alloys. Some representative analyses of various grades are given in Table 4.

*Chromium alloys* can be categorized as nickel-chromium, cobalt-chromium and iron-nickel-chromium alloys. Some representative analyses are given in Table 5.

A range of chromium-containing alloys is used for surgical implants. Specifications of the American Society for Testing and Materials for such alloys are given in Table 6.

**Table 3. Composition of typical ferrochromium and chromium metals[a]**

| Grade | Chromium | Silicon | Carbon | Sulfur (max) | Phosphorus (max) |
|---|---|---|---|---|---|
| High-carbon | 65-70 | 1-2 | 5-6.5 | 0.04 | 0.03 |
| Charge chromium: | | | | | |
| 50-55% chromium | 50-55 | 3-6 | 6-8 | 0.04 | 0.03 |
| 66-70% chromium | 66-70 | 3 | 5-6.5 | 0.04 | 0.03 |
| Low-carbon: | | | | | |
| 0.025% carbon | 67-75 | 1 | 0.025 | 0.025 | 0.03 |
| 0.05% carbon | 67-75 | 1 | 0.05 | 0.025 | 0.03 |
| Ferrochromium-silicon | | | | | |
| 36/40 grade | 35-37 | 39-41 | 0.05 | - | - |
| 40/43 grade | 39-41 | 42-45 | 0.05 | - | - |

[a]From Morning (1975)

**Table 4. Elemental analysis of representative grades of stainless steel[a]**

| Grade of steel | Elements in presence of iron (weight %) | | | | | | | | |
|---|---|---|---|---|---|---|---|---|---|
| | Cr | Ni | Mn | Mo | C | Si | S | P | N |
| Austenitic | | | | | | | | | |
| AISI-201 | 16.0-18.0 | 3.5-5.5 | 5.5-7.5 | - | 0.15 | 1.0 | 0.03 | 0.06 | 0.25 |
| AISI-302 | 17.0-19.0 | 8.0-10.0 | 2.0 | - | 0.15 | 1.0 | 0.03 | 0.05 | - |
| AISI-304 | 18.0-20.0 | 8.0-10.5 | 2.0 | - | 0.08 | 1.0 | 0.03 | 0.05 | - |
| AISI-316 | 16.0-18.0 | 10.0-14.0 | 2.0 | 2.0-3.0 | 0.08 | 1.0 | 0.03 | 0.05 | - |
| Ferritic | | | | | | | | | |
| AISI-405 | 11.5-14.5 | - | 1.0 | - | 0.08 | 1.0 | 0.03 | 0.04 | - |
| AISI-430 | 16.0-18.0 | - | 1.0 | - | 0.12 | 1.0 | 0.03 | 0.04 | - |
| AISI-442 | 18.0-23.0 | - | 1.0 | - | 0.20 | 1.0 | 0.03 | 0.04 | - |
| Martensitic | | | | | | | | | |
| AISI-403 | 11.5-13.0 | - | 1.0 | - | 0.15 | 0.50 | 0.03 | 0.04 | - |
| AISI-440 A | 16.0-18.0 | - | 1.0 | 0.75 | 0.60-0.75 | 1.0 | 0.03 | 0.04 | - |

[a]From Nickel Development Institute (1987a)

Table 5. Elemental analyses of representative chromium alloys (weight %)

| Alloy | Cr | Ni | Co | Fe | Mo | W | Ta | Nb | Al | Ti | Mn | Si | C | B | Zr |
|---|---|---|---|---|---|---|---|---|---|---|---|---|---|---|---|
| Nickel base | | | | | | | | | | | | | | | |
| Cast alloys | | | | | | | | | | | | | | | |
| Cast alloy 625 | 21.6 | 63.0 | – | 2.0 | 8.7 | – | – | 3.9 | 0.2 | 0.2 | 0.06 | 0.20 | 0.20 | – | – |
| Nimocast alloy 263 | 20.0 | 55.0 | 20.0 | 0.5 | 5.8 | – | – | – | 0.5 | 2.2 | 0.50 | – | 0.06 | 0.008 | 0.04 |
| Udimet 500 | 18.0 | 52.0 | 19.0 | – | 4.2 | – | – | – | 3.0 | 3.0 | – | – | 0.07 | 0.007 | 0.05 |
| Wrought alloys | | | | | | | | | | | | | | | |
| Hastelloy alloy X | 22.0 | 47.0 | 1.5 | 18.5 | 9.0 | 0.6 | – | – | – | – | 0.50 | 0.50 | 0.10 | – | – |
| Inconel alloy 617 | 22.0 | 54.0 | 12.5 | – | 9.0 | – | – | – | 1.0 | – | – | – | 0.07 | – | – |
| Nimonic alloy PE 16 | 16.5 | 43.5 | – | 34.4 | 3.2 | – | – | – | 1.2 | 1.2 | – | – | 0.05 | 0.003 | 0.04 |
| Cobalt base | | | | | | | | | | | | | | | |
| Cast alloys | | | | | | | | | | | | | | | |
| Haynes alloy 1002 | 22.0 | 16.0 | Bal. | 1.5 | – | 7.0 | 3.8 | – | 0.3 | 0.2 | 0.70 | 0.40 | 0.60 | – | 0.30 |
| WI-52 | 21.0 | – | 63.0 | 2.0 | – | 11.0 | – | 2.0 | – | – | 0.25 | 0.25 | 0.45 | – | – |
| Wrought alloy | | | | | | | | | | | | | | | |
| Haynes alloy 188 | 22.0 | 22.0 | 39.0 | 3.0 (max) | – | 14.0 | – | – | – | – | 1.25 (max) | 0.40 | 0.10 | – | – |
| Iron-nickel base | | | | | | | | | | | | | | | |
| Wrought alloys | | | | | | | | | | | | | | | |
| Haynes alloy 556 | 22.0 | 20.0 | 20.0 | 29.0 | 3.0 | 2.5 | 0.9 | 0.1 | 0.3 | – | 1.50 | 0.40 | 0.10 | – | – |
| Incoloy alloy 800 | 21.0 | 32.5 | – | 46.0 | – | – | – | – | 0.4 | 0.4 | 0.80 | 0.50 | 0.05 | – | – |

[a]From Nickel Development Institute (1987b); Bal, balance

**Table 6. Composition specifications for four representative chromium–containing alloys used in surgical implants (weight %)[a]**

| Alloy | Cr | Mo | Ni | Fe | C | Si | Mn | N | P | S | Ti | W | Co |
|-------|------|------|----------|---------|------------|----------|---------|----------|-----------|----------|---------|---------|---------|
| A | 27.0–30.0 | 5.0–7.0 | 1.0 max | 0.75 max | 0.35 max | 1.0 max | 1.0 max | NA | NA | NA | NA | NA | Balance |
| B | 19.0–21.0 | 9.0–10.5 | 33.0–37.0 | 1.0 max | 0.025 max | 0.15 max | 0.15 max | NA | 0.015 max | 0.01 max | 1.0 max | NA | Balance |
| C | 18.0–22.0 | 3.0–4.0 | 15.0–25.0 | 4.0–6.0 | 0.05 max | 0.50 max | 1.0 max | NA | NA | 0.01 max | 0.5–3.5 | 3.0–4.0 | Balance |
| D | 26.0–30.0 | 5.0–7.0 | 1.0 max | 0.75 max | 0.35 max | 1.0 max | 1.0 max | 0.25 max | NA | NA | NA | NA | Balance |

[a]From American Society for Testing and Materials (1984a, 1987a,b, 1988a)

NA, not applicable

*(c)    Chromium [III] compounds*

*Basic chromic sulfate* is produced by one company in the UK, as 67% basic chromic sulfate and 25-37% sodium sulfate (British Chrome & Chemical Ltd, 1988).

*Chromic acetate* is available as a 50% green aqueous solution with the following typical analysis; chromium, 11.4%; sulfate, less than 0.2%; chloride, less than 0.1% (McGean-Rohco, 1984).

*Chromic chloride* hexahydrate is available as a 62% green aqueous solution, typically containing 12% chromium and less than 0.2% sulfate (McGean-Rohco, 1984).

*Chromic nitrate* is available as a hydrate ($Cr(NO_3)_3.7.5-9H_2O$) in granules; 12.5-13.5% chromium and as the nonahydrate in liquid form (6.5-10.9% chromium) (McGean-Rohco, 1984).

*Chromic oxide* is available in several grades depending on its use in metallurgical and refractory industries. A typical analysis of a metallurgical grade is 99.4% chromium (as chromic oxide) and less than 0.1% moisture. A typical analysis of a refractory grade is 98.5-99.4% chromium (as chromic oxide), 0.1% alkali metals (as sodium oxide), 0.1% other metal oxides (mainly aluminium, iron and magnesium), and average particle size, 0.5-3.5 μm (American Chrome & Chemicals, undated a,b,c,d). Chromic oxide pigment (dark chromium oxide) typically contains > 99.0% chromium as chromic oxide (Mineral Pigments Corp., undated a).

*Chrome base spinels* are part of the family of mixed metal oxide organic coloured pigments. Two such pigments are (i) chromium iron nickel black spinel, the composition of which may include any one or a combination of cupric oxide, manganese oxide and manganese sesquioxide as modifiers, and (ii) chrome manganese zinc brown spinel, which may contain any one or a combination of aluminium oxide, nickel monoxide, silicon dioxide, stannous oxide and titanium dioxide as modifiers (Dry Color Manufacturers' Association, 1982).

*Chromic phosphate* tetrahydrate is available with a purity of 99.9% (National Chemical Co., undated a).

Analytical reagent-grade *chromium sulfate* hydrate is available with the following impurities: ammonium, 0.01% max; chloride, 0.002% max; insoluble matter, 0.01% max; and iron, 0.01% max. Analytical reagent-grade *potassium chromic sulfate* dodecahydrate is available at a purity greater than 98.0%. Potassium chromic sulfate with various degrees of hydration is available commercially as Chrome Alum Crystal (violet crystals) containing 10% chromium and Chrome Alum 0% Basicity (green powder) containing 15.4% chromium (McGean-Rohco, 1984).

### (d) Chromium[VI] compounds

*Ammonium dichromate* is available as analytical reagent-grade crystals (99.5%) and as purified-grade crystals and granules with the following impurities: chloride, 0.005% max; fixed alkalis (as sulfate), 0.1-0.2% max; insoluble matter, 0.005% max; and sulfate, 0.005% max.

*Calcium chromate* is available at a purity of 96% min (Barium & Chemicals, 1988a). When used as a pigment for primer applications, it has the following typical analysis: chromium oxide, 45%; calcium oxide, 44%; chloride, less than 0.001%; sulfate, less than 0.001%; and moisture, 0.01% (National Chemical Co., undated b).

*Chromium trioxide* is available commercially at a purity of 99.9% (McGean-Rohco, 1984; Occidental Chemical Corp., 1987a; American Chrome & Chemicals, undated e). Two grades available from one company in Europe contain maxima of 20 and 100 mg/kg metallic impurities.

Analytical reagent-grade *potassium chromate* (crystals) is available at a purity of 99.0%. *Potassium dichromate* is available at a purity of 99.8% (Occidental Chemical Corp., 1987b).

Technical-grade anhydrous *sodium chromate* is available at a purity of 99.5% (Occidental Chemical Corp., 1987c). *Sodium dichromate* dihydrate is available at a purity of 100.0% (American Chrome & Chemicals, undated f). Anhydrous sodium dichromate is available at a purity of 99.70% (American Chrome & Chemicals, undated g).

*Barium chromate* is available at a purity of 98.5-99% (Atomergic Chemetals Corp., 1980; Barium & Chemicals, 1988b; National Chemical Co., undated c).

The term '*zinc chromate*' is a generic term for a series of commercial products with three kinds of molecular structure: (i) 'zinc chromate' type (like $ZnCrO_4$); (ii) 'basic zinc chromate' type (like zinc tetrahydroxychromate ($ZnCrO_4.4Zn(OH)_2$); and (iii) '(basic) zinc potassium chromate' type (like $3ZnCrO_4.Zn(OH)_2.K_2CrO_4.2H_2O$). Several different commercial 'zinc chromates' are also referred to as 'zinc yellow'.

Analytical reagent-grade *lead chromate* powder is available at a purity of >98%. The commercial lead chromate pigments, Primrose Chrome Yellow, Light Chrome Yellow and Medium Chrome Yellow, contain 65-89% lead chromate (Mineral Pigments Corp., undated b,c; National Chemical Co., undated d).

*Molybdenum orange* is described as a complex of lead molybdate, lead chromate and lead sulfate (National Chemical Co., undated e). One composition comprises 65% lead, 12% chromium and 3% molybdenum (Wayne Pigment Corp., 1985a,b).

*Strontium chromate* is available at a purity of 99% (National Chemical Co., undated f). A strontium chromate pigment is available with a typical analysis of 41.4% strontium and 46.7-47.3% chromium (Mineral Pigments Corp., undated d).

# 2. Production, Use, Occurrence and Analysis

The early history of chromium compounds, including synthetic methods used in their preparation, has been reviewed (Mellor, 1931).

## 2.1 Production

Chromium was first isolated and identified as a metal by the French chemist, Vauquelin, in 1798, working with a rare mineral, Siberian red lead (crocoite, $PbCrO_4$).

A generalized flow diagram for the production processes used now to lead from chromite ore to the major products containing chromium is shown in Figure 1.

### (a) Chromite ore

Although chromium is found in various minerals, chromite is the sole source of chromium used commercially (Stern, 1982). From 1797 until 1827, chromite from the Ural Mountains of Russia was the principal source of world supply, primarily for chemical use. After chromite ore was discovered in the USA in 1827, that country became the principal source for the limited world demand; it no longer produces it. Large Turkish deposits were developed in 1860 to supply the world market. Table 7 presents world production figures by region in 1976, 1982 and 1987.

### (b) Metallic chromium and chromium alloys

*Chromium metal* is made commercially in the USA by two processes: (i) an electrolytic method in which a chromium-containing electrolyte, prepared by dissolving a high-carbon ferrochromium in a solution of sulfuric acid and chromium potassium sulfate, is subjected to electrolysis; and (ii) an aluminothermic reduction method in which chromic oxide is reduced with finely divided aluminium (Bacon, 1964; Papp, 1983).

In 1970, US production of chromium metal and metal alloys, other than ferrochromium alloys, was 14 thousand tonnes (about 75% by the electrolytic method; IARC, 1980a); this had increased to 18 thousand tonnes by 1976 (Morning, 1978). Production included chromium briquets, exothermic chromium additives and miscellaneous chromium alloys, in addition to chromium metal. By 1987, US production of chromium metal and ferrochromium-silicon (including exothermic chro-

**Fig. 1. Simplified flow chart for the production of metallic chromium, chromium compounds and selected products from chromite ore. Processes for which occupational exposure levels to chromium are available are indicated by ▲[a]**

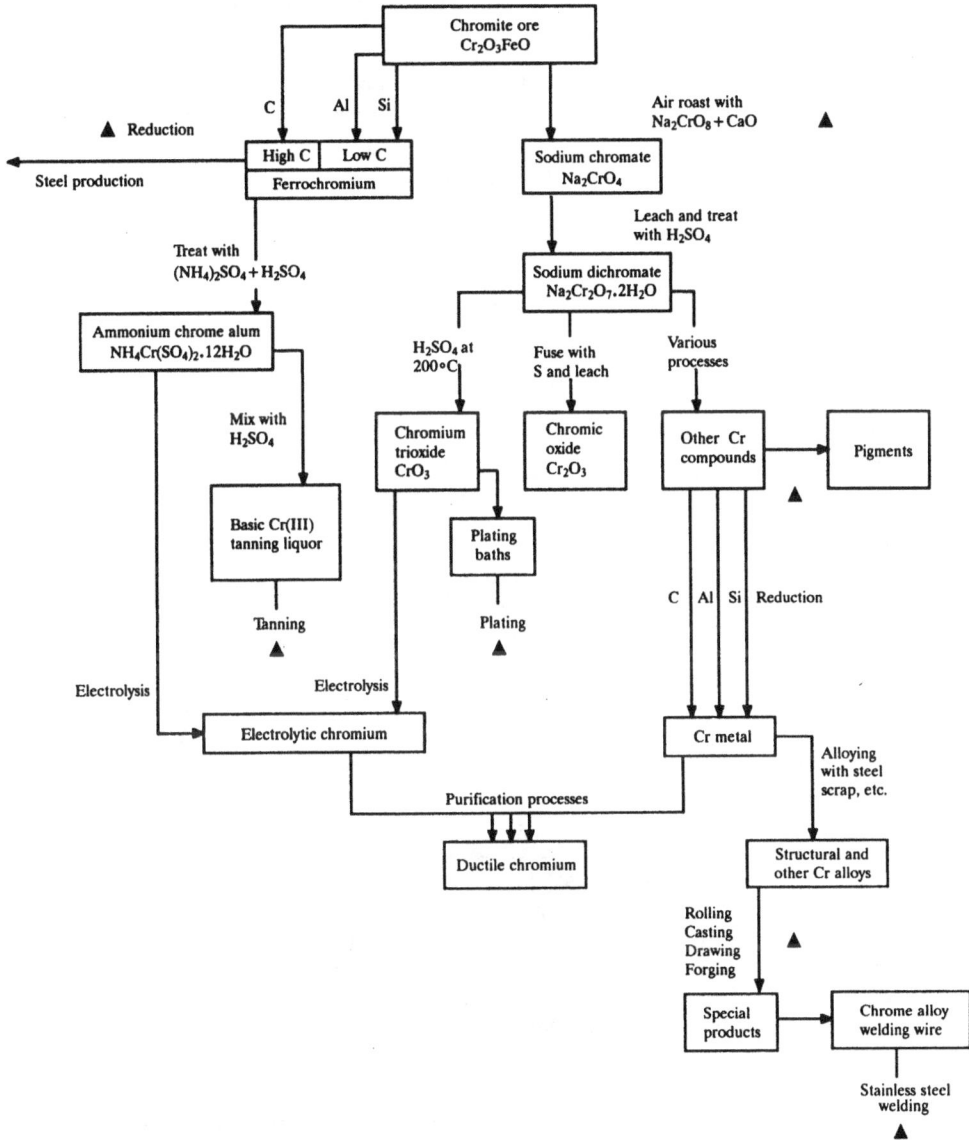

Chromite ore
$Cr_2O_3FeO$

C    Al    Si

▲ Reduction

Steel production

Air roast with
$Na_2CrO_8 + CaO$    ▲

High C    Low C
Ferrochromium

Sodium chromate
$Na_2CrO_4$

Treat with
$(NH_4)_2SO_4 + H_2SO_4$

Leach and treat
with $H_2SO_4$

Sodium dichromate
$Na_2Cr_2O_7.2H_2O$

Ammonium chrome alum
$NH_4Cr(SO_4)_2.12H_2O$

$H_2SO_4$ at
$200 °C$

Fuse with
S and leach

Various
processes

Mix with
$H_2SO_4$

Chromium
trioxide
$CrO_3$

Chromic
oxide
$Cr_2O_3$

Other Cr
compounds

Pigments

▲

Basic Cr(III)
tanning liquor

Plating
baths

C    Al    Si    Reduction

Tanning    Plating
▲          ▲

Electrolysis          Electrolysis

Electrolytic chromium          Cr metal

Alloying
with steel
scrap, etc.

Purification processes

Ductile chromium          Structural and
other Cr alloys

Rolling
Casting
Drawing
Forging    ▲

Special
products

Chrome alloy
welding wire

Stainless steel
welding
▲

[a]From Stern (1982)

mium additives and other miscellaneous chromium alloys) had dropped to 1900 tonnes (Papp, 1988).

**Table 7. World mine production of chromite ore by region (thousand tonnes)[a]**

| Region[b] | 1976 | 1982 | 1987 |
|---|---|---|---|
| Albania | 794 | 675 | 830 |
| Brazil | 172 | 276 | 227 |
| Cuba | 32 | 27 | 122 |
| Cyprus | 9 | 3 | 0 |
| Egypt | 1 | 0 | 0 |
| Finland | 414 | 345 | 712 |
| France (New Caledonia) | 10 | 50 | 62 |
| Greece | 27 | 29 | 64 |
| India | 401 | 364 | 522 |
| Iran | 160 | 41 | 56 |
| Japan | 22 | 11 | 12 |
| Madagascar | 221 | 44 | 100 |
| Oman | 0 | 0 | 6 |
| Pakistan | 11 | 4 | 8 |
| Philippines | 427 | 322 | 172 |
| South Africa | 2409 | 2431[c] | 3787[c] |
| Sudan | 22 | 19 | 8 |
| Turkey | 740 | 453 | 599 |
| USSR | 2120 | 2939 | 3148 |
| Viet Nam | 9 | 16 | 15 |
| Yugoslavia | 2 | 0 | 0 |
| Zimbabwe | 608 | 432 | 540 |
| Total | 8611 | 8481 | 10 990 |

[a]From Morning (1978); Papp (1987, 1988)

[b]In addition to the regions listed, Argentina, Bulgaria, China, Colombia, the Democratic Republic of Korea and Thailand may also have produced chromite ore, but output was not reported quantitatively and available general information was inadequate for formulation of reliable estimates of production.

[c]Includes production by Bophuthatswana

Chromium metal has been produced in Japan since 1956, where it is manufactured by two companies by electrolysis of an ammonium chromic sulfate solution. About 9000 tonnes were produced in 1977; there were no reported imports or exports (IARC, 1980a).

*Ferrochromium* is produced by treatment of chromite ore in electric furnaces using coke as a reducing agent. Worldwide production figures for all grades of ferrochromium are summarized in Table 8.

**Table 8. World production of ferrochromium (all grades, in thousands of metric tonnes)[a]**

| Country | 1983 | 1985 | 1987 |
|---|---|---|---|
| Albania | 35 | 13 | 35 |
| Brazil | 80 | 136.2 | 113.5 |
| Finland | 58.7 | 133 | 143 |
| France | 18.1 | 0 | 0 |
| Germany, Federal Republic of | 45 | 70 | 23 |
| Greece | 18.5 | 45 | 45 |
| India | 53.5 | 78.5 | 122.1 |
| Italy | 45.4 | 57.6 | 59 |
| Japan | 329.1 | 379.7 | 291 |
| Philippines | 27 | 51 | 59 |
| South Africa | 699.5 | 851 | 948 |
| Spain | 18 | 30 | 17.6 |
| Sweden | 119.4 | 135 | 110 |
| Turkey | 30.1 | 53.3 | 54 |
| USA[b] | 33 | 99.7 | 106.7 |
| USSR | 634 | 415 | NA |
| Yugoslavia | 68 | 73 | 80 |
| Zimbabwe | 140 | 180 | 185 |

[a]From Chromium Association (1989)
[b]Includes L and HC ferrochromium, FeSiCr, Cr metal and other miscellaneous alloys
NA, not available

*Chromium-containing steels* (stainless steels and others) are produced by melting cast iron and adding ferrochromium and/or steel scraps in large electric furnaces. The melt is transferred to a refining vessel to adjust the carbon content and impurity levels and is then cast into ingots or continuously into casting shapes. Defects in the cast steel are repaired by cutting or scarfing or by chipping or grinding. The desired shapes are produced primarily by rolling, and their surfaces are conditioned by a variety of operations, including grinding, polishing and pickling (Warner, 1984).

Production figures are given in Table 9.

*Chromium alloys* are produced by technology very similar to that used for steel production, except that the melting and decarburizing units are generally smaller

and greater use is made of vacuum melting and remelting (Warner, 1984). No data
were available on production volumes of these alloys.

**Table 9.  Stainless-steel production in selected countries[a]**
**(in thousands of metric tonnes)**

| Country | 1987 | 1988 |
|---|---|---|
| Austria | 54 | 67 |
| Belgium | 182 | 254 |
| Finland | 189 | 206 |
| France | 720 | 784 |
| Germany, Federal Republic of | 957 | 1186 |
| Italy | 550 | 623 |
| Japan | 2722 | 3161 |
| Spain | 327 | 426 |
| Sweden | 457 | 482 |
| UK | 393 | 427 |
| USA | 1840 | 1995 |
| Yugoslavia | 30 | 30 |

[a]From ERAMET-SLN (1989)

Cobalt-chromium alloys were first made in 1907 by fusion of cobalt with
10-60% chromium (Haynes, 1907). Commercial production began shortly thereafter, and since 1920 more than 75% of the cobalt used in the USA has been for the
manufacture of alloys with chromium (Sibley, 1976).

Eight US companies produced chromium alloys in 1975, but separate data on
the quantity of cobalt-chromium alloys produced were not available (Morning,
1978). Stellite (usually 53% Co, 35% Cr and the remainder tungsten) has been produced by one company in the UK (Roskill Information Services, 1974).

### (c)   Chromium [III] compounds

Solutions of *chromic acetate* are produced by dissolving freshly prepared hydrous chromic oxide in acetic acid (IARC, 1980a). Commercial mixtures of chromic
acetate with sodium acetate have been prepared by reduction of sodium dichromate with glucose or corn sugar in the presence of acetic acid (Copson, 1956).

Chromic acetate was produced by five companies in the USA, but no data on
volumes were available (IARC, 1980a); it is now produced by one company (Chemical Information Services Ltd, 1988). Annual production in Japan has been about 30
tonnes (IARC, 1980a). Chromic acetate is currently produced by two companies
each in Japan and the UK and one each in Australia, Canada and Italy (Chemical
Information Services Ltd, 1988).

*Chromic chloride* hexahydrate is prepared by dissolving freshly prepared chromium hydroxide in hydrochloric acid. Anhydrous chromic chloride can be produced by passing chlorine over a mixture of chromic oxide and carbon (Sax & Lewis, 1987). Chromic chloride has been produced by two companies in the USA, but no data on volumes were available.

In Japan, chromic chloride has been produced from chromic sulfate by converting it to purified chromic carbonate, which is treated with hydrochloric acid. About 100 tonnes of chromic chloride were produced by one Japanese company in 1977; there were no reported imports or exports. Four companies currently produce chromic chloride in Japan (Chemical Information Services Ltd, 1988).

Chromic chloride is also produced by three companies in the UK, two in the Federal Republic of Germany and one each in Australia and the German Democratic Republic (Chemical Information Services Ltd, 1988).

*Chromic hydroxide* is produced by adding a solution of ammonium hydroxide to the solution of a chromium salt (Sax & Lewis, 1987). It is produced by one company each in Argentina, Brazil, France, Japan and Turkey, two each in Austria, Spain, the UK and the USA and four in India (Chemical Information Services Ltd, 1988).

*Chromic nitrate* may be produced by the action of nitric acid on chromium hydroxide (Sax & Lewis, 1987). It is produced by three companies each in Japan, the UK and the USA, two each in Italy and Spain and one in the Federal Republic of Germany (Chemical Information Services Ltd, 1988).

Anhydrous *chromic oxide* is produced commercially by heating chromic hydroxide, by heating dry ammonium dichromate, or by heating sodium dichromate with sulfur and washing out the sodium sulfate (Sax & Lewis, 1987). The hydrated material is made commercially by calcining sodium dichromate with boric acid and hydrolysing chromic borate (IARC, 1980a).

Chromic oxide was produced by six companies in the USA in 1977. US production of the most important type of chromic oxide, chromic oxide green, was reported to be about 6000 tonnes in 1971 (IARC, 1980a), about 3700 tonnes in 1976 and 2700 tonnes in 1977 (Hartford, 1979). It is now produced by one company in the USA (Chemical Information Services Ltd, 1988). Chromic oxide has been produced in Japan by two companies, either by heating hydrous chromic oxide or chromium trioxide or by reducing sodium dichromate with carbon. An estimated 2700 tonnes were produced in 1977 (IARC, 1980a). It is also produced by two companies each in the Federal Republic of Germany and the UK and one each in France, India, Italy, Spain and Switzerland (Chemical Information Services Ltd, 1988).

A violet hexahydrate form of *chromic phosphate* is formed by mixing cold solutions of potassium chromium sulfate (chrome alum) with disodium phosphate. A green crystalline dihydrate is obtained by boiling the violet hexahydrate with acetic anhydride or by heating it in dry air (Udy, 1956).

Chromic phosphate is produced by two companies in the USA and one each in Australia, Austria, the Federal Republic of Germany, India, Japan and the UK (Chemical Information Services Ltd, 1988).

Solutions of mixed hydrated *chromic sulfates* are obtained by dissolving chromic oxide in concentrated sulfuric acid and allowing it to stand until crystals of the hydrated chromic sulfate separate. The anhydrous form is produced by heating any of the hydrates to 400°C in air or to 280°C in a stream of carbon dioxide (IARC, 1980a). Mixtures of *basic chromic sulfates* (containing mainly $Cr(OH)SO_4$) with sodium sulfate are produced commercially by the organic reduction (with such substances as molasses) of a solution of sodium dichromate in the presence of sulfuric acid or by reduction of dichromate solutions with sulfur dioxide (Copson, 1956).

Two companies in the USA produce chromium sulfate and one produces basic chromic sulfate, but no data on volumes were available (Chemical Information Services Ltd, 1988).

Both chromium sulfate and basic chromic sulfate have been produced in Japan since about 1950, by reduction of sodium dichromate with glucose. The combined production of the two producers in 1977 (which are still operating) was about 2000 tonnes basic chromic sulfate and about 120 tonnes chromium sulfate (IARC, 1980a).

Chromium sulfate is also produced by one company each in Brazil, France, India and New Zealand, two each in the Federal Republic of Germany and Spain and three in the UK. Basic chromic sulfate is also produced by one company each in Australia, Brazil, Colombia, Italy, Mexico, Pakistan, Turkey and the USSR, two each in China and India and three in the UK (Chemical Information Services Ltd, 1988).

*Potassium chromic sulfate dodecahydrate* (potassium chrome alum) is produced commercially by the reduction of potassium dichromate with sulfur dioxide (Copson, 1956). One company in the USA currently produces potassium chromic sulfate, but no data on volumes were available (Chemical Information Services Ltd, 1988). It was produced commercially in Japan before 1940. Production reached about 20-30 tonnes in 1970; subsequently, the annual quantity produced decreased rapidly, and only about one tonne was produced in 1977 (IARC, 1980a).

Potassium chromic sulfate is also produced by one company in Brazil and one company in Czechoslovakia (Chemical Information Services Ltd, 1988).

### (d)   Chromium[VI] compounds

Hexavalent chromium compounds that are commonly manufactured include sodium chromate, potassium chromate, potassium dichromate, ammonium dichromate and chromium trioxide. Other materials that contain chromium[VI] are paint and primer pigments, graphic art supplies, fungicides, wood preservatives and corrosion inhibitors (National Institute for Occupational Safety and Health, 1975). Each chromate-producing process involves the roasting of chromite ore with soda and lime at about 1100°C in a furnace or rotary kiln (Gafafer, 1953). Water-soluble hexavalent chromium compounds do not occur in the ore but comprise part of roast, residue and product materials (Kuschner & Laskin, 1971). The presence of lime ensures that aluminium and silicon oxides in the ore are converted to insoluble compounds, the soluble sodium chromate being recovered by a leaching and crystallization process (National Institute for Occupational Safety and Health, 1975). Chromium trioxide is produced by acidifying the leachate solution with sulfuric acid (Gafafer, 1953). In the manufacture of pigments, chromium trioxide or alkali chromates are reacted with soluble compounds of zinc, lead, iron, molybdenum, strontium and other metals (Stern, 1982). The insoluble precipitates are washed, filtered and dried in the wet department of the processing plant and then ground, blended and packed in the dry departments, where conditions are often dustiest (Gafafer, 1953).

*Ammonium dichromate* is produced by a crystallization process involving equivalent amounts of sodium dichromate and ammonium sulfate. When low alkali salt content is required, it can be prepared by the reaction of ammonia with chromium trioxide (Hartford, 1979).

Ammonium dichromate is produced by one company each in Argentina, Australia, Brazil, France, Japan, Spain and Switzerland, by two each in the Federal Republic of Germany and India, by four in the USA, and by five in the UK (Chemical Information Services Ltd, 1988).

*Calcium chromate* is produced commercially by the reaction of calcium chloride with sodium chromate. Hydrated forms can be made, but the anhydrous salt is the only product of commercial significance (IARC, 1980a).

Calcium chromate is currently produced by three companies in the USA, but no data on volumes were available (Chemical Information Services Ltd, 1988). Calcium chromate was formerly produced in Japan at an annual rate of about 100 tonnes, but it has been produced recently in only small amounts for reagent use (IARC, 1980a). It is also produced by one company each in Australia and the UK and two in France (Chemical Information Services Ltd, 1988).

*Chromium trioxide* is produced commercially by the reaction of sodium dichromate with concentrated sulfuric acid (Hartford, 1979). In 1978, there were two US producers of chromium trioxide, each with a capacity to produce 18 thousand tonnes per year (Anon., 1978). Annual US production in 1977 was in the range of 26 thousand tonnes (Hartford, 1979). In 1988, there were six US producers (Chemical

Information Services Ltd, 1988) with a combined capacity of 52 thousand tonnes per year (Anon., 1988a).

Commercial production in Japan was started before 1940. In 1977, three companies produced a total of 8300 tonnes, of which 1200 tonnes were exported; there were no reported imports (IARC, 1980a). Four companies currently produce chromium trioxide in Japan (Chemical Information Services Ltd, 1988).

Chromium trioxide is also produced by four companies each in the Federal Republic of Germany, India and the UK, three in China, two each in Argentina, Brazil and Mexico and one each in France, Italy, Pakistan, Poland and the USSR (Chemical Information Services Ltd, 1988).

*Potassium chromate* is produced by the reaction of potassium dichromate with potassium hydroxide or potassium carbonate (Hartford, 1979).

There was one US producer in 1977, but no data on volumes were available; combined US imports of potassium chromate and potassium dichromate in that year were 2.7 tonnes (US Department of Commerce, 1978). There are currently two US producers, but no data on volumes were available (Chemical Information Services Ltd, 1988). Combined US imports of the two compounds in 1985, 1986 and 1987, respectively, were 580, 750 and 1000 tonnes from the UK (52%), the USSR (22%), the Federal Republic of Germany (13%) and Canada (11%); combined US exports for the same years were 64, 19 and 9 tonnes to the Philippines (40%), the Republic of Korea (30%) and Panama (30%) (Papp, 1988).

The two Japanese producers made about one tonne in 1977 for reagent uses; there were no reported imports or exports (IARC, 1980a). One company currently produces potassium chromate in Japan (Chemical Information Services Ltd, 1988). It is also produced by five companies in the UK, four in Brazil, three each in India and Italy, and one each in Argentina, Canada, the Federal Republic of Germany, Spain and Switzerland (Chemical Information Services Ltd, 1988).

*Potassium dichromate* is produced industrially by roasting chrome ore with potassium carbonate (IARC, 1980a), or, preferably, by reacting sodium dichromate with potassium chloride (Hartford, 1979). Combined US production of potassium dichromate and potassium chromate in 1966 was estimated to be 2600-3800 tonnes, the potassium dichromate believed to be the more important industrially (IARC, 1980a).

Three companies in the USA produce potassium dichromate (Chemical Information Services Ltd, 1988). Current information on imports/exports is given above. Potassium dichromate was first produced commercially in Japan before 1940. Production by two companies in 1978 amounted to about 1000 tonnes, well below the 3200 tonnes level of 1972 and below the 1977 level of 1400 tonnes. Exports are believed to be minor (IARC, 1980a).

Potassium dichromate is also produced by six companies in India, five in the UK, four in Brazil, two each in the Federal Republic of Germany and Italy, and one each in Argentina, Romania, Spain, Switzerland, Turkey, Yugoslavia and the USSR (Chemical Information Services Ltd, 1988).

*Sodium chromate* is produced commercially by roasting chromite ore with sodium carbonate, or with sodium carbonate and calcium oxide, and leaching to dissolve the sodium chromate. After treatment to remove hydrated alumina, the sodium chromate solution is either marketed directly or evaporated to produce hydrated or anhydrous crystals (Hartford & Copson, 1964). Sodium chromate may also be produced from sodium dichromate by treatment with sodium hydroxide.

Two companies produced sodium chromate in the USA in 1978. The combined US production of sodium chromate and sodium dichromate increased from 123 thousand tonnes in 1967 to 144 thousand tonnes in 1977 (Hartford, 1979), and was 159 thousand tonnes in 1978. Currently, three companies in the USA have been reported to produce sodium chromate, but data on production volumes were not available (Chemical Information Services Ltd, 1988).

Commercial production in Japan started before 1940. Production in 1977 by the two producing companies was less than 10 tonnes (IARC, 1980a); two companies currently produce this compound (Chemical Information Services Ltd, 1988). It is also produced by five companies in India, four in Brazil, three in the UK, two in the Federal Republic of Germany and one in Spain (Chemical Information Services Ltd, 1988).

*Sodium dichromate* is produced commercially by the reaction of sulfuric acid with sodium chromate (Hartford, 1979). Three companies in the USA produced this compound in 1976. In 1988, two of five companies that produced it (Chemical Information Sciences Ltd, 1988) had a combined capacity of 144 thousand tonnes per year (Anon., 1988b).

Sodium dichromate was first produced commercially in Japan in about 1908. In 1978, the combined production of two companies was estimated to be 20.7 thousand tonnes, slightly below the 1977 level of 21 thousand tonnes (IARC, 1980a). Three companies currently produce it in that country (Chemical Information Services Ltd, 1988).

Sodium dichromate is also produced by five companies in India, four each in Brazil and the UK, three in China, two each in the Federal Republic of Germany and Turkey, and one each in Argentina, Czechoslovakia, Italy, Mexico, Pakistan, Poland, Romania, Spain, Switzerland and the USSR (Chemical Information Services Ltd, 1988).

*Barium chromate* is produced commercially by the reaction of barium chloride with sodium chromate (Copson, 1956). Five companies in the USA produced this chemical in 1977 (IARC, 1980a), and now there are four (Chemical Information Services Ltd, 1988), but no data on volumes were available. Barium chromate is produced by one company in Japan (Chemical Information Services Ltd, 1988). Production in 1977 was estimated to have been less than 50 tonnes; there were no reported imports or exports (IARC, 1980a). It is also produced by four companies in France, two in the UK, and one each in Australia, Austria, Belgium, the Federal Republic of Germany, India, Italy and Spain (Chemical Information Services Ltd, 1988).

*Basic lead chromate* (Chrome Orange) is produced by the reaction of lead oxide with sodium dichromate in the presence of acetic acid or by the reaction of lead nitrate with sodium chromate in the presence of sodium carbonate (Chalupski, 1956). No information on production of this compound in the USA was available, but combined production of Chrome Yellow and Chrome Orange, containing various proportions of basic lead chromate, amounted to 32.1 thousand tonnes in 1976 and 28.2 thousand tonnes in 1977 (Hartford, 1979). Basic lead chromate is also produced by one company each in Argentina, Colombia, the Federal Republic of Germany, Italy, Japan, Poland and Spain (Chemical Information Services Ltd, 1988).

*Lead chromate* (Chrome Yellow) can be produced by reacting sodium chromate with lead nitrate, or by reacting lead monoxide with chromic acid solution. By varying the proportion of reactants, either lead chromate ($PbCrO_4$) or lead chromate oxide (basic lead chromate; $PbO.PbCrO_4$) can be produced. High lead chromate content is associated with yellow pigments; increasing the lead chromate oxide content gives orange colours; and mixing with lead molybdate gives red pigments (Chalupski, 1956).

No information on production of this compound in the USA was available, but combined production of Chrome Yellow and Chrome Orange pigments was 32.1 thousand tonnes in 1976 and 28.2 thousand tonnes in 1977 (Hartford, 1979). Assuming an average of 70% lead chromate in these pigments, about 20 thousand tonnes of lead chromate were produced in the USA or imported for use in these pigments in that year. Lead chromate is currently produced by five companies in the USA (Chemical Information Services Ltd, 1988).

Commercial production in Japan was started in about 1910, and there were three major producers and one minor producer in 1977. Production in 1977 was 10.8 thousand tonnes and exports were 1800 tonnes. Six companies currently produce lead chromate in Japan (Chemical Information Services Ltd, 1988). Production of Chrome Yellow in 1984, 1985 and 1986, respectively, was 9900, 8500 and 7900 tonnes (Sasaki, 1985, 1986, 1987).

Lead chromate is also produced by six companies in Spain, five in Italy, three in Belgium, two each in Argentina, Austria, Canada, China, the Federal Republic of

Germany, France, the Netherlands and Turkey, and one each in Australia, Colombia, Mexico, Poland, Taiwan and the UK (Chemical Information Services Ltd, 1988).

*Molybdenum orange* pigments are variable complexes of lead sulfate, lead chromate and lead molybdate, made by pouring sodium dichromate, sulfuric acid and sodium molybdate into excess lead nitrate, preferably cold, at pH3. An ageing step is required in precipitation to permit development of the orange tetragonal form (Hartford, 1979).

Molybdenum orange is currently produced by four companies in the USA (Chemical Information Services Ltd, 1988). US imports for 1985, 1986 and 1987, respectively, were 980, 750 and 1100 tonnes from Canada (78%), the Federal Republic of Germany (16%) and Japan (6%) (Papp, 1988). Four companies currently produce molybdenum orange and molybdenum red in Japan (Chemical Information Services Ltd, 1988), and production of molybdenum red in 1984, 1985 and 1986, respectively, was 2900, 2600 and 2200 tonnes (Sasaki, 1985, 1986, 1987).

Molybdenum orange (including molybdenum red) is also produced by one company each in Australia, Austria, Canada, Colombia, India, Italy, Mexico and Taiwan, two each in Belgium, the Federal Republic of Germany, France and the Netherlands and four in Spain (Chemical Information Services Ltd, 1988).

*Strontium chromate* is prepared by adding a solution of a strontium salt to a solution of sodium chromate (Lalor, 1973).

Production of strontium chromate by three companies in the USA in 1970 was estimated to be 680 tonnes (Lalor, 1973). US imports in 1977 were 242 tonnes, mostly from Canada (US Department of Commerce, 1978). It is currently produced by five companies in the USA, but no data on volumes are available (Chemical Information Services Ltd, 1988). US imports for 1985, 1986 and 1987, respectively, were 390, 120 and 120 tonnes from France (61%), the Federal Republic of Germany (15%) and Canada (11%) (Papp, 1988).

Production in Japan began after 1940. The combined production of three companies in 1977 was about 600 tonnes, comparable with that of the previous seven years; there were no reported imports or exports (IARC, 1980a). Two companies currently produce strontium chromate in that country (Chemical Information Services Ltd, 1988).

Strontium chromate is also produced by four companies in France, two each in Australia, Italy, Spain and the UK and one each in Austria, Belgium, Brazil and the Federal Republic of Germany (Chemical Information Services Ltd, 1988).

*Zinc chromates* have been produced commercially since about 1940. Basic zinc chromates (including 'zinc chromates') are prepared by reaction between a solution of chromium trioxide and a slurry of zinc oxide. Zinc potassium chromates are prepared by a reaction between a solution of sodium dichromate, a slurry of zinc oxide and a solution of potassium chloride (Lalor, 1973).

Zinc chromate (zinc tetroxychromate) is currently produced by three companies each in Belgium, France, Italy, Japan, Spain and the USA, two each in Argentina and Austria, and one each in Australia, Canada, Colombia, India, the Netherlands, Norway, Poland, Taiwan, Turkey and the UK. Zinc potassium chromate is produced by two companies in Austria, one each in Belgium, France, Italy, Norway, Turkey and the USA (Chemical Information Services Ltd, 1988), and probably elsewhere. Production of 'zinc chromate' in Japan in 1984, 1985 and 1986 was 1530, 1280 and 1000 tonnes, respectively (Sasaki, 1985, 1986, 1987).

### (e) Other chromium compounds

*Chromium carbonyl* is produced by the reaction of carbon monoxide with chromic chloride and aluminium metal (IARC, 1980a). Two companies in the USA produce this chemical, but no data on volumes are available. Chromium carbonyl is also produced by one company in the Federal Republic of Germany (Chemical Information Services Ltd, 1988).

## 2.2 Use

An early use of chromium compounds was as pigments, particularly chrome yellow. Basic chromic sulfate was used in tanning hides, as the reaction of chromium with collagen raises the hydrothermal stability of the leather and renders it resistant to bacterial attack. The most important use of chromium, namely as an alloying element, developed gradually during the nineteenth century and led to the introduction of chromium steels (Westbrook, 1979).

Chromium is currently used in such widely diversified products as stainless, tool and alloy steels, heat- and corrosion-resistant materials, special purpose alloys, alloy cast iron, pigments, metal plating, leather tanning, chemicals, and refractory materials for metallurgical furnaces. It is used in the metallurgical industry to enhance such properties as hardenability (response to quenching), creep (unit stress that will produce plastic deformation at a specified rate and temperature), strength and impact strength and resistance to corrosion, oxidation, wear and galling; its major use is in the production of stainless steel. Chromium pigments represent the largest use of chromium in the chemical industry (Papp, 1983).

### (a) Chromite ore

Use of chromite ore in the USA decreased from 1.3 million tonnes in 1974 to 912 thousand tonnes in 1976, when utilization by the three consuming industries was as follows: metallurgical, 59.3%; refractory, 20.1%; and chemical, 20.6% (Morning, 1978). US consumption of chromite ore (and concentrate) was 504 thousand tonnes in 1987, 91% of which was used by the chemical and metallurgical industries and 9% by the refractory industry (Papp, 1988).

The metallurgical grade is used primarily to produce ferrochromium alloys, which are used in the production of stainless and other special steels (Bacon, 1964). The major use of chromite refractory materials in 1974 was in iron and steel processing, nonferrous alloy refining, glass making and cement processing (Morning, 1975); in 1987, the primary use was in refractory bricks to line metallurgical furnaces (Papp, 1988). Chemical-grade chromite ore is converted (by a series of operations involving roasting with soda ash and/or lime and leaching, with appropriate control of acidity) to sodium dichromate, used as such and in the production of many other chromium chemicals (Copson, 1956).

The major use of chromite ore in Japan has been in the production of ferrochromium (90%), the balance being used in the manufacture of refractory materials (6%), chromium compounds (3%) and chromium metal (1%) (IARC, 1980a).

### (b) Metallic chromium and chromium alloys

*Chromium metal* (pure) is used to prepare alloys with high purity specifications. Chromium is thus an important and widely used alloying element in ferrous and nonferrous alloys, including those based on nickel, iron-nickel, cobalt, aluminium, titanium and copper. In alloys based on nickel, iron-nickel and cobalt, chromium is used primarily to confer oxidation and corrosion resistance. In alloys of aluminium, titanium and copper, chromium is used to control microstructure. Stainless steel contains at least 12% and may contain up to 36% chromium. Chromium-containing tool steels contain 1-12% chromium. Most full alloy steels contain 0.5-9% chromium, but some grades contain up to 28%. Cast irons contain 0.5-30% chromium (Papp, 1983).

In 1976, 70% (170 thousand tonnes) of all US chromium metal and metal alloys were used in the production of stainless steel. Of the total of chromium metal and alloys used in the production of commercial alloys, about 60% was in high-carbon ferrochromium, 11% in low-carbon ferrochromium, 21% in ferrochromium-silicon and 7.4% in other alloys, chromium briquets, exothermic additives and chromium metal (Morning, 1978). In 1987, 82% (330 thousand tonnes) of all US chromium ferroalloys, metal and other chromium-containing materials were used in the production of stainless steel. Of the total of chromium metal and alloys used in the production of commercial alloys, about 88% was in high-carbon ferrochromium, 6.5% in low-carbon ferrochromium, 4% in ferrochromium-silicon, 0.5% in other alloys and 1% in chromium metal (Papp, 1988).

*Chromium-containing steels* are widely used in, for instance, general engineering, architectural panels and fasteners, pollution control equipment, chemical equipment, cryogenic uses, hospital equipment, domestic equipment, automotive parts, engine components and food processing (Eurométaux, 1986).

*Chromium alloys* are used in a large variety of applications, including jet engine parts, nuclear plants, high-temperature reaction vessels, chemical industry equipment, high temperature-resistant equipments, coinage, desalinization plants, ships' propellers, acid-resistant equipment, cutting tools and implants (National Research Council, 1974).

Cobalt-chromium alloys were originally developed for use in cutting tools. Subsequently, because of their corrosion resistance, they were also used for equipment in contact with acids and other chemicals. They are used for facing valves and seats in internal combustion engines; wearing surfaces or cutting edges of hot shears, trimming dies, cam gauges, punches and turbine blades; pipeline linings; and pumps for corrosive liquids (Cobalt Development Institute, 1985). Stellite alloys are used in high-temperature applications. The superalloys are used for turbine discs and blades and nozzle vanes in jet engines; grates and quenching baskets in furnaces; and high-temperature springs and fasteners (Roskill Information Services, 1974). Vitallium alloy (27 wt% Cr, 5% Mo, 0.5% C, balance Co) is most commonly used as a denture alloy (Sullivan *et al.*, 1970).

### (c)   Chromium[III] compounds

*Chromic acetate* is used in printing and tanning, as a textile mordant, a polymerization and oxidation catalyst, and an emulsion hardener (Hartford, 1979; Sax & Lewis, 1987). Most of the chromic acetate produced in Japan has been used in dyeing processes (IARC, 1980a).

*Chromic chloride* is used for the production of commercial solutions of the basic chlorides ($Cr(OH)_2Cl$) by reaction with sodium hydroxide. These solutions have been reported to have minor special applications, such as use as a mordant for alizarin dyes on cotton yarn and certain cyamine dyes on silk. In Japan, they are also used for decorative chromium plating (IARC, 1980a).

Anhydrous chromic chloride has been used as a catalyst for polymerizing olefins, for chromium plating (including vapour plating), for preparing sponge chromium and other chromium salts, as an intermediate, and for waterproofing (Sax & Lewis, 1987).

*Chromic hydroxide* has been used as a catalyst, a tanning agent, a mordant, and in the preparation of Guignet's green (hydrated chromic oxide green) (Sax & Lewis, 1987).

*Chromic nitrate* has been used as a catalyst and a corrosion inhibitor (Sax & Lewis, 1987). It has also been used in textiles and in the manufacture of chromium dioxide (Hartford, 1979).

Most *chromic oxide* (anhydrous and hydrated) is used as a pigment. A substantial portion is also used in metallurgy in the manufacture of chromium metal and aluminium-chromium master alloys and, to a lesser extent, as a catalyst, in refractory brick, and as a chemical intermediate (IARC, 1980a; Sax & Lewis, 1987).

Anhydrous chromic oxide is the most stable green pigment known and is used in applications requiring resistance to heat, light and chemicals (e.g., in glass and ceramics). It is used in dyeing polymers, and its resistance to alkali makes it a valuable colourant for latex paints. It has special use in colouring cement and granules for asphalt roofing and in camouflage paints. Metallurgical-grade anhydrous chromic oxide is used in the manufacture of chromium metal and aluminium-chromium master alloys. It is used as a catalyst in the preparation of methanol, butadiene and high-density polyethylene. Chromic oxide is also used in refractory brick as a minor component to improve performance. When used as a mild abrasive for polishing jewellery and fine metal parts, it is known as 'green rouge' (IARC, 1980a).

Hydrated chromic oxide is also used as a green pigment, especially for automotive finishes (IARC, 1980a).

In Japan, chromic oxide has been used for the production of refractory materials (36%), pigments (35%), abrasives (15%) and other uses, such as glaze for glass (14%) (IARC, 1980a).

*Chromic phosphate* is used in pigments, phosphate coatings and wash primers, and as a catalyst (Hartford, 1979; Sax & Lewis, 1987).

*Chromic sulfate* is used in chrome plating, chromium alloys, green paints and varnishes, green inks, ceramic glazes, and as a mordant for textile dyeing. Basic chromic sulfate is the principal chemical used in leather tanning (Sax & Lewis, 1987).

*Potassium chromic sulfate* (chrome alum) has been reported to be used as a mordant prior to application of mordant dyes. It is also used to treat cotton that has been dyed with certain direct cotton dyes and sulfur dyes, rendering the dyed textile faster to washing. Another important application is in the preparation of hydrous chromic oxide, which, in turn, is used to make many of the trivalent chromium mordants (Howarth, 1956). It has also been used in chrome-tan liquors for tanning, in photographic fixing baths, and in ceramics (Sax & Lewis, 1987).

*(d)   Chromium[VI] compounds*

*Ammonium dichromate* has a variety of uses, including a mordant for dyeing; in pigments; in the manufacture of alizarin, potassium chromic sulfate and catalysts; in oil purification; in pickling; in leather tanning; in synthetic perfumes; in photography; in process engraving and lithography; and in pyrotechnics (Sax & Lewis, 1987).

*Calcium chromate* is largely used as a corrosion inhibitor and as a depolarizer in batteries (Hartford, 1979). Its addition to protective coatings for steel and light metals is sometimes reported as a pigment use, but its primary function in these products is to inhibit corrosion. It is also used in ceramics and in paint pigments (Barium & Chemicals, undated). The use of calcium chromate as a pigment was discontinued in Japan some years ago (IARC, 1980a).

A major use of *chromium trioxide* has been in chromium plating, particularly in the production of automobiles. Uses in other metal-finishing operations include aluminium anodizing, particularly on military aircraft; chemical conversion coatings, which provide both decoration and corrosion protection; and the production of phosphate films on galvanized iron or steel (IARC, 1980a). Other uses of chromium trioxide are as a wood preservative (Anon., 1988a), as a corrosion inhibitor for ferrous alloys in recirculating water systems, as an oxidant in organic synthesis and in catalyst manufacture. Small amounts are used to modify the properties of basic magnesite refractories (IARC, 1980a).

US demand for chromium trioxide was 31.5 thousand tonnes in 1978 (Anon., 1978) and 57 thousand tonnes in 1988 (Anon., 1988a). The pattern of use in the USA in 1978 was as follows: metal treating and plating, 80%; wood treatment, 10%; chemical manufacturing, 5%; and other, 5% (Anon., 1978). The pattern of use in the USA in 1988 was: wood treatment, 63%; metal finishing, 22%; other (including water treatment, magnetic particles and catalysts), 7% (Anon., 1988a).

In Japan, the major use of chromium trioxide (90%) has been in chromium plating; 3% is used in pigments and 7% in other uses such as abrasives. The total used in Japan dropped from 11 800 tonnes in 1972 to 8300 tonnes in 1977 (IARC, 1980a).

*Potassium chromate* has limited applications in the textile industry — when a potassium rather than a sodium salt is essential or when differences in solubility or other physical properties make its use desirable (Howarth, 1956). Among these uses are as a mordant for wool, in dyeing nylon and wool with mordant acid dyes, in oxidizing vat dyes and indigosol dyes on wool, in dyeing with chromate colours, in treating direct dyes and some sulfur dyes on cotton to render them faster to washing, in oxidizing aniline black, and in stripping dyed wool (IARC, 1980a).

*Potassium dichromate* was once the most important commercial chromium compound, but it has largely been replaced in many applications by sodium dichromate. It is used in many small-volume applications such as photomechanical processing, chrome-pigment production and wool preservative formulations. The major use for potassium dichromate in Japan has been pigment production (54%); dye manufacture consumes an estimated 22%, with the remaining 24% used as an oxidizing agent in miscellaneous uses (as a catalyst and in other applications) (IARC, 1980a).

*Sodium chromate* is used in inks, leather tanning, wood preservation, corrosion inhibition, as a pigment in paint, water treatment, drilling muds, textile dyeing, cutting oils, catalysts, and as a raw material for the production of other chromium compounds (Sax & Lewis, 1987; American Chrome & Chemicals, undated h,i). In Japan, its principal use is as a mordant in dyeing operations (IARC, 1980a).

*Sodium dichromate* is the primary base material for the manufacture of chromium chemicals, which are used in leather tanning, metal treatment, drilling muds, textile dyes, catalysts, and wood and water treatment (Papp, 1983).

Demand for sodium dichromate in the USA was 146 thousand tonnes in 1978 (Anon., 1979) and 149 thousand tonnes in 1988 (Anon., 1988b). The pattern of use in 1978 was as follows: manufacture of chromium trioxide, 28%; manufacture of pigments, 24%; manufacture of leather tanning chemicals, 17%; corrosion control, 7%; metal treatment, drilling muds and textiles, 8%; and other (including chemical manufacture, catalysts, and wood preservation), 8% (Anon., 1979). The pattern of use in the USA in 1988 was as follows: manufacture of chromium trioxide, 54%; leather tanning, 9%; manufacture of chromium oxide, 9%; manufacture of pigments, 8%; wood preservation, 5%; and other (including drilling muds, catalysts, water treatment and metal finishing), 5% (Anon., 1988b).

*Barium chromate* is used in pyrotechnics, in high-temperature batteries, in safety matches, as a corrosion inhibitor in metal-joining compounds, as a pigment in paints, in ceramics, in fuses, in metal primers, and in ignition control devices (Hartford, 1979; Sax & Lewis, 1987). In Japan, the principal use was reported to be in explosive fuses (IARC, 1980a).

*Chrome orange pigments*, consisting largely of basic lead chromate, have been widely used in paints, metal protective primers and linoleum (Chalupski, 1956). In the early 1970s, use of chrome oranges in the USA was decreasing, although they were still being used in tints and rust-inhibiting paints (Schiek, 1973).

*Lead chromate* is used to make pigments for paints to be applied to both wood and metal. Chrome yellows (containing 52-98% lead chromate) are considered to be the most versatile of the inorganic pigments and are therefore found in many formulations designed for a wide spectrum of uses. The largest use of chrome yellows in the early 1970s was in paint for automotive finishes, farm machinery, architectural and air-dried finishes, and water-thinned coatings for exterior and interior use. Medium chrome yellow paints make up about 30% of the paint used for traffic control. Chrome yellows are also used as colourants in vinyls, rubber and paper. The second largest use of chrome yellows is in printing inks (Schiek, 1973).

The major use for lead chromate in Japan is in the production of pigments for paint and inks (85%); other uses are as a colourant for synthetic resins (14%) and miscellaneous applications (1%) (IARC, 1980a).

*Molybdenum orange* pigments are used in coatings, inks and plastics (National Chemical Company, undated e).

*Strontium chromate* was first used commercially (near the end of the nineteenth century) as a colourant in artists' paints, under the name 'citron yellow'. It was replaced for this use by organic pigments in 1936, at which time it was also being used for corrosion resistance on aluminium and magnesium alloys. Later, it was used in chemical-resistant coatings because of its low reactivity, and in epoxy polyamide vehicles and vinyl sheeting because of its heat-resistant properties. In 1973, some strontium chromate was still being used in vinyl sheeting and chemical-resistant coatings and in primer coatings for water tanks, but most of it was used, either alone or in combination with basic zinc chromate, in wash primers or in aluminium flake coatings (Lalor, 1973). Strontium chromate has also been used as an additive to control the sulfate content of solutions in electrochemical processes (Hartford & Copson, 1964). In Japan, the only known use has been as a corrosion inhibitor (IARC, 1980a).

*Zinc chromates* are used as pigments in paints, varnishes and oil colours. Many of them are used as a corrosion-resisting primer coatings and in metal conditioners (wash primers) applied before priming; in this case, they are used more for their chemical characteristics than their hue (Lalor, 1973; Windholz, 1983).

### (e)   Other chromium compounds

*Chromium carbonyl* has reportedly been used as an isomerization and polymerization catalyst, as a gasoline additive, and as a chemical intermediate (Sax & Lewis, 1987). It has also been used in the synthesis of 'sandwich' compounds (Hartford, 1979) from aromatic hydrocarbons, such as dibenzene(chromium) from benzene. Some of these compounds have been investigated as possible sources of vapour-deposited chromium and for the production of carbides.

### 2.3   Occurrence

The occurrence and distribution of chromium in the environment has been reviewed (Sayato & Nakamuro, 1980; Sequi, 1980; Balsberg-Påhlsson *et al.*, 1982; Cary, 1982; Filiberti *et al.*, 1983; Fishbein, 1984; Gauglhofer, 1984; Jin & Hou, 1984; Barceló *et al.*, 1986; Poschenrieder *et al.*, 1986; Camusso & Montesissa, 1988; Nriagu & Nieboer, 1988).

### (a)   Natural occurrence

Chromium is widely distributed in the earth's crust but is concentrated in the ultrabasic rocks. At an overall crust concentration of 125 mg/kg Cr (National Research Council, 1974), it is the twentieth most abundant element, ranking with vanadium, zinc, nickel, copper and tungsten (Westbrook, 1979). Only the trivalent and hexavalent compounds are detected in the environment in significant quantities (Fishbein, 1976). In reducing environments, chromium[VI] is unstable relative to chromium[III]. The average concentration of chromium in basalt, shale and granite has been reported to be 200, 100 and 20 ppm (mg/kg), respectively. The world average concentration of chromium in ultramafic, mafic, intermediate and felsic rock has been reported to be 2000, 200, 50 and 25 ppm (mg/kg), respectively. Concentrations in rock samples from Hawaiian lavas, from the Skaergaard intrusion in Greenland and from tertiary lavas of northeastern Ireland ranged from less than 1 ppm to 1750 ppm (mg/kg) chromium (Cary, 1982).

Chromium is found in nature only in the combined state and not as the free metal. It exists mainly as chromite, which has the idealized composition $FeO.Cr_2O_3$, although this composition has been found in nature only in meteorites. Chromite is a mixed metal oxide spinel containing iron, chromium, magnesium and aluminium in various proportions (Hartford, 1963) and as such is found in considerable quantities in Zimbabwe, the USSR, South Africa, New Caledonia and the Philippines (National Research Council, 1974; World Health Organization, 1988); it contains 40-50% chromium (Bidstrup & Case, 1956).

Of the chromium chemicals (other than chromite ore) included in this monograph, only two are known to occur in nature in mineral form: lead chromate as crocoite and potassium dichromate as lopezite (Hartford, 1963).

### (b) Occupational exposures

Occupational exposures to a number of specific chromium compounds have been reported. With respect to hexavalent compounds, the most important exposures are to sodium, potassium, calcium and ammonium chromates and dichromates during chromate production, to chromium trioxide during chrome plating, to insoluble chromates of zinc and lead during pigment production and spray painting, to water-soluble alkaline chromates during steel smelting and welding and to other chromates during cement production and use. Trivalent compounds that are common in work place air include chromite ore during chromate production and in the ferrochromium industry, chromic oxide during pigment production and use, and chromic sulfate during leather tanning. In addition, occupational exposures to airborne dusts containing chromium metal may occur during production, welding, cutting and grinding of chromium alloys (Stern, 1982; Nieboer et al., 1984; World Health Organization, 1988; see the monograph on welding, pp. 463-474). A schematic diagram of the production processes for some important commercial chromium compounds was given in Figure 1, on which those operations for which exposure data are available are indicated.

Potential occupational exposure to chromium occurs through inhalation, ingestion or skin contact (National Research Council, 1974). The US National Institute for Occupational Safety and Health (1977) estimated that about two million workers are exposed to chromium and chromium compounds. Chromium ulcers or chromate dermatitis, which are indicative of occupational exposure, have been reported in numerous occupations, involving manual handling of cement, leather, plastics, dyes, textiles, paints, printing inks, cutting oils, photographic materials, detergents, wood preservatives, anticorrosion agents and welding rods (Pedersen, 1982; Burrows, 1983; Polak, 1983; Nieboer et al., 1984; Table 10; see also section 3.3(b), p. 182).

**Table 10. Occupations with potential exposure to chromium[a]**

| | |
|---|---|
| Abrasives manufacturers | Jewellers |
| Acetylene purifiers | Laboratory workers |
| Adhesives workers | Leather finishers |
| Aircraft sprayers | Linoleum workers |
| Alizarin manufacturers | Lithographers |
| Alloy manufacturers | Magnesium treaters |
| Aluminium anodizers | Match manufacturers |
| Anodizers | Metal cleaners |
| Battery manufacturers | Metal workers |
| Biologists | Milk preservers |
| Blueprint manufacturers | Oil drillers |
| Boiler scalers | Oil purifiers |
| Candle manufacturers | Painters |
| Cement workers | Palm-oil bleachers |
| Ceramic workers | Paper waterproofers |
| Chemical workers | Pencil manufacturers |
| Chromate workers | Perfume manufacturers |
| Chromium-alloy workers | Photoengravers |
| Chromium-alum workers | Photographers |
| Chromium platers | Platinum polishers |
| Copper etchers | Porcelain decorators |
| Copper-plate strippers | Pottery frosters |
| Corrosion-inhibitor workers | Pottery glazers |
| Crayon manufacturers | Printers |
| Diesel locomotive repairmen | Railroad engineers |
| Drug manufacturers | Refractory-brick manufacturers |
| Dye manufacturers | Rubber manufacturers |
| Dyers | Shingle manufacturers |
| Electroplaters | Silk-screen manufacturers |
| Enamel workers | Smokeless-powder manufacturers |
| Explosives manufacturers | Soap manufacturers |

**Table 10 (contd)**

| | |
|---|---|
| Fat purifiers | Sponge bleachers |
| Fireworks manufacturers | Steel workers |
| Flypaper manufacturers | Tanners |
| Furniture polishers | Textile workers |
| Fur processors | Wallpaper printers |
| Glass-fibre manufacturers | Wax workers |
| Glass frosters | Welders |
| Glass manufacturers | Wood-preservative workers |
| Glue manufacturers | Wood stainers |
| Histology technicians | |

ªFrom National Research Council (1974)

This section summarizes data on exposure to chromium in air and the results of biological monitoring in various industries and occupations. The biological indicator levels are influenced by the solubility of chromium compounds and by the time of sampling. It should be noted that the chromium compounds, the timing of collection of biological samples (normally at the end of a shift) and the analytical methods used differ from study to study, and elevated levels of chromium in biological fluids and tissue samples are mentioned only as indications of uptake of chromium. (See also section 3.3(*b*) and the monographs on nickel and nickel compounds, and on welding.)

(i) *Ferrochromium steel and high chromium alloy production*

During the electrothermal reduction of chromite ore with coke for the production of ferrochromium, workers in the area near the furnaces are exposed to fumes containing 0.1-10% chromium (Stern, 1982).

In 1959, an industrial hygiene survey was carried out in a US plant producing ferrochromium, ferrosilicon and chromium alloys in electric furnaces. The mean concentrations of chromium trioxide [values for chromium calculated by the Working Group in square brackets] in the air were 1 [< 1] $\mu g/m^3$ in the maintenance shop, 266 [140] $\mu g/m^3$ in the charging area, 317 [160] $\mu g/m^3$ in the casting area and 2470 [1300] $\mu g/m^3$ in the finishing area. The overall mean of 127 samples was 452 $\mu g/m^3$ chromium trioxide [230 $\mu g/m^3$ chromium] (Princi *et al.*, 1962).

In 1973, workplace concentrations of hexavalent chromium were reported to be 30-60 $\mu g/m^3$ during the production of ferrochromium in the USSR (World Health Organization, 1988).

Concentrations of total dust and chromium in 1975 in a Norwegian ferrochromium plant are shown in Table 11. In various occupations, the mean level of total

**Table 11. Air concentrations of total dust and chromium in a Norwegian ferro-chromium plant**[a]

| Occupation or area | No. of samples | Mean and range of dust concentration (mg/m³) | Mean and range of chromium concentration (μg/m³) |
|---|---|---|---|
| Potmen | 20 | 6.3 (4.0-15.7) | 40 (20-70) |
| Cleaner-balers | 5 | 18.2 (10.5-23.9) | 90 (50-130) |
| Crane drivers | 10 | 4.6 (3.1-7.6) | 40 (10-50) |
| Packers | 10 | 4.9 (2.3-8.3) | 290 (50-1300) |
| Maintenance workers | 9 | 15.6 (4.0-46.0) | 90 (20-370) |
| Transport workers | 9 | 12.8 (5.6-30.1) | 10 (10-30) |
| Charge floor | 5 | 4.8 (2.8-8.4) | 50 (30-70) |
| Top electrode | 3 | 15.5 (13.9-17.8) | 170 (150-190) |
| Packing area | 18 | 1.9 (0.3-5.5) | 190 (10-1340) |

[a]From Langård et al. (1980)

chromium was 10-290 μg/m³, about 11-13% of which was water-soluble (Langård et al., 1980).

Among Swedish ferrochromium workers, exposure to hexavalent chromium was estimated at 250 μg/m³ during arc-furnace operations and 10-50 μg/m³ during transport, metal grinding, maintenance and sample preparation. The total concentration of metallic and trivalent chromium at the work sites was 500-2500 μg/m³ (Axelsson et al., 1980).

In an Italian ferrochromium plant, dust samples contained 0.9-3.8% chromium, and airborne levels of total chromium were 20-158 μg/m³. The concentration of hexavalent chromium was below 1 μg/m³. Levels of urinary chromium measured at the beginning and end of a work shift were low (less than 5 μg/g creatinine), although the results indicated absorption of chromium in some groups of workers (Foa et al., 1988).

In ten steel, 15 iron and 11 copper alloy foundries in Finland in 1973 and 1974, furnacemen and casters were exposed to a mean level of 1-6 μg/m³ acid-soluble chromium (Tossavainen, 1976).

During the production of chromium carbide powder in the USSR, dust concentrations were 11-20 mg/m³ during weighing of chromium[III] oxide, 260-640 mg/m³ during milling and 24-200 mg/m³ during loading, screening and packing of the product (Brakhnova, 1975). In open-hearth steel works, concentrations of chromium trioxide in work place air were 13-37 μg/m³ [7-20 μg/m³ chromium] (Belitskaya, 1981).

In Sweden, the tissue concentrations of chromium in the lungs of 20 deceased smelter workers were three to four times higher than those of eight control subjects (median level, 0.29 and 0.08 µg/g wet tissue, respectively) (Brune *et al.*, 1980).

In Finland, fumes and dusts contained 6-15% chromium during ferrochromium smelting, 1.5-5% during stainless-steel smelting, 0.2-0.3% during continuous casting and 1.6-13% during grinding of stainless steel (Koponen *et al.*, 1981). Air concentrations of total chromium were 200 µg/m³ during ferrochrome smelting and 10 µg/m³ during continuous casting of stainless steel. The mean concentration of hexavalent chromium during the production of stainless steel was 1.5 µg/m³ (Koponen, 1985).

In France, air concentrations of total chromium ranged from 15 to 300 µg/m³ in a steel production plant (Klein, 1985).

Triebig *et al.* (1987) measured the exposure of 230 workers in high-alloy steel plants to chromium in the Federal Republic of Germany. Levels of chromium trioxide [chromium] in the air were 10-2280 [5-1200] µg/m³. Urinary levels of chromium were 0.1-79 µg/g creatinine, indicating some exposure to metal fumes and dusts in steel smelting, cutting and grinding.

### (ii) *Production of chromates and of chromate pigments*

Airborne concentrations of chromates [chromium] in four US chromate plants over the period 1941-47 were 10-4600 [5-2300 µg/m³] at kilns and mills, 40-340 [20-170] µg/m³ at dryers, 200-21 000 [100-11 000] µg/m³ in packing areas and 3-2170 [2-1100] µg/m³ in other parts of the factories (Machle & Gregorius, 1948). Workplace air concentrations of chromium[III], chromium[VI] and total chromium during various operations in chromite ore processing were reported for a plant in Ohio (USA) which produced sodium dichromate (Bourne & Yee, 1950) and for a chromate production plant in the UK (Buckell & Harvey, 1951; see Table 12).

**Table 12. Air concentrations of chromium[III] and chromium[VI] in US[a] and UK[b] chromate factories**

| Operation | Chromium[III] (mg/m³) | | Chromium[VI] (mg/m³) | |
|---|---|---|---|---|
| | USA | UK | USA | UK |
| Chromite and lime mixing | 1.52 | 2.14 | 0.03 | 0.005 |
| Roasting | 0.39 | 0.17 | 0.26 | 0.029 |
| Filtering | 0.12 | 0.037 | 0.08 | 0.52 |
| Shipping | 0.30 | 0.005 | 0.2 | 0.88 |

[a]From Bourne & Yee (1950)
[b]From Buckell & Harvey (1951)

In a chromate production plant in the USA, the levels of water-soluble hexavalent chromium were 100-900 $\mu$g/m$^3$ in 1945-49 and 5-100 $\mu$g/m$^3$ in 1950-59 (Braver *et al.*, 1985). In 1953, the US Public Health Service studied the health hazards associated with the chromate-producing industry. Six plants were directly involved in the production of alkaline chromates and dichromates from chromite ore. One of the plants also manufactured chromium pigments. In about 1600 air samples, the weighted average exposures by occupational groups were 7-890 $\mu$g/m$^3$ insoluble chromium as chromite, 5-170 $\mu$g/m$^3$ water-soluble chromium[VI] and 10-470 $\mu$g/m$^3$ acid-soluble, water-insoluble chromium (Gafafer, 1953).

Concentrations of soluble and acid-insoluble chromium in lung tissues of 16 chromate manufacturing workers in the USA ranged from 3 to 161 $\mu$g/g dry tissue and 5 to 402 $\mu$g/g dry tissue, respectively; the workers had been exposed to chromite ore, sodium chromate, potassium dichromate and various intermediate chromium compounds for 1.5-42 years (Baetjer *et al.*, 1959a).

In Italy, chromic acid and alkaline chromate production workers were exposed to mean levels of 110-150 $\mu$g/m$^3$ chromates [60-80 $\mu$g/m$^3$ hexavalent chromium] (Vigliani & Zurlo, 1955). More recently, dust exposures and urinary excretion of chromium were studied in another Italian factory that produces potassium dichromate and chromic sulfate. A group of 22 potassium dichromate workers was exposed to levels of 10-100 $\mu$g/m$^3$ chromium[III] and 8-212 $\mu$g/m$^3$ water-soluble chromium[VI] (Mutti *et al.*, 1984), and their mean urinary concentration of total chromium was 31.5 $\mu$g/l (Cavalleri & Minoia, 1985). A group of 15 chromic sulphate workers were exposed to levels of 46-1689 $\mu$g/m3 chromium[III] and 2-23 $\mu$g/m$^3$ chromium[VI] (Mutti *et al.*, 1984); their urinary chromium concentrations averaged 24.7 $\mu$g/l. Chromium levels in serum and erythrocytes were also increased among exposed workers (Cavalleri & Minoia, 1985).

In Japan, air concentrations of total chromium during sodium and potassium dichromate and chromium trioxide production in one plant ranged from 19 to 219 $\mu$g/m$^3$; in 1960, levels of chromium trioxide [chromium] were 390-20 170 [180-10 000] $\mu$g/m$^3$ in this factory, where enclosures and local exhausts were not properly used. Chromium content was measured in several organs of six chromate workers who had been exposed for over ten years and had died of lung cancer; the chromium concentration in the lungs averaged 51.1 $\mu$g/g wet weight, while in unexposed controls it averaged 0.31 $\mu$g/g wet weight (Kishi *et al.*, 1987). In six Japanese studies, the chromium contents of the lungs of chromate workers were 0.5-132 $\mu$g/g wet weight and 14-2368 $\mu$g/g dry weight, as compared to 0.05-3.72 $\mu$g/g wet weight and 0.47-5.14 $\mu$g/g dry weight in men without occupational exposure (Adachi, 1987). High concentrations of chromium were found in the respiratory organs of chromate workers who had died of cancer, and in the spleen, liver, kidney, brain, heart, bone marrow and skin (Hyodo *et al.*, 1980; Teraoka, 1987). In 1957, chromium trioxide [chromium] concentrations in the plant ranged from 40-8430 [20 to 4300] $\mu g/m^3$, with a mean of 520 [260] $\mu g/m^3$ (Hyodo *et al.*, 1980).

Chromate pigment workers are exposed primarily to zinc and lead chromates although they may also be exposed to other compounds, such as chromium trioxide, sodium chromate and dichromate and zinc oxide (Davies, 1984a).

In three Norwegian pigment plants producing zinc and lead chromates, workers mixing raw materials and filling sacks were exposed to mean concentrations of 1.2-9.8 $mg/m^3$ total dust and 10-1350 $\mu g/m^3$ chromium. The chromium levels to which foremen are exposed were taken as a measure of general exposure in the plants; in one plant it was 40 $\mu g/m^3$, in another it was 190 $\mu g/m^3$ (Langård & Norseth, 1975).

In India, the concentration of chromium in the urine of workers exposed to chromates in two paint manufacturing factories was about ten fold that of unexposed persons (Tandon *et al.*, 1977).

In almost all positions at a US chromate pigment plant, production workers were exposed to hexavalent chromium in the form of zinc and lead chromates. Concentrations of airborne chromium were estimated to be more than 2 $mg/m^3$ for highly exposed workers, between 0.5 and 2 $mg/m^3$ for moderately exposed workers and less than 0.1 $mg/m^3$ for the low-exposure category (Sheffet *et al.*, 1982).

(iii)  *Leather tanning* (see also IARC, 1981)

The most common tanning process involves the use of basic chromic sulfate liquor. Tanning is accomplished in large vats where the hides are soaked with dehairing, neutralizing, pickling, colouring and finishing chemicals. In the two-bath method, the hides are first immersed in a bath of hexavalent chromium salts (potassium or sodium dichromate), sodium chloride and sulfuric acid, and then removed and placed in a reduction bath to reduce the dichromate to trivalent chromic sulfate. An exothermic reaction takes place with a reduction agent such as sugar, starch or sulfur dioxide. The majority of tanneries do not produce their own tanning liquors, and a large number of proprietary products are available for direct use. Occupational exposure to chromium in the tanning industry may occur through contact with the trivalent chromium solutions. Wet, freshly tanned skins contain 1-2% chromium by weight, and dry leather powder contains 2-6% depending on the method and degree of tanning (Stern, 1982; Stern *et al.*, 1987).

Airborne levels of 20-50 $\mu g/m^3$ trivalent chromium were measured in 1975 in an Italian tannery when tanning baths were emptied (IARC, 1980a).

Air concentrations of trivalent chromium in a Finnish tannery were 1-29 $\mu g/m^3$ (personal samples). Two press operators were exposed to a mean level of 13 $\mu g/m^3$, and their urinary chromium excretion varied during one working week from 5 to 62 µg/l. A diurnal variation was evident, with the highest values occurring in post-shift samples. Blood samples contained 10-22 µg/l chromium in the plasma and 4.7-11 µg/l in whole blood; plasma levels were < 1 µg/l in workers who were less exposed to tanning liquors. During press operations, splashes are common, and absorption from the gastrointestinal tract was suggested to be the main route of exposure (Aitio *et al.*, 1984).

Urine samples were collected from 34 male tannery workers in Turkey. The mean urinary concentration of chromium was 6.6 µg/l (5.6 µg/g creatinine) in tannery workers, 2.3 µg/l (1.9 µg/g creatinine) in office and kitchen workers at the same factory and 0.22 µg/l (0.26 µg/g creatinine) in unexposed controls (Saner *et al.*, 1984).

In two leather tanning facilities in the USA, the total concentration of chromium in work place air was 0.2-54 µg/m³, with a mean of 39 µg/m³ (Stern *et al.*, 1987).

### (iv)   *Chromium plating*

There are two types of chromium electroplating: decorative ('bright') and hard chromium plating. In decorative plating, a thin (0.5-1 µm) layer of chromium is deposited over nickel or nickel-type coatings to provide protective, durable, non-tarnishable surface finishes. Hard chromium plating produces a thicker (5-10 µm) coating, usually directly on the base metal, to increase its heat, wear and corrosion resistance. Plating baths contain chromium trioxide (250-350 g/l) and sulfuric acid (2.5-3.5 g/l) or a mixture of sulfuric acid and fluoride or fluorosilicate, as well as various organic additives. Electrolysis emits bubbles of oxygen and hydrogen that generate chromium trioxide mist by bursting at the liquid surface. Surfactants and floating balls may be used to control the mist emission (Guillemin & Berode, 1978; Stern, 1982; Sheehy *et al.*, 1984). Exposure to substances other than chromium occurs in a number of pretreatment and finishing operations: acid and alkali mists, nitrogen oxides, cyanide and solvents may be released during pickling, acid dipping, stripping and degreasing processes, and metal and abrasive dusts are released from grinding and polishing. In some plants, decorative-chrome platers also perform nickel plating (Sheehy *et al.*, 1984).

Air measurements made in metal plating plants since 1928 are summarized in Table 13. It is apparent that exposures to chromium have been markedly reduced with modern technology. In most studies, the levels were measured as total water-soluble chromium or hexavalent chromium and reported as a chromium trioxide concentration.

**Table 13. Workplace levels of hexavalent chromium during metal plating**

| Reference and country | Process and sampling data | Chromium oxide (chromium VI) concentration ($\mu g/m^3$) |
|---|---|---|
| Bloomfield & Blum (1928) USA | Chromium plating 6 plants, 19 samples | 120-6900 [60-3800] |
| Riley & Goldman (1937) USA | Chromium plating with no local exhaust with low local exhaust with high local exhaust | 2780-3680 [1440-1910] 11 200 [580] 340 [180] |
| Gresh (1944) USA | Chromium plating 7 samples | 90-1200 [45-600] |
| Molos (1947) USA | Chromium plating with local exhaust with plastic beads on the bath with plastic beads and local exhaust | 4500-5000 [2300-2500] 1900-3000 [950-1500] 20-50 [10-25] |
| Sheehy et al. (1984) USA | Chromium plating with no local exhaust with local exhaust with local exhaust and plastic beads on the bath | [140-2960] [0.5-270] [0.5-5] |
| Lumio (1953) Finland | Chromium plating 16 plants | < 3 [ < 1.5] |
| Hama et al. (1954) USA | Decorative chromium plating 4 plants | 2-60 [1-30] |
| Kleinfeld & Rosso (1965) USA | Decorative chromium plating with no local exhaust with local exhaust | 180-1400 [90-730] 2-9 [2-5] |
| Hanslian et al. (1967) Czechoslovakia | Chromium plating 8 plants | 23-681 [12-330] |
| Mitchell (1969) UK | Chromium plating (stripping) with no local exhaust  with local exhaust | 240-21 300 [120-10 600] 10-30 [5-15] |
| Gomes (1972) Brazil | Chromium plating 8 hard chromium plants 63 decorative chromium plants | < 100-1400 [ < 50-700] < 100-700 [ < 50-350] |

**Table 13 (contd)**

| Reference and country | Process and sampling data | Chromium oxide (chromium VI) concentration ($\mu g/m^3$) |
|---|---|---|
| National Institute for Occupational Safety and Health (1973-81) (reviewed by Sheehy et al., 1984) USA | Hard chromium plating | |
| | plant 1 | [1.1-48.6] |
| | plant 2 | [0.8-9.6] |
| | plant 3 | [3.6-66.0] |
| | plant 4 | [3-6] |
| | Decorative chromium plating | |
| | plant 5 | [<0.5-3] |
| | plant 6 | [0.2-5.9] |
| | plant 7 | [0.2-9.0] |
| | plant 8 | [<3] |
| | Nickel-chromium plating | |
| | plant 9 | [2.9] |
| | Zinc plating | |
| | plant 10 | [<1.2-3.6] |
| | plant 11 | [0.3] |
| Royle (1975a) UK | Chromium plating | |
| | 40 plants | <30 [<15] |
| | 2 plants | >30 [>15] |
| Yunusova & Pavlovskaya (1975) [quoted by the World Health Organization, 1988] USSR | Chromium plating | |
| | 8 plants | [40-400] |
| Michel-Briand & Simonin (1977) France | Chromium plating | 5-15 [2.5-7.5] |
| Guillemin & Berode (1978) Switzerland | Hard chromium plating | |
| | 6 plants, 23 samples | 2-655 [1-330] |
| | Bright chromium plating | |
| | 6 plants, 11 samples | 2-26 [1-13] |
| Ekholm et al. (1983) Sweden | Hard chromium plating | |
| | 4 plants | <1-46 |
| | Decorative chromium plating | |
| | 9 plants | <1-2 |
| Mutti et al. (1984) Italy | Chromium plating | |
| | 24 hard chromium platers | [4-146] |
| | 16 bright chromium platers | [0-31] |

**Table 13 (contd)**

| Reference and country | Process and sampling data | Chromium oxide (chromium VI) concentration ($\mu$g/m$^3$) |
|---|---|---|
| Sheehy et al. (1984) USA | Chromium, nickel, zinc, copper, cadmium and silver plating, 8 plants | |
| | 53 personal samples | [< 1-14] |
| | 293 tank area samples | [< 1-11 000] |
| | 39 general area samples | [< 1-31] |
| Sorahan et al. (1987) UK | Decorative chromium plating | |
| | 60 samples before 1973 | 0-8000 [0-4000] |
| | numerous samples after 1973 | < 50 [< 25] |

Typical levels of chromium in post-shift urine samples from electroplaters are given in Table 14. In one study of 21 electroplaters, chromium levels in serum were 0.2-1.3 $\mu$g/l (Verschoor et al., 1988). High concentrations of chromium were found in the respiratory organs of two chromium platers as well as in the spleen, liver, kidney and heart (Teraoka, 1987).

**Table 14. Urinary concentrations of chromium in electroplaters**

| Reference and country | Type of workers (no.) | Mean and range of chromium concentrations in urine ($\mu$g/l or $\mu$g/g creatinine) |
|---|---|---|
| Franzen et al. (1970) Federal Republic of Germany | Chromium platers (133) | < 4-32 $\mu$g/l |
| Schaller et al. (1972) Federal Republic of Germany | Chromium platers (12) | 9.7 (1.4-24.6) $\mu$g/l |
| Guillemin & Berode (1978) Switzerland | Hard chromium platers[a] (21) | 23 $\mu$g/l (18 $\mu$g/g) |
| | Bright chromium platers[a] (16) | 5.6 $\mu$g/l (5.3 $\mu$g/g) |
| Sarto et al. (1982) Italy | Bright chromium platers (17) | 6.1 $\mu$g/g |
| | Hard chromium platers (21) | 10.0 $\mu$g/g |
| Lindberg & Vesterberg (1983) Sweden | Chromium platers (90) | [< 0.3-98 $\mu$g/l] Calculated by the Working Group from plots |

**Table 14 (contd)**

| Reference and country | Type of workers (no.) | Mean and range of chromium concentrations in urine (μg/l or μg/g creatinine) |
|---|---|---|
| Mutti et al. (1984) Italy | Hard chromium platers[a] (24) | 15.3 μg/g |
| | Bright chromium platers[a] (16) | 5.8 μg/g |
| Verschoor et al. (1988) Netherlands | Chromium platers (21) | 9 (1-34) μg/g |
| Nagaya et al. (1989) Japan | Chromium platers (44) | 0.25 (0.05-1.54 μmol/l) [13 (3-80) μg/l] |

[a]Corresponding air concentrations can be found in Table 13.

### (v)  Welding

Welding produces particulate fumes that have a chemical composition reflecting the elemental content of the consumable used. For each couple of process/material of application, there is a wide range of concentrations of the elements present in the fume. Chromium and nickel are found in significant concentrations in fumes from welding by manual metal arc, metal inert gas and tungsten inert gas processes on stainless and alloy steels. Typical ranges of total fume, total chromium and hexavalent chromium found in the breathing zone of welders are presented in Table 15. Certain special process applications not listed can also produce high chromium and nickel concentrations, and welding in confined spaces produces significantly higher concentrations of total fume and elemental constituents. Exposure to welding fumes that contain nickel and chromium can lead to elevated levels of these elements in tissues, blood and urine (see monograph on welding for details).

### (vi)  Other occupations

During the production of trivalent chromium compounds (chromic oxide and chromic sulfate) in the Federal Republic of Germany, work place air contained 180-13 200 μg/m³ chromic oxide and 850-2700 μg/m³ chromic sulfate during filtering, drying and unloading operations (Korallus et al., 1974a).

Exposures of spray painters to solvents and paint mists have been measured in a variety of industries by the US National Institute for Occupational Safety and Health. Air concentrations of total chromium in breathing zone samples were 1600 μg/m³ during aircraft painting, 220 μg/m³ during railroad car painting and 5-9 μg/m³ during metal furniture painting (O'Brien & Hurley, 1981). At a US plant manu-

**Table 15. Total fume and chromium concentrations found in the breathing zone of welders**[a]

| Process[b] | Total fume[c] (mg/m$^3$) | Total Cr ($\mu$g/m$^3$) | Cr(VI) ($\mu$g/m$^3$) |
|---|---|---|---|
| MMA/SS | 2-40 | 30-1600 | 25-1500[d] |
| MIG/SS | 2-3 | 60 | < 1 |
| TIG/SS | 1-3 | 10-55 | < 1 |

[a]From van der Wal (1985)

[b]MMA, manual metal arc; SS, stainless steel; MIG, metal inert gas; TIG, tungsten inert gas

[c]50%-90% range

[d]50%-90% Cr(VI) from MMA/SS is soluble in water (Stern, 1982).

facturing truck bodies and refuse handling equipment, breathing zone concentrations of paint mists ranged from 4.8 to 47 mg/m$^3$ total dust and 10 to 400 $\mu$g/m$^3$ chromium (Vandervort & Cromer, 1975). Personal air samples had concentrations of hexavalent chromium ranging from 30 to 450 $\mu$g/m$^3$ with a mean of 230 $\mu$g/m$^3$ during spray painting of buses (Zey & Aw, 1984), 13 to 2900 $\mu$g/m$^3$ with a mean of 607 $\mu$g/m$^3$ during spray painting of aircraft wheels (Kominsky *et al.*, 1978) and 10 to 40 $\mu$g/m$^3$ with a mean of 20 $\mu$g/m$^3$ during spray painting of bridge girders (Rosensteel, 1974).

Breathing zone samples were also taken in a small automotive body repair workshop in the USA. One of the eight samples contained 490 $\mu$g/m$^3$ chromium; the others were below the detection limit (Jayjock & Levin, 1984).

In a Swedish study, mean chromium levels of 1300 $\mu$g/m$^3$ were measured during car painting and 500 $\mu$g/m$^3$ during industrial painting, while work place levels averaged 300 $\mu$g/m$^3$ during grinding activities (Elofsson *et al.*, 1980). Low overall levels were found for spray painters working in a fireplace manufacturing plant; the concentrations of total dust and chromium oxide [unspecified] were 1700 and 5-8 $\mu$g/m$^3$ [chromium, 3-4 $\mu$g/m$^3$], respectively (Hellquist *et al.*, 1983).

In Italy, 12 spray painters using lead and zinc chromate paints were exposed to levels of 450-1450 $\mu$g/m$^3$ insoluble hexavalent chromium, and their mean urinary excretion was 13.2 $\mu$g/g creatinine at the end of a work shift (Mutti *et al.*, 1984).

At the largest wood treatment plant in Hawaii, air concentrations of 2-9 $\mu$g/m$^3$ chromium were measured. Urinary excretion of 89 workers using chromated copper arsenate wood preservatives did not differ from that of controls (Takahashi *et al.*, 1983).

In a cement-producing factory in the USSR, concentrations of hexavalent chromium in work place air varied from 5 to 8 µg/m³, measured as chromium trioxide (Retnev, 1960). Hexavalent chromium was found in 18 of 42 US cement samples at concentrations ranging from 0.1 to 5.4 µg/g, with a total chromium content of 5-124 µg/g (Perone et al., 1974). Portland cement contains 41.2 ppm (mg/kg) chromium (range, 27.5-60), due to the presence of chromium in limestone. Soluble chromium in cement averaged 4.1 mg/kg (range, 1.6-8.8), of which 2.9 mg/kg (range, 0.03-7.8) was hexavalent chromium (Fishbein, 1976). Analysis of 59 samples of Portland cement from nine European countries showed concentrations of 1-83 µg/g hexavalent chromium and 35-173 µg/g total chromium (Fregert & Gruvberger, 1972). In France and Belgium, cements manufactured in 11 plants contained 8-49 µg/g total chromium, originating from limestone, clay, gypsum, fly ash and slag used in the manufacture as well as from the refractory kiln materials (Haguenoer et al., 1982). Cement in Iceland contained 5.8-9.5 mg/kg hexavalent chromium (Rafnsson & Jóhannesdóttir, 1986).

In open-cast chromium mining in the USSR, concentrations of total airborne dust ranged from 1.3 to 16.9 mg/m³; in the crushing and sorting plant, dust levels were 6.1-188 mg/m³. The chromium content of settled dust varied from 3.6 to 48% (calculated as chromic oxide). No hexavalent chromium was found in the dust (Pokrovskaya et al., 1976; World Health Organization, 1988).

During the manufacture of chromium[III] lignosulfonate in Finland, five packing workers were exposed to dust containing about 2% trivalent chromium. The product contained 6% trivalent chromium attached to wood lignin. In personal samples, the concentration of chromium in the air was 2-230 µg/m³, and three-day averages ranged from 11 to 80 µg/m³. Urinary levels in samples from workers were 0.01-0.59 µmol/l (0.5-30 µg/l), and mean excretion was 0.02-0.23 µmol/l (1-12 µg/l). It was concluded that chromium occurred exclusively in a trivalent state in both dust and urine (Kiilunen et al., 1983).

(c)   *Air*

Chromium is generally associated with particulates in ambient air at concentrations of 0.001-0.1 µg/m³ (Fishbein, 1976; O'Neill et al., 1986). In the USA in 1966, only seven of 58 cities in the National Air Sampling Network had annual average chromium levels of 0.01 µg/m³ or more, and only 16 had maximal single values above that level. In approximately 200 urban stations in the USA during 1960-69, annual mean concentrations were 0.01-0.03 µg/m³ (minimal level detectable, 0.01 µg/m³). In nonurban areas, the level of chromium was less than 0.01 µg/m³. Levels of 0.9-21.5 µg/m³ were reported in 23 localities in northern England and Wales in 1956-58 (Fishbein, 1976). In 1957-74, the amount of chromium in the atmospheric aerosol at a rural site in the UK declined at an average yearly rate of 11.3% (Salmon *et al.*, 1977).

During the period May 1972-April 1975, the range of average levels of chromium determined at 15 stations in Belgium was 0.01-0.04 µg/m³ (maximal value, 0.54 µg/m³). The values were stated to reflect background pollution and levels representative of those in air inhaled by the majority of the population. Sampling station locations were selected to avoid, as much as possible, a direct influence of local sources (Kretzschmar *et al.*, 1977).

Coal from many sources can contain as much chromium as soils and rocks, i.e., up to 54 ppm (mg/kg); consequently, the burning of coal can contribute to chromium levels in air, particularly in cities (Fishbein, 1976; Merian, 1984). Particulates emitted from coal-fired power plants contained 2.3-31 ppm (mg/kg) chromium, depending on the type of boiler firing; the emitted gases contained 0.22-2.2 mg/m³. These concentrations were reduced by fly ash collection to 0.19-6.6 ppm (mg/kg) and 0.018-0.5 mg/m³, respectively (Fishbein, 1976). Fly ash has been shown to contain 1.4-6.1 ppm (mg/kg) chromium[VI] (Stern *et al.*, 1984).

Mean concentrations in the air of US cities with metallurgical chromium or chromium chemical producers or with refractories were 0.012-0.016 µg/m³, all of which were higher than the US national average. Cement-producing plants are probably an additional source of chromium in the air. When chromate chemicals are used as rust inhibitors in cooling towers, they are dissolved in recirculating water systems, which continually discharge about 1% of their flow to waste. Additionally, chromate and water are lost to the atmosphere (Fishbein, 1976).

The concentration of chromium in the air at the South Pole was reported to be 0.005 ng/m³. Concentrations in samples taken over the Atlantic Ocean ranged from 0.007 to 1.1 ng/m³. Airborne chromium concentrations were reported to be 0.7 ng/m³ in the Shetland Islands and Norway, 0.6 in northwestern Canada, 1-140 in Europe, 1-300 in North America, 20-70 in Japan and 45-67 in Hawaii, USA (Cary, 1982).

### (d)  Water

Naturally occurring chromium concentrations in water arise from mineral weathering processes, soluble organic chromium, sediment load and precipitation (Cary, 1982).

Concentrations of chromium in rivers have been found to be 1-10 µg/l. Chromium (both hexavalent and trivalent) is generally found at lower concentrations in seawater (well below 1 µg/l) than in rivers and wells. It has been estimated that 6.7 million kg of chromium are added to the oceans every year. As a result, much of the chromium lost from the land by erosion and mining is eventually deposited on the ocean floor (Fishbein, 1976).

The mean chromium concentration in ocean water in 1979 was 0.3 µg/l, with a range of 0.2-50 µg/l. Samples taken from the first 100 m of water from several areas of the Pacific Ocean contained about 0.12 µg/l chromium, about 83% being hexavalent chromium; below 100 m, total chromium increased to about 0.16 µg/l, with hexavalent chromium accounting for 90%. In saline waters of Australia, 62-87% of the labile chromium present ( < 1 µg/l) was hexavalent (Cary, 1982).

Of 1500 samples of US surface waters taken between 1960 and about 1968, 24.5% contained chromium detectable spectrographically; the maximal and mean levels observed were 112 and 9.7 µg/l, respectively (Kroner, 1973). A survey of chromium content of 15 North American rivers showed levels of 0.7-84 µg/l, with most in the range of 1-10 µg/l (Hartford, 1979). Levels in 3834 samples of tap water taken from 35 regions of the USA in 1974-75 ranged from 0.4 to 8 µg/l chromium, with the median 1.8 µg/l (US Environmental Protection Agency, 1984).

Of 170 samples taken from lakes in the higher Sierra Mountains of California, USA, in 1968, only two contained as much as 5 µg/l chromium. Chromium concentrations in 1977 in the Amazon (Brazil) and Yukon (USA) Rivers were 2.0 and 2.3 ppb (µg/l), respectively; the two rivers were considered to represent unpolluted systems draining watersheds of a wide variety of mineral types from extremely different climates. The concentration of chromium in 96% of the 4342 samples of stream- and river-water in Canada was less than 10 µg/l; about 2% of the samples contained 15-500 µg/l chromium (Cary, 1982).

The mean concentration of dissolved chromium compounds in the Rhine River during 1975 was 6.5 µg/l with a range of 3.7-11.4 µg/l; the concentration in drinking-water was 0.29 µg/l (Nissing, 1975). The concentration of chromium compounds in Austrian medicinal and table waters was determined as 1.2-4.2 µg/l (Sontag *et al.*, 1977). The average levels of chromium in three tributaries of the Han River in the Republic of Korea were found to be 96, 106 and 65 µg/l (Min, 1976).

Municipal sewage sludge can contain chromium at levels up to 30 000 mg per kg dry sludge (Pacyna & Nriagu, 1988).

Surface waters and groundwaters contaminated with wastewaters from electroplating operations, leather tanning and textile manufacturing, or through deposition of airborne chromium, may also be sources of chromium exposure. Other sources are solid wastes resulting from the roasting and leaching steps of chromate manufacture and improper disposal of municipal incineration wastes in landfill sites (Beszedits, 1988; Calder, 1988; Handa, 1988).

*(e)  Soil and plants*

Chromium is present in the soil at levels which vary from traces to 250 mg/kg (as chromic[III] oxide) (Davis, 1956) and is particularly prevalent in soil derived from basalt or serpentine (US Environmental Protection Agency, 1984).

Virtually all plants contain detectable levels of chromium, taken up by the roots or through the leaves. Vegetables from 25 botanical families were found to contain chromium in amounts varying from 10-1000 µg/kg of dry matter, with most samples in the range of 100-500 µg/kg (Davis, 1956). Strong seasonal variations in chromium levels were found in three kinds of grass (World Health Organization, 1988).

The chromium content of mosses and liverworts collected in 1951 in a remote rural area in Denmark was compared with that in the same plants collected in 1975: an increase of about 62% was observed, which coincided with increases in industrial activity and fossil fuel combustion (Rasmussen, 1977).

The chromium content of cigarette tobacco from different sources has been reported as follows: Iraq, 8.6-14.6 mg/kg (two varieties); Iran, 4.3-6.2 mg/kg (two brands); and the USA, 0.24-6.3 mg/kg (Al Badri *et al.*, 1977).

*(f)  Food*

The chromium content of most foods is extremely low; small amounts were found in vegetables (20-50 µg/kg), fruits (20 µg/kg) and grains and cereals (excluding fats, 40 µg/kg). The mean daily intakes of chromium from food, water and air have been estimated to be 280, 4 and 0.28 µg, respectively (Fishbein, 1976). Hartford (1979) indicated that nearly all foodstuffs contain chromium in the range of 20-590 µg/kg, resulting in a daily intake for humans of 10-400 µg, with an average of about 80 µg. In a more recent study, the mean daily intake of chromium for 22 healthy subjects was about 24.5 µg (Bunker *et al.*, 1984).

*(g)  Animal tissues*

Table 16 summarizes data on chromium levels in tissues from various food and feral animals.

The report of the US National Status and Trends Program for Marine Environmental Quality, conducted by the National Oceanic and Atmospheric Administration (1987), gave concentrations of chromium at 0.1-11.0 µg/g (dry weight) in mussels and oysters collected in 1986 at East, West, and Gulf Coast sites, and 0.02-1.4 µg/g (dry weight) in livers of ten species of fish collected in 1984 throughout the USA.

**Table 16. Chromium levels found in food and feral animals**

| Animal | Tissue | Range (mean) (μg/kg) | Comments | Reference |
|--------|--------|----------------------|----------|-----------|
| Largemouth bass | Muscle | 1-2 | Collected near Savannah | Koli & |
| Bluegill | | 1 | River, SC, USA, nuclear | Whitmore |
| Catfish | | 1 | plant | (1983) |
| Redbreast sunfish | | 1 | | |
| Crappie, American eel | | 2 | | |
| Spotted sunfish | | 1-2 | | |
| American shad | Gonad | ND-180 | Collected in 1979, USA | Eisenberg |
| | Flesh | ND | | & Topping |
| Finfish | Flesh | ND-1900 | Collected in 1978-79 | (1986) |
| Striped bass | Gonad | ND | Collected in 1978-79 | |
| | Liver | ND | Collected in 1978-79 | |
| | Flesh | ND | Collected in 1978-79 | |
| Striped bass | Liver | 2600-9800 (6000) | Collected from | Heit (1979) |
| | Muscle | 2700-9500 (5000) | Chesapeake Bay, MD, USA | |
| Cattle | Blood | (25/10) | Grazed on pasture | Fitzgerald |
| | Bone | (614/934) | treated/untreated with | et al. (1985) |
| | Brain | (209/306) | sludge (from Chicago, | |
| | Diaphragm | (206/215) | IL, USA) | |
| | Heart | (172/434) | | |
| | Kidney | (231/390) | | |
| | Liver | (186/365) | | |
| | Milk | (248/160) | | |
| Cattle | Liver | 200-3000 | | Stowe et al. (1985) |
| Cattle | Kidney | < 10-30 | Collected from slaugh- | Kramer |
| | Liver | < 10-910 (10) | ter-houses in Queens- | et al. (1983) |
| | Muscle | < 10-100 | land, Australia | |
| Cattle | | | Oklahoma, USA | Kerr & |
| | Blood | 6-66 (22) | Unexposed animals | Edwards |
| | | 1080 | Animal found dead near an oil-well drilling site | (1981) |
| | Kidney | 500-6200 (2970) | Unexposed animals | |
| | | 15 800 | Animal found dead near a recently completed oil well | |

**Table 16 (contd)**

| Animal | Tissue | Range (mean) (μg/kg) | Comments | Reference |
|---|---|---|---|---|
| Clam | Body | (2100-3800) | Collected from Lake | Byrne & |
| American oyster | | (1300) | Pontchartrain, LA, USA | DeLeon (1986) |
| Pike-perch | Body | 10-20 (10) | The Netherlands Hollands Diep | Vos et al. (1986) |
| Cod | | 10-20 (10) | Collected near the coast | |
| Baltic herring | | 10-70 (20) | | |
| Sole | | 10-20 (20) | | |
| Eel | | 20-340 (80) | Collected from Lake | |
| Pike-perch | | 10-70 (20) | Ijssel | |
| Blue mussel | | 210-810 (430) | Collected from Eastern Scheldt | |
| Shrimp | | 100-710 (260) | Collected from Western Wadden Sea | |
| Killifish | Body | (3600-7600) | Collected near electro- | Custer et al. |
| Common tern | Liver | ND-18 310 | plating industry, RI, USA | (1986) |
| Cape oyster | Body | < 100-4600 | Collected along the coast of South Africa | Watling & Watling (1982) |
| Sponge | Body | 1 000 000-2 000 000 (1 520 000) | Collected near the Tarapur coast, India | Patel et al. (1985) |
| Snapping turtle | Kidney | (930-1260) | Collected from uncon- | Albers et al. |
| | Liver | (100-1970) | taminated areas of MD, USA | (1986) |
| | Kidney | (1130-2970) | Collected from contami- | |
| | Liver | (360-600) | nated areas of NJ, USA | |
| Crab | Body | 40-200 (120) | Collected in sewage out- | Sadiq et al. |
| Shrimp | | 29-133 (59) | fall area of the Arabian Gulf, Saudi Arabia | (1982) |
| Pacific oyster | Body | (93 000, 113 000) | Collected from two cul- | Wong et al. |
| | Gills | (40 000, 170 000) | ture beds in Deep Bay, | (1981) |
| | Intestine | (42 000, 106 000) | Hong Kong | |
| | Mantle | (47 000, 188 000) | | |
| | Muscle | (35 000, 111 000) | | |

ND, none detected

*(h)    Human tissues and secretions*

As with most metals that occur in trace quantities, the normal concentrations of chromium in human tissues are usually reported wrongly because of extraneous additions during sampling and analysis. However, recent developments in the analytical chemistry of chromium permit the reliable routine determination of nanogram quantities in biological samples (Nieboer & Jusys, 1988). Selected current reference values for chromium concentrations in a few biological materials are presented in Table 17.

**Table 17.  Chromium concentrations in specimens from non-occupationally exposed persons**[a]

| Sample | Median | Range |
|--------|--------|-------|
| Serum  | 0.19 μg/l | 0.12-2.1 μg/l |
| Blood  | < 0.5 μg/l | - |
| Urine  | 0.4 μg/l | 0.24-1.8 μg/l |
| Liver  | [c] | 8-72 ng/g wet weight |
| Lung[b] | 204 ng/g wet weight | 29-898 ng/g wet weight |

[a]From Iyengar & Woittiez (1988), except when noted
[b]From Raithel *et al.* (1987)
[c]Too few measurements to determine median values

*(i)    Regulatory status and guidelines*

The 1970 WHO European and 1978 Japanese standard for chromium[VI] in drinking-water (World Health Organization, 1970; Ministry of Health & Welfare, 1978) and the European standard for total chromium in surface water intended for the abstraction of drinking-water (Commission of the European Communities, 1975) are 0.05 mg/l. The US Environmental Protection Agency (1988) has established the same maximal contaminant level for chromium in drinking-water, as the maximal permissible level in water delivered to any user of a public water system.

The US Environmental Protection Agency (1979) also established pretreatment standards that limit the concentration of chromium that may be introduced into a publicly owned wastewater treatment facility by leather tanning and finishing plants. The maximal total chromium permitted in existing sources on any one day is 6 mg/l, and the average daily values for 30 consecutive days must not exceed 3 mg/l.

Table 18 gives occupational exposure limits for airborne chromium in various forms.

**Table 18. Occupational exposure limits for airborne chromium in various forms[a]**

| Country or region | Year | Form of chromium | Concen-tration (mg/m³) | Interpre-tation[b] |
|---|---|---|---|---|
| Austria | 1987 | Cr, soluble compounds (as Cr) | 0.1 | TWA |
| Belgium | 1987 | Cr, compounds (as Cr) | 0.05 | TWA |
| | | Cr, soluble compounds (as Cr) | 0.1 | TWA |
| Brazil | 1987 | Cr, compounds (as Cr) | 0.04 | TWA |
| Bulgaria | 1987 | Cr, compounds (as Cr) | 0.1 | TWA |
| Chile | 1987 | Cr, compounds (as Cr) | 0.04 | TWA |
| China | 1987 | Cr, compounds (as $CrO_3$), chromium trioxide, chromates, dichromates (as $CrO_3$) | 0.5 | TWA |
| Czechoslovakia | 1987 | Cr, compounds (as Cr) | 0.05 | Average |
| | | Cr, compounds (as Cr) | 0.1 | Maximum |
| Denmark | 1988 | Cr and inorganic Cr compounds, except those mentioned below | 0.5 | TWA |
| | | Chromates, chromium trioxide (as Cr) | 0.02 | TWA |
| Egypt | 1987 | Cr, compounds (as Cr) | 0.1 | TWA |
| Finland | 1987 | Cr, Cr[II] and Cr[III] compounds (as Cr) | 0.5 | TWA |
| | | Cr[VI] compounds (as Cr) | 0.05 | TWA |
| France | 1986 | Cr[VI] and derivatives | 0.05 | TWA |
| German Democratic Republic | 1987 | Cr, compounds, except those mentioned below | 0.5 | TWA |
| | | | 1.0 | STEL |
| | | Chromium trioxide, chromates, dichromates (as $CrO_3$) | 0.1 | TWA |
| | | | 0.1 | STEL |
| Hungary | 1987 | Cr, compounds (as Cr) | 0.05 | TWA |
| | | | 0.1 | STEL |
| India | 1987 | Cr, compounds (as Cr) | 0.05 | TWA |
| | | Cr, soluble compounds (as Cr) | 0.5 | TWA |
| Indonesia | 1987 | Cr, compounds (as Cr) | 0.1 | TWA |
| Italy | 1987 | Cr, compounds (as Cr) | 0.05 | TWA |
| | | Cr, soluble compounds (as Cr) | 0.5 | TWA |
| Japan | 1987 | Cr, compounds (as Cr) | 0.1 | TWA |
| Korea, Republic of | 1987 | Cr, compounds (as Cr) | 0.05 | TWA |
| Mexico | 1987 | Chromite ore (as Cr) | 0.05 | TWA |
| | | Cr, compounds (as Cr); insoluble, soluble Cr[II], Cr[III], Cr[VI] compounds (as Cr) | 0.5 | TWA |

**Table 18 (contd)**

| Country or region | Year | Form of chromium | Concentration (mg/m³) | Interpretation[b] |
|---|---|---|---|---|
| Netherlands | 1986 | Cr, soluble compounds (as Cr) | 0.5 | TWA |
| | | Chromyl chloride | 0.15 | TWA |
| | | Cr, insoluble compounds; chromium trioxide (as Cr) | 0.05 | TWA |
| Norway | 1981 | Cr, Cr[II] and Cr[III] compounds (as Cr) | 0.5 | TWA |
| | | Chromates, chromium trioxide (as Cr) | 0.02 | TWA |
| Sweden | 1987 | Cr and inorganic Cr compounds, except those mentioned below | 0.5 | TWA |
| | | Chromates, chromium trioxide (as Cr) | 0.02 | TWA |
| Switzerland | 1987 | Cr, compounds (as Cr); Cr, soluble compounds (as Cr) | 0.5 | TWA |
| | | Cr[II] and Cr[III] soluble compounds; chromium oxychloride dust (as Cr) | 0.05 | TWA |
| Taiwan | 1987 | Cr and compounds (as Cr) | 0.1 | TWA |
| UK | 1987 | Cr, Cr[II] and Cr[III] compounds (as Cr) | 0.5 | TWA |
| | | Cr[VI] compounds (as Cr) | 0.05 | TWA |
| USA[c] | | | | |
| ACGIH | 1988 | Zinc chromates (as Cr) | 0.01 | TWA |
| | | Chromite ore (chromate) (as Cr); water-soluble and certain (confirmed human carcinogens) water-insoluble Cr[VI] compounds (as Cr); lead chromate (as Cr) | 0.05 | TWA |
| | | Chromium metal, Cr[II] and Cr[III] compounds (as Cr) | 0.5 | TWA |
| NIOSH | 1988 | Carcinogenic Cr[VI] | 0.001 | TWA |
| | | Other Cr[VI]; chromic acid | 0.025 | TWA |
| | | (as noncarcinogenic Cr[VI]) | 0.05 | Ceiling (15 min) |
| OSHA | 1987 | Soluble chromium, chromic and chromous salts | 0.5 | TWA |
| | | Chromium metal and insoluble salts | 1.0 | TWA |
| USSR | 1987 | Cr and compounds (as Cr) | 0.01 | MAC |
| | | Chromium phosphate uni-substituted (as Cr[III]) | 0.02 | MAC |

**Table 18 (contd)**

| Country or region | Year | Form of chromium | Concentration (mg/m³) | Interpretation[b] |
|---|---|---|---|---|
| Yugoslavia | 1987 | Cr and compounds (as Cr) | 0.1 | TWA |

[a]From Arbeidsinspectie (1986); Institut National de Recherche et de Sécurité (1986); Arbetarskydds-styrelsens (1987); Cook (1987); Health and Safety Executive (1987); US Occupational Safety and Health Administration (1987); Työsuojeluhallitus (1987); American Conference of Governmental Industrial Hygienists (1988); Arbejdstilsynet (1988); National Institute for Occupational Safety and Health (1988)

[b]TWA, time-weighted average; STEL, short-term exposure limit; MAC, maximum allowable concentration

[c]ACGIH, American Conference of Governmental Industrial Hygienists; NIOSH, National Institute for Occupational Safety and Health; OSHA, Occupational Safety and Health Administration

## 2.4 Analysis

Numerous analytical methods have been developed for the qualitative and quantitative determination of chromium in a wide variety of matrices. Methods for analysing urban, industrial and work-place air, fresh water, sea-water, sewage effluents, sediments, soil, foodstuffs, crops, plants and biological materials such as human milk, blood, serum, urine and faeces and human and animal tissues, have been reviewed (National Research Council, 1974; Whitney & Risby, 1975; US Environmental Protection Agency, 1977, 1978; Slavin, 1981; Torgrimsen, 1982; Love, 1983; Nieboer *et al.*, 1984; US Environmental Protection Agency, 1984; O'Neill *et al.*, 1986; Harzdorf, 1987; Cornelis, 1988; World Health Organization, 1988).

Typical methods for the analysis of chromium are summarized in Table 19.

Most instrumental procedures are not specific for the oxidation states of chromium and are suitable for total chromium determinations only, unless accompanied by prior separations or supportive qualitative analyses. The reagent *sym*-diphenylcarbazide forms a violet complex with chromium[VI] but not with other chromium compounds, and the stability of the colour contributes to the high sensitivity of the analysis of soluble chromate in aerosols, water, cement and other materials. Interfering, reducing or oxidizing substances, if present in the sample, must be taken into account, since they tend to cause erroneous results during sampling, sample storage and preparation and spectrometric measurement (National Institute for Occupational Safety and Health, 1975). The chromium content of single particles can be determined by electron microscopy combined with X-ray microanalysis. Electron spectroscopy can be used to measure the valency state of chromium in thin surface layers of solid samples (Lautner *et al.*, 1978).

**Table 19. Analytical methods for chromium and chromium compounds**

| Sample matrix | Sample preparation | Assay procedure[a] | Limit of detection[b] | Reference |
|---|---|---|---|---|
| **Formulations** | | | | |
| Tanning liquors (trivalent chromium) | Oxidize to Cr[VI] (dichromate) with ammonium persulfate (oxidant) and cupric sulfate-cobaltous nitrate mixture (catalyst) | IT | NR | Makarov-Zemly-anskii et al. (1978) |
| Pigments | Dissolve in hydrofluoric acid | EAAS | 0.1 mg/kg | Kolihova et al. (1978) |
| **Air** | | | | |
| Total chromium | Collect particulate sample on polystyrene filter; irradiate for 5 min at a flux of $2 \times 10^{12}$ neutrons/ $cm^2 \times sec$; count with a Ge(Li) detector | NAA | 0.02 μg | Dams et al. (1970) |
| Total chromium | Extract collection filter with mixture of hot hydrochloric and nitric acids; concentrate extraction liquid; hold overnight; dilute | AAS | NR | Smith et al. (1976) |
| Total chromium | Collect particulate sample on acetate fibre superfilter; use filter as thin target sample and bombard in a proton beam for 10 min | X-REA | 0.01 μg | Li et al. (1979) |
| Total chromium | Collect particulate sample on 0.8 μm cellulose ester membrane; extract with hydrochloric and nitric acids; dilute | AAS | 0.06 μg | National Institute for Occupational Safety and Health (1984a); Eller (1984) [Method 7024] |
| Total chromium | Extract collection filter with mixture of concentrated nitric and perchloric acids; evaporate to dryness; redissolve in dilute nitric/perchloric acid mixture | ICP/AES | 1 μg | Eller (1984) [Method 7300]; O'Neill et al. (1986) |

**Table 19 (contd)**

| Sample matrix | Sample preparation | Assay procedure[a] | Limit of detection[b] | Reference |
|---|---|---|---|---|
| Total chromium | Collect particulate sample on cellulose nitrate membrane; extract with nitric acid; dilute | EAAS | 0.09 μg | Kettrup et al. (1985) |
| Hexavalent chromium | Extract collection filter with 0.5 N sulfuric acid; filter to remove suspended dust; add sym-diphenylcarbazide | VIS | 0.05 μg | Eller (1984) [Method 7600]; O'Neill et al. (1986) |
| Hexavalent chromium | Extract collection filter with hot 2% sodium hydroxide/3% sodium carbonate solution; add 6 N sulfuric acid and sym-diphenylcarbazide | VIS | 0.05 μg | Eller (1984) [Method 7600]; O'Neill et al. (1986) |
| Hexavalent chromium | Collect particulate sample on 5.0-μm polyvinylchloride membrane; extract with sulfuric acid or with sodium hydroxide-sodium carbonate solution; add sym-diphenylcarbazide; measure absorption at 540 nm | VIS | 0.05 μg | Abell & Carlberg (1974); Carelli et al. (1981); Bhargava et al. (1983); National Institute for Occupational Safety and Health (1984b) |
| Soluble chromium compounds | Collect aerosol sample compounds in sodium hydroxide solution with a midget impinger; oxidize Cr[III] compounds with bromine; add sym-diphenylcarbazide; measure absorption at 540 nm | VIS | 2.3 μg/m³ | Kettrup et al. (1985) |
| Chromic acid | Collect aerosol sample on a cellulose ester membrane; chelate Cr[VI] with ammonium pyrrolidine dithiocarbamate; extract with methyl isobutyl ketone | EAAS | 0.2 μg | National Institute for Occupational Safety and Health (1973) |

**Table 19 (contd)**

| Sample matrix | Sample preparation | Assay procedure[a] | Limit of detection[b] | Reference |
|---|---|---|---|---|
| **Water** | | | | |
| Wastewaters<br>Total chromium<br>Hexavalent chromium | – | PP | 0.04 mg/l<br>0.01 mg/l | Heigl (1978) |
| River water | Separate suspended particles by centrifugation; add diethyldithiocarbamate; filter through acetate superfilter; use filter as thin target sample and bombard in a proton beam for 10 min | X-REA | NR | Li *et al.* (1979) |
| Seawater<br>Hexavalent and total chromium | Extract with ammonium pyrrolidine dithiocarbamate into chloroform at pH 2 | IDMS | 0.001 μg/l | Osaki *et al.* (1976) |
| Hexavalent and trivalent chromium, selective | Extract hexavalent chromium with Aliquat-336 (a mixture of methyl tri-*n*-alkyl ammonium chlorides) at pH 2; extract trivalent chromium by adding thiocyanate to at least 1M; adjust pH to 6-8 | EAAS | 0.01 μg/l [VI]<br>0.03 μg/l [III] | de Jong & Brinkman (1978) |
| Drinking-water, surface water, groundwater, domestic and industrial wastewaters<br>Total chromium | Various acidification/evaporation/dilution steps, depending on specific matrix and method | AAS | 0.05 mg/l | US Environmental Protection Agency (1983, 1986) [Methods 218.1, 218.3, 3005, 3010, 7190] |
| | | ICP/AES | 7 μg/l | [Methods 200.7, 6010] |
| | | EAAS | 1 μg/l | [Methods 218.2, 3020, 7191] |
| Hexavalent chromium | Acidify to pH 3.5 with acetic acid; add lead nitrate, glacial acetic acid and ammonium sulfate; centrifuge and discard supernatant; dissolve precipitate in concentrated nitric acid | EAAS | 2 μg/l | US Environmental Protection Agency (1983, 1986) [Methods 218.5, 7195] |

**Table 19 (contd)**

| Sample matrix | Sample preparation | Assay procedure[a] | Limit of detection[b] | Reference |
|---|---|---|---|---|
| Hexavalent chromium | Chelate with ammonium pyrrolidine dithiocarbamate or pyrrolidine dithiocarbamic acid in chloroform; extract with methyl isobutyl ketone | AAS | NR | US Environmental Protection Agency (1983, 1986) [Methods 218.4, 7197] |
| Hexavalent chromium | Use ammonium hydroxide/ammonium chloride as supporting electrolyte | DPP | 10 µg/l | US Environmental Protection Agency (1986) [Method 7198] |
| Hexavalent chromium | Remove interfering metals by adding aluminium sulfate; filter; add sodium hypochlorite solution; add phosphoric acid solution and sodium chloride; add sym-diphenylcarbazide | VIS | NR | Deutsches Institut für Normung (1987) [DIN 38405]; (see also US Environmental Protection Agency (1986) [Method 7196] |
| Oily waste samples: oils, greases, waxes, crude oil (soluble chromium) | Dissolve in xylene or methyl isobutyl ketone | AAS | 0.05 mg/l | US Environmental Protection Agency (1986) [Methods 3040, 7190] |
| | | ICP | 7 µg/l | [Method 6010] |
| Sediments, sludges, soils and solid wastes (total chromium) | Digest with nitric acid and hydrogen peroxide; dilute with dilute hydrochloric or nitric acid | AAS | 0.05 mg/l | US Environmental Protection Agency (1986) [Methods 3050, 7190] |
| | | ICP | 7 µg/l | [Method 6010] |
| | | EAAS | 1 µg/l | [Methods 3050, 7191] |
| Sediments | Activate with neutrons for 6 h | NAA | 1.5 mg/kg | Ackermann (1977) |
| **Food** | | | | |
| Tinned foods | Oxidize to hexavalent chromium with hydrogen peroxide; treat with sym-diphenylcarbazide | VIS | 0.05 mg/kg | Il'inykh (1977) |

**Table 19 (contd)**

| Sample matrix | Sample preparation | Assay procedure[a] | Limit of detection[b] | Reference |
|---|---|---|---|---|
| **Biological samples** | | | | |
| SRM 1569 brewers' yeast; SRM 1577 bovine liver; SRM 1570 spinach; human hair and nails | Chemical procedures developed for digestion of biological matrices and separation of chromium without large analytical blanks or significant losses by volatilization | IDMS | 1 µg | Dunstan & Garner (1977) |
| Blood, plasma, urine | Dilute with Triton X100 solution; standard addition method | EAAS | NR | Morris et al. (1989) |
| Tissue | Digest sample with nitric and sulfuric acids with a defined time-temperature programme; dilute with water; standard addition method | EAAS | 0.3 µg/g wet wt | Raithel et al. (1987) |
| Serum | – | NAA | NR | Versieck et al. (1978) |
| Serum, human milk, urine | Dilute with water | EAAS | 0.05 ng/ml (urine, serum) 0.1 ng/ml (milk) | Kumpulainen et al. (1983) |
| Blood or tissue | Digest with mixture of nitric, perchloric and sulfuric acids; heat for 4-5 h; cool; dilute with deionized water or add yttrium internal standard | ICP/AES | 0.01 µg/g blood 0.2 µg/g tissue | Eller (1985) [Method 8005] |
| Blood erythrocytes | Wash with isotonic saline; dilute with Triton X100 solution | EAAS | 1 µg/l | Lewalter et al. (1985) |
| Human urine  Total chromium | Adjust pH to 2.0 with sodium hydroxide; add polydithiocarbamate resin; filter, saving filtrate and resin; adjust filtrate to pH 8.0 and add more resin; ash filters and resins; add nitric/perchloric acid mixture and warm | ICP/AES | 0.1 µg | Eller (1984) [Method 8310] |

**Table 19 (contd)**

| Sample matrix | Sample preparation | Assay procedure[a] | Limit of detection[b] | Reference |
|---|---|---|---|---|
| Total chromium | Dilute and acidify with nitric acid | EAAS | 0.1-0.5 μg/l | Nise & Vesterberg (1979); Kiilunen et al. (1987); Angerer & Schaller (1988) |
| Plant materials | Dry in an oven at 120°C for 2-4 h; ash in a muffle furnace at 550°C for 6 h | ES | 2 mg/kg | Dixit et al. (1976) |
| **Airborne chromium** | | | | |
| Welding fumes Hexavalent chromium | Extract with sodium carbonate; remove precipitate by filtration; add sym-diphenylcarbazide; measure absorption at 540 nm | EAAS | 0.8 μg | Thomsen & Stern (1979) |
| Total and hexavalent chromium | Extract with sodium hydroxide and carbonate or fuse with sodium carbonate; remove precipitate by filtration; acidify with sulfuric acid; add sym-diphenylcarbazide; measure absorption at 540 nm | VIS | 1 μg/m³ | Moreton et al. (1983) |
| Hexavalent and trivalent chromium | Collect on polycarbonate membranes | ESCA, NAA | 0.001 μg | Lautner et al. (1978) |
| Total, hexavalent and trivalent chromium | Collect on cellulose ester membranes | PIXE, ESCA, TEM, EDXA | 0.0001-0.01 μg | Bohgard et al. (1979) |
| Welding fumes; complex matrices with redox systems | | | | |
| Insoluble and total hexavalent chromium | Add sodium carbonate; warm; remove precipitate by filtration | AAS | 1 μg/m³ | Thomsen & Stern (1979) |
| Total chromium | Add phosphoric acid:sulfuric acid (3:1) | AAS | 1 μg/m³ | Pedersen et al. (1987) |
| Welding and brazing fumes | Sample on cellulose ester membrane filter; load sample and irradiate | XRF | 2 μg | Eller (1984) [Method 7200] |

**Table 19 (contd)**

| Sample matrix | Sample preparation | Assay procedure[a] | Limit of detection[b] | Reference |
|---|---|---|---|---|
| Cement (hexavalent chromium) | Extract with water; add ammonium acetate and ethylene diamine | DPP | 0.3 μg/g | Vandenbalck & Patriarche (1987) |
| Grinding dusts | Collect particulate sample on polycarbonate membrane | SEM, EDXA | NR | Koponen (1985) |
| Paint aerosols (hexavalent chromium) | Extract with a sodium hydroxide—sodium carbonate solution; dilute with buffer solution | IC | 0.003 μg | Molina & Abell (1987) |

[a]Abbreviations: IT, iodometric titration; EAAS, electrothermal atomic absorption spectrometry; NAA, neutron activation analysis; AAS, atomic adsorption spectrometry; X-REA, X-ray emission analysis; ICP/AES, inductively coupled argon/plasma/atomic emission spectroscopy; VIS, visible absorption spectrometry; PP, pulse polarography; IDMS, isotope dilution mass spectrometry; DPP, differential pulse polarography; ES, emission spectrography; ESCA, electron spectroscopy for chemical analysis; PIXE, proton induced X-ray emission; TEM, transmission electron microscopy; EDXA, energy dispersive X-ray analysis; XRF, X-ray fluorescence; SEM, scanning electron microscopy; IC, ion chromatography

[b]NR, not reported

The American Society for Testing and Materials (ASTM) has established standard methods for determining the chromium (or chromium compound) content of various commercial products. These include methods for the chemical analysis of chromium-containing refractory materials and chromium ore (ASTM C572-81), for chromium in water (ASTM D1687-86), for strontium chromate pigment (ASTM D1845-86) and for chromic oxide in leather that has been partly or completely tanned with chromium compounds (ASTM D2807-78); a colorimetric method for the determination of soluble chromium (trivalent and hexavalent chromium) in workplace atmospheres (ASTM D3586-85); methods for the determination of chromium (including chromium oxide) in the solids of liquid coatings (paint) or in dried films obtained from previously coated substrates (ASTM D3718-85a), for chromium in residues obtained by air sampling of dusts of lead chromate and lead silicochromate-type pigments (ASTM D4358-84), for chromium and ferrochromium (ASTM E363-83), for chromium oxide in chromium ores (ASTM E342-71), for yellow, orange and green pigments containing lead chromate and chromium oxide green (ASTM D126-87) and for zinc yellow pigment (zinc chromate yellow) (ASTM D444-88) (American Society for Testing and Materials, 1971, 1978, 1981, 1983, 1984b, 1985a,b, 1986a,b, 1987c, 1988b).

# 3. Biological Data Relevant to the Evaluation of Carcinogenic Risk to Humans

## 3.1 Carcinogenicity studies in animals[1]

The carcinogenicity of chromium and chromium-containing compounds in experimental animals has been reviewed recently (Yassi & Nieboer, 1988; Fairhurst & Minty, 1990).

The description and evaluation of the available carcinogenicity studies in experimental animals have been subdivided into four subsections, mainly according to the chemical and physical properties of different chromium-containing materials: (*a*) Metallic chromium; (*b*) chromium [III] compounds; (*c*) chromium [VI] compounds; and (*d*) other chromium compounds. Chromium-containing alloys used in implants will be considered in a subsequent volume of *IARC Monographs* (Volume 52), in a monograph on cobalt and cobalt compounds.

### (*a*) Metallic chromium

#### (i) Intrapleural administration

*Mouse*: No tumour was observed after 14 months in a group of 50 male C57Bl mice, approximately six weeks of age, that received six intrapleural injections of 10 µg chromium powder in 0.2 ml of a 2.5% gelatin-saline solution every other week. A total of 32 mice lived for up to 14 months (Hueper, 1955).

*Rat*: Groups of 17 female and eight male Osborne-Mendel rats, approximately four months old, were given six monthly intrapleural injections of 16.8 mg chromium powder in 50 µl lanolin; and 25 male Wistar rats, of approximately the same age, received six weekly intrapleural injections of 0.5 mg chromium powder suspended in 0.1 ml of a 2.5% gelatin-saline solution. Six Osborne-Mendel rats survived up to 19-24 months and 12 Wistar rats up to 25-30 months. Three female Osborne-Mendel rats developed adenofibromas of the thoracic wall; in addition, one rat also had a retroperitoneal haemangioma. Two other rats [group unspecified] had a haemangioma and an angiosarcoma, and another rat [group unspecified] had an intra-abdominal round-cell sarcoma. Of 12 male Wistar rats receiving gelatin alone, three developed intra-abdominal round-cell sarcomas (Hueper, 1955).

---

[1]The Working Group was aware of carcinogenicity studies in progress with sodium chromate by intraperitoneal administration in mice and rats, with calcium chromate and chromite ore residue by inhalation in rats and with chromium by intratracheal administration in hamsters (IARC, 1988).

(ii)   *Intramuscular administration*

*Rat*: A group of 24 male Fischer rats, eight weeks of age, received a single intra-muscular injection of 2 mg chromium dust (elemental Cr, 65%, chromium oxides as $Cr_2O_3$, 35%; Ni, Al, Cu, Mn and Co, < 0.1%; mean particle diameter, 1.6 μm) sus-pended in 0.5 ml penicillin G procaine. No local tumour was reported in the 22 survivors at 24 months (Sunderman *et al.*, 1974). [The Working Group noted that only a single low dose was given.]

Two groups of 18 and 20 male Fischer-344 rats, aged eight weeks, received a single intramuscular injection of 4.4 mg chromium dust (Cr, 76%; $O_2$, 24%; Mn, 0.2%; median particle diameter, 1.4 μm) suspended in 0.2 ml penicillin G procaine. The study was terminated at two years, when 13/18 and 0/20 were still alive in the two groups, respectively; the low survival in the second group was due to an epidem-ic of pulmonary pneumonia. No local tumour developed in either group (Sunder-man *et al.*, 1980). [The Working Group noted that only a single dose was given.]

A group of 25 male and 25 female weanling Fischer-344 rats received monthly intramuscular injections of 100 mg chromium powder (99.9% pure) in 0.2 ml tri-caprylin. Treatment was continued until definite nodules appeared at the injection site in more than one animal [time unspecified]. The study was terminated at 644 days [survival figures not given]. A single injection-site fibrosarcoma was reported in a male rat. No local tumour was seen in 50 vehicle-control rats (Furst, 1971).


(iii)   *Intraperitoneal administration*

*Mouse*: A group of 50 male C57Bl mice, approximately six weeks old, was given weekly intraperitoneal injections for four consecutive weeks of 10 μg chromium powder (diameter, > 100 μm to colloidal particle size) suspended in 0.2 ml of a 2.5% gelatin-saline solution. Forty mice survived up to 21 months, at which time the ex-periment was terminated. One mouse developed a myeloid leukaemia; no other tumour was noted (Hueper, 1955). [The Working Group noted the low dose given.]

*Rat*: A group of 25 male Wistar rats, three to four months old, was given weekly intraperitoneal injections for six consecutive weeks of 50 μg chromium powder in 0.1 ml of a 2.5% gelatin-saline solution. One rat developed a scirrhous carcinoma of the caecal submucosa, two rats developed intra-abdominal round-cell sarcomas, one rat had both a sarcoma of the leg of cartilaginous osteoid origin and an insulin-oma of the pancreas, and one rat had an insulinoma (Hueper, 1955). [The Working Group noted that no vehicle control group was reported and that the authors stated that, although round-cell sarcomas also occurred in controls, insulinomas were found only in treated rats.]

(iv)  *Intravenous administration*

*Mouse*: A group of 25 C57Bl mice [sex unspecified], about eight weeks of age, received six weekly injections into the tail vein of 2.5 µg chromium powder (particle size, ≤4 µm) in 0.05 ml of a gelatin-saline solution. Six animals lived up to 12 months, but none to 18 months. No tumour was observed (Hueper, 1955).

*Rat*: A group of 25 male Wistar rats, approximately seven months of age, was given six weekly injections of 90 µg chromium powder in 0.18 ml of a 2.5% gela-tin-saline solution into the left vena saphena. Fifteen were still alive at one year and 13 at two years, at which time the study was terminated. Round-cell sarcomas were observed in four rats - three in the ileocaecal region and one in the intrathoracic region. One rat had a haemangioma of the renal medulla, and two rats had papillary adenomas of the lungs, one of which showed extensive squamous-cell carcinoma-tous changes. Use of vehicle-treated controls was not reported. The author stated that, although round-cell sarcomas also occurred in groups of control rats in this series of studies, lung adenomas were found only in treated rats (Hueper, 1955).

*Rabbit*: Eight albino rabbits [sex unspecified], approximately six months of age, received six weekly intravenous injections of 25 mg/kg bw chromium powder in 0.5 ml of a 2.5% gelatin-saline solution into the ear vein; the same course of treat-ment was given four months later; and, three years after the first injection, a third series of injections was given to the three surviving rabbits. Four rabbits given in-travenous injections of the vehicle alone served as controls. One of three rabbits that survived six months after the last injection developed a tumour of uncertain origin (apparently an immature carcinoma) involving various lymph nodes, but no tumour occurred in controls (Hueper, 1955).

(v) *Intrafemoral administration*

*Rat*: A group of 25 male Wistar rats, approximately five months old, received an injection into the femur of 0.2 ml of a 50% (by weight) suspension of chromium powder (approximately 45 mg) in 20% gelatin-saline and was observed for 24 months; 19 survived over one year. No tumour developed at the injection site. Simi-larly, a group 25 male Osborne-Mendel rats, approximately five months of age, was injected in the femur with a similar dose of chromium powder in 0.2 ml lanolin and observed for 24 months; 14 survived for one year, and one rat developed a fibroma at the injection site (Hueper, 1955).

[The Working Group noted that many of the above studies suffered from vari-ous limitations, including the use of low doses, low effective numbers of animals and inadequate reporting.]

### (vi)  *Administration with known carcinogens*

*Rat*: Groups of 35-62 female Wistar rats, four to six weeks old, were given one intratracheal instillation of 10 mg powdered chromium (purity, 99.4%; diameter, 1-3 μm) in combination with 1 or 5 mg 20-methylcholanthrene (MC) or MC alone in saline and were killed at various intervals up to 12 weeks. Squamous-cell carcinomas of the lung developed 12 weeks after treatment in 7/12 (58%) rats given Cr + 5 mg MC, in 3/12 (25%) given Cr + 1 mg MC, in 3/7 (43%) given 5 mg MC alone, in 1/8 (12.5%) given 1 mg MC alone and in 0/12 given Cr alone (Mukubo, 1978.) [The Working Group noted the short duration of the study.]

### (b)  *Chromium[III] compounds*

#### (i)  *Intratracheal instillation*

*Rat*: Random-bred and Wistar rats [age, sex and distribution unspecified] were given single intratracheal instillations of 50 and 20 mg chromic oxide, respectively. Malignant lung tumours developed in 7/34 and 6/18 animals; and four and five of these, respectively, were lung sarcomas, which appeared between 11 and 22 months after treatment (Dvizhkov & Fedorova, 1967). [The Working Group noted that use of controls was not reported and other details were not given.]

#### (ii)  *Intrabronchial administration*

*Rat*: A group of 98 rats [strain, age and sex unspecified] received implants of intrabronchial stainless-steel mesh pellets (5 × 1 mm) loaded with 3-5 mg of a 50:50 mixture of chromic oxide with a cholesterol binder. Animals were observed up to 136 weeks. No lung tumour was found in treated or in 24 cholesterol binder-treated controls (Laskin *et al.*, 1970).

Groups of 100 male and female Porton-Wistar rats received intrabronchial pellets loaded with 2 mg chromite ore [purity not given], 2 mg chromic oxide (metallurgical-grade, 99-100% pure), 2 mg chromic chloride hexahydrate (95% pure) or 2 mg chrome tan ($Cr_2(OH)_2(SO_4)_2Na_2SO_4 \cdot xH_2O$ [purity not given]) suspended 50:50 in cholesterol. The incidence of squamous metaplasia in the left bronchus of treated animals was similar to that in controls. An increased incidence was seen with all five Cr[VI] compounds examined in the same study (see p. 125; Levy & Venitt, 1986).

In a second study using the same technique, no lung tumour was seen in a group of 101 rats treated with high silica chrome ore (TSS 695, containing 46.1% chromic oxide) (Levy *et al.*, 1986).

#### (iii)  *Oral administration*

*Mouse*: Groups of 54 male and 54 female weanling Swiss mice received 5 mg/l chromic acetate in drinking-water for life. No difference was found in the survival of treated females compared with controls, but treated males died earlier than control males (mean survival, 831 *versus* 957 days); only 60% of males survived 18 months. The incidence of tumours in treated animals was no greater than that in controls (Schroeder *et al.*, 1964).

*Rat*: Chromic acetate was given in drinking-water at a level of 5 mg/l to 46 male and 50 female weanling Long Evans rats for life. At least 70% of the animals survived for up to two years; treated females lived as long as control females, but treated males lived up to 100 days longer than control males. The incidences of tumours at various sites in rats of either sex were not significantly different from those in controls. The total numbers of autopsied animals with tumours were: 16/39 treated males, 18/35 treated females, 9/35 male controls and 15/35 female controls (Schroeder *et al.*, 1965).

Chromic oxide (green) obtained by the reduction of chromate at 600°C was baked in bread with other nutrients at levels of 1, 2 and 5%, and the bread was fed to groups of 60 male and female inbred BD rats, 100 days of age, on five days per week for two years. At the high-dose level, the total dose consumed was about 1800 g/kg bw. Average survival times were 860-880 days. Mammary fibroadenomas were found in three rats given 1%, in one given 2% and in three given 5%. One mammary carcinoma and two fibroadenomas were detected in controls (Ivankovic & Preussmann, 1975).

### (iv)  *Intrapleural administration*

*Mouse*: Only granulomas were produced when 10 mg chromite ore dust [$FeO(CrAl)_2O_3$] particles (average diameter, 1 µm; range, 0.1-5 µm) were injected intrapleurally in 0.5 ml distilled water into 25 Balb/c mice [sex and age unspecified]. Animals were killed at intervals from two weeks to 18 months after the injection (Davis, 1972). [The Working Group noted the lack of detailed reporting.]

*Rat*: A group of 14 male and 11 female Osborne-Mendel rats, four months of age, received six monthly intrapleural injections of 37 mg chromite ore suspended in 0.05 ml lanolin. Thirteen survived one year and all animals were dead at 24 months. One thoracic tumour (fibrosarcoma) was found in a treated animal but none in 25 controls (Hueper, 1955).

A group of 34 rats [strain, sex and age unspecified] received intrapleural implantations of chromic acetate [dose unspecified] in sheep fat. Eighteen rats were still alive at 15 months and 15 at 21 months. One implantation-site tumour [type unspecified] was seen. Of 34 control rats administered sheep fat alone, 30 were alive at one year and 11 at 21 months; none developed a tumour (Hueper, 1961).

A group of 42 Bethesda Black [NIH Black] rats [sex unspecified], approximately three months of age, received eight intrapleural implantations over 13 months of 25 mg chromic acetate in gelatin capsules. No implantation-site tumour was seen after two years (Hueper & Payne, 1962). [The Working Group noted the lack of controls.]

### (v)  Intramuscular administration

*Rat*: A group of 34 rats [sex, age and strain unspecified] received intramuscular implantations of chromic acetate [dose unspecified]. Thirty were still alive at one year and 17 at 21 months. One animal developed an injection-site tumour [type unspecified]. Of 32 controls given implants of sheep fat alone 30 were alive at one year and ten at 21 months. None developed a local tumour (Hueper, 1961).

A group of 35 Bethesda Black [NIH Black] rats [sex unspecified], approximately three months of age, received an intramuscular implantation of 25 mg chromic acetate in a gelatin capsule; a further seven intramuscular implantions were made over a period of 24 months, at which time the rats were sacrificed. One spindle-cell sarcoma was observed at the site of implantation (Hueper & Payne, 1962). [The Working Group noted that no control group was reported.]

### (vi)  Intraperitoneal administration

*Mouse*: In a strain A mouse assay for lung adenomas, three groups of ten male and ten female strain A/Strong mice, six to ten weeks of age, were given intraperitoneal injections of chromic sulfate suspended in tricaprylin three times a week for eight weeks (total doses, 480, 1200 and 2400 mg/kg bw). Animals were killed 30 weeks after the first injection. No significant increase in the incidences of pulmonary adenomas over those in 20 vehicle-treated or 20 untreated control mice of each sex was observed (Stoner *et al.*, 1976; Shimkin *et al.*, 1977). [The Working Group noted the small number of animals used.]

*Rat*: In experiments with Wistar and random-bred rats [sex, age and distribution unspecified], 4/20 animals developed lung sarcomas 16-19 months after a single intraperitoneal injection of 20 mg chromic oxide (Dvizhkov & Fedorova, 1967). [The Working Group noted that no control group was reported.]

### (vii)  Intravenous administration

*Mouse*: Strain A mice in a group of 25 males and 25 females [age unspecified] were each given an intravenous injection into the tail vein of 5 mg chromite ore (39-60% chromic oxide; particle size, 1.6 μm) suspended in saline. The animals were killed at three, 4.5 and six months. There was no difference in the incidence of pulmonary adenomas between treated mice and 75 untreated controls (Shimkin & Leiter, 1940; Shimkin *et al.*, 1977).

*Rabbit*: A group of six female albino rabbits, six months of age, received six weekly intravenous injections of 25 mg chromite ore suspended in 5 ml of a 2.5% gelatin-saline solution; treatment was repeated in four of the six rabbits nine months later. The six rabbits died or were killed at 13, 20, 22, 22, 48 and 48 months.

No tumour was observed during these periods (Hueper, 1955). [The Working Group noted the small number of animals used and the lack of controls.]

### (viii)  *Intrafemoral administration*

*Rat*: A group of 15 male and 10 female Osborne-Mendel rats, five months of age, each received an injection into the femur of 0.05 ml of a 50% (by volume) suspension containing about 58 mg chromite ore (44% chromic oxide) in lanolin; 13 survived one year. No tumour developed at the injection site (Hueper, 1955).

### (ix)  *Administration with known carcinogens*

*Rat*: Groups of 15 male Fischer 344 rats, seven weeks of age, received drinking-water (distilled) containing 0 or 500 mg/l $N$-nitrosoethylhydroxyethylamine (NEHEA) for two weeks. Thereafter, rats received drinking-water alone or drinking-water containing 600 mg/l chromic chloride hexahydrate (98% pure) for 25 weeks, when the study was terminated. There was no significant increase in the incidence of renal-cell tumours in the group receiving NEHEA and chromic chloride (6/15) over that in the group given NEHEA alone (2/15). No renal tumour was reported in the group receiving chromic chloride alone (Kurokawa *et al.*, 1985). [The Working Group noted that the experiment was not intended as a test for the overall carcinogenicity of chromic chloride.]

### (c)  *Chromium[VI] compounds*

### (i)  *Inhalation*

*Mouse*: Groups of 136 C57Bl/6 mice of each sex, eight weeks old, were exposed by inhalation to calcium chromate dust (reagent grade; particle size, 99.9% < 1.0 $\mu$m) at 13 mg/m$^3$ for 5 h per day on five days per week over their lifespan. The median survival time was 93 weeks for treated and 80 weeks for control mice. Six lung adenomas appeared in treated males and eight in females, compared with three and two in the 136 respective controls [$p = 0.04$ for males and females combined]. No carcinoma was seen; no information was given on the occurrence of tumours at other sites (Nettesheim *et al.*, 1971).

A group of 50 female ICR/JcI mice [age unspecified] was exposed by inhalation to chromic acid (chromium trioxide) mist (particle size, 84.5% > 5 $\mu$m) generated by a miniaturized electroplating system at a chromium concentration of 3.63 mg/m$^3$ for 30 min per day on two days per week for up to 12 months. Mice surviving at that time were maintained for a further six months; two groups of ten mice killed at 12 and 18 months served as controls. A single lung adenoma was reported in 1/15 mice that died or were killed between six and nine months; lung adenomas occurred in 3/14 mice that died between ten and 14 months; and 1/19 adenoma and 2/19 adenocarcinomas in mice that died at 15-18 months. In the control groups, no lung tumour was reported in ten mice killed at 12 months, but 2/10 adenomas occurred in those killed at 18 months. The authors observed nasal perforations in six mice exposed for more than ten months and time-related inflammatory changes, including squamous metaplasia, in the trachea and bronchus of exposed mice (Adachi *et al.*, 1986). [The Working Group noted the incomplete reporting of lesions.]

A group of 43 female C57Bl mice [age unspecified] was exposed by inhalation to chromic acid (chromium trioxide) mist (85% of particles > 5 μm) generated by a miniaturized electroplating system at a chromium concentration of 1.81 mg/m³ for 120 min twice a week for 12 months, at which time 23 mice were killed. The remaining 20 were killed six months after the last exposure. Nasal perforation was seen in 3/23 and 3/20 mice killed at 12 and 18 months, respectively; 0/23 and 6/20 nasal papillomas occurred in these groups. A single lung adenoma was reported in the group killed at 18 months. No nasal inflammatory change or lung tumour was seen in a group of 20 untreated control mice (Adachi, 1987). [The Working Group noted the inadequate reporting of lesions.]

*Rat*: Groups of 20 male TNO-W74 Wistar rats, six weeks of age, were exposed by inhalation to sodium dichromate at 25, 50 or 100 μg/m³ Cr (average mass median diameter, 0.36 μm), produced from an aqueous sodium dichromate solution, for 22-23 h per day on seven days per week for 18 months. The rats were then held for a further 12 months, at which time the study was terminated. A control group consisted of 40 untreated male rats. Survival was about 90% at 24 months; at termination at 30 months, survival was 65, 55, 75 and 57.5% in the 25, 50, 100 μg/m³ and control groups respectively. In rats that survived 24 or more months, lung tumours occurred in 0/37, 0/18, 0/18 and 3/19 in the control, 25, 50 and 100 μg/m³ groups, respectively. The three lung tumours were two adenomas and an adenocarcinoma; a squamous carcinoma of the pharynx was also reported in this group. The incidence of treatment-related tumours was not increased at other sites (Glaser *et al.*, 1986). [The Working Group noted the small number of animals used.]

(ii)  *Intratracheal instillation*

*Mouse*: A group of 62 strain A mice [sex unspecified], ten to 11 weeks of age, received six intratracheal injections of 0.03 ml of a 0.2% saline suspension of zinc chromate [basic potassium zinc chromate, $K_2O.4ZnO.4CrO_3.3H_2O$ (Baetjer *et al.*, 1959b)] at six-week intervals and were observed until death. No pulmonary carcinoma was found; pulmonary adenomas occurred in 31/62 exposed, in 7/18 untreated control and 3/12 zinc carbonate-treated control animals (Steffee & Baetjer, 1965).

Groups of 40 male and 40 female Sprague-Dawley rats, ten weeks of age, received intratracheal instillations of 1 ml/kg bw sodium dichromate (99.95% pure) or calcium chromate (chemically pure) in 0.9% sodium chloride solution once a week or five times a week. Equal numbers of male and female rats were used as vehicle and untreated controls. Administered doses and schedules are given in Table 20. Treatment and study of all groups was continued for 30 months; median survival was approximately 800 days in the sodium dichromate-treated groups. [The Working Group noted that survival was not reported for the calcium chromate-treated groups.] No lung tumour was reported in the groups treated five times weekly with sodium dichromate. Among animals treated weekly with sodium dichromate, 14/80, 1/80 and 0/80 animals developed lung tumours in the groups receiving 1.25, 0.25 and 0.05 mg/kg bw, respectively, with 0/80 in controls [$p < 0.001$, Cochran-Armitage test for trend]. Of the 14 animals that developed lung tumours after receiving 1.25 mg/kg bw sodium dichromate weekly 12 had adenomas and eight had malignant lung tumours, described as two adenocarcinomas (bronchioalveolar) and six squamous-cell carcinomas. The authors noted that two of the tumours were questionable and that the majority of the observed lung tumours were small, non-metastasizing, non-fatal and co-existed with scarring and other treatment-related inflammatory changes not seen in animals treated five times a week with lower doses. In the groups receiving calcium chromate, similar findings were made, with a total of six lung tumour-bearing rats (five adenomas ($p < 0.01$) and one squamous-cell carcinoma) in the group receiving 0.25 mg/kg bw five times a week, and 13 lung-tumour-bearing rats (11 adenomas ($p < 0.01$) and three with two squamous-cell carcinomas and one adenocarcinoma ($p < 0.01$)) in the group receiving 1.25 mg/kg bw once a week. [The Working Group assumed that one rat had both an adenoma and a squamous-cell carcinoma.] The authors noted that one of the squamous-cell carcinomas may have been a metastasis from a primary tumour of the jaw (Steinhoff *et al.*, 1986).

*Hamster*. Groups of 35 male Syrian golden hamsters, about six weeks old, received weekly intratracheal instillations of 0.1 mg calcium chromate in 0.2 ml saline for 56 weeks and were maintained for a further 44 weeks. No lung tumour was reported (Reuzel *et al.*, 1986).

*Guinea-pig*. Groups of 21 or 13 guinea-pigs [sex and strain unspecified], three months of age, received six intratracheal instillations of 0.3 ml of a 1% suspension in saline of 3 mg zinc chromate as basic potassium zinc chromate (Baetjer *et al.*, 1959b) or 3 mg lead chromate, at three-monthly intervals. The animals were observed until death. A single pulmonary adenoma was seen in the group given zinc chromate, but no pulmonary carcinoma. No pulmonary adenoma was seen in the lead chromate group or in 18 vehicle controls (Steffee & Baetjer, 1965). [The Working Group noted the limited reporting of the study.]

*Rabbit*. Groups of seven rabbits [sex and strain unspecified], four months of age, received three to five intratracheal instillations of 1 ml of a suspension in saline of 1% (10 mg) zinc chromate (basic potassium zinc chromate, Baetjer *et al.*, 1959b) or lead chromate at three-monthly intervals. No lung tumour was reported in

Table 20. Protocol and results of test by intratracheal instillation of various chromium[VI] compounds to rats[a]

| Compound | No. of animals | | Dose (mg/kg bw) | Schedule | No. of lung tumours | | Total no. of tumour-bearing animals |
|---|---|---|---|---|---|---|---|
| | Males | Females[b] | | | Benign | Malignant | |
| Sodium dichromate | 40 | 50 | 0.25 | 5 × weekly | – | – | – |
| Sodium dichromate | 40 | 45 | 0.05 | 5 × weekly | – | – | – |
| Sodium dichromate | 40 | 45 | 0.01 | 5 × weekly | – | – | – |
| Sodium dichromate | 40 | 40 | 1.25 | 1 × weekly | 12* | 8* | 14 |
| Sodium dichromate | 40 | 40 | 0.25 | 1 × weekly | – | 1 | 1 |
| Sodium dichromate | 40 | 40 | 0.05 | 1 × weekly | – | – | – |
| Calcium chromate | 40 | 50 | 0.25 | 5 × weekly | 5* | 1 | 6 |
| Calcium chromate | 40 | 40 | 1.25 | 1 × weekly | 11* | 3* | 13 |
| Benzo[a]pyrene | 0 | 10 | 5.0 | 1 × weekly | | | |
| Dimethyl carbamoyl chloride | 10 | 10 | 1.0 | 1 × weekly | | | |
| Sodium chloride (0.9%) | 40 | 50 | 1 ml/kg | 5 × weekly | – | – | – |
| Sodium chloride (0.9%) | 40 | 40 | 1 ml/kg | 1 × weekly | – | – | – |
| Untreated | 40 | 50 | – | – | – | – | – |

[a]From Steinhoff et al. (1986)

[b]Only 40 females used for carcinogenicity tests (five to ten extra in test groups)

*Significant at $p < 0.01$

treated animals or in five saline-treated controls (Steffee & Baetjer, 1965). [The Working Group noted the limited reporting of the study.]

### (iii) *Intrabronchial administration*

*Rat*: A group of 100 rats [strain, sex and age unspecified] received intrabronchial implantations of stainless-steel mesh pellets (5 × 1 mm) loaded with 3-5 mg of a 50:50 mixture of calcium chromate with a cholesterol binder. Six squamous-cell carcinomas and two adenocarcinomas of the lung were found in animals observed up to 136 weeks. The median time to appearance of tumours was 540 days. A group of 100 rats similarly treated with chromium trioxide and observed up to 136 weeks had no such tumour, nor did 24 controls treated with cholesterol binder (Laskin *et al.*, 1970). [Although the incidence of lung tumours was not statistically significant, the Working Group noted the probable biological significance of these tumours.]

Groups of approximately 50 male and 50 female Porton-Wistar rats, six to eight weeks old, received intrabronchial implantations into the left lung of stainless-steel mesh pellets (5 × 1 mm) loaded with about 2 mg of a series of chromium-containing test materials suspended 50:50 in cholesterol. Groups of approximately 75 male and 75 female rats receiving blank pellets or pellets loaded with cholesterol alone acted as negative controls. Animals were maintained for 24 months, at which time the study was terminated and all lungs and abnormal tissues examined. [The Working Group noted that survival was not reported]. No lung tumour was seen in either control group or among rats receiving pellets loaded with sodium dichromate (99-100% pure) or sodium chromate (98-99% pure); a single squamous-cell carcinoma of the left lung was seen in the group treated with chromic acid (chromium trioxide; 99-100% pure) and eight squamous-cell carcinomas ($p < 0.05$) of the left lung in the group treated with calcium chromate (95% pure). There was a significant increase in the incidence of bronchial squamous metaplasia of the left lung in rats without lung tumours in all treatment groups when compared to the groups receiving cholesterol or a blank pellet. Of animals that received intrabronchial pellets loaded with zinc potassium chromate ($K_2CrO_4.3ZnCrO_4.Zn(OH)_2$, 99-100% pure) suspended in cholesterol, 3/61 developed squamous-cell carcinomas of the left lung (Levy & Venitt, 1986).

In a second study using the techniques and protocol described above, the incidences of squamous-cell carcinomas of the left lung in groups of animals given a range of lead chromates, zinc chromates and strontium chromates were as shown in Table 21. Significance was calculated by comparing the incidence of bronchial carcinomas in each test group with that in a reference group comprising the two negative control groups and all groups treated with chromium-containing materials. Survival was 96% at 400 days and 54% at 700 days. Calcium chromate (96.7% pure), included as a positive control, induced 25/100 left-lung bronchial carcinomas

(24 squamous-cell carcinomas and one adenocarcinoma); chromium trioxide (99.9% pure) induced 2/100 left-lung bronchial carcinomas (one squamous-cell carcinoma and one anaplastic carcinoma); sodium dichromate dihydrate (TSS 612; 99.7% pure) gave 1/100 left-lung squamous-cell carcinoma; and a residue material (vanadium solids) from the bichromate production process, containing 5.3% calcium chromate and 17.2% sodium dichromate, induced 1/100 squamous-cell carcinoma of the left lung. No bronchial carcinoma was seen in the 100 rats given cholesterol alone; and 22/48 bronchial carcinomas (21 squamous-cell carcinomas and one anaplastic carcinoma) were seen in a positive control group receiving 20-methylcholanthrene (Levy *et al.*, 1986).

**Table 21. Incidence of bronchial carcinomas in rats administered various chromium[VI] compounds by intrabronchial implantation into the left lung**[a]

| Compound | Composition | Incidence of bronchial carcinomas |
|---|---|---|
| Lead chromates | | |
|    Lead chromate (99.8% pure) | Pb, 64%; $CrO_4$, 35.8% | 1/98 |
|    Primrose chrome yellow | Pb, 62.1%; Cr, 12.6% | 1/100 |
|    Molybdate chrome orange[b] | | 0/100 |
|    Light chrome yellow | Pb, 62.1%; Cr, 12.5% | 0/100 |
|    Supra (70 FS) LD chrome yellow | PbO, 61.5%; $CrO_3$, 26.9% | 1/100 |
|    Medium chrome yellow | Pb, 60.2%; Cr, 16.3% | 1/100 |
|    Silica encapsulated medium chrome yellow | Pb, 40.4%; Cr, 10.5% | 0/100 |
| Barium chromate (98% pure) | Ba, 54.1%; $CrO_4$, 42.1% | 0/101 |
| Zinc chromate IW (low water solubility) | ZnO, 39.4%; $CrO_3$, 40.8% | 5/100[c] [$p = 0.004$] |
| Zinc chromate (Norge composition) | ZnO, 39.2%; $CrO_3$, 43.5% | 3/100[c] [$p = 0.068$] |
| Zinc tetroxychromate | Zn, 56.6%; Cr, 8.8% | 1/100 |
| Strontium chromate | Sr, 42.2%; $CrO_4$, 54.1% | 43/99 |
| Strontium chromate | Sr, 43.0%; Cr, 24.3% | 62/99 |
| Cholesterol control | | 0/100 |
| 20-Methylcholanthrene control | | 22/48 |

[a]From Levy *et al.* (1986)

[b]Composition incompletely described by Levy *et al.* (1986); it is a mixture of lead chromate, lead sulfate and lead molybdate (Pb, 62.9%; Cr, 12.9%; Mo, 4.2%).

[c]Significance for each treatment group based on a reference group composed of a combination of the negative control group and all groups treated with chromate-containing materials, except those treated with calcium or strontium chromate

(iv) *Intrapleural administration*

*Rat*: A number of chromium[VI] compounds [doses unspecified] administered to rats [sex, age and strain unspecified] by intrapleural implantation in experiments lasting 27 months gave the following numbers of implantation-site tumours [type unspecified]: strontium chromate, 17/28 (nine alive at one year); barium chromate, 1/31 (30 alive at one year); lead chromate, 3/34 (32 alive at one year); zinc yellow [unspecified composition], 22/33 (11 alive at one year); calcium chromate, 20/32 (none alive at one year); sintered calcium chromate, 17/33 (nine alive at one year, one alive at 21 months); and sodium dichromate, 0/26 (20 alive at one year, none alive at 18 months). None of 34 control rats had tumours (30 alive at one year, five alive at two years) (Hueper, 1961).

Groups of 20 male and 19 female Bethesda Black [NIH Black] rats, three months of age, received 16 monthly intrapleural injections of 2 mg sodium dichromate in gelatin and were observed for up to two years. One adenocarcinoma of the lung was observed; no tumour at the injection site was observed in 60 control rats treated with gelatin solution. After intrapleural implantation of 12.5 mg calcium chromate in a gelatin capsule to 14 rats, eight developed malignant tumours [type unspecified] at the site of implantation after two years compared with none in 35 controls (Hueper & Payne, 1962).

(v) *Subcutaneous administration*

*Mouse*: A group of 26 female and 26 male C57Bl mice received calcium chromate or sintered calcium chromate (prepared by heating calcium chromate with less than 1% impurities to about 1100°C for about 1 h) by subcutaneous injection of 10 mg chromium compound in tricaprylin, and the animals were observed for 18-26 months. One sarcoma was observed in 13 mice treated with calcium chromate that lived longer than six months, but none was seen at the injection site in the other treated groups or in vehicle controls. Histologically, the injection-site tumours were spindle-cell sarcomas or fibrosarcomas (Payne, 1960a).

*Rat*: Groups of 40 male and female Sprague-Dawley rats, 13 weeks of age, received a single subcutaneous injection of 30 mg lead chromate (chromium yellow) or basic lead chromate (chromium orange) in water. Sarcomas (rhabdomyosarcomas and fibrosarcomas) developed at the injection site in 26/40 and 27/40 animals, respectively, within 117-150 weeks. No local tumour occurred in 60 vehicle-control rats, and a single local sarcoma occurred in 80 control rats that received comparable subcutaneous injections of iron yellow or iron red (Maltoni, 1974, 1976; Maltoni *et al.*, 1982).

Groups of 20 male and 20 female Sprague-Dawley rats, 13 weeks of age, received single subcutaneous injections of 30 mg zinc yellow (basic zinc chromate) at 20% or 40% $CrO_3$ in 1 ml saline. Local sarcomas (rhabdomyosarcomas and fibrosarcomas) were seen in 6/40 and 7/40 rats given 20% and 40% $CrO_3$ at 110 and 137 weeks, respectively. No local tumour had occurred in the 40 control animals by 136 weeks (Maltoni et al., 1982).

A further group of 20 male and 20 female Sprague-Dawley rats received single subcutaneous injections of 30 mg molybdenum orange (described as a mixture of lead chromate, sulfate and molybdate) in 1 ml saline. At termination of the study at 117 weeks, 36/40 rats had injection-site sarcomas; no local tumour occurred in 45 male and 15 female untreated controls (Maltoni, 1974; Maltoni et al., 1982).

### (vi)  *Intramuscular administration*

*Mouse*:  Groups of 26 female and 26 male C57Bl mice [age unspecified] received calcium chromate or sintered calcium chromate (prepared by heating calcium chromate with less than 1% impurities to about 1100°C for about 1 h) by intramuscular implantation of 10 mg of the chromium compound mixed with 20 mg sheep fat. Animals were observed for a total of 14 months. Nine implantation-site sarcomas were observed among 46 mice given sintered calcium chromate that lived longer than six months; one sarcoma was observed in 50 mice given non-sintered calcium chromate; and no sarcoma was found among 50 control mice that lived six months or more (Payne, 1960a).

A group of 25 female NIH-Swiss weanling mice was given intramuscular injections of 3 mg lead chromate in trioctanoin every four months. Two lymphomas were seen within 16 months and three lung adenocarcinomas within 24 months among 17 mice that were necropsied. The incidences of these tumours were 1/15 and 1/15 in untreated control mice and 2/22 and 1/22 among vehicle-injected control mice (Furst et al., 1976).

*Rat*:  Groups of 35 Bethesda Black [NIH Black] male and female rats, approximately three months of age, received an intramuscular implantation of pellets containing 25 mg calcium chromate (99% pure), 25 mg sintered calcium chromate or 25 mg sintered chromium trioxide, all in 50 mg sheep fat. Sarcomas (spindle-cell sarcomas and fibrosarcomas) at the implantation site were seen after 12-14 months in 8/35 rats given calcium chromate, 8/35 given sintered calcium chromate and 15/35 given sintered chromium trioxide. No local tumour was seen in 35 controls or in groups of 20 males and 15 females given implants of 25 mg barium chromate (99% pure) in 50 mg sheep fat (Hueper & Payne, 1959). [The Working Group noted that sintered chromium trioxide at 1100°C would contain appreciable amounts of chromic chromate; it also noted the short duration of the experiment.]

In groups of 32-34 rats [sex, strain and age unspecified] that received intramuscular implantation of various chromium compounds in sheep fat [doses unspecified], the following incidences of implantation-site tumours [type unspecified] were recorded after 27 months: calcium chromate, 9/32 (22 alive at one year, seven alive at two years); sodium dichromate, 0/33 (25 alive at one year, 16 alive at 18 months); sintered calcium chromate, 12/34 (22 alive at one year, none alive at two years); strontium chromate, 15/33 (20 alive at one year); barium chromate, 0/34 (30 alive at one year); lead chromate, 1/33 (28 alive at one year); and zinc yellow [composition unspecified], 16/34 (22 alive at one year). None of 32 control rats given implants of sheep fat alone developed local tumours (30 alive at one year, six alive at two years) (Hueper, 1961).

A group of 20 male and 19 female Bethesda Black [NIH Black] rats, three months of age, was given 16 intramuscular injections of 2 mg sodium dichromate in gelatin at monthly intervals and observed for two years (17 alive at 16 months). No tumour appeared at the injection site. After intramuscular implantation of 12.5 mg calcium chromate in a gelatin capsule to eight rats, four malignant tumours developed at the implantation site in animals observed for two years; compared with none in 35 controls (Hueper & Payne, 1962).

Each of a group of 24 male CB stock rats, five to six weeks of age, was given an intramuscular injection of calcium chromate in arachis oil (total dose, 19 mg) once a week for 20 weeks. Eighteen developed spindle-cell or pleomorphic-cell sarcomas at the injection site, none of which metastasized [$p < 0.01$]. The mean time to tumour appearance was 323 days (duration of experiment, 440 days). No tumour developed in 15 control rats given arachis oil only that were alive at 150 days (Roe & Carter, 1969).

Groups of 25 male and 25 female weanling Fischer-344 rats received intramuscular injections of 8 mg lead chromate suspended in trioctanoin once a month for nine months or 4 mg calcium chromate in the same vehicle once a month for 12 months. Lead chromate induced 14 fibrosarcomas and 17 rhabdomyosarcomas at the site of injection in 31/47 rats. In addition, renal carcinomas were observed in 3/23 male rats at 24 months. Calcium chromate induced tumours (three fibrosarcomas, two rhabdomyosarcomas) in 5/45 animals. No such tumour appeared in a group of 22 controls injected with the vehicle (Furst et al., 1976). [The Working Group noted that the renal tumours might be attributable to the lead content of the compound (IARC, 1980b)].

(d)   *Other chromium compounds*

(i)   *Inhalation*

*Mouse*: Groups of mice, eight to ten weeks of age, were exposed in dust chambers for 4 h per day on five days per week to a mixed chromium dust[1] containing 1-2 mg/m³ soluble chromium (as chromium trioxide) until they died or were killed (total dose of chromium trioxide inhaled, 272-1330 mg-h): 127 Swiss females were exposed for up to 58 weeks, ten Swiss males and 11 Swiss females for up to 39 weeks, 34 strain A females for 16 weeks, 45 strain A females for 24 weeks, 110 strain A females for 38 weeks, 52 strain A males for 46 weeks, 50 C57Bl males for 42 weeks and 61 C57Bl females for 41 weeks. No lung carcinoma was observed, and the incidence of lung adenomas did not significantly exceed that in control mice in any strain. The experiment lasted for up to 101 weeks (Baetjer *et al.*, 1959b). [The Working Group noted the low doses and the small numbers of animals used.]

*Rat*: A group of 78 Wistar rats [sex unspecified], six to eight weeks of age, was exposed by inhalation to a mixed chromium dust[1] for 4-5 h per day on four days a week for life, to give an average chromium trioxide concentration of 3-4 mg/m³. No significant difference in tumour incidence was observed between treated and control groups. A group of 38 Sherman rats [sex unspecified], six to eight weeks of age, received 16 monthly intratracheal injections of 0.1 ml of a suspension consisting of 0.5% mixed chromium dust plus 0.6% potassium dichromate, equivalent to 0.07 mg chromium/dose. No lung tumour occurred (Steffee & Baetjer, 1965).

A group of 20 male TNO-W74 Wistar rats, six weeks of age, was exposed by inhalation to 100 µg/m³ pyrolysed Cr[VI]/Cr[III] oxides (3:2; average mass median diameter, 0.39 µm) for 22-23 h per day on seven days a week for 18 months. The rats were then held for a further 12 months. A control group consisted of 40 untreated male rats. Survival was over 90% at 24 months and at 30 months was 50% and 42% in treated and controls, respectively. A single lung adenoma was found in the treated group and none in the controls (Glaser *et al.*, 1986). [The Working Group noted the small number of animals used].

---

[1]The Working Group noted that, in the publications of Baetjer *et al.*, the mixed chromium dust used was prepared by grinding to a fine powder the roast that is produced when chromite ore is heated at a high temperature with sodium carbonate and calcium hydroxide. The mixture contained approximately 12% chromium, consisting of water-soluble sodium chromate (chromium[VI]), water-insoluble but acid-soluble chromium[VI] and [III] chemicals and some unchanged chromite ore; to this mixture was added 1% potassium bichhromate. The final analysis of the dust gave 13.7% chromium trioxide and 6.9% chromic oxide. The Working Group commented that this roasted mixture, known as 'frit', is the product of the first stage of the bichromate production process prior to leaching. This first-stage process may or may not involve the addition of calcium hydroxide or limestone.

Groups of 120 male and 120 female Sprague-Dawley rats, six to seven weeks of age, were exposed by inhalation to 0.5 mg/m³ 'unstabilized', 0.5 or 25 mg/m³ 'stabilized' chromium[IV] dioxide particles (mass median aerodynamic diameter, 2.6-2.8 μm) for 6 h a day on five days per week for two years. Ten rats from each group were killed at 12 months for interim observation. Between 101 and 108 lungs were examined for each group exposed up to 24 months. [The Working Group noted that no survival data were reported.] In the 25 mg/m³ stabilized group, there was treatment-related alveolar bronchiolization. In addition, lung adenomas occurred in 1/106 males and 1/108 females in this group, and keratin cysts and 'cystic keratinized squamous-cell carcinomas' in 108 females. The authors considered that the cystic keratinized squamous-cell carcinomas were related to a dust reaction alone and were not true malignant tumours (Lee *et al.*, 1988). [The Working Group noted that similar lesions of the lung were described in a previous *IARC Monograph* on titanium dioxide (IARC, 1989).]

*Guinea-pig*: Three-month-old guinea-pigs [sex unspecified] were exposed by inhalation to a combination of mixed chromium dust[1] for 4-5 h per day on four days per week for lifespan (average dose, 3-4 mg/m³ chromic trioxide); 3/50 developed pulmonary adenomas. No pulmonary adenoma occurred in 44 controls (Steffee & Baetjer, 1965).

*Rabbit*: Eight rabbits [sex and strain unspecified], four months of age, were exposed by inhalation for 4-5 h per day on four days per week for up to 50 months to mixed chromium dust[1] according to a complex dosage schedule (average dose, 3-4 mg/m³ chromium trioxide). No pulmonary tumour was seen (Steffee & Baetjer, 1965).

### (ii) *Intratracheal instillation*

*Mouse:* Five to six intratracheal instillations of a mixed chromium dust[1], equivalent to 0.04 mg chromium trioxide per instillation, were given either to 14 and 20 Swiss males, which were then observed for 26 and 32 weeks, respectively; to 45 and 110 Swiss females, observed for up to 32 and 48 weeks, respectively; to 28, 52, 77 and 48 strain A females observed for up to 31, 37, 43 and 52 weeks respectively; to 17 strain A males observed for up to 52 weeks; or to 48 C57Bl males and 47 C57Bl females observed for up to 32 weeks. Treated animals developed no more lung tumours than did untreated control animals (Baetjer *et al.*, 1959b).

*Guinea–pig:* Groups of 19 guinea–pigs [sex unspecified], three months old, were given six intratracheal instillations of 0.3 ml of a 1% suspension in saline of a mixed chromium dust[1] or a pulverized residue dust (roast material from which solu-

---

[1]See footnote on p. 130

ble chromates had been leached) at intervals of three months. The animals were observed until they died. No pulmonary carcinoma developed in any experimental group or in 18 vehicle controls (Steffee & Baetjer, 1965).

*Rabbit:* Groups of rabbits received three to five intratracheal injections of 1 ml of a 1% suspension in saline of mixed chromium dust (ten rabbits) or 'pulverized residue dust' (roast material from which soluble chromates had been leached) (seven rabbits) at intervals of three months. No pulmonary tumour was seen in either group (Steffee & Baetjer, 1965).

### (iii)    *Intrabronchial administration*

*Rat:* A group of 100 rats [strain, sex and age unspecified] received intrabronchial implants of stainless-steel mesh pellets (5 × 1 mm) loaded with 3-5 mg of a 50:50 mixture of a chromate process residue (an intermediate process residue from the bichromate-producing industry, which may have contained up to 3% calcium) with a cholesterol binder. Animals were observed up to 136 weeks. One squamous-cell carcinoma was observed after 594 days in 1/93 rats that lived more than 150 days. No lung tumour was seen in 24 cholesterol binder-treated controls (Laskin *et al.*, 1970).

In a study using intrabronchial implantation, described previously (p. 125), no bronchial tumour was seen in five groups of 100 Porton-Wistar rats that received pellets loaded with five residues from bichromate production: Bolton high lime residue, residue after alumina precipitation, residue from slurry tank (free of soluble chromium), residue from vanadium filter and residue from slurry disposal tank. All five materials contained less than 5% hexavalent chromium (Levy & Venitt, 1986; Levy *et al.*, 1986).

In a second study using the technique described above, but examining bichromate production residues containing lime, the following incidences of squamous-cell carcinomas of the left lung were seen: high lime residue from old tip (TSS 643D; $Cr_2O_3$, 2.4%; $CaCrO_4$, 2.7%; $Na_2CrO_4$, 1.0%), 1/99; kiln frit (TSS 643B, with 2% limestone added to feedmix; $Cr_2O_3$, 13.0%; $Na_2CrO_4$, 29.0%), 2/100; and recycled residue (TSS 643C, with 2% limestone added to feedmix; $Cr_2O_3$, 20.4%; $Na_2CrO_4$, 2.2%), 0/100 (Levy *et al.*, 1986).

### (iv)    *Intrapleural administration*

*Mouse:* Groups of 30 male and 25 female strain A mice, eight to ten weeks of age, were given four intrapleural injections of 0.05 ml of a 2 or 4% suspension of mixed chromium dust[1] in olive oil at intervals of four to six weeks. The incidence of

---

[1]See footnote on p. 130.

lung tumours during an observation period of 38 weeks was similar to that in a control group of 23 males and 18 females (Baetjer *et al.*, 1959b).

*Rat*: A group of 25 male Bethesda Black [NIH Black] rats, three months of age, received sheep-fat cubes containign 25 mg roasted chromite ore implanted into the pleural cavity. Squamous-cell carcinomas of the lungs were observed in 2/24 rats that survived 19-24 months. One lung adenoma occurred in the 4/15 female controls given an implant of sheep fat that survived this period (Hueper, 1958). [The Working Group noted that the roasted chromite ore tested in this study was a process-derived material that contained unspeciated chromium compounds formed during oxidative heating of a chromium ore that had been subjected to alkaline leaching. Hueper sometimes referred to this material as 'chromate' and sometimes as 'chromite'.]

Of a group of 32 rats [age, sex and strain unspecified] that received intrapleural implantations of chromite roast residue [amount unspecified], 5/32 (28 alive at one year, ten alive at 24 months) developed malignant tumours at the implantation site. In a group of 34 rats given chromic chromate [precise chemical nature unspecified], 25 tumours developed at the implantation site. None of 34 control rats had a tumour (30 alive at one year, five alive at 24 months) (Hueper, 1961).

When 25 mg roasted chromite ore in 50 mg sheep fat (equivalent to 2 mg Cr) were implanted intrapleurally into 15 male and 20 female Bethesda Black rats [age unspecified], implantation-site sarcomas occurred in three rats over 17 months. No tumour was seen in 35 rats injected intrapleurally with the sheep-fat vehicle only (Payne, 1960b)

### (v)  *Intramuscular administration*

*Mouse*: A group of 26 male and 26 female C57Bl mice [age unspecified] was given intramuscular implantations of 10 mg roasted chromite ore (equivalent to 0.79 mg chromium) in sheep fat. None developed tumours at the implantation site within 22 months. No local tumour developed in 52 controls treated with sheep fat alone (Payne, 1960b). [The Working Group noted that no data on survival were reported.]

*Rat*: A group of 31 female Bethesda Black [NIH Black] rats, approximately three months old, was given intramuscular implants of small cubes composed of 25 mg roasted chromite ore suspended in 75 mg sheep fat. Three rats developed fibrosarcomas at the site of implantation within 24 months. No implantation-site tumour occurred in 15 vehicle-treated controls (Hueper, 1958).

In a group of 34 rats [age, sex and strain unspecified] that received intramuscular implantations of chromite roast residue, 1/34 (32 alive at one year, two alive at 27 months) developed a malignant tumour at the injection site [type unspecified]. In a further group of 22 rats given intramuscular implantations of chromic chromate [precise chemical nature unspecified], 24 local tumours were observed after 24 months. None of 32 controls given implants of sheep fat alone developed local tumours (30 alive at one year, six alive at 24 months) (Hueper, 1961).

(vi)   *Injections into subcutaneously implanted tracheal grafts*

*Rat*: Seventy-two tracheal rings excised from female Wistar-Lewis rats were implanted subcutaneously into the backs of 13 rats of the same strain (weighing 100-150 g at the start of the experiment). Two weeks later, the grafts were filled by injection with 0.05 ml of an agar suspension of 2.5 mg chromium carbonyl with or without 2.5 mg benzo[*a*]pyrene. Biopsies were performed at intervals. Ten squamous-cell carcinomas developed in 24 tracheas that received the mixture, and two carcinomas developed in 22 tracheas treated with chromium carbonyl alone. Three of the tracheal carcinomas produced by the mixture metastasized within nine months. The time to appearance of the tumours was four to 14 months. No tumour occurred in the four trachea that received the vehicle only (Lane & Mass, 1977).

The experiments described in section 3.1 are summarized in Table 22, by compound.

**Table 22. Summary of studies used to evaluate the carcinogenicity to experimental animals of metallic chromium and chromium compounds**

| Compound | Route | Species (No. at start) | Tumour incidence[a] | Reference |
|---|---|---|---|---|
| *Metallic chromium* | | | | |
| Chromium | Intratracheal | Rat (53) | 0/12 | Mukubo (1978) |
| Chromium | Intrapleural | Mouse (50) | 0/50 | Hueper (1955) |
| Chromium | Intrapleural | Rat/2 groups (25; 25) | A few tumours, also in controls | Hueper (1955) |
| Chromium | Intramuscular | Rat (24) | 0/22 local tumour | Sunderman et al. (1974) |
| Chromium | Intramuscular | Rat (38) | 0/38 local tumour | Sunderman et al. (1980) |
| Chromium | Intramuscular | Rat (50) | 1/50 *vs* 0/50 | Furst (1971) |
| Chromium | Intraperitoneal | Mouse (50) | 0/50 local tumour | Hueper (1955) |
| Chromium | Intraperitoneal | Rat (25) | 5/25 (mixed) | Hueper (1955) |
| Chromium | Intravenous | Mouse (25) | 0/25 | Hueper (1955) |
| Chromium | Intravenous | Rat (25) | 6/25 (mixed) | Hueper (1955) |
| Chromium | Intravenous | Rabbit (8) | 1/3 *vs* 0/4 | Hueper (1955) |
| Chromium | Intrafemoral | Rat/2 groups (25; 25) | 0/25; 1/25 local tumour | Hueper (1955) |

**Table 22 (contd)**

| Compound | Route | Species (No. at start) | Tumour incidence[a] | Reference |
|---|---|---|---|---|
| *Chromium[III] compounds* | | | | |
| Chromic acetate | Drinking-water | Mouse (108) | M 6/39 vs 11/44 F 9/29 vs 22/60 | Schroeder et al. (1964) |
| Chromic acetate | Drinking-water | Rat (96) | M 16/39 vs 9/35 F 18/35 vs 15/35 | Schroeder et al. (1965) |
| Chromic acetate | Intrapleural | Rat (34) | 1/34 vs 0/34 | Hueper (1961) |
| Chromic acetate | Intrapleural | Rat | 0/42 local tumour | Hueper & Payne (1962) |
| Chromic acetate | Intramuscular | Rat (34) | 1/34 vs 0/32 local tumour | Hueper (1961) |
| Chromic acetate | Intramuscular | Rat (35) | 1/35 local tumour | Hueper & Payne (1962) |
| Chromic oxide | Oral (in bread) | Rat (3 groups of 60) | As controls | Ivankovic & Preussman (1975) |
| Chromic oxide | Intratracheal | Rat (?) | Malignant lung tumours 7/34 (50 mg) and 6/18 (20 mg) | Dvizhkov & Fedorova (1967) |
| Chromic oxide | Intrabronchial | Rat (98) | 0/98 vs 0/24 | Laskin et al. (1970) |
| Chromic oxide | Intrabronchial | Rat (100) | 0/100 vs reference[b] | Levy & Venitt (1986) |
| Chromic oxide | Intraperitoneal | Rat (?) | Lung sarcomas 4/20 | Dvizhkov & Fedorova (1967) |
| Chromic chloride hexahydrate | Intrabronchial | Rat (100) | 0/100 vs reference[b] | Levy & Venitt (1986) |
| Chromic chloride | Drinking-water | Rat (15) | 0/15 | Kurokawa et al. (1985) |
| Chrome tan | Intrabronchial | Rat (100) | 0/100 vs reference[b] | Levy & Venitt (1986) |
| Chromic sulfate | Intraperitoneal | Mouse (10 per group; 3 dose levels) | As controls | Stoner et al. (1976) |
| Chromite | Intrabronchial | Rat (100) | 0/100 vs reference[b] | Levy & Venitt (1986) |

**Table 22 (contd)**

| Compound | Route | Species (No. at start) | Tumour incidence[a] | Reference |
|---|---|---|---|---|
| Chromite (high silica chrome ore TSS 645) | Intrabronchial | Rat | 0/99 vs reference[b] | Levy et al. (1986) |
| Chromite | Intrapleural | Mouse (25) | 0/25 | Davis (1972) |
| Chromite | Intrapleural | Rat (25) | 1/25 vs 0/25 | Hueper (1955) |
| Chromite | Intravenous | Mouse (50) | As controls | Shimkin & Leiter (1940) |
| Chromite | Intravenous | Rabbit (6) | 0/6 | Hueper (1955) |
| Chromite | Intrafemoral | Rat (25) | 0/25 local tumour | Hueper (1955) |
| *Chromium[VI] compounds* | | | | |
| Calcium chromate | Inhalation | Mouse (136) | Lung adenomas M 6/136 vs 3/136 F 8/136 vs 2/136 | Nettesheim et al. (1971) |
| Calcium chromate | Intrabronchial | Rat (100) | Bronchial carcinomas 8/100 vs 0/24 (NS) | Laskin et al. (1970) |
| Calcium chromate | Intrabronchial | Rat (100) | Squamous-cell carcinomas 8/84 vs reference[b] $p < 0.05$ | Levy & Venitt (1986) |
| Calcium chromate | Intrabronchial | Rat (100) | Bronchial carcinomas 25/100 ($p < 0.01$) positive control | Levy et al. (1986) |
| Calcium chromate | Intratracheal | Rat (80) | Lung: 5 x weekly; 0.25 mg/kg 6/80 vs 0/80 ($p < 0.01$) Lung: 1 x weekly; 1.25 mg/kg 13/80 vs 0/80[c] ($p < 0.01$) | Steinhoff et al. (1986) |
| Calcium chromate | Intratracheal | Hamster (35) | No lung tumour | Reuzel et al. (1986) |
| Calcium chromate | Intramuscular | Mouse (52) | 1/50 vs 0/50 local tumour (NS) | Payne (1960a) |
| Calcium chromate sintered | Intramuscular | Mouse (52) | 9/46 vs 0/50 local tumours [$p < 0.01$)] | Payne (1960a) |
| Calcium chromate | Intramuscular | Rat | 9/32 vs 0.32 local tumours [$p < 0.01$] | Hueper (1961) |
| Calcium chromate sintered | Intramuscular | Rat | 12/34 vs 0/32 local tumours [$p < 0.01$] | Hueper (1961) |

**Table 22 (contd)**

| Compound | Route | Species (No. at start) | Tumour incidence[a] | Reference |
|---|---|---|---|---|
| Calcium chromate | Intramuscular | Rat (50) | 5/45 vs 0/22 local tumours (NS) | Furst et al. (1976) |
| Calcium chromate | Intramuscular | Rat (8) | 4/8 vs 0/35 local tumours | Hueper & Payne (1962) |
| Calcium chromate | Intramuscular | Rat (24) | 18/24 vs 0/15 local tumours [$p < 0.01$] | Roe & Carter (1969) |
| Calcium chromate | Intramuscular | Rat (35) | 8/35 vs 0/35 [$p < 0.01$] | Hueper & Payne (1959) |
| Calcium chromate sintered | Intramuscular | Rat (35) | 8/35 vs 0/35 [$p < 0.01$] | Hueper & Payne (1959) |
| Calcium chromate | Intraperitoneal | Rat (14) | 8/14 vs 0/35 local tumours | Hueper & Payne (1962) |
| Calcium chromate | Intraperitoneal | Rat (?) | 20/32 vs 0/34 [$p < 0.01$] | Hueper (1961) |
| Calcium chromate sintered | Intraperitoneal | Rat (?) | 17/33 vs 0/34 [$p < 0.01$] | Hueper (1961) |
| Calcium chromate | Subcutanous | Mouse (52) | 1/13 vs 0/52 (NS) | Payne (1960a) |
| Calcium chromate sintered | Subcutaneous | Mouse (52) | 0/31 vs 0/52 | Payne (1960a) |
| Chromic acid (chromium trioxide) | Inhalation | Mouse (50) | Lung adenomas, 10-14 months: 3/14 vs 0/10 (NS) Adenomas, 15-18 months: 1/19 vs 2/10 Adenocarcinoma: 2/19 vs 0/10 (NS) | Adachi et al. (1986) |
| Chromic acid (chromium trioxide) | Inhalation | Mouse (43) | Nasal papilloma, 18 months: 6/20 vs 0/20 ($p < 0.05$); 1/20 adenoma of lung | Adachi (1987) |
| Chromic acid (chromium trioxide) | Intrabronchial | Rat (100) | Squamous-cell carcinoma: vs reference[b] (NS) | Levy & Venitt (1986) |
| Chromic acid (chromium trioxide) | Intrabronchial | Rat (100) | Bronchial carcinoma: 2/100 vs 0/100 (NS) | Levy et al. (1986) |
| Chromic acid (chromium trioxide) | Intrabronchial | Rat (100) | Lung: 0/100 vs 0/24 | Laskin et al. (1970) |
| Chromic oxide sintered | Intramuscular | Rat (35) | 15/35 local tumours | Hueper & Payne (1959) |

**Table 22 (contd)**

| Compound | Route | Species (No. at start) | Tumour incidence[a] | Reference |
|---|---|---|---|---|
| Sodium dichromate | Inhalation | Rat (20 per group) | Lung tumours: controls, 0/37 25 μg, 0/18 50 μg, 0/18 100 μg, 3/19 (2 adenomas) 1 adenocarcinoma + 1 squamous-cell carcinoma of pharynx | Glaser *et al.* (1986) |
| Sodium dichromate | Intrabronchial | Rat (100) | 0/89 *vs* reference[b] | Levy & Venitt (1986) |
| Sodium dichromate | Intrabronchial | Rat (100) | Bronchial carcinoma: 1/100 *vs* 0/100 (NS) | Levy *et al.* (1986) |
| Sodium dichromate | Intratracheal | Rat (80) | 5 × weekly: 0/80 in all groups 1 × weekly: control, 0/80; 0.05 mg/kg, 0/80; 0.25 mg/kg, 1/80; 1.25 mg/kg, 14/80[c] ($p < 0.01$) | Steinhoff *et al.* (1986) |
| Sodium dichromate | Intrapleural | Rat (39) | Lung adenocarcinoma: 1/34 | Hueper & Payne (1962) |
| Sodium dichromate | Intrapleural | Rat (?) | 0/26 *vs* 0/34 local tumour | Hueper (1961) |
| Sodium dichromate | Intramuscular | Rat (39) | 0/39 local tumour | Hueper & Payne (1962) |
| Sodium dichromate | Intramuscular | Rat | 0/33 *vs* 0/32 local tumour | Hueper (1961) |
| Sodium chromate | Intrabronchial | Rat (100) | Lung: 0/89 *vs* reference[b] | Levy & Venitt (1986) |
| Bichromate residue (vanadium solids) | Intrabronchial | Rat (100) | Bronchial carcinoma: 1/100 *vs* reference[b] | Levy *et al.* (1986) |
| *Zinc chromates* | | | | |
| Basic potassium zinc chromate | Intratracheal | Mouse (62) | Pulmonary adenomas: 31/62 *vs* 7/18 | Steffee & Baetjer (1965) |
| Basic potassium zinc chromate | Intratracheal | Guinea-pig (21) | Pulmonary adenomas: 1/21 *vs* 0/18 | Steffee & Baetjer (1965) |

**Table 22 (contd)**

| Compound | Route | Species (No. at start) | Tumour incidence[a] | Reference |
|---|---|---|---|---|
| Basic potassium zinc chromate | Intratracheal | Rabbit (7) | 0/7 $vs$ 0/5 | Steffee & Baetjer (1965) |
| Zinc potassium chromate | Intrabronchial | Rat (100) | Squamous-cell carcinoma: 3/61 $vs$ reference ($p < 0.05$) | Levy & Venitt (1986) |
| Zinc chromate (IW) | Intrabronchial | Rat (100) | Lung: 5/100 $vs$ reference[b] [$p = 0.004$] | Levy et al. (1986) |
| Zinc chromate (Norge) | Intrabronchial | Rat (100) | 3/100 $vs$ reference[b] [$p = 0.068$] NS according to authors | Levy et al. (1986) |
| Zinc tetroxychromate | Intrabronchial | Rat (100) | 1/100 $vs$ reference[b] (NS) | Levy et al. (1986) |
| Zinc yellow | Intrapleural | Rat | 22/33 $vs$ 0/34 | Hueper (1961) |
| Zinc yellow | Subcutaneous | Rat (40) | Local tumours: control, 0/40 20% $CrO_3$, 6/40 40% $CrO_3$, 7/40 | Maltoni et al. (1982) |
| Zinc yellow | Intramuscular | Rat | 16/34 $vs$ 0/32 | Hueper (1961) |
| *Lead chromates* | | | | |
| Lead chromate | Intrabronchial | Rat (100) | Bronchial carcinoma: 1/98 $vs$ 0/100 (NS) | Levy et al. (1986) |
| Primrose chrome yellow | Intrabronchial | Rat (100) | 1/100 $vs$ reference[b] (NS) | Levy et al. (1986) |
| Molybdate chrome orange | Intrabronchial | Rat (100) | 0/100 | Levy et al. (1986) |
| Molybdenum orange | Subcutaneous | Rat (40) | 36/40 $vs$ 0/60 | Maltoni (1974); Maltoni et al. (1982) |
| Light chrome yellow | Intrabronchial | Rat (100) | 0/100 | Levy et al. (1986) |
| Supra LC chrome yellow | Intrabronchial | Rat (100) | 1/100 $vs$ reference[b] (NS) | Levy et al. (1986) |
| Medium chrome yellow | Intrabronchial | Rat (100) | 1/100 $vs$ reference[b] | Levy et al. (1986) |
| Silica encapsulated | Intrabronchial | Rat (100) | 0/100 (NS) | Levy et al. (1986) |
| Lead chromate | Intratracheal | Guinea-pig (13) | 0/13 | Steffee & Baetjer (1965) |

**Table 22 (contd)**

| Compound | Route | Species (No. at start) | Tumour incidence[a] | Reference |
|---|---|---|---|---|
| Lead chromate | Intrapleural | Rat | 3/34 vs 0/34 | Hueper (1961) |
| Lead chromate | Intramuscular | Mouse (25) | Lymphoma, lung adenocarcinoma: not different from controls | Furst et al. (1976) |
| Lead chromate | Subcutaneous | Rat (40) | 26/40 vs 0/60 and 1/80 local tumours | Maltoni (1974, 1976); Maltoni et al. (1982) |
| Basic lead chromate | Subcutaneous | Rat (40) | 27/40 vs 0/60 and 1/80 local tumours | Maltoni (1974, 1976); Maltoni et al. (1982) |
| Lead chromate | Intramuscular | Rat (50) | 31/47 vs 0/22 local tumours and 3/23 M vs 0/22 renal carcinomas | Furst et al. (1976) |
| Lead chromate | Intramuscular | Rat | 1/33 vs 0/32 local tumour | Hueper (1961) |
| Barium chromate | Intrabronchial | Rat (101) | 0/101 | Levy et al. (1986) |
| Barium chromate | Intrapleural | Rat (?) | 1/31 vs 0/34 | Hueper (1961) |
| Barium chromate | Intramuscular | Rat (?) | 0/34 vs 0/32 local tumour | Hueper (1961) |
| Barium chromate | Intramuscular | Rat (35) | 0/35 | Hueper & Payne (1959) |
| Strontium chromate | Intrabronchial | Rat (100) | Bronchial carcinoma: 43/99 vs reference[b] | Levy et al. (1986) |
| Strontium chromate | Intrabronchial | Rat (100) | Bronchial carcinoma: 64/99 vs reference[b] | Levy et al. (1986) |
| Strontium chromate | Intrapleural | Rat (?) | 17/28 vs 0/34 | Hueper (1961) |
| Strontium chromate | Intramuscular | Rat | 15/33 vs 0/32 local tumour | Hueper (1961) |

*Other chromium compounds and chromium-containing mixtures*

| | | | | |
|---|---|---|---|---|
| Mixed chromium dust | Inhalation | Mouse (500) | As controls | Baetjer et al. (1959b) |
| Mixed chromium dust | Inhalation | Rat (78) | As controls | Steffee & Baetjer (1965) |

**Table 22 (contd)**

| Compound | Route | Species (No. at start) | Tumour incidence[a] | Reference |
|---|---|---|---|---|
| Mixed chromium dust | Inhalation | Guinea-pig (50) | Pulmonary adenomas: 3/50 *vs* 0/44 | Steffee & Baetjer (1965) |
| Mixed chromium dust | Inhalation | Rabbit (8) | 0/8 local tumour | Steffee & Baetjer (1965) |
| Mixed chromium dust | Intratracheal | Mouse (506) | As controls | Baetjer *et al.* (1959b) |
| Mixed chromium dust | Intratracheal | Guinea-pig (19) | 0/19 *vs* 0/18 | Steffee & Baetjer (1965) |
| Mixed chromium dust plus $K_2Cr_2O_4$ | Intratracheal | Rat (38) | 0/38 local tumour | Steffee & Baetjer (1965) |
| Mixed chromium dust | Intratracheal | Rabbit (10) | 0/10 local tumour | Steffee & Baetjer (1965) |
| Mixed chromium dust | Intrapleural | Mouse (55) | As controls | Baetjer *et al.* (1959b) |
| Residue dust | Intratracheal | Guinea-pig (19) | 0/19 *vs* 0/18 | Steffee & Baetjer (1965) |
| Residue dust | Intratracheal | Rabbit (7) | 0/7 local tumour | Steffee & Baetjer (1965) |
| Roasted chromite ore | Intrapleural | Rat (25) | Bronchial carcinoma: 2/24 | Hueper (1958) |
| Roasted chromite ore | Intrapleural | Rat (35) | 3/35 *vs* 0/35 | Payne (1960b) |
| Roasted chromite ore | Intramuscular | Mouse (52) | 0/52 local tumour | Payne (1960b) |
| Roasted chromite ore | Intramuscular | Rat (31) | 3/31 *vs* 0/15 | Hueper (1958) |
| Roasted chromite residue | Intrapleural | Rat (32) | 5/32 *vs* 0/34 | Hueper (1961) |
| Roasted chromite residue | Intramuscular | Rat (34) | 1/34 vs 0/32 | Hueper (1961) |
| Chromate process residue | Intrabronchial | Rat (100) | 1/93 *vs* 0/24 | Laskin *et al.* (1970) |

**Table 22 (contd)**

| Compound | Route | Species (No. at start) | Tumour incidence[a] | Reference |
|---|---|---|---|---|
| Bichromate production residues (all with <5% Cr[VI]) | Intrabronchial | | | Levy & Venitt (1986); Levy et al. (1986) |
|   Bolton high lime residue | | Rat (100) | 0/100 | |
|   Alumina precipitation residue | | Rat (100) | 0/100 | |
|   Slurry tank residue | | Rat (100) | 0/100 | |
|   Vanadium filter residue | | Rat (100) | 0/100 | |
|   Slurry disposal residue tank | | Rat (100) | 0/100 | |
| Bichromate production residues with lime | | | | |
|   High lime residue (TSS 643D) | Intrabronchial | Rat (99) | Bronchial carcinoma: 1/99 (NS) | Levy et al. (1986) |
|   Kiln frit (CTSS 643B) +2% limestone | Intrabronchial | Rat (100) | 2/100 (NS) | Levy et al. (1986) |
|   Recycled residue (CTSS 643C) +2% limestone | Intrabronchial | Rat (100) | 0/100 | Levy et al. (1986) |
| Pyrolysed Cr[VI]/ Cr[III] 3:2 oxide | Inhalation | Rat (20) | Lung adenoma: 1/20 vs 0/40 | Glaser et al. (1986) |
| Chromium[IV] dioxide | Inhalation | Rat | | |
|   Unstabilized (0.5 mg/m³) | | (240) | 0/240 vs 0/240 | Lee et al. (1988) |
|   Stabilized (0.5 and 25 mg/m³) | | (480) | 2/210 adenomas 6/108 keratin cysts 2/108 cystic keratin squamous lesions | |

[a]NS, not significant

[b]p-Value calculated by comparing the incidence of bronchial carcinomas in each test group with that in a reference group comprising the two negative control groups and all the groups receiving chromium-containing materials

[c]No. of tumour-bearing animals

## 3.2 Other relevant data in experimental systems

### (a) Absorption, distribution, excretion and metabolism

The metabolism of chromium has been reviewed (Aitio *et al.*, 1988; Nieboer & Jusys, 1988; World Health Organization, 1988). De Flora and Wetterhahn (1990) have specifically reviewed the redox chemistry of chromium[VI] with respect to cellular metabolism; a metabolic model has been suggested by Elinder *et al.* (1988).

#### (i) Metallic chromium and chromium alloys

Chromium-cobalt alloys appear to release chromium[VI] after intramuscular implantations in rats (Wapner *et al.*, 1986). Chromium metal powder released chromium[VI] when incubated in aerated phosphate buffer, Ringer's solution, phosphate buffer with added bicarbonate and Locke's physiological buffer (Grogan, 1957).

#### (ii) Chromium[III] compounds

In contrast to chromium[VI] compounds, less than 1% of chromium[III] is absorbed from the gastrointestinal tract of animals (Mertz, 1969).

Four hours after intratracheal instillation of chromic chloride in rabbits, 85% of the chromium remained in the lungs and 8% was found in the urine; after uptake, chromium was confined mainly to plasma, and the peak concentration was reached after 20 min (Wiegand *et al.*, 1984a).

After exposure of rats by inhalation to chromic chloride particles (mass median aerodynamic diameter (MMAD), 1.8 and 1.5 μm; 19 and 27% less than 1 μm; 8-10.7 mg chromium/m$^3$), only one clearance phase was demonstrated, with a half-time of about 160 h (Suzuki *et al.*, 1984). As with chromium[VI] compounds, the highest organ concentrations in both rats and rabbits were found in the kidney and liver after exposure to chromic chloride by the pulmonary route, although the concentrations found were lower than those after a corresponding exposure to chromium[VI] (Suzuki *et al.*, 1984; Wiegand *et al.*, 1984a).

Chromium (especially trivalent chromium) strongly accumulated in the interstitial tissues of the gonads of male mice, but not in seminiferous epithelium (Danielsson *et al.*, 1984).

Little chromium[III] is taken up by cells (Aaseth *et al.*, 1982; Nieboer & Jusys, 1988), but more of some organic chromium[III] complexes may be taken up (Yamamoto *et al.*, 1981; Norseth *et al.*, 1982).

After parenteral administration of chromium[III] to rats (as with chromium[VI]), chromium is excreted predominantly in the urine (National Research Council, 1974; Langård, 1980, 1982). Less than 2% of an intravenous dose of chromic chloride was found in the faeces of rats 8 h after injection (Hopkins, 1965). In a subsequent study, seven days after intraperitoneal injection of chromic chloride to mice, the cumulated amounts excreted in faeces and urine were about equal (Bryson & Goodall, 1983).

Studies on the mechanism of excretion of chromium[III] by the kidneys indicate that glomerular filtration is the major mechanism (Donaldson et al., 1986).

As with chromium[VI], biliary excretion of chromic chloride has been demonstrated in rats (Cikrt & Bencko, 1979; Norseth et al., 1982); less than 1% of an intravenously injected dose of chromic chloride was excreted in 5 h (Norseth et al., 1982).

The elimination curve for chromium, as measured by whole-body determination, has an exponential form. In rats, three different components of the curve have been identified, with half-times of 0.5, 5.9 and 83.4 days after intravenous injection of chromic chloride at 1 µg/kg bw Cr (Mertz et al., 1965).

In contrast to results with hexavalent chromium, a single intraperitoneal injection of chromic chloride to mice resulted in 45% retention of chromium three weeks after the injection (Bryson & Goodall, 1983).

In mice administered sodium dichromate, chromium was shown to cross the placenta throughout gestation; transfer was more effective than with chromic chloride, which was not detectably transferred during early gestation, although placental transfer of chromium[III] did occur during late gestation (Danielsson et al., 1982).

A total of 25-30% of chromium administered as chromic chloride to pregnant rats on days 17-20 of gestation was transferred to the placental-fetal unit (Wallach & Verch, 1984). Groups of ICR mice were given a single intraperitoneal injection of [51Cr]chromic chloride on day 8 of gestation and were sacrificed 4, 8 and 12 h after injection. The radioactivity in the fetus increased with time since injection, whereas maternal blood levels decreased (Iijima et al., 1983a).

### (iii)   Chromium[VI] compounds

Gastrointestinal absorption of chromates has been reported. In a review, 3-6% of an administered dose was reported to appear in the urine of rats; this may be an underestimate of the absorption from the gastrointestinal tract, which also takes part in chromium excretion (Mertz, 1969). The absorption of chromates depends on the degree of reduction of chromium[VI] to chromium[III], which is poorly absorbed from the gastrointestinal tract (Donaldson & Barreras, 1966; De Flora et al., 1987a).

Following intratracheal administration of sodium chromate solution to rabbits, about 45% (as Cr) remained in the lungs 4 h after instillation; 15% was excreted in urine. The highest concentration of chromium[VI] was reached in red cells after about 3 h, and the corresponding plasma concentration at that time was about one-third of that in red cells (Wiegand et al., 1984a). Absorption from the lungs may be decreased by extracellular reduction of the hexavalent form (Suzuki, 1988).

Zinc chromate was absorbed in rats exposed to known atmospheric concentrations (6.3-10.7 mg/m³, equivalent to 1.3-2.2 mg/m³ Cr) in an inhalation chamber: a five-fold increase in the blood chromium level was observed after 100 min of exposure by inhalation, and this level increased at a similar rate during the next 150 min (Langård et al., 1978).

Suzuki et al. (1984) exposed rats by inhalation to potassium dichromate particles (MMAD, 1.6-2.0 µm: 12-25% of particles < 1 µm; determined by multistage impactor (Andersen Sampler) and controlled by electron microscopy). A two-phase clearance pattern for chromium was demonstrated, the smaller particles having half-times of 30 h and 700 h; for larger particles, a single phase with a half-time of 160 h was demonstrated. [The Working Group noted that no statistical evaluation of the differences is given in the paper.] The authors stated that there might also be an undetected rapid component for the larger particles and noted that reduction of the hexavalent form may explain the two-phase clearance from the respiratory tract after exposure to chromium[VI]. This reduction was demonstrated by Suzuki (1988).

Sodium chromate (69 µg Cr), zinc chromate (66 µg Cr) and lead chromate (38 µg Cr), all at 20 µl, were injected intratracheally into Wistar rats; 30 min later, 36, 25 and 81% of the doses, respectively, were still present in the lungs. From 30 min and up to six days, lung clearance followed first-order kinetics, with half-times of 2.4 days for sodium chromate, 1.9 days for zinc chromate and 1.8 days for lead chromate. Limited amounts of chromium were found in blood and organs after exposure to lead chromate; the concentrations found were similar with sodium and zinc chromates. At ten days, 20% of the dose of sodium and zinc chromates had been excreted in the urine; negligible amounts of lead chromate were found. After exposure to lead chromate, about 80% of the chromium was excreted in faeces during the same interval (Bragt & van Dura, 1983).

Percutaneous absorption of labelled sodium chromate occurred in guinea-pigs (Wahlberg & Skog, 1963): a maximum of 4% of the dose applied on the skin disappeared within 5 h, and labelled chromium was detected in a number of organs.

Following administration of chromium[VI], most of the chromium found in the blood is bound to red blood cells (Mutti et al., 1979; Suzuki et al., 1984; Wiegand et al., 1984a). After exposure of rats by inhalation to potassium dichromate or of rabbits by inhalation to sodium dichromate, the highest concentrations were found in the kidney and liver (Suzuki et al., 1984; Wiegand et al., 1984a). The spleen also contained high concentrations of chromium after subcutaneous administration of potassium dichromate to rats (Mutti et al., 1979). The organ concentrations after exposure to chromium[VI] were always much higher than after a corresponding exposure to chromium[III] (Suzuki et al., 1984; Wiegand et al., 1984a).

After parenteral administration of chromium[VI] to rats, chromium was excreted predominantly in the urine (National Research Council, 1974; Langård, 1980, 1982). Seven days after intraperitoneal injection of potassium chromate to mice, urinary excretion was twice as high as faecal excretion; following administration of chromium[III], faecal excretion was three times as high as urinary excretion (Bryson & Goodall, 1983).

Subcutaneous injections of 3 mg/kg bw potassium dichromate were given to rats every other day for eight weeks. Urinary elimination of chromium increased steadily during the experiment and was correlated with the concentration of chromium in the renal cortex (Franchini et al., 1978).

Elimination of chromium from the blood of rats exposed by inhalation to zinc chromate was slow: the blood chromium level fell by less than 50% during the first three days after exposure; and after 18 and 37 days 20% and 9% of the initial concentration, respectively, remained. Excretion occurred mainly via the urine (Langård et al., 1978).

Biliary excretion of chromium following administration of sodium dichromate has been demonstrated in rats (Cikrt & Bencko, 1979; Norseth et al., 1982); 6-8% of an intravenous dose of sodium dichromate was excreted in 5 h (Norseth et al., 1982).

Three weeks after a single intraperitoneal injection of potassium dichromate to mice, 7.5% chromium was retained. After repeated weekly intraperitoneal injections of potassium dichromate, about 3% of chromium was retained eight weeks after the first injection. In both cases, this level is about one-sixth of that observed after administration of chromium[III] (Bryson & Goodall, 1983).

Chromium[VI] (tested as sodium dichromate and as an unspecified chromate in vitro) was transported effectively through mammalian cell membranes by the carboxylate, sulfate and phosphate carrier systems; the kinetics of uptake also involve intracellular reduction to the trivalent form (Sanderson, 1976; Wetterhahn-Jennette, 1981; Aaseth et al., 1982; Alexander et al., 1982). Chromium[VI] (tested as sodium dichromate) was rapidly reduced to chromium[III] after cellular uptake, but such reduction may also take place outside the cell, with decreased uptake as a result (De Flora et al., 1987a; Suzuki, 1988). Glutathione seems to be the most important factor for intracellular reduction of chromium[VI], but ascorbic acid, microsomes in the presence of NAD/NADH microsomal cytochrome P450, mitochondria and proteins such as haemoglobin and glutathione reductase in red blood cells may also be active in the reduction process (Connett & Wetterhahn, 1983; Ryberg & Alexander, 1984; Wiegand et al., 1984b; Connett & Wetterhahn, 1985; De Flora & Wetterhahn, 1990). Once absorbed and retained in biological tissue, chromium compounds occur in the trivalent form (Mertz, 1969). Initial binding may involve the pentavalent form (Rossi & Wetterhahn, 1989). When the reducing capacity of liver cells is decreased, the hexavalent form may be found in bile (Norseth *et al.*, 1982).

After treatment of rats with sodium dichromate at 20 mg/kg bw intraperitoneally (134 μmol/kg bw Cr), more of the chromium associated with chromatin was bound to DNA than was the case after chromic chloride treatment (Cupo & Wetterhahn, 1985a).

The intracellular reduction of hexavalent chromium implies the generation of short-lived species of pentavalent and tetravalent chromium with affinities that differ from that of the trivalent form (Connett & Wetterhahn, 1983). The pentavalent form is stabilized by increased amounts of glutathione (Kitagawa *et al.*, 1988). The reduction process thus serves as a detoxification process even intracellularly, when it takes place at a distance from the target site for toxic or genotoxic effect; it serves to activate if it takes place near the cell nucleus, presumably of target organs (De Flora & Wetterhahn, 1990). It has been suggested that phagocytosis may be important for the uptake of hexavalent compounds — in particular soluble forms — as it would allow the slow intracellular release of chromate ions over a long time (Norseth, 1986).

### (b)   Toxic effects

As a general rule, chromium[VI] is much more toxic than chromium[III] when administered to animals, and very marked differences in the cytotoxicity of compounds of the two oxidation states have been observed *in vitro*. Effects on the kidney and the respiratory organs are the most important (for reviews, see Nieboer & Jusys, 1988; World Health Organization, 1988).

The mean intravenous lethal dose in mice is 85 mg/kg bw chromic sulfate, 400-800 mg/kg bw chromic chloride and 2290 mg/kg bw chromic acetate (National Research Council, 1974). The $LD_{50}$ in rats for potassium dichromate administered by stomach tube was reported to be 177 mg/kg for males and 149 mg/kg for females (World Health Organization, 1988).

### (i)   Chromium[III] compounds

Morphological changes in rabbit alveolar macrophages occurred after exposure by inhalation to chromic nitrate (0.6 mg/m³ Cr) for four to six weeks. Fewer macrophages were obtained by lavage than with chromium[VI], but only chromium[III] caused functional changes in macrophages, measured by increased metabolic activity and reduced phagocytotic activity. The authors speculated that these effects may be due to the release of chromium[III] ions from phagocytized particles, with subsequent binding to macromolecules in the cell. Such particles were not seen after exposure to chromium[VI] (Johansson *et al.*, 1986).

Chromium[III] has been found in ribonucleic acids from all sources examined. It is possible that chromium helps stabilize the structure of RNA (Wacker & Vallee,

1959). Chromium bound to only a limited extent to chromatin and DNA from the liver and kidney of rats treated intraperitoneally with chromic chloride at 80 mg/kg bw (290 μmol/kg bw Cr), as indicated in a study by Tsapakos et al. (1983a); DNA damage, as measured by alkaline elution, was not demonstrable in kidney after injection of chromium[III]. The binding of chromic nitrate to denatured or native DNA was limited and relatively unaffected by the presence of microsomes and NADPH (Tsapakos & Wetterhahn, 1983).

Chromic chloride was 100 times less effective than chromium[VI] in inhibiting DNA synthesis (Levis et al., 1978a). A large difference in cytotoxic activity between chromium[VI] and chromium[III] was also noted when the effects of 11 water-soluble chromium compounds on BHK cells were compared: of the chromium[III] compounds, only chromic nitrate appeared to be cytotoxic, but it was contaminated with chromium[VI] at about 0.2% (Levis & Majone, 1979).

Chromic chloride inhibited the uptake of ribo- and deoxyribonucleosides by BHK cells (Levis et al., 1978a). In contrast to chromium[VI], chromic chloride inhibited the plasma membrane $Mg^{2+}$-ATPase activity of BHK cells only when it was present in the incubation medium and not when cells were pretreated with it (Luciani et al., 1979).

Chromic oxide particles are taken up by cells by phagocytosis; chromium[III] may thus reach its target sites even if it is not derived from intracellular chromate ion. An inhibitory effect on cell cycle progression in Chinese hamster cells was demonstrated after exposure to crystalline chromic oxide (particle size, 91% < 1 μm; purity, 99.8%) at concentrations ranging from 50 to 200 μg/ml (Elias et al., 1986). Chromic chloride does, however, stimulate RNA synthesis both in vitro and in vivo in mouse liver and in regenerating rat liver (Okada et al., 1981, 1983, 1984).

### (ii)  Chromium[VI] compounds

Renal lesions in animals are confined to the proximal convoluted tubules (for review, see National Research Council, 1974; Aitio et al., 1988; World Health Organization, 1988). In rats exposed to a single subcutaneous dose of 15 mg/kg bw potassium dichromate, increases in urinary β-glucuronidase, lysozyme, glucose and protein as well as morphological changes in renal tubules were observed, although the glomerular filtration rate was unchanged (Franchini et al., 1978).

Ngaha (1981) demonstrated that urinary volume was increased with increased amounts of acid and alkaline phosphatases in the urine in rats after subcutaneous injection of potassium dichromate at 25 mg/kg. The concentrations of the phosphatases and of lactate dehydrogenase in kidney tissue decreased. No significant change in the levels of these enzymes in liver tissue was demonstrated.

Morphological changes occurred in rabbit alveolar macrophages after exposure by inhalation to sodium chromate (0.9 mg/m$^3$ Cr) for four to six weeks. Significantly more macrophages were present in the lavage fluid from the chromium[VI]-exposed animals than in those exposed to chromium[III], but functional changes in macrophages were observed after exposure to chromium[III] and not after exposure to chromium[VI] (Johansson *et al.*, 1986). Activation of phagocytosis was demonstrated in rat alveolar macrophages after exposure to 25-50 μg/m$^3$ sodium dichromate by inhalation for 28 days; exposure to 200 μg/m$^3$ for the same interval inhibited phagocytotic function. Lung clearance of inhaled [$^{59}$Fe] iron oxide was significantly decreased after exposure to the high dose of sodium dichromate. The antibody response to sheep red blood cells and the mitogen-stimulated T-lymphocyte response were stimulated at the low doses but inhibited at the high dose (Glaser *et al.*, 1985).

Exposure of cats by inhalation to 11-23 mg/m$^3$ chromium[VI] as dichromate for 2-3 h/day during five days caused bronchitis and pneumonia. In rabbits exposed similarly, no effect was observed. Mixed dusts containing chromates (7 mg/m$^3$ as chromium trioxide) were fatal to mice when inhaled for 37 h over ten days; whereas no marked effect was noted in rabbits or guinea-pigs that inhaled 5 mg/m$^3$ (as chromium trioxide) for 4 h/day on five days/week for one year (National Research Council, 1974). Increased subepithelial connective tissue and flattened epithelium in the large bronchi were observed in mice exposed to chromate (Nettesheim *et al.*, 1971).

In chronically treated cell cultures, chromium[VI] was much more active than chromium[III] in reducing cell growth and survival, independently of the particular compound used (Bianchi *et al.*, 1980). Chromium bound to chromatin and DNA from liver and kidney of rats treated intraperitoneally with sodium dichromate (140 μmol [7.2 mg]/kg as Cr) (Tsapakos *et al.*, 1983a) Binding of chromium to nucleic acids *in vitro* depends on the reduction of the chromium[VI] to chromium[III]. In contrast to chromium[III], binding to denaturated or native DNA was demonstrated with potassium dichromate only in the presence of the complete microsomal reducing system (Tsapakos & Wetterhahn, 1983).

Potassium dichromate induced a rapid blockage of DNA replication in Syrian hamster fibroblasts (BHK line), whereas RNA and protein synthesis were inhibited secondarily (Levis *et al.*, 1978b). It also reduced the colony-forming ability of BHK cells at $10^{-7}$-$10^{-4}$M. It facilitated the uptake of ribo- and deoxyribonucleosides in BHK cells (Levis *et al.*, 1978a). The effect of potassium dichromate on the nucleoside pool in BHK cells could not be explained solely by changes in transport (Bianchi *et al.*, 1979). Plasma membrane $Mg^{2+}$-ATPase activity of BHK cells was inhibited when the cells were pretreated with potassium dichromate, even when chromate was absent from the assay medium (Luciani *et al.*, 1979). Mitochondrial respiration was inhibited by about 50% by the addition of 25 $\mu$M [1.3 mg] sodium chromate in rat liver (Ryberg & Alexander, 1984).

### (c)    Effects on reproduction and prenatal toxicity

#### (i)    Chromium[III] compounds

Treatment of sea-urchin sperm with potassium chromic sulfate or chromic nitrate ($5 \times 10^{-5}$-$5 \times 10^{-4}$ M [2.6-26 mg]) before fertilization failed to induce larval malformation (Pagano et al., 1983).

In cultured mouse embryos, chromium nitrate (0.02-2 $\mu$g/ml Cr) caused less impairment of blastocyst formation and inhibition of hatching from the zona pellucida to the formation of the inner cell mass than the chromium[VI] salts tested (Jacquet & Draye, 1982).

In contrast to chromium[VI], chromic chloride showed no overt cytotoxicity in chick limb bud mesenchymal cells in vitro (Danielsson et al., 1982).

Groups of 30 pregnant ICR mice were given a single intraperitoneal injection of [$^{51}$Cr]chromic chloride (19.5 mg/kg bw Cr) on day 8 of gestation and were sacrificed at intervals of 4-192 h after injection. More pyknotic cells were observed in the neural plate of experimental embryos than controls [percentages not given], especially by 8 h after injection (Iijima et al., 1983a).

A dose-dependent increase in the frequency of rib fusion in fetuses (6-16%, depending on dose) and exencephaly and anencephaly were seen occasionally at higher dose levels following intraperitoneal injection of 9.8-24.4 mg/kg bw chromic chloride to mice on day 8 of gestation. Maternal effects were not described (Matsumoto et al., 1976).

#### (ii)    Chromium[VI] compounds

Treatment of sea-urchin sperm with sodium chromate before fertilization resulted in a number of abnormal larvae, depending on length of exposure and concentration. Sea-urchin embryos reared in the presence of chromate at $5 \times 10^{-5}$-$5 \times 10^{-4}$ M had retarded differentiation of the gut and skeleton (Pagano et al., 1983).

Cultured mouse embryos at the two-cell stage were incubated in Brinster's medium with potassium chromate or calcium chromate (0.02-2 $\mu$g/ml Cr). Blastocyst formation was damaged, and hatching of the blastocyst from the zona pellucida to the formation of the inner cell mass was inhibited (Jacquet & Draye, 1982).

As reported in an abstract, male mice were administered $3 \times 10^{-3}$ M [882 mg] potassium bichromate by either intratesticular or intraperitoneal injection, then mated weekly. A decrease in the number of sperm was seen after three weeks of treatment, and abnormalities in shape reached about 50% of the total sperm after four weeks of treatment. Decreases in the number of implantation sites, in litter size and in fetal body weight were observed. No conspicuous malformation of fetuses was detected. None of the females became pregnant after three weeks of treatment of males (Yasuda, 1980).

Sodium chromate inhibited chondrogenesis in chick limb bud mesenchymal cells *in vitro* at concentrations of about 0.1 µg/ml Cr (Danielsson *et al.*, 1982).

Chromium trioxide dissolved in saline was injected into the air sacs of embryonated chicken eggs at doses of 0.002-0.05 mg/egg on days 0-4 of incubation. Control eggs were injected with a comparable volume of saline. All embryos were examined on day 8, and malformations, such as short and twisted limbs, microphthalmia, exencephaly, short and twisted neck, everted viscera, oedema and reduced body size, were observed in treated eggs. Most embryos showed unilateral or bilateral limb defects (Gilani & Marano, 1979).

Chromium trioxide was administered intravenously at doses of 5, 7.5, 10 or 15 mg/kg bw to groups of ten pregnant golden hamsters early on day 8 of gestation. Fetuses were collected on gestation days 12, 14 and 15 and were examined for frequency and types of malformations. In the different dose groups, 6-40% of the fetuses were resorbed and 1-100% of fetuses had growth retardation; 2% of control fetuses were resorbed. Maternal toxicity (mortality, decreased weight gain, kidney tubular necrosis) was seen in treated animals. Cleft palate occurred in 34-85% of exposed fetuses (2% in controls) and defects in skeletal ossification in up to 96% (Gale, 1978). On comparing five strains of hamsters (ten animals per group, exposure to 8 mg/kg bw on day 8), different susceptibilities were observed: three strains were very susceptible to the embryotoxic effects, while the others were more resistant. In the more susceptible strains, the percentage of resorption sites was 13-28%, whereas in the less susceptible strains it was 7-11%. External abnormalities observed were cleft palate (0-30%) and hydrocephalus. Maternal toxicity (decreased weight gain) was seen in all groups. The time of administration of the chromium trioxide was important: cleft palate was induced only when chromium was administered on day 7, 8 or 9 of gestation and not when it was given on day 10 or 11 (Gale & Bunch, 1979; Gale, 1982).

### (d)   Genetic and related effects

The activity of chromium and chromium compounds in tests for genetic and related effects was evaluated in previous *IARC Monographs* (1980a, 1982, 1987a,b). Moreover, a number of reviews on this subject are available in the literature (e.g., Heck & Costa, 1982a,b; Léonard & Lauwerys, 1980; Petrilli & De Flora, 1980; Paschin & Kozachenko, 1981; Levis & Bianchi, 1982; Petrilli & De Flora, 1982; Baker, 1984; Bianchi & Levis, 1984; Hansen & Stern, 1984; Bianchi & Levis, 1985; Petrilli *et al.*, 1986a,b; Sunderman, 1986; Venitt, 1986; Bianchi & Levis, 1987, 1988; Nieboer & Shaw, 1988; World Health Organization, 1988; De Flora *et al.*, 1990).

Over 600 reports have been published on 32 chromium compounds of various oxidation states and solubilities, and the data base covers 125 experimental systems with different endpoints and/or targets. The studies described below are summarized in Appendix 1 to this volume.

### (i)  Metallic chromium

Metallic chromium was assayed for the ability to induce cell transformation (anchorage-independent growth) in Syrian hamster BHK fibroblasts. Although chromium particles were phagocytized by cells, no significant increase in the number of cell foci growing in soft agar was observed (Hansen & Stern, 1985). [See General Remarks, p. 44, for concerns about this assay.]

As reported in an abstract, male Sprague-Dawley rats were exposed to chromium fumes generated from powders of chromium metal by a plasma flame sprayer at concentrations of $1.84 \pm 0.55$ mg/m$^3$ or $0.55 \pm 0.07$ mg/m$^3$ fume for 5 h/day on five days a week for one week or two months. Significant increases in the frequencies of sister chromatid exchange and of chromosomal aberrations were observed in peripheral blood lymphocytes, whereas chromosomal aberration frequencies in bone-marrow cells were unchanged (Koshi et al., 1987). [The Working Group noted that some oxidation of metallic chromium may have occurred during generation of the fumes.]

### (ii)  Chromium[III] compounds

Twelve chromium[III] compounds of various water solubilities were assayed in a number of short-term tests, often at the same time as chromium compounds of other oxidation states. They included: (a) highly soluble compounds, such as chromic chloride, chromic acetate, chromic nitrate, chromic sulfate and chromic potassium sulfate; (b) sparingly soluble products, such as basic chromic sulfate or neochromium, chromium alum and chromic phosphate; and (c) almost insoluble compounds, such as chromic hydroxide, chromic oxide, chromite ore and cupric chromite. In addition, several reports dealt with the activity of chromium[III] tannins and of chromium[III] compounds bound to organic ligands, as described below. In evaluating the results, summarized in Appendix 1, it should be noted that some of the positive results, obtained with both pure laboratory compounds and industrial products, might be due to contamination by traces of chromium[VI] (indicated as [+] in Appendix 1); therefore, reported positive results with chromium[III] compounds should be interpreted with caution, particularly for those studies in which the purity of test compounds was not checked.

In several studies, the activity of chromic chloride in acellular (i.e., purified nucleic acids) or subcellular (i.e., cell nuclei) systems was investigated. Depurination of calf thymus DNA did not occur, as shown by the unchanged release of adenine detectable by thin-layer chromatography. In addition, it did not induce mutation of single-stranded φ X 174 *am*3 DNA, transfected into *Escherichia coli* spheroplasts and then tested for reversion in a progeny phage assay (Schaaper *et al.*, 1987). As reported previously, chromium[VI] trioxide was also inactive in this system; chromic chloride, however, induced *lacZα* forward mutation in double-stranded M13mp2 DNA, transfected into JM101 *E. coli* (Snow & Xu, 1989). Moreover, chromic chloride suppressed the infectivity of tobacco mosaic virus RNA, probably by nonenzymic cleavage of internucleotide phosphodiester bonds (Huff *et al.*, 1964). Assessments of viscosity, ultraviolet absorption spectra and thermal denaturation of purified DNA and RNA showed that, at variance with chromium[VI] which (as an oxidizing agent) breaks the polynucleotide chain (see potassium dichromate), chromium[III] is responsible for physicochemical alterations of nucleic acids by interacting with the phosphate groups and nitrogen bases (Tamino & Peretta, 1980; Tamino *et al.*, 1981). As evaluated by nucleotide incorporation into calf thymus DNA in the presence of *E. coli* DNA polymerase, chromic chloride inhibited DNA synthesis more potently than chromium[VI] (potassium dichromate); however, at levels below the inhibitory concentration, it enhanced nucleotide incorporation (Nishio & Uyeki, 1985). Like chromium[VI] (potassium dichromate), chromic chloride increased misincorporation of nucleotide bases into daughter DNA strands synthesized from a synthetic polynucleotide template, poly[d(A-T)], in the presence of avian myeloblastosis virus or *E. coli* DNA polymerases (Sirover & Loeb, 1976; Tkeshelashvili *et al.*, 1980). The misincorporated bases were present as single-base substitutions (Tkeshelashvili *et al.*, 1980). In contrast to chromium[VI] salts (potassium chromate and potassium dichromate), chromic chloride favoured cross-links between *E. coli* DNA and bovine serum albumin, as assessed by checking [3]H-DNA-bovine serum albumin binding in a filtration assay (Fornace *et al.*, 1981). The same chromium[III] compound produced DNA fragmentation (alkaline elution technique), as determined by single-strand breaks and cross-links in isolated calf thymus nuclei (Beyersmann & Köster, 1987) and in purified DNA from V79 cells (Bianchi *et al.*, 1983). DNA-protein cross-links were also detected by exposing nuclei of mouse leukaemia L1210 cells to chromic chloride; chromium[VI] (potassium chromate) was inactive (Fornace *et al.*, 1981).

Most studies in which the activity of chromium[III] compounds was evaluated in prokaryotes yielded negative results. Chromic chloride did not induce λ prophage in *E. coli* WP2$_s$(λ) (Rossman *et al.*, 1984) after overnight incubation at concentrations near the growth inhibitory concentration of the compound. No SOS response was induced in *E. coli* GC2375, UA4202 or PQ30 by chromic chloride, chromic nitrate or chromic acetate (Llagostera *et al.*, 1986), or in strain PQ37 by chromic potassium sulfate (De Flora *et al.*, 1985a) or chromic chloride (Olivier & Marzin, 1987). Chromic nitrate, chromic chloride and chromic potassium sulfate were confirmed to be inactive in strain PQ37, whereas chromic acetate produced a low but significant increase in SOS-inducing activity (Venier *et al.*, 1989).

In differential killing assays with *E. coli*, chromic chloride was equally toxic in the wild strain AB1157 and in the repair-deficient strains AB1886 (*uvrA6*⁻), GW801 (*recA56*⁻), GW802 (*recA56⁻uvrA6*⁻), PAM AA34 (*recA56⁻lexA2*⁻) and PAM5717 (*lexA2*⁻) (Warren *et al.*, 1981).

Chromic chloride, chromic phosphate and chromic oxide (spotted in powder form) were equally toxic in *E. coli* WP2 (wild strain) and in the repair-deficient strains WP2 *uvrA* (*uvrA*⁻), CM571 (*rec A*⁻) and WP100 (*uvrA*⁻ *rec A*⁻), as assessed by the streak method on agar and, in the case of chromic phosphate, by means of a test-tube assay (Yagi & Nishioka, 1977).

Chromic chloride and chromic acetate were equally toxic to WP2 and to the repair-deficient strains WP67 (*uvrA⁻polA*⁻) and CM871 (*uvrA⁻recA⁻lexA*⁻) when assayed in the treat-and-plate test, but these compounds, chromic nitrate and chromic potassium sulfate were more toxic in the repair-deficient strains when assayed by a liquid micromethod (De Flora *et al.*, 1984a). Four conditions were required to elicit this unusual positivity of chromium[III] in this system: (a) performance of the test in a liquid medium, (b) long contact between chromium[III] and bacteria (at least 6-8 h), (c) a physiological pH (7.0-7.4) and (d) the presence of high, subtoxic concentrations (0.2-0.3 M) of phosphate (De Flora *et al.*, 1990). Chromic chloride, chromic sulfate and chromic potassium sulfate did not induce differential killing of *S. typhimurium* TA1978 (wild strain) or TA1538 (*rec*⁻) (Gentile *et al.*, 1981). In the *rec* assay in *Bacillus subtilis* H17 (wild strain) and M45 (*rec*⁻), negative results were obtained with chromic chloride (Nishioka, 1975; Nakamuro *et al.*, 1978; Matsui, 1980; Gentile *et al.*, 1981), chromic sulfate and chromic potassium sulfate (Kada *et al.*, 1980; Kanematsu *et al.*, 1980; Gentile *et al.*, 1981). Positive results were obtained in this system, using the spot test procedure, with chromic acetate and chromic nitrate. Chromic acetate also gave positive results in the *arg*⁻ → *arg*⁺ reversion test in *E. coli* Hs30R (Nakamuro *et al.*, 1978).

No reversion of *trp*⁻ → *trp*⁺ was produced in *E. coli* by chromic chloride or chromic acetate (strains WP2 and WP2*uvrA*) (Petrilli & De Flora, 1982) or by chromic sulfate (strain DG1153) (Arlauskas *et al.*, 1985). In a *lacI*⁺ /*lacI*⁻ forward mutation assay in *E. coli* KMBL3835, chromic chloride yielded unclear results (Zakour & Glickman, 1984).

In more than 30 reports (see Appendix 2), highly soluble or sparingly soluble chromium[III] compounds were inactive in the *his*⁻ → *his*⁺ reversion test in several strains of *Salmonella typhimurium* (TA1535, TA1537, TA1538, TA92, TA94, TA97, TA98, TA100 and TA102) in the absence of exogenous metabolic systems (Tamaro *et al.*, 1975; Petrilli & De Flora, 1977, 1978a; De Flora, 1981a; Tso & Fung, 1981; Venier *et al.*, 1982; Bennicelli *et al.*, 1983; Bianchi *et al.*, 1983; De Flora *et al.*, 1984a,b;

Arlauskas *et al.*, 1985; Langerwerf *et al.*, 1985; Loprieno *et al.*, 1985; Marzin & Phi, 1985; Petrilli *et al.*, 1985). Chromic chloride, chromic nitrate, chromic potassium sulfate, chromium alum and neochromium were still not mutagenic in the presence of metabolic systems, including post-mitochondrial supernatants of rat liver, lung or muscle, rat muscle mitochondria (with or without ATP), human erythrocyte lysates and oxidized glutathione. Mutagenic effects were produced by all these compounds only in the presence of a strong oxidizing agent, such as potassium permanganate (Petrilli & De Flora, 1978a). The inactivity of chromic sulfate was unaffected by the presence of nitrilotriacetic acid (NTA) (Loprieno *et al.*, 1985). Surprisingly, high amounts of chromic chloride [unspecified source and purity] were reported to be weakly mutagenic to strains TA98 and TA94 in one study (Langerwerf *et al.*, 1985). Other positive results can be ascribed to contamination with traces of chromium[VI], in a chromic nitrate sample (Venier *et al.*, 1982; Bianchi *et al.*, 1983) and in an industrial chromite sample (Petrilli & De Flora, 1978a; De Flora, 1981a; Venier *et al.*, 1982; Bianchi *et al.*, 1983).

Chromic chloride was reported to induce mitotic gene conversion at the *trp5* locus and point reverse mutation at the *ilv* locus in strain D7 of *Saccharomyces cerevisiae*. Such activity, usually detected when the yeast was in the logarithmic growth phase, was very weak, was obtained only with high doses of chromium[III] and occurred only in the presence of 0.1 M phosphate; no activity was seen when 0.05 M Tris-hydrochloric acid was used as the buffer (Galli *et al.*, 1985; Bronzetti *et al.*, 1986).

Chromic potassium sulfate gave weakly positive results in an unscheduled DNA synthesis assay in mature pollen of *Petunia hybrida* (W166K) (Jackson & Linskens, 1982). [The Working Group noted that the effect was very weak and that the existence of a dose-response relationship was not investigated.] Chromic nitrate induced chromosomal aberrations in the root tips of *Vicia faba* (Gläss, 1955).

A study of the cytotoxic effects produced in Syrian hamster BHK monolayers and of mitotic cycle alterations in human epithelial-like heteroploid HEp2 cells produced by chromic chloride, chromic sulfate, chromium alum, neochromium and chromium[VI]-contaminated chromite provided evidence that chromium[III] is far less active than chromium[VI] (Levis & Majone, 1981). Chromic chloride did not induce unscheduled DNA synthesis in mouse kidney A18BcR cells (Raffetto *et al.*, 1977) or human heteroploid EUE cells (Bianchi *et al.*, 1983). It did not inhibit DNA synthesis in Syrian hamster BHK fibroblasts, even when the cells were reversibly permeabilized in hypertonic medium (Bianchi *et al.*, 1984), or in mouse L cells unless they were permeabilized with detergents (Nishio & Uyeki, 1985).

Chromic chloride did not induce DNA fragmentation in mouse leukaemia 1210 cells (Fornace *et al.*, 1981), in Chinese hamster V79 cells (Bianchi *et al.*, 1983) or in human embryo lung IMR-90 fibroblasts (Fornace *et al.*, 1981), as assessed by alkaline elution, or in human white blood cells, as assessed by the alkaline unwinding technique (McLean *et al.*, 1982). Similarly, chromic nitrate, even at concentrations up to 25 times those of chromium[VI] compounds needed to damage DNA, did not produce DNA fragmentation (alkaline elution) in chicken embryo hepatocytes (Tsapakos *et al.*, 1983b). In contrast, a sample of cupric chromite induced DNA-protein cross-links in Novikoff ascites hepatoma cells, as evaluated by high-speed centrifugation of detergent-treated cells followed by polyacrylamide gel electrophoresis; chromous chloride was inactive in this test (Wedrychowski *et al.*, 1986a).

Using the *hprt* forward mutation assay, negative results were obtained with chromic sulfate in mouse mammary carcinoma Fm3A cells (8-azaguanine resistance) (Nishimura & Umeda, 1978 [Abstract]), with chromic acetate in Chinese hamster V79/4 cells (8-azaguanine resistance) (Newbold *et al.*, 1979) and in CHO cells (6-thioguanine resistance) (Bianchi *et al.*, 1983). In V79 cells, a sample of chromic oxide, uncontaminated with chromium[VI] was phagocytized, as shown by electron microscopic detection of intracytoplasmic vacuoles containing crystalline chromic oxide particles, after an 18-h exposure of cells; it also induced 6-thioguanine resistance (Elias *et al.*, 1986).

Mostly negative results have been reported with regard to the induction of sister chromatid exchange by chromium[III] compounds in various types of cultured mammalian cells (Table 23). Both positive and negative results have been reported in the literature concerning the ability of these compounds to induce chromosomal aberrations in mammalian cells (Table 24). In parallel assays, aberrations were induced more frequently than sister chromatid exchange by chromium[III] compounds, but much higher concentrations of chromium[III] than chromium[VI] were generally needed to induce chromosomal aberrations, due perhaps to an indirect effect of high doses, such as the release of lysosomal nucleases (Levis & Majone, 1981). The decreased frequency of chromium[III]-induced chromosomal aberrations in the presence of superoxide dismutase, copper (salicylate), copper (tyrosine), catalase and mannitol suggests the involvement of active oxygen species (Friedman *et al.*, 1987). The occasional finding of both sister chromatid exchange and chromosomal aberrations in CHO cells was ascribed by the authors to contamination of their chromium[III] samples with traces of chromium[VI] (Levis & Majone, 1979; Bianchi *et al.*, 1980; Venier *et al.*, 1982).

Chromic chloride inhibited spindle formation in human skin fibroblasts, but only at the highest concentration tested (100 μM), which was several orders of magnitude higher than the concentration required for chromium[VI] compounds (sodium chromate and calcium chromate) to produce the same effect (Nijs & Kirsch-Volders, 1986).

**Table 23. Induction of sister chromatid exchange by chromium[III] compounds in cultured mammalian cells**

| Chromium compound | Cell line | Result and comments | Reference |
|---|---|---|---|
| Chromic acetate | Chinese hamster CHO | - | Levis & Majone (1979) |
| | | - | Bianchi et al. (1980) |
| | Mouse macrophage P388D₁ | + | Andersen (1983) |
| | Human peripheral lymphocytes | + | Andersen (1983) |
| Chromic chloride | Mouse primary lymphocytes (BALB/c) | - | Venier et al. (1982) |
| | | - | Majone et al. (1983) |
| | | - | Bianchi et al. (1983) |
| | Mouse primary lymphocytes (BALB/Mo) | - | Venier et al. (1982) |
| | | - | Majone et al. (1983) |
| | | - | Bianchi et al. (1983) |
| | Mouse LSTRA lymphocytes | - | Bianchi et al. (1983) |
| | Syrian hamster embryo primary | - | Tsuda & Kato (1977) |
| | Chinese hamster CHO | - | Macrae et al. (1979) |
| | | - | Levis & Majone (1979) |
| | | - | Levis & Majone (1981) |
| | | - | Majone & Rensi (1979) |
| | | - | Bianchi et al. (1980) |
| | | - | Bianchi et al. (1983) |
| | | - | Venier et al. (1982) |
| | | - | Uyeki & Nishio (1983) |
| | | + (48-h incubation) | Venier et al. (1985a) |
| | Chinese hamster lung Don | - | Koshi (1979) |
| | | + | Ohno et al. (1982) |
| | BHK fibroblasts | - | Bianchi et al. (1984) |
| | BHK fibroblasts (permeabilized) | - | Bianchi et al. (1984) |
| | Human peripheral lymphocytes | - | Ogawa et al. (1978) |
| | | - | Stella et al. (1982) |
| | Chinese hamster V79 | + (300 × dose needed for Cr[VI]) | Elias et al. (1983) |
| Chromic nitrate | Chinese hamster CHO | - | Levis & Majone (1979) |
| | | - | Bianchi et al. (1980) |
| | | - | Venier et al. (1982) |

**Table 23 (contd)**

| Chromium compound | Cell line | Result and comments | Reference |
|---|---|---|---|
| Chromic potassium sulfate | Chinese hamster CHO | - | Levis & Majone (1979) |
| | | - | Bianchi et al. (1980) |
| Chromic sulfate | Chinese hamster CHO | - | Levis & Majone (1981) |
| | | - | Loprieno et al. (1985) |
| | Chinese hamster lung Don | - | Ohno et al. (1982) |
| Chromium alum | Chinese hamster CHO | - | Levis & Majone (1981) |
| | | - | Venier et al. (1982) |
| Neochromium | Chinese hamster CHO | - | Levis & Majone (1981) |
| Chromic oxide | Mouse macrophage P388D₁ | - (taken up by cells after 48 h) | Andersen (1983) |
| | Chinese hamster V79 | + (1000 × dose needed for Cr[VI]) | Elias et al. (1983) |

Chromic chloride (Bianchi et al., 1983; Hansen & Stern, 1985) and chromic oxide (Hansen & Stern, 1985) did not induce anchorage-independent growth in Syrian hamster BHK fibroblasts (see General Remarks, p. 44, for concern about this assay). Chromic chloride was reported to produce morphological transformation of mouse fetal cells (Raffetto et al., 1977), but it did not transform Syrian hamster embryo primary cells nor, in contrast to chromium[VI] (potassium chromate), did it affect the transforming capacity of benzo[a]pyrene (Rivedal & Sanner, 1981).

In vivo, intraperitoneal injection of chromic chloride did not induce DNA fragmentation in rat liver or kidney cells (Tsapakos et al., 1983b; Cupo & Wetterhahn, 1985a), as assessed by the alkaline elution technique in the same laboratory from which positive results were reported with chromium[VI] (see sodium dichromate). The number of micronucleated erythrocytes in bone-marrow cells of BALB/c mice was not increased after intraperitoneal injection of 250-500 mg/kg bw chromic nitrate, which contrasts with the positive result recorded with a soluble chromium[VI] compound (potassium dichromate) at ten-fold lower doses (Fabry, 1980).

**Table 24. Induction of chromosomal aberrations by chromium[III] compounds in cultured mammalian cells**

| Chromium compound | Cell line | Result | Reference |
|---|---|---|---|
| Chromic acetate | Chinese hamster CHO | + | Levis & Majone (1979) |
| | | + | Bianchi et al. (1980) |
| | Human peripheral lymphocytes | + | Nakamuro et al. (1978) |
| Chromic chloride | Mouse fetal | + | Raffetto et al. (1977) |
| | Syrian hamster embryo | - | Tsuda & Kato (1977) |
| | Chinese hamster CHO | + | Levis & Majone (1979) |
| | | + | Levis & Majone (1981) |
| | | + | Majone & Rensi (1979) |
| | | + | Bianchi et al. (1980) |
| | | + | Venier et al. (1982) |
| | Human peripheral lymphocytes | - | Nakamuro et al. (1978) |
| | | - | Sarto et al. (1980) |
| | | + | Kaneko (1976) |
| | | + | Stella et al. (1982) |
| Chromic nitrate | Chinese hamster CHO | - | Levis & Majone (1979) |
| | | - | Bianchi et al. (1980) |
| | | - | Venier et al. (1982) |
| | Human peripheral lymphocytes | - | Nakamuro et al. (1978) |
| Chromic potassium sulfate | Chinese hamster CHO | + | Levis & Majone (1979) |
| | | + | Bianchi et al. (1980) |
| Chromic sulfate | Mouse mammary carcinoma Fm3A | - | Umeda & Nishimura (1979) |
| | Syrian hamster embryo primary | - | Tsuda & Kato (1977) |
| | Chinese hamster CHO | + | Levis & Majone (1981) |
| | Chinese hamster 237-2a | + | Rössner et al. (1981) |
| Chromium alum | Chinese hamster CHO | + | Levis & Majone (1981) |
| Neochromium | Chinese hamster CHO | + | Levis & Majone (1981) |
| Chromic oxide | Chinese hamster CHO | [+] | Levis & Majone (1981) |
| | | [+] | Venier et al. (1982) |

The results of these studies with pure and industrial chromium[III] products are summarized in Appendix 1. Data on the genotoxicity of chromium tanning liquors used in the hide and leather industry, most of which are composed of almost insoluble sulfates, are also available. None of 17 tanning liquors, dissolved in water, acids or alkali, reverted *his⁻ S. typhimurium* strains; however, the frequency of sister chromatid exchange was increased by eight (including chromium alum) of 13 tannins tested in Chinese hamster CHO cells. Contamination with chromium[VI] was detected in four of the active compounds (Venier et al., 1982, 1985a).

The marked differences in potency seen in parallel assays with chromium[III] and chromium[VI] compounds have already been commented upon. The positive results sometimes obtained with chromium[III] compounds (46 positive and 141 negative results) can be ascribed to a variety of factors, which emerged from analyses of the literature (Levis et al., 1978b; Levis & Bianchi, 1982). These include unquantified contamination with trace amounts of chromium[VI], nonspecific effects of very high doses, and penetration of chromium[III] by endocytosis following long exposure in vitro or under special treatment conditions, such as exposure to detergents or to subtoxic concentrations of phosphate. In addition, a technical artefact may result from interaction of chromium[III] with DNA released from disrupted cells during extraction procedures.

### Chromium[III] complexes

Unlike chromium[VI] (potassium chromate), a chromic glycine complex did not produce unscheduled DNA synthesis in cultured human skin fibroblasts (Whiting et al., 1979). In a differential killing assay with E. coli AB1157 (wild strain) and various repair-deficient strains and in the S. typhimurium his⁻ reversion test, four of 17 hexacoordinate chromium[III] compounds gave positive results only in the DNA repair test and four in both tests (Warren et al., 1981). The most active complexes were those containing aromatic amine ligands, like 2,2'-bipyridine and 1,10-phenanthroline. [The Working Group noted that the genotoxicity of these ligands was not checked.] Complexation with salicylate and citrate (but not with NTA, ethylenediaminetetraacetic acid, Tiron, glucose, glycine, pyrophosphate or acetate) rendered chromic chloride weakly active in the rec assay with B. subtilis (Gentile et al., 1981). The mutagenicity of [Cr(bipy)$_2$Cl$_2$]Cl and [Cr(phen)$_2$Cl$_2$]Cl was confirmed in S. typhimurium TA100 (Beyersmann et al., 1984). Water-soluble complexes of chromium[III] (chromic sulfate and chromic chloride) with five amino acids (arginine, aspartic acid, glycine, hydroxyproline and lysine) or with salicylic acid or ascorbic acid did not revert various his⁻ S. typhimurium strains (Langerwerf et al., 1985). Initial observations were reported in an abstract concerning the ability of [Cr(bipy)$_2$Cl$_2$]Cl to induce predominantly extragenic suppressors in TA103 (Vieux et al., 1986). This complex was shown in the same laboratory to revert his⁻ S. typhimurium TA92, TA100 and TA98 (Warren et al., 1981). In a further abstract (Rogers et al., 1987), the same compound was reported to revert TA102 and TA104, with an appreciable reduction of activity under anaerobiosis and in the presence of the hydroxyl ion scavenger mannitol. Exposure of calf thymus nuclei to Cr(glycine)$_3$ produced DNA-protein cross-links as well as DNA strand-breaks, i.e., the same type of lesions caused by hexahydrated chromic chloride (Beyersmann & Köster,

1987). In the same study, [Cr(phen)$_2$Cl$_2$]Cl also produced DNA fragmentation, but with a lower fraction of cross-links, when applied to intact Chinese hamster V79 cells; this phenanthroline complex, in contrast to Cr(glycine)$_3$, also induced 6-thioguanine resistance. No mutagenic effect was detected in *his⁻ S. typhimurium* with a commercial preparation of glucose tolerance factor, a yeast-extracted natural complex of chromium[III] with nicotinic acid, glycine, glutamic acid and cysteine, which is prescribed as a dietary supplement in cases of deficient chromium[III] intake with food and impaired glucose tolerance (De Flora *et al.*, 1989a). Cr(maltolate)$_3$, a chromium[III] complex with a low lipophilic ligand, did not induce gene mutations in *S. typhimurium* TA92, TA98, TA100 or TA104 nor sister chromatid exchange in mammalian cell culture (CHO line), whereas a complex with a high lipophilic ligand, Cr(acetyl acetonate)$_3$, although inactive to TA92, TA98 and TA100 strains, was clearly mutagenic to strain TA104 and increased the frequency of sister chromatid exchange (Gava *et al.*, 1989a).

### (iii)   *Chromium[VI] compounds*

*Potassium dichromate, sodium dichromate, ammonium dichromate, potassium chromate, sodium chromate, ammonium chromate and chromium trioxide*

Highly soluble chromium[VI] compounds were assayed in several acellular systems. Potassium dichromate did not induce cross-links of *E. coli* [³H]DNA to bovine serum albumin (Fornace *et al.*, 1981). It inhibited DNA synthesis by decreasing nucleotide incorporation into calf thymus DNA in the presence of *E. coli* DNA polymerase (Nishio & Uyeki, 1985). Potassium dichromate (Sponza & Levis, 1980 [Abstract]; Bianchi *et al.*, 1983) and chromium trioxide (Sirover & Loeb, 1976; Tkeshelashvili *et al.*, 1980) decreased the fidelity of DNA synthesis by altering the ratio of incorporation of radiolabelled complementary to noncomplementary nucleotides. In these studies, the synthetic polynucleotide poly[d(A-T)] was used as a template in the presence of viral (avian myeloblastosis virus), bacterial (*E. coli*) and mammalian (calf thymus) DNA polymerase (Miyaki *et al.*, 1977). Chromium trioxide induced depurination in calf thymus DNA by enhancing the release of guanine, whereas no effect was produced on the release of adenine (Schaaper *et al.*, 1987). Potassium dichromate induced breakage in the polynucleotide chain of purified DNA and RNA, as inferred from studies of viscosity, ultraviolet absorption spectra and thermal denaturation patterns (Tamino & Peretta, 1980; Tamino *et al.*, 1981). Sodium chromate induced single-strand breaks in supercoiled circular DNA of the bacterial phage PM2, but only when combined with glutathione. Of two purified reaction products, the chromium[V] complex Na$_4$(glutathione)$_4$CrV.8H$_2$O cleared supercoiled PM2 DNA, whereas the final product, the chromium[III]-glutathione complex was inactive (Kortenkamp *et al.*, 1989). A positive (Tkeshelashvili *et al.*, 1980) and a negative result (Schaaper *et al.*, 1987) were reported for the recovery of viral infectivity of single-stranded φX174 DNA which, following treatment with chromium trioxide, was transfected into *E. coli* spheroplasts (*am3* reversion). Potassium chromate induced *lacZα* forward mutation in double-stranded M13mp2 DNA transfected into JM101 *E. coli* (Snow & Xu, 1989). Gel electrophoresis analysis demonstrated production of oligonucleotides from [$^{32}$P-5']-end-labelled DNA fragments treated with sodium chromate only in the presence of hydrogen peroxide (Kawanishi *et al.*, 1986). Several of these studies showed that chromium[VI] compounds are less active than chromium[III] compounds in simplified systems (See General Remarks, p. 43, for a discussion of the biological activity of chromium[VI] and chromium[III] compounds.)

DNA-damaging effects were observed by treating bacteria with highly soluble chromium[VI] compounds. Thus, potassium dichromate produced DNA fragmentation in strain WP2 of *E. coli*; this effect, detected by alkaline sucrose gradient sedimentation, was attenuated by α-tocopherol (Kalinina & Minseitova, 1983a,b). λ Prophage was induced by potassium chromate in *E. coli* WP2$_s$ (Rossman *et al.*, 1984). An SOS response, inferred from induction of an SOS operator gene coupled with a gene coding for β-galactosidase in *E. coli*, was elicited by sodium dichromate in strain PQ37 (De Flora *et al.*, 1985a), by potassium dichromate, potassium chromate and chromium trioxide in strains GC2375, UA4202 and PQ30 (Llagostera *et al.*, 1986), and by potassium dichromate and potassium chromate in strain PQ37 (Venier *et al.*, 1989) and in strains PQ35 and PQ37 (Olivier & Marzin, 1987). Potassium dichromate also showed SOS-inducing activity in strain TA1535/pSK1002 of *S. typhimurium* (Nakamura *et al.*, 1987).

As shown by means of various techniques (spot test, streak method, treat-and-plate test, liquid test), soluble chromium[VI] compounds induce nonreparable DNA damage in repair-deficient bacteria. In particular, potassium dichromate, sodium dichromate, ammonium dichromate, potassium chromate, sodium chromate, ammonium chromate and chromium trioxide were active in the *rec* assay in *B. subtilis* in strains H17 (wild-type) and M45 (*rec⁻*) (Nishioka, 1975; Nakamuro *et al.*, 1978; Kada *et al.*, 1980; Kanematsu *et al.*, 1980; Matsui, 1980; Gentile *et al.*, 1981). Potassium dichromate, sodium dichromate, ammonium dichromate, sodium chromate and chromium trioxide were more toxic in strain TA1538 (*rec⁻*) than in the parental strain (TA1978) of *S. typhimurium* (Gentile *et al.*, 1981). Potassium dichromate, ammonium dichromate and potassium chromate were equally toxic in wild strain WP2 and in WP2*uvrA* (*uvrA-*) but more toxic in CM571 (*recA⁻*) and in WP100 (*uvrA⁻recA⁻*) than in WP2 (Yagi & Nishioka, 1977). Sodium dichromate was more toxic in TM1080 (*polA⁻ lexA⁻* R factor) and CM871 (*uvrA⁻recA⁻lexA⁻*) than in the *E. coli* wild strain (WP2). No lethality was observed in WP2*uvrA* (*uvrA⁻*) or WP67 (*uvrA⁻polA⁻*) (Petrilli & De Flora, 1982). The lethality of sodium dichromate, potassium chromate, ammonium chromate and chromium trioxide to the triple mutant CM871 (*uvrA⁻recA⁻lexA⁻*) was greater than to WP2; this was not the case for WP67 (*uvrA⁻polA⁻*) (De Flora *et al.*, 1984a). [The Working Group noted that these results indicate the importance of the *rec* and *lex* SOS functions, rather than of the polymerase mechanism and *uvr* excision repair system, in repairing DNA damage produced by chromium[VI] in bacteria.]

Reversion to luminescence (bioluminescence test) was induced by potassium dichromate in strain Pf-13 of *Photobacterium fischeri* (Ulitzur & Barak, 1988). Reversion to *arg* autotrophy was induced by potassium dichromate and potassium chromate in *E. coli* strain Hs30R (Nakamuro *et al.*, 1978), and by sodium chromate in K12-343-113(λ) (Mohn & Ellenberger, 1977). The ability of soluble chromium[VI] compounds to revert *E. coli* to *trp* auxotrophy was reported by Venitt and Levy (1974) for sodium chromate (strains WP2 and WP2*uvrA*) and potassium chromate (WP2, WP2*uvrA* and WP2*exrA*), by Nishioka (1975) for potassium dichromate (WP2 and WP2*uvrA*, CM871 being insensitive), by Green *et al.* (1976) for potassium chromate (WP2), by Nestmann *et al.* (1979) for chromium trioxide (WP2*uvrA*, but only in a fluctuation test), by Petrilli and De Flora (1982) for sodium dichromate (WP2 and WP2*uvrA*), by Venitt and Bosworth (1983) for potassium dichromate (WP2*uvrA*, further increased under anaerobic growth conditions) and by Venier *et al.* (1987) for potassium dichromate (WP2*uvrA*, further increased by NTA). The only negative result was reported by Kanematsu *et al.* (1980), who identified potassium dichromate as a mutagen (in WP2*hcr⁻* only, WP2 *try⁻* being insensitive) but failed to detect the mutagenicity of chromium trioxide (in either WP2 or WP2*hcr⁻*). Potassium chromate had no effect on ultraviolet-induced mutagenesis in WP2 (Rossman & Molina, 1986).

The mutagenicity of soluble chromium[VI] compounds in *his- S. typhimurium* and its modulation were investigated in a large number of laboratories, using various techniques (spot test, spiral test, plate test and preincubation test). A number of studies yielded positive results (Tamaro *et al.*, 1975; Petrilli & De Flora, 1977; De Flora, 1978; Petrilli & De Flora, 1978b; Nestmann *et al.*, 1979; De Flora, 1981a,b; Tso & Fung, 1981; Petrilli & De Flora, 1982; Venier *et al.*, 1982; Bennicelli *et al.*, 1983; Bianchi *et al.*, 1983; Beyersmann *et al.*, 1984; De Flora *et al.*, 1984a,b; Arlauskas *et al.*, 1985; Langerwerf *et al.*, 1985; Loprieno *et al.*, 1985; Marzin & Phi, 1985; LaVelle, 1986a,b; Vieux *et al.*, 1986 [Abstract]; Farrell *et al.*, 1989). Negative results were reported in all the strains tested in one study only (Kanematsu *et al.*, 1980) [doses were not reported]. Using the replicate plate technique, Pedersen *et al.* (1983) claimed that a high proportion of *S. typhimurium his⁺* revertant colonies were false, but this conclusion was criticized by Baker *et al.* (1984), using the same technique. In general, with the exception of TA1535, all *his S. typhimurium* strains tested were reverted by chromium[VI]. The following ranking of sensitivity was reported:

TA102 > TA100 > TA97 > TA92 > TA1978 > TA98 > TA1538 > TA1537 (Bennicelli *et al.*, 1983). Other sensitive strains included TA103 (Gava *et al.*, 1989b), TA104 (De Flora *et al.*, 1988; Gava *et al.*, 1989b), TA94 (Langerwerf *et al.*, 1985), TS26 (LaVelle, 1986a) and GV19 (LaVelle, 1986b). The nitroreductase-deficient derivative strain TA100NR was even more sensitive than TA100, which suggests a diminution of the mutagenicity of chromium[VI] by bacterial nitroreductases (De Flora *et al.*, 1989b). Reversion patterns indicate that chromium[VI] induces frameshift errors in bacterial DNA and, to a greater extent, base-pair substitution at both GC base-pairs (TA100) and AT base-pairs (TA102, TA104). The latter two strains are known to be sensitive to oxidative mutagens. In any case, the presence of plasmid pKM101 in the most sensitive strains indicates that the mutagenicity of chromium[VI] is amplified through error-prone DNA repair pathways, which is consistent with the results of the DNA-repair tests reported above. The potency of chromium[VI] compounds correlated with their chromium[VI] content, being in the range of a few revertants per nanomole chromium[VI] in TA100 and TA102 (De-Flora, 1981a; De Flora *et al.*, 1984a,b). Since the potency of mutagens of various chemical classes tested in the same laboratory varied between $2 \times 10^{-6}$ and $1.4 \times 10^{4}$ revertants/nmol ($6.8 \times 10^{9}$-fold range), chromium[VI] compounds can be classified as mutagens of medium potency in this test system (De Flora *et al.*, 1984b).

The bacterial mutagenicity of potassium dichromate was also confirmed in forward mutation assay in *E. coli*, testing acquired resistance to rifampicin in AB1157 and derived *recA⁻*, *recB⁻*, *recC⁻*, *recF⁻* and *sbc⁻* strains (Kalinina & Minseitowa, 1983b,c), *lacI⁺/lacI⁻* mutation in strain KMBL3835 (Zakour & Glickman, 1984), and replication of integrated λ genes in strain CHY832 (RK test) (Hayes *et al.*, 1984). Chromium trioxide induced Ara^r forward mutation in strains BA9 and BA13 of *S. typhimurium* (Ruiz-Rubio *et al.*, 1985). Potassium chromate did not induce forward or back mutations in a fluctuation test with K-12-derived *E. coli* strains but enhanced the frameshift mutagenicity of 9-aminoacridine (LaVelle, 1986a).

Reducing chemicals (ascorbic acid and sodium sulfite) and glutathione, NADH and NADPH decreased the bacterial mutagenicity of various chromium[VI] compounds (Petrilli & De Flora, 1978b; De Flora *et al.*, 1985b; Petrilli *et al.*, 1986a). A similar reducing effect was induced by other sulfur compounds, such as *N*-acetylcysteine (De Flora *et al.*, 1984c), cysteine (Petrilli *et al.*, 1986a) and dithiothreitol (Rogers *et al.*, 1987 [Abstract]). The mutagenicity of potassium dichromate was also considerably decreased by anaerobic growth conditions, but not by addition of the hydroxyl ion scavenger mannitol (Rogers *et al.*, 1987 [Abstract]). The mutagenicity of soluble chromium[VI] compounds was not affected or was poorly affected by addition of soda ash, diethyl ether, prostaglandin or ethylenediaminetetraacetic acid (Petrilli & De Flora, 1982; Petrilli *et al.*, 1986a) or complex mixtures (crude oil, oil dispersants) (Petrilli *et al.*, 1980; De Flora *et al.*, 1985a), whereas it was inhibited by other metals (Sokolowska & Jongen, 1984 [Abstract]). Sodium dichromate and unfractionated cigarette smoke condensate had antagonistic mutagenic effects (Petrilli & De Flora, 1982). The mutagenicity of potassium dichromate was increased by nitrilotriacetic acid (Gava *et al.*, 1989a). Potassium chromate decreased the mutagenicity of ethyl methanesulfonate and increased that of sodium azide (LaVelle & Witmer, 1984) and of its metabolite azidoalanine (LaVelle, 1986b); more than additive effects were observed with 9-aminoacridine (LaVelle, 1986a).

The mutagenicity of soluble chromium[VI] compounds in *S. typhimurium* was consistently decreased by rat liver post-mitochondrial supernatant in all studies in which this aspect was evaluated (De Flora, 1978; Löfroth, 1978; Petrilli & De Flora, 1978b; Nestmann *et al.*, 1979; Petrilli & De Flora, 1980; De Flora, 1981a; Petrilli & De Flora, 1982; Venier *et al.*, 1982; Bianchi *et al.*, 1983; De Flora *et al.*, 1984a; Loprieno *et al.*, 1985; Petrilli *et al.*, 1986b). The polychlorinated biphenyl Aroclor 1254 was the most efficient inducer of this effect, followed in activity by phenobarbital and 3-methylcholanthrene (Petrilli *et al.*, 1985). Pretreatment of rats with *N*-acetylcysteine also stimulated reduction of chromium[VI] by liver and lung post-mitochondrial supernatant (De Flora *et al.*, 1985c). The effect of the rat liver fraction on the mutagenicity of various chromium[VI] compounds was inhibited by dicoumarol, a specific inhibitor of the cytosolic enzyme DT diaphorase (De Flora *et al.*, 1987b); purified DT diaphorase itself decreased the mutagenicity of sodium dichromate (De Flora *et al.*, 1988). The mutagenicity of sodium dichromate was also decreased by liver preparations from other animal species, including fish (*Salmo gairdneri*) (De Flora *et al.*, 1982), chicken, hamster (De Flora *et al.*, 1985d), Pekin duck (De Flora *et al.*, 1989a), mouse (De Flora, 1982), woodchuck (De Flora *et al.*, 1987c, 1989c) and humans (De Flora, 1982). Moreover, mutagenicity was decreased by thermostable components of human gastric juice (De Flora & Boido, 1980; De Flora *et al.*, 1987a), with peaks of reducing activity during post-meal periods following stimulation of gastric secretion (De Flora *et al.*, 1987a). Human erythrocyte lysates decreased the mutagenicity of chromium[VI] (Petrilli & De Flora, 1978b); human and rat pulmonary alveolar macrophages were particularly efficient (Petrilli *et al.*, 1986c). Human peripheral lung parenchyma decreased the mutagenicity of chromium[VI] more efficiently than a post-mitochondrial supernatant of bronchial tree (Petruzzelli *et al.*, 1989); as assessed from 71 surgical specimens from cancer and noncancer patients, the ability of lung parenchyma to decrease the mutagenicity of chromium[VI] was significantly enhanced in cigarette smokers (De Flora *et al.*, 1987d). In rats, the inhibitory effect of lung was autoinduced by repeated intratracheal instillations of sodium dichromate (Petrilli *et al.*, 1985). Comparative assays provided evidence that the reducing capacity of rat tissue post-mitochondrial supernatant ranked as follows: liver > adrenal > kidney >

testis > stomach and lung; preparations of skeletal muscle, spleen and intestine had no effect on the mutagenicity of chromium[VI] (Petrilli & De Flora, 1978b, 1980, 1982). Further assays confirmed the negligible effect of rat muscle (which is a typical target of the carcinogenicity of chromium[VI] in bioassays) in decreasing the mutagenicity of chromium[VI], as compared to liver and, to a lesser extent, to cutis and subcutis (De Flora *et al.*, 1989a). The selective loss of chromium[VI] mutagenicity was accompanied by the disappearance of measurable chromium[VI] in the presence of various body fluids and cell and tissue preparations. [The Working Group interpreted these findings as indicating mechanisms that limit the activity of chromium[VI] compounds *in vivo*.]

Forward mutation and mitotic gene conversion were induced by potassium dichromate in the yeast *Schizosaccharomyces pombe* (Bonatti *et al.*, 1976). The same compound induced reversion ($ilv^- \rightarrow ilv^+$) and mitotic gene conversion in strain D7 of *Saccharomyces cerevisiae* (Singh, 1983; Galli *et al.*, 1985; Kharab & Singh, 1985). Conversely, chromium trioxide elicited gene conversion and mitotic crossing-over but failed to revert the same yeast strain (Fukunaga *et al.*, 1982). Potassium dichromate slightly enhanced recombination frequency in strain D1513 of *Saccharomyces cerevisiae* and produced disomic and diploid gametes (Sora *et al.*, 1986), but it did not induce mitochondrial 'petite' mutants in strain D7 (Kharab & Singh, 1987).

Neither potassium chromate nor chromium trioxide induced micronuclei in pollen mother cells of *Tradescantia paludosa* (Ma *et al.*, 1984). In contrast, further studies indicated a dose-dependent increase in the induction of micronuclei by chromium trioxide, which was significantly inhibited by cysteine (Zhang *et al.*, 1984).

In *Drosophila melanogaster*, sodium dichromate gave positive results in a somatic eye-colour test (*zeste* mutation) (Rasmuson, 1985). Both potassium dichromate and chromium trioxide induced sex-linked recessive lethal mutations, but only potassium dichromate induced non-disjunction and X-Y chromosome loss at a dose corresponding to the $LD_{50}$ (Rodriguez-Arnaiz & Molina Martinez, 1986). The induction of sex-linked recessive lethal mutations by potassium dichromate was enhanced by NTA (Gava *et al.*, 1989b).

A variety of genetic and related endpoints were explored in cultured mammalian cells. Potassium dichromate produced alterations of the mitotic index and of mitotic phases in human epithelial-like heteroploid HEp-2 cells (Majone, 1977; Levis & Majone, 1981) and NHIK 3025 cervix tissue cells (Bakke *et al.*, 1984), and imbalance of the endogenous adenylate pool in Syrian hamster BHK fibroblasts (Levis *et al.*, 1978b; Bianchi *et al.*, 1982a). It inhibited DNA synthesis, as evaluated by [3]H-thymidine incorporation, in mouse L cells (Nishio & Uyeki, 1985), in BHK fibroblasts and in HEp-2 cells (Levis *et al.*, 1977, 1978a,b), in which a secondary inhibition of RNA and protein syntheses was also observed (Levis *et al.*, 1978b).

Inhibition of DNA synthesis was further enhanced following reversible permeabilization of cells in hypertonic medium (Bianchi *et al.*, 1984). Potassium dichromate also reduced the colony-forming ability of BHK cells by a multi-hit mechanism of cell inactivation (Levis *et al.*, 1978a). Unscheduled DNA synthesis was induced by potassium dichromate in mouse kidney A18BcR cells (Raffetto *et al.*, 1977) but not in human EUE heteroploid cells (Bianchi *et al.*, 1982b, 1983); potassium chromate induced unscheduled DNA synthesis in human skin fibroblasts (Whiting *et al.*, 1979). Chromium trioxide inhibited repair of γ-ray-induced chromosome breaks in human peripheral blood lymphocytes (Morimoto & Koizumi, 1981).

DNA fragmentation and cross-links were produced by soluble chromium[VI] compounds in a number of cultured mammalian cell lines, as assessed by various techniques, including alkaline elution, alkaline sucrose gradient, nucleoid sedimentation, alkaline unwinding, the nick translation assay, and polyacrylamide gel electrophoresis (Table 25). An exception was a study by alkaline elution in Chinese hamster V79 cells with potassium dichromate (Bianchi *et al.*, 1983).

In the *hprt* forward mutation assay, potassium chromate did not induce 8-azaguanidine–resistant mutants in mouse mammary carcinoma FM3A cells, in contrast to the activity of potassium dichromate and chromium trioxide in the same system (Nishimura & Umeda, 1978 [Abstract]). An unspecified chromate induced 6-thioguanine resistance in Chinese hamster V79 cells (Beyersmann & Köster, 1987). Potassium dichromate induced 8-azaguanidine resistance and 6-thioguanidine resistance in Chinese hamster V79 cells (Newbold *et al.*, 1979; Rainaldi *et al.*, 1982; Paschin *et al.*, 1981; Bianchi *et al.*, 1983); its mutagenic activity was decreased by thiotepa (Paschin & Kozachenko, 1982), unaffected by nitrilotriacetic acid (Celotti *et al.*, 1987) and enhanced by nickel[II] (Hartwig & Beyersmann, 1987). In comparative assays, Chinese hamster V79 cells were found to be more sensitive to chromium[VI] than Chinese hamster CHO cells (Paschin *et al.*, 1983). The combined use of selective 8-azaguanidine-resistant and ouabain-resistant systems showed that potassium dichromate can also induce base-pair substitutions in the DNA of V79 cells (Rainaldi *et al.*, 1982). Potassium dichromate and potassium chromate induced forward mutation at the thymidine kinase locus in mouse lymphoma L5178Y cells (Oberly *et al.*, 1982). As assessed in an assay for the synthesis of P-100$^{gag-mos}$ viral proteins, sodium chromate induced expression of the *v-mos* gene in MuSVts110-infected rat kidney 6m2 cells (Biggart & Murphy, 1988).

Soluble chromium[VI] compounds consistently increased the frequency of sister chromatid exchange (Table 26). The highest frequency of induction was observed in the early S-phase of the human lymphocyte cycle (Stella *et al.*, 1982).

**Table 25. Studies in which DNA fragmentation and DNA–DNA and DNA–protein cross–linking were induced in cultured mammalian cells by soluble chromium[VI] compounds**

| Chromium compound | Cell line | Comment | Reference |
|---|---|---|---|
| Potassium dichromate | Mouse L1210 leukaemia | | Fornace et al. (1981) |
| | Novikoff ascitic hepatoma | | Wedrychowski et al. (1986a) |
| | Chinese hamster CHO | | Brambilla et al. (1980) [Abstract]; Hamilton–Koch et al. (1986) |
| | Human foreskin HSBP fibroblasts | Detected by alkaline sucrose gradient but not nick translation, nucleoid sedimentation or alkaline un-winding | Hamilton–Koch et al. (1986); Snyder (1988) |
| | | Enhanced by glutathione, unaffected by hydroxyl radical scavengers (mannitol, iodine), diminished by superoxide dismutase and catalase | |
| | Human white blood | | McLean et al. (1982) |
| Sodium dichromate | Rat primary hepatocytes | | Sina et al. (1983) |
| Potassium chromate | Mouse L1210 leukaemia | | Fornace et al. (1981) |
| | Chinese hamster CHO fibroblasts | DNA–protein cross–linkage, probably due to chromium[III] | Miller & Costa (1988, 1989) |
| | Human embryo lung IMR–90 fibroblasts | | Fornace et al. (1981) |
| | Human skin fibroblasts | At 7th–8th passage | Whiting et al. (1979) |
| | Human CRL1223 fibroblasts | | Fornace (1982) |
| | Human AG1522 fibroblasts | | Fornace (1982) |
| | Human XP12BE fibroblasts | Similar effect in normal xeroderma pigmentosum cells | Fornace (1982) |
| | Novikoff ascitic hepatoma | | Wedrychowski et al. (1986b) |
| | Human bronchial epithelium | | Fornace et al. (1981) |

**Table 25 (contd)**

| Chromium compound | Cell line | Comment | Reference |
|---|---|---|---|
| Sodium chromate | Chick embryo hepatocytes | Related to glutathione and cytochrome P450 metabolism | Tsapakos et al. (1983b); Cupo & Wetterhahn (1984, 1985b) |
| | Chinese hamster V79 | Decreased by α-tocopherol; increased by riboflavin and sodium sulfite; DNA–protein breaks recognized by poly(ADT–ribose)polymerase | Sugiyama et al. (1987, 1988) |
| Chromium trioxide | Novikoff ascitic hepatoma | | Wedrychowski et al. (1986a) |

**Table 26. Studies in which sister chromatid exchange was induced in cultured mammalian cells by chromium[VI] compounds**

| Chromium compound | Cell line | Comment[a] | Reference |
|---|---|---|---|
| Potassium dichromate | Mouse lymphocytes LSTRA BALB mouse primary lympho- cytes | BALB cells carrying endogenized Moloney leukaemia virus more sensitive than uninfected cells | Bianchi et al. (1983) Bianchi et al. (1983); Majone et al. (1983) |
| | Mouse macrophage P388D, Mouse embryo blastocytes Chinese hamster CHO | | Andersen (1983) Iijima et al. (1983b) Levis & Majone (1979); Majone & Levis (1979); Bianchi et al. (1980); Levis & Majone (1981); Majone et al. (1982); Venier et al. (1982); Majone et al. (1982); Uyeki & Nishio (1983); Loprieno et al. (1985); Montaldi et al. (1987b) |
| | Chinese hamster V79 Chinese hamster lung Don Syrian hamster BHK fibroblasts Human peripheral blood lym- phocytes | Increased in permeabilized cells | Rainaldi et al. (1982) Ohno et al. (1982) Bianchi et al. (1984) Ogawa et al. (1978); Gómez-Arroyo et al. (1981); Imreh & Radulescu (1982 [Ab- stract]); Stella et al. (1982); Andersen (1983) |
| | Human skin fibroblasts | | Macrae et al. (1979) |
| Sodium dichromate | Chinese hamster CHO Chinese hamster V79 | | Levis & Majone (1979); Majone & Levis (1979); Bianchi et al. (1980) Elias et al. (1983) |
| Potassium chromate | Chinese hamster CHO | | Levis & Majone (1979); Macrae et al. (1979); Majone & Rensi (1979); Bianchi et al. (1980); Majone et al. (1982) |
| | Chinese hamster V79 | | Price-Jones et al. (1980); Elias et al. (1983) |

**Table 26 (contd)**

| Chromium compound | Cell line | Comment[a] | Reference |
|---|---|---|---|
| Potassium chromate (contd) | Chinese hamster lung Don | | Ohno et al. (1982) |
| | Human skin fibroblasts | | Macrae et al. (1979) |
| | Human peripheral blood lymphocytes | | Douglas et al. (1980) |
| Sodium chromate | Chinese hamster CHO | | Levis & Majone (1979); Bianchi et al. (1980) |
| | Chinese hamster V79 | | Elias et al. (1983) |
| Chromium trioxide | Chinese hamster CHO | | Levis & Majone (1979); Bianchi et al. (1980) |
| | Chinese hamster lung Don | | Koshi (1979); Ohno et al. (1982) |
| | Human peripheral blood lymphocytes | | Gómez-Arroyo et al. (1981) |
| Calcium chromate | Chinese hamster CHO | Increased in presence of NTA | Venier et al. (1985b); Sen & Costa (1986) |
| Lead chromate | Human peripheral blood lymphocytes | Dissolved in NaOH | Douglas et al. (1980) |
| Strontium chromate | Chinese hamster CHO | Increased in presence of NTA | Venier et al. (1985b) |
| Zinc chromates | Chinese hamster CHO | Increased in presence of NaOH or NTA | Levis & Majone (1981); Venier et al. (1985b) |
| | Chinese hamster V79 | | Elias et al. (1983) |
| Basic zinc chromates | Chinese hamster CHO | Increased in presence of NaOH or NTA | Levis & Majone (1981); Venier et al. (1985b) |
| Zinc chromate | Chinese hamster CHO | Increased in presence of NTA | Venier et al. (1985b) |
| Barium chromate | Chinese hamster CHO | Increased in presence of NTA | Venier et al. (1985b) |

**Table 26 (contd)**

| Chromium compound | Cell line | Comment[a] | Reference |
|---|---|---|---|
| Lead chromate | Chinese hamster CHO | Increased in presence of NTA | Montaldi et al. (1987a,b) |
| | Chinese hamster CHO | Increased in presence of NTA | Loprieno et al. (1985) |
| | Human peripheral blood lymphocytes | Dissolved in NaOH | Douglas et al. (1980) |
| Chromium yellow | Chinese hamster CHO | Increased in presence of NTA | Venier et al. (1985b) |
| | Chinese hamster CHO | Increased in presence of NaOH | Levis & Majone (1981) |
| Chromium orange | Chinese hamster CHO | Increased in presence of NaOH | Levis & Majone (1981) |
| | Chinese hamster CHO | | Loprieno et al. (1985) |
| Molybdenum orange | Chinese hamster CHO | Increased in presence of NTA | Venier et al. (1985b) |
| | Chinese hamster CHO | Increased in presence of NaOH | Levis & Majone (1981) |

[a]NTA, nitrilotriacetic acid

As reported in an abstract, potassium dichromate also increased the frequency of micronucleated cells in human lymphocytes cultured *in vitro* (Imreh & Radulescu, 1982).

In many studies, the induction of chromosomal aberrations was investigated, often in parallel with assessments of the frequency of sister chromatid exchange; all of them gave positive results (Table 27). Chromatid-type aberrations, mainly gaps, breaks and chromatid exchanges, were the most frequently reported aberrations (Levis & Bianchi, 1982).

Two studies dealt with the induction of aneuploidy by soluble chromium[VI] salts in cultured mammalian cells: no increase in the number of aneuploids or polyploids was detected following treatment of Chinese hamster V79 cells with potassium chromate (Price-Jones *et al.*, 1980). Sodium chromate, however, exhibited spindle-modifying properties in human skin fibroblasts, as assessed by means of a differential staining technique for chromosomes and spindles, alterations in which may represent one of the major causes of aneuploidy (Nijs & Kirsch-Volders, 1986).

The majority of studies provided evidence that soluble chromium[VI] salts can induce cell transformation in different experimental systems. In particular, as evaluated by means of the soft agar assay, potassium dichromate produced anchorage-independent growth of Syrian hamster BHK fibroblasts (Bianchi *et al.*, 1983; Hansen & Stern, 1985), which was further enhanced in the presence of NTA (Lanfranchi *et al.*, 1988). [See General Remarks, p. 44, for concern about this assay.] The same compound induced morphological transformation of Syrian hamster embryo (SHE) primary cells (Tsuda & Kato, 1977; Hansen & Stern, 1985) and of mouse fetal cells at the third passage (Raffetto *et al.*, 1977), whereas a negative result was reported in mouse embryo C3H10T1/2 cells (Patierno *et al.*, 1988). [See General Remarks, p. 44, for concerns about this assay.] Sodium chromate also induced morphological transformation of SHE primary cells (DiPaolo & Casto, 1979), but potassium chromate did not, although it potentiated the transforming capacity of benzo[a]pyrene (Rivedal & Sanner, 1981); it also enhanced the morphological transformation induced by the simian adenovirus SA7 in SHE primary cells (Casto *et al.*, 1979).

Several studies were also carried out with soluble chromium[VI] compounds *in vivo*. Following intraperitoneal injection to Sprague-Dawley rats, sodium dichromate induced a selective DNA fragmentation in different tissues, as assessed by means of the alkaline elution technique. In particular, liver nuclei contained protein-associated DNA single-strand breaks as well as DNA-protein cross-links, whereas kidney nuclei contained mainly DNA-protein cross-links (Tsapakos *et al.*, 1981) and lung nuclei contained both DNA interstrand and DNA-protein cross-links (Tsapakos *et al.*, 1983a). These lesions were repaired most rapidly in the liver, which may provide a partial explanation of the differential toxicity of

**Table 27. Studies in which chromosomal aberrations were induced in cultured mammalian cells by chromium[VI] compounds**

| Chromium compound | Cell line | Comment[a] | Reference |
|---|---|---|---|
| Potassium dichromate | Mouse tertiary fetal | | Raffetto et al. (1977) |
| | Mouse mammary carcinoma Fm3A | | Umeda & Nishimura (1979) |
| | Rat peripheral blood lymphocytes | | Newton & Lilly (1986) |
| | Rat embryo fibroblasts | | Bigaliev et al. (1977a) |
| | Syrian hamster embryo primary | Inhibited by sodium sulfite | Tsuda & Kato (1977) |
| | Chinese hamster CHO | | Levis & Majone (1979); Majone & Levis (1979); Bianchi et al. (1980); Levis & Majone (1981); Venier et al. (1982) |
| | Chinese hamster V79 | | Newbold et al. (1979) |
| | Human peripheral blood lymphocytes | | Nakamuro et al. (1978); Imreh & Radulescu (1982 [Abstract]); Stella et al. (1982) |
| Sodium dichromate | Chinese hamster CHO | | Levis & Majone (1979); Majone & Levis (1979); Bianchi et al. (1980) |
| | Human peripheral blood lymphocytes | | Sarto et al. (1980) |
| Potassium chromate | Mouse mammary carcinoma Fm3A | | Umeda & Nishimura (1979) |
| | Chinese hamster CHO | | Levis & Majone (1979); Majone & Rensi (1979); Bianchi et al. (1980) |
| | Chinese hamster lung Don | | Koshi & Iwasaki (1983) |
| | Human skin fibroblasts | | Macrae et al. (1979) |
| | Human peripheral blood lymphocytes | | Nakamuro et al. (1978); Douglas et al. (1980) |
| Sodium chromate | Chinese hamster CHO | | Levis & Majone (1979); Bianchi et al. (1980) |

**Table 27 (contd)**

| Chromium compound | Cell line | Comment[a] | Reference |
|---|---|---|---|
| Chromium trioxide | Mouse mammary carcinoma Fm3A | | Umeda & Nishimura (1979) |
| | Syrian hamster embryo primary | | Tsuda & Kato (1977) |
| | Chinese hamster CHO | | Levis & Majone (1979); Bianchi et al. (1980) |
| | Chinese hamster lung Don | | Koshi (1979) |
| | Human peripheral blood lymphocytes | | Kaneko (1976) |
| Calcium chromate | Mouse embryo C3H10T1/2 | Random damage | Sen et al. (1987) |
| | Chinese hamster CHO | Random damage | Levis & Majone (1979); Sen et al. (1987) |
| | Chinese hamster lung Don | | Koshi & Iwasaki (1983) |
| Basic zinc chromates | Chinese hamster CHO | Increased in presence of NaOH | Levis & Majone (1981) |
| Zinc chromate | Chinese hamster lung Don | | Koshi & Iwasaki (1983) |
| Lead chromate | Chinese hamster CHO | Increased in presence of NaOH or NTA | Levis & Majone (1981); Montaldi et al. (1987b) |
| | Chinese hamster lung Don | | Koshi & Iwasaki (1983) |
| | Human peripheral blood lymphocytes | Increased in presence of NaOH | Douglas et al. (1980) |

[a]NTA, nitrilotriacetic acid

chromium[VI] in these organs (Tsapakos et al., 1983a). Following its injection onto the inner shell membrane of eggs, sodium dichromate produced single-strand breaks in blood cells and DNA cross-links in liver cells of chicken embryos (Hamilton & Wetterhahn, 1986). Intraperitoneally injected potassium dichromate inhibited DNA repair synthesis in rat lymphocytes (Rudnykh & Saichenko, 1985); it was active in a mammalian spot test in C57Bl/6J/BOM mice, but only when administered at 10 mg/kg and not at 20 mg/kg (Knudsen, 1980).

Intraperitoneal injection of potassium dichromate or potassium chromate to Chinese hamsters induced sister chromatid exchange in bone-marrow cells and an increased frequency of micronucleated polychromatic erythrocytes (Kaths, 1981). Micronucleated polychromatic erythrocytes were also enhanced by potassium dichromate in BALB/c mice (Fabry, 1980) and in CBA × C57Bl/6J mice (Paschin & Toropsev, 1982, 1983) and by potassium chromate in NMRI mice (Wild, 1978), ms and ddY mice, the former strain being more sensitive (Hayashi et al., 1982). Comparative trials in various mouse strains showed no important sex-related variation in induction of micronucleated cells by chromium[VI] and confirmed the different susceptibilities of different strains (rank of sensitivity: ms > BDF1 > CD-1 > ddY) (Collaborative Study Group for the Micronucleus Test, 1986, 1988).

Chromosomal aberrations were induced in gill tissue cells of *Boleophthalmus dussumieri* fish by intramuscular injection or addition to water of sodium dichromate (Krishnaja & Rege, 1982). Potassium dichromate induced chromosomal rearrangements and aneuploidy in rat bone–marrow cells when given orally or intratracheally (Bigaliev et al., 1977b). Following intraperitoneal or intravenous injection, it produced chromosomal aberrations in lymphocytes and bone-marrow cells (Newton & Lilly, 1986). Intraperitoneal injection of potassium dichromate was also clastogenic to bone-marrow cells of BALB/c mice (Léonard & Deknudt, 1981 [Abstract]), but no increase in chromosomal aberrations was observed in CBA × C57Bl/6J hybrid mice (Paschin et al., 1981). In the same animals, dominant lethal effects were produced at 2 mg/kg bw (21 doses) and 20 mg/kg bw (single dose) (Paschin et al., 1982) but not at 0.5-1.5 mg/kg bw (single dose) (Paschin et al., 1981). At 20 mg/kg bw, potassium dichromate reduced the rate of pregnancies in BALB/c mice (Léonard & Deknudt, 1981 [Abstract]; Deknudt, 1982 [Abstract]) but failed to produce dominant lethal effects (Léonard & Deknudt, 1981 [Abstract]).

*Calcium chromate, strontium chromate, basic zinc chromate*

Calcium chromate, strontium chromate and the industrial product, basic zinc chromate or zinc yellow [$ZnCrO_4.Zn(OH)_2$ plus 10% $CrO_3$], are generally completely dissolved in the media used in short-term tests. The results obtained in a variety of experimental systems thus virtually overlap with those reported for highly soluble chromium[VI] compounds.

Calcium chromate failed to induce an SOS response in strain PQ37 of *E. coli* (Brams *et al.*, 1987). In contrast, it was active in a differential killing assay in *E. coli* WP2, using the triple mutant CM871 (*uvrA⁻ recA⁻ lexA⁻*) (De Flora *et al.*, 1984a), and in the $trp^- \rightarrow trp^+$ reversion test with strains WP2 (Venitt & Levy, 1974) and WP2*uvrA* (Dunkel *et al.*, 1984). In the $his^- \rightarrow his^+$ reversion test in *S. typhimurium*, positive results were reported with calcium chromate (Petrilli & De Flora, 1977; De Flora, 1981a; Bennicelli *et al.*, 1983; Haworth *et al.*, 1983; De Flora *et al.*, 1984a, 1987b; Dunkel *et al.*, 1984; Petrilli *et al.*, 1985; Venier *et al.*, 1985b), strontium chromate (Venier *et al.*, 1985b) and zinc yellow (Petrilli & De Flora, 1978b; De Flora, 1981a). The potency, spectrum of sensitivity of *S. typhimurium* strains and behaviour in the presence of in-vitro metabolic systems were comparable to those reported for highly soluble chromium[VI] compounds. However, toxic effects of calcium chromate hampered the detection of forward and back mutations in the DNA of phage T4 grown in *E. coli* BB (Corbett *et al.*, 1970).

Calcium chromate induced 'petite' mutants in mitochondria of 19 haploid strains of *Saccharomyces cerevisiae* (Egilsson *et al.*, 1979) and produced differential chromosome breakage in excision-repair-deficient females of *Drosophila melanogaster* (*mei-9ª* test), with complete loss of the X or Y and partial loss of the Y chromosome (Zimmering, 1983).

Zinc yellow produced alterations of the mitotic cycle in human epithelial-like heteroploid HEp-2 cells (Levis & Majone, 1981). Calcium chromate stimulated DNA repair replication in Syrian hamster embryo primary cells, as evaluated by caesium chloride gradient density sedimentation (Robison *et al.*, 1984). It also produced DNA single-strand breaks, DNA interstrand and DNA-protein cross-links (alkaline elution technique) in mouse embryo C3H10T1/2 cells, Chinese hamster CHO cells and human osteosarcoma cells, the maximal sensitivity being recorded in early S-phase (Sugiyama *et al.*, 1986a,b); human cells were more sensitive than mouse or hamster cells (Sugiyama *et al.*, 1986b). In Chinese hamster CHO cells, calcium chromate produced single-strand breaks, induced alkali-labile sites (Cantoni & Costa, 1984) and, as assessed by alkaline sucrose gradient, decreased the DNA molecular weight (Robison *et al.*, 1982). DNA cross-links were more pronounced and only partially repaired in a repair-deficient line (EM9) as compared with CHO wild-type cells (AA8). Conversely, repair of single-strand breaks was similar in the two cell lines (Christie *et al.*, 1984). Calcium chromate produced strand breaks, detected by nucleoid gradient sedimentation, when applied to intact cells, but no breakage was observed when nucleoids were exposed directly to chromium[VI] (Robison *et al.*, 1984).

Calcium chromate induced forward mutation at the thymidine kinase locus in mouse lymphoma L5178Y cells, with no change (Myhr & Caspary, 1988) or decreased activity (McGregor *et al.*, 1987; Mitchell *et al.*, 1988) in the presence of rat liver post-mitochondrial supernatant. This salt induced dose-dependent cytotoxicity and forward mutation to 6-thioguanine resistance in Chinese hamster CHO cells but no mutation to ouabain resistance in the same cells or in mouse embryo C3H10T1/2 cells (Patierno et al., 1988).

The frequency of sister chromatid exchange was increased in Chinese hamster CHO cells by all three compounds (Table 26). In contrast to nickel, no predominance of sister chromatid exchange was observed in heterochromatic regions (Sen & Costa, 1986). Chromosomal aberrations, with a random distribution of chromosomal damage, were produced by calcium chromate and zinc yellow (Table 27). Aberrant division patterns and spindle modifications were also caused by calcium chromate in human skin fibroblasts (Nijs & Kirsch-Volders, 1986).

Several authors reported that calcium chromate could determine cell transformation in vitro in different systems: anchorage-independent growth of Syrian hamster BHK fibroblasts in carboxymethylcellulose, after several passages of treated cells (Fradkin et al., 1975) or in soft agar (Bianchi et al., 1983; Hansen & Stern, 1985), with an enhancing effect in the presence of NTA (Lanfranchi et al., 1988), attachment-independence of virus-infected rat embryo 2 $FR_4$ 50 cells (Traul et al., 1981) [see General Remarks for concern about this assay], morphological transformation of mouse BALB/3T3 cells, R-MulV-infected rat embryo cells and Syrian hamster embryo primary cells (Dunkel et al., 1981); and enhancement of morphological transformation in the same cells by the simian adenovirus SA7 (Casto et al., 1979). As reported for potassium dichromate, calcium chromate did not induce morphological transformation in mouse embryo C3H10T1/2 cells (Patierno et al., 1988).

Conflicting results were reported in studies in vivo with calcium chromate. It increased the frequency of sister chromatid exchange in bone-marrow cells of intraperitoneally injected Chinese hamsters (Kaths, 1981), whereas it failed to increase micronuclei in bone-marrow polychromatic erythrocytes of intraperitoneally injected BALB/c mice (Fabry, 1980) or Chinese hamsters (Kaths, 1981), and did not induce dominant lethal mutations in BALB/c mice (Léonard & Deknudt, 1981 [Abstract]).

*Zinc chromate, barium chromate, lead chromate and derived pigments (chromium orange, chromium yellow and molybdenum orange)*

An extensive data base is available concerning chromium[VI] compounds with poor solubility under the conditions used in experimental systems. These are zinc chromate, chromium orange or basic lead chromate [(PbCrO$_4$.PbO)], molybdenum orange (PbCrO$_4$.PbSO$_4$.PbMoO$_4$), barium chromate, chromium yellow (PbCrO$_4$.PbSO$_4$.SiO$_2$.Al$_2$O$_3$) and lead chromate, which is one of the most insoluble salts. As is to be expected, their activity in short-term tests was related to the availability of chromate to target cells, which was often achieved by artificial solubilization in acids or alkali, except in mammalian cells, where some penetration of insoluble compounds is likely to occur by phagocytosis.

Lead chromate did not induce differential killing in *E. coli* W3110 or P3478 (*polA⁻*), even when dissolved in sodium hydroxide (Nestmann *et al.*, 1979); this result parallels those reported with soluble chromium[VI] compounds in *polA⁻* strains. It was equally toxic in WP2 and in CM871 (*uvrA⁻ recA⁻ lexA⁻*), unless dissolved in NTA (Venier *et al.*, 1987). Lead chromate did not elicit the SOS response in *E. coli* PQ37, unless it was solubilized by NTA (Venier *et al.*, 1989).

Lead chromate reverted *E. coli* (*trp⁻ → trp⁺*), when assayed in a fluctuation test after preliminary solubilization in sodium hydroxide (Nestmann *et al.*, 1979) and in both the spot test and a fluctuation test when dissolved in NTA (Venier *et al.*, 1987). In the *his⁻ → his⁺* reversion test in *S. typhimurium*, zinc chromate was active in aqueous medium, and its mutagenicity was increased in the presence of sodium hydroxide or NTA (Venier *et al.*, 1985b). Chromium orange was mutagenic when spotted directly on the centre of agar plates and also became active in the plate test when dissolved in sodium hydroxide (Petrilli & De Flora, 1978b; De Flora, 1981a) or in NTA (Venier *et al.*, 1985b; Loprieno *et al.*, 1985). Likewise, molybdenum orange was mutagenic when spotted in solid form and in the plate test when dissolved in sodium hydroxide (De Flora, 1981a). Barium chromate was inactive unless dissolved in NTA (Venier *et al.*, 1985b). Lead chromate, tested following solubilization in acid or alkali, was mutagenic to the same strains that are sensitive to soluble chromium[VI] compounds (Nestmann *et al.*, 1979; Petrilli & De Flora, 1982). When tested in aqueous suspension, it was not mutagenic, but mutagenic chromate was released when it was dissolved in sodium hydroxide or NTA (Loprieno *et al.*, 1985; Venier *et al.*, 1985b, 1987). Its inactivity in strain TA102 was unaffected by the presence of oil dispersants (De Flora *et al.*, 1985a). Highly insoluble chromium yellow was inactive even when spotted in solid form; it became mutagenic in the plate test only when dissolved in sodium hydroxide (De Flora, 1981a; Petrilli & De Flora, 1982). In the *gal⁺/gal⁻* forward mutation test in strain K-12/343/113 (λ) of *E. coli*, lead chromate was inactive even when dissolved in sodium hydroxide (Nestmann *et al.*, 1979).

Lead chromate, dissolved in hydrochloric acid, induced mitotic recombination in strain D5 of *Saccharomyces cerevisiae*; the effect was decreased in the presence of rat liver post-mitochondrial supernatant (Nestmann *et al.*, 1979). It induced sex-linked recessive lethal mutations in *Drosophila melanogaster* only when dissolved in NTA (Costa *et al.*, 1988).

Alterations in the mitotic cycle were induced by the lead chromate-containing pigments, chromium orange, molybdenum orange and chromium yellow, in human epithelial-like heteroploid HEp-2 cells following a 48-h incubation in cell growth medium (Levis & Majone, 1981). Lead chromate, even when dissolved in sodium hydroxide, did not induce DNA fragmentation in Chinese hamster CHO cells, as evaluated by alkaline sucrose gradient (Douglas *et al.*, 1980), and it was not mutagenic in these cells, as evaluated in both 6-thioguanine- and ouabain-resistant systems; it did not induce ouabain or 6-thioguanine resistance in mouse embryo C3H10T1/2 cells (Patierno *et al.*, 1988). In the *hprt* assay in Chinese hamster V79 cells, lead chromate gave negative results both for 8-azaguanine resistance (Newbold *et al.*, 1979) and 6-thioguanine resistance, unless it was dissolved in NTA (Celotti *et al.*, 1987).

In aqueous suspension, all of these poorly soluble chromium[VI] compounds induced sister chromatid exchange in mammalian cells (Table 26). In human peripheral blood lymphocytes, lead chromate also induced micronuclei, with an enhancing effect following addition of an equimolar concentration of NTA (Montaldi *et al.*, 1987b). Aqueous suspensions of lead chromate, of all three derived pigments and of zinc chromate were clastogenic in mammalian cells (Table 27).

Zinc chromate and lead chromate induced anchorage-independent growth of Chinese hamster BHK fibroblasts in the soft agar assay (Hansen & Stern, 1985). [See General Remarks, p. 44, for concern about this assay.] Only lead chromate (which was phagocytized) induced morphological transformation in mouse embryo C3H10T1/2 cells, which contrasted with the lack of transforming ability of potassium dichromate, calcium chromate and strontium chromate observed in the same study (Patierno *et al.*, 1988). Both lead chromate (Casto *et al.*, 1979; Hatch & Anderson, 1986) and zinc chromate (Casto *et al.*, 1979) enhanced viral transformation in Syrian hamster embryo primary cells.

Lead chromate increased the frequency of micronuclei in polychromatic erythrocytes and decreased the polychromatic/normochromatic erythrocyte ratio in bone-marrow cells of intraperitoneally treated C57Bl/6N mice (Watanabe *et al.*, 1985).

### Chromyl chloride

Chromyl chloride [$Cl_2CrO_2$], a volatile liquid chromium[VI] compound, reverted *his⁻ S. typhimurium* in the plate test; its potency, the spectrum of sensitivity of bacterial strains and the attenuating effect of rat liver post-mitochondrial supernatant were similar to those seen for soluble chromium[VI] compounds. Moreover, as assessed by suitable modifications of the standard *Salmonella* test, its vapours were also mutagenic (De Flora *et al.*, 1980; De Flora, 1981a).

### (iv)   *Other chromium compounds*

The water-soluble chromium[II] salt, chromous chloride [$CrCl_2$], which readily oxidizes to chromium[III] in contact with air, induced infidelity of DNA synthesis, with poly[d(A-T)] as a template in the presence of avian myeloblastosis virus DNA polymerase (Sirover & Loeb, 1976). Chromium[II] was inactive, however, in all assays with cellular systems, including production of DNA fragmentation in Novikoff ascites hepatoma cells (Wedrychowski *et al.*, 1986a), of chromosomal aberrations and sister chromatid exchange in Syrian hamster embryo primary cells (Tsuda & Kato, 1977), and of aneuploidy in human skin fibroblasts (Nijs & Kirsch-Volders, 1986).

Chromium carbonyl [$Cr(CO)_6$], a hexacoordinated compound with oxidation state 0 (dissolved in ether due to its insolubility in water), was inactive in a differential killing test in *E. coli* (WP2 *vs.* WP67 and CM871) (De Flora *et al.*, 1984a) and in the reversion test in various *his⁻ S. typhimurium* strains (De Flora, 1981a; De Flora *et al.*, 1984a).

In contrast to a purple, anionic chromium[III]-glutathione complex, a green sodium chromium[V]-glutathione complex ($Na_4(GSH)_4Cr(V).8H_2O$) cleaved super-coiled DNA of the bacteriophage $PM_2$ (Kortenkamp *et al.*, 1989). Similarly, in contrast to chromium[VI] and [III], the chromium[V] complex *trans*-bis[2-ethyl-2-hydroxybutanoato(2-)]oxochromate[V] cleaved covalently closed, circular plasmid puc9 DNA. In addition, it reverted strain TA100 of *S. typhimurium* with a potency comparable to that of potassium dichromate (Farrell *et al.*, 1989).

### 3.3  Other relevant data in humans

### (a)  *Absorption, distribution, excretion and metabolism*

#### (i)  *Chromium[III] compounds*

More than 99% of administered chromium was recovered in faeces following oral administration of chromic chloride to humans; about 94% was recovered after duodenal administration. In both cases, about 0.5% was excreted in urine (Donaldson & Barreras, 1966). After exposure to chromium[III] by inhalation, urinary concentrations of chromium were somewhat increased, indicating respiratory absorption (Aitio *et al.*, 1984; Foa *et al.*, 1988). Pulmonary uptake of chromium[III] is influenced by the nature of the compound; uptake and excretion of chromium[III] lignosulfonate dust by industrial workers was similar to that of water-soluble chromium[VI] (Kiilunen *et al.*, 1983). A study of tannery workers indicated two half-times — one in the order of hours, the other in the order of several days — for urinary excretion of chromium[III] (Aitio *et al.*, 1988).

After one volunteer had immersed his hand in tanning liquor for 1 h, monitoring of blood and urine for 24 h failed to detect dermal absorption of chromic sulfate (Aitio *et al.*, 1984). However, a fatal chromium intoxication, due to skin absorption, was described after accidental submersion of a worker in hot (70°C) chromic sulfate tanning liquor (Kelly *et al.*, 1982).

(ii)  *Chromium[VI] compounds*

Following oral administration of sodium chromate in tracer doses to humans, faecal excretion of chromium indicated that about 10% of the administered dose had been absorbed from the gastrointestinal tract. After duodenal administration, approximately half of the administered radioactivity appeared to have been absorbed on the basis of faecal excretion, while 10% appeared in the urine during the first 24 h. Reduction of chromium[VI] to the trivalent form was demonstrated (Donaldson & Barreras, 1966). Circadian monitoring showed post-meal peaks of chromium[VI] reducing activity that may correspond to several tens of milligrams per day (De Flora *et al.*, 1987a).

Correlation between respiratory exposure to chromium[VI] and urinary excretion of chromium has been demonstrated in welders and in workers in the plating industry (Lindberg & Vesterberg, 1983; Aitio *et al.*, 1988). The respiratory uptake rate is unknown, but it depends on the solubility of the chromium compound (for review, see Aitio *et al.*, 1988). Chromium[VI] is reduced in the lower respiratory tract by the epithelial lining fluid and by pulmonary alveolar macrophages. At equivalent numbers of cells, the reducing efficiency of alveolar macrophages by biochemical mechanisms was significantly greater in smokers than in nonsmokers (Petrilli *et al.*, 1986c).

In contrast to chromium[III], which is bound to plasma proteins such as transferrin, chromium[VI] entering the blood stream is taken up selectively by erythrocytes, reduced, and bound predominantly to haemoglobin (Gray & Sterling, 1950; Aaseth *et al.*, 1982; Kitagawa *et al.*, 1988; see also the section on genetic and related effects). Reduction of chromium[VI] during transport in the blood is consistent with the finding that chromium is present in urine only in its reduced form (Mertz, 1969; Nomiyama *et al.*, 1980).

Aitio *et al.* (1988) reviewed the results of biological monitoring of chromium exposure to estimate biological half-times for excretion; the most data were available for manual metal arc stainless-steel welders exposed to soluble chromium[VI]. Three half-times — 7 h, 15-30 days and three to five years — were identified. The best estimates for the sizes of the different compartments are 40%, 50% and 10%, respectively. Lindberg and Vesterberg (1983) also found a correlation between exposure and urinary excretion of chromium in platers.

Retention of chromium on the skin was observed following topical application of sodium chromate (Baranowska-Dutkiewicz, 1981).

*(b)  Toxic effects*

In adults, the lethal oral dose of chromates is considered to be 50-70 mg/kg bw. The clinical features of acute poisoning are vomiting, diarrhoea, haemorrhagic diathesis and blood loss into the gastrointestinal tract, causing cardiovascular shock

(Sharma *et al.*, 1978; World Health Organization, 1988). If the patient survives for more than about eight days, the major effects are liver necrosis and tubular necrosis of the kidneys (World Health Organization, 1988).

Chronic ulcers of the skin and acute irritative dermatitis have been reported consistently in workers exposed to chromium-containing materials (World Health Organization, 1988). Chromates and chromium[VI] released from alloys and chromium-plated objects have been associated with the induction of allergic contact dermatitis. It is generally assumed that chromium[VI] is necessary for the sensitization, while both chromium[VI] and chromium[III] may cause dermatitis in sensitized individuals (see review by Haines & Nieboer, 1988). Intracellular reduction of chromium[VI] to the trivalent form seems to be a prerequisite for the effect (Polak *et al.*, 1973). In a study conducted in Finland, 2% of men and 1.5% of women showed a positive patch-test reaction to potassium dichromate (Pelkonen & Fräki, 1983). Chromium ulcers and chromate dermatitis have been reported in people in numerous occupations that involve manual handling of products containing chromium (Pedersen, 1982; Burrows, 1983; Polak, 1983; Nieboer *et al.*, 1984). The role of chromium[III] compounds in causing skin ulcers and acute irritative dermatitis is unclear (World Health Organization, 1988).

Inhalation of chromium[VI] compounds may give rise to necrosis in the nasal septum, leading to perforation. Lindberg and Hedenstierna (1983) found nasal irritation in chrome plating workers exposed by inhalation to chromium trioxide ( > 1 $\mu g/m^3$ Cr) and nasal perforation in two-thirds of workers with exposure to peak levels above 20 $\mu g/m^3$ Cr. Decreased respiratory function has been reported in platers exposed to chromates (Bovet *et al.*, 1977; Lindberg & Hedenstierna, 1983). Similar effects have been observed in welders and ferrochromium workers, although the role of chromium is uncertain as such persons have mixed exposures (World Health Organization, 1988).

Bronchial asthma may occur as a result of inhalation of chromate dust or chromium trioxide fumes (Meyers, 1950). Asthma among chromium platers, welders and ferrochromium workers has been reported to be due to exposure to chromates, among other compounds (Haines & Nieboer, 1988).

Franchini *et al.* (1978) reported on the excretion of β-glucuronidase, protein and lysozyme in the urine of 99 workers exposed to chromium compounds. No abnormal level was found among 39 stainless-steel welders; eight of 36 workers using special electrodes when welding on armoured steel had increased urinary levels of β-glucuronidase, and three of these workers had proteinuria. Among 24 workers engaged in chrome plating, nine had increased β-glucuronidase levels and four had elevated levels of protein in urine. The increased excretion of enzymes found in these workers was corroborated by exposing rats to potassium dichromate by subcutaneous injection (1.5 mg/kg bw as a single injection or 0.3 mg/kg bw every other day for two weeks); furthermore, a correlation between chromium in the renal cortex and an increase in chromium clearance was reported. Verschoor *et al.* (1988) investigated a number of parameters of kidney function in chrome platers, welders, boiler-makers and an unexposed reference group. Urinary chromium values ranged from 0.3 to 62 μg/g creatinine (0.1-2 μg/g among controls). Renal function was not related to urinary chromium or to chromium clearance, but chromium clearance was increased in the two groups with the highest exposure (platers and welders).

### (c)  *Effects on reproduction and prenatal toxicity*

In a review, Clarkson *et al.* (1985) found no report in the literature of an effect of any chromium compound on reproduction or prenatal development in humans.

### (d)  *Genetic and related effects*

The studies described below are summarized in Appendix 1 to this volume.

#### (i)  *Chromium[III] compounds*

In a comparison of 17 healthy tannery workers with continuous exposure for 13.4 ± 8.2 years to chrome alum and 13 external employees matched for social status, age, sex and years of service, no increase in the frequency of chromosomal aberrations was seen (Hamamy *et al.*, 1987). Average chromium levels of exposed persons were 0.12 μg/l plasma and 0.14 μg/l urine; these values were not considered to be different from those of controls. The level of chromium in air ranged from 15 (day) to 47 (night) μg/m³. [The Working Group noted that exposure was estimated by correlation with a parallel study.] When the data were analysed according to smoking habit, workers who smoked had higher frequencies of chromosome-type aberrations per cell (0.035) than either nonsmoking workers (0.011; $p < 0.01$) or control smokers (0.016; $p < 0.05$). The authors commented that the values for controls were relatively high in comparison with those in other cytogenetic studies reported in the literature.

In the study described below, enhanced levels of chromosomal aberrations, correlated with exposure duration, were observed in workers exposed to 'chromoxide' (Bigaliev *et al.*, 1977a). [The Working Group was unclear whether or not this was a chromium[III] compound.]

#### (ii)  *Chromium[VI] compounds*

Bigaliev *et al.* (1977a) examined peripheral lymphocytes from 132 workers in chromium production who were exposed to one of five chromium compounds and compared them with 37 healthy, unexposed workers. Significant increases in the frequency of chromosomal aberrations over control values of 1.88 ± 0.74% meta-phases with aberrations were observed, as follows: monochromate (sodium chro-mate), with a dose-related trend (correlation with exposure duration) ranging from 3.6 to 8.2% aberrant metaphases; sodium chrompik (sodium dichromate), with a dose-related trend ranging from 4.5 to 5.7% aberrant metaphases; potassium dich-romate, with a dose-related trend ranging from 3.6 to 9.0%; chromoxide (as re-ported in the preceding section), with a dose-related trend ranging from 4.5 to 7.2%; and chromanhydride (chromium trioxide), with a dose-effect trend ranging from 5.4 to 9.4%. [The Working Group noted that no information was provided on exposure levels or on selection criteria, but the overall sample size was large.] When chromo-somal aberrations were examined in detail (Bigaliev *et al.*, 1977b,c; Bigaliev, 1981), increased frequencies were found for single and double fragments, for transloca-tions and for aneuploidy, consisting mainly of chromosome loss. Dose-responses were observed overall, and for each type of damage. In a later study (Bigaliev *et al.*, 1979), elongated cell-cycle times were seen for cultured peripheral lymphocytes from a group of chromium workers with five or more years' exposure, compared with a control group registered at the city blood transfusion station. An effect of duration of exposure was reported in a further analysis (Bigaliev *et al.*, 1977c; Bigal-iev, 1981).

Several studies have been carried out on chromium platers. Increased fre-quencies of sister chromatid exchange were found in a study of male chromium platers exposed to chromium trioxide fumes (Stella *et al.*, 1982). Mean sister chro-matid exchange values of 8.08 ± 2.67 ($p < 0.001$) were observed in exposed workers *versus* 6.31 ± 1.56 in ten healthy male donors aged 20-35 who had not been exposed to ionizing radiation. The authors noted particularly that the seven youngest work-ers, although the most recently engaged in chromium plating, showed significantly increased sister chromatid exchange frequencies. An effect of age on the induction of sister chromatid exchange was noted in the control group. [The Working Group noted that details were not provided on exposure, or on confounding factors].

Sarto *et al.* (1982) analysed sister chromatid exchange and chromosomal aber-rations in peripheral blood lymphocytes of chrome platers in four factories in the same region, grouped by type of exposure and factory: groups 1 (eight persons) and 2 (nine persons) used a 'bright plating' process and were exposed to chromium trioxide and nickel; groups 3 (12 persons) and 4 (nine persons) used a 'hard plating' process and were exposed only to chromium trioxide. Controls were 35 healthy male sanitary workers who had not been exposed to occupational or diagnostic ion-izing radiation for at least five years and had not knowingly been exposed to either occupational mutagens or mutagenic drugs. Their mean ages and smoking habits were similar to those of the exposed workers. The average ages in the four exposed groups were 39, 42, 24 and 34 years, respectively; urinary chromium levels (μg/g creatinine) in the four groups were $5.1 \pm 1.8$, $7.1 \pm 3.3$, $11.8 \pm 8.7$ and $6.8 \pm 3.7$, respectively, *versus* $1.9 + 1.4$ for controls. Sister chromatid exchange frequencies in the 'hard plating' groups were increased ($p < 0.001$) from $6.60 \pm 0.80\%$ in controls to $8.30 \pm 1.80\%$; however, when the values were analysed by age, a significant increase in sister chromatid exchange was observed only in the group of younger workers (group 3). A correlation was observed between sister chromatid exchange frequency and both age and urinary chromium levels (more sister chromatid exchange in younger workers with higher levels of chromium). A significant increase in the frequency of chromosomal aberrations, mostly of the chromosome type, was observed, from $1.7\%$ of metaphases in controls to $3.8$ ($p < 0.001$) in 'bright' platers and $2.8$ ($p < 0.01$) in 'hard' platers. Chromatid-type aberrations were observed only in the 'bright' platers. The correlation between urinary chromium levels and chromosomal aberrations was poor.

No increase in the frequency of sister chromatid exchange was observed in a group of 24 male chromium platers exposed to chromium in air for 0.5-30.5 (mean, $11.6 \pm 7.5$) years, when compared with a group of office workers matched for sex, age and smoking habit (Nagaya, 1986). Smokers and nonsmokers were analysed separately for each group, and a smoking-related increase in the frequency of sister chromatid exchange was observed for both exposed (smokers, $10.7 \pm 1.7\%$; nonsmokers, $9.0 \pm 1.0\%$) persons and controls (smokers, $10.6 \pm 2\%$; nonsmokers, $8.9 \pm 1.2\%$). No correlation was seen between sister chromatid exchange frequencies and urinary chromium levels ($13.1 \pm 16.7$ μg/l for exposed persons, none detected for controls). In a further study of a larger group (Nagaya *et al.*, 1989), essentially the same results were obtained. The authors speculated that the chromium exposure may have been too low to affect circulating lymphocytes. [The Working Group noted that high control values were observed in both studies.]

Choi *et al.* (1987) compared two groups of metal platers, consisting of seven workers in chromium surface treatment (group 1) and 25 workers in chromium plating (group 2), with 15 non-plating workers matched for age, sex and length of career. Exposures to chromium in air and urine were 0.027 (0.021-0.034) mg/m³ and $24.0 \pm 7.8$ μg/l, respectively, for group 1, and 0.008 (0.005-0.012) mg/m³ and $15.2 \pm 5.9$ μg/l, respectively, for group 2. Sister chromatid exchange frequency was increased from $3.6 \pm 1.5$ (controls) to $6.9 \pm 1.8$ ($p < 0.05$) in group 1 and to $5.4 \pm 2.1$ ($p < 0.05$) in group 2. A dose-effect relationship was observed with urinary chromium levels ($p < 0.01$). No effect of smoking was observed in exposed workers or controls.

Deng *et al.* (1983, 1988) observed significant increases in the frequencies of sister chromatid exchange and of chromosomal aberrations (gaps, breaks, fragments; $5.7\%$ *versus* $0.8\%$ in controls) in lymphocytes of seven chromium platers. Details of the study are provided in the monograph on nickel and nickel compounds, p. 389.

Several studies of occupational exposures to chromium during welding are described in the monograph on welding, pp. 487-489. Both enhancement (Koshi *et al.*, 1984) and lack of enhancement (Husgafvel-Pursiainen *et al.*, 1982; Littorin *et al.*, 1983) of sister chromatid exchange and chromosomal aberrations were reported in exposed workers.

As reported in an abstract (Imreh & Radulescu, 1982), 18 workers in a bichromate producing plant with a mean duration of exposure of 21.3 years (19-26 years) showed significantly elevated frequencies of chromosomal and chromatid-type aberrations and micronuclei when compared with eight mechanics from the same plant and with 34 healthy external controls. Sister chromatid exchange frequencies were not significantly greater than in the mechanics.

### 3.4 Case reports and epidemiological studies of carcinogenicity to humans

Epidemiological studies on chromium have been reviewed extensively (see, e.g., Sunderman, 1976; Norseth, 1980; Anon., 1981; Norseth, 1981; Sunderman, 1984, 1986; Adachi & Takemoto, 1987; Fan & Harding-Barlow, 1987; Hayes, 1988; World Health Organization, 1988; Yassi & Nieboer, 1988). Epidemiological studies on welders exposed to chromium and its compounds are summarized in the monograph on welding (see pp. 489-505).

Epidemiological studies of cancer in workers in industries in which exposure to chromium compounds could occur are summarized in Tables 28-31. Standardized mortality ratios (SMRs) and confidence intervals (CIs), assuming Poisson distribution, are given in square brackets when they were calculated by the Working Group.

(*a*)   *Chromate production*

(i)   *Case reports*

Many case reports of lung cancer have been published in relation to work in chromate production. Many of these were reviewed by a Working Group for the IARC (1980a); further case reports were made by Pfeil (1935), Alwens and Jonas (1938), Zober (1979), Hyodo *et al.* (1980), Abe *et al.* (1982), Tsuneta (1982) and Nishiyama *et al.* (1985, 1988). After having seen five cases of gastrointestinal cancer among 44 deceased chromate workers, Teleky (1936) drew attention to the possibility that chromate exposure could also be associated with an increased risk for cancer of the gastrointestinal tract.

(ii)   *Epidemiological studies*

The Working Group considered six studies covering several partially overlapping populations in seven plants producing chromate from chemical-grade chromite ore (Brinton *et al.*, 1952) in the USA; the degree of overlap could not be ascertained.

**Table 28. Epidemiological studies of cancer in workers in chromate-producing industries**

| Study population | Reference population | Cancer of respiratory organs | | | Cancer at other sites | | | Reference |
|---|---|---|---|---|---|---|---|---|
| | | Site | Number | Estimated relative risk | Site | Number | Estimated relative risk | |
| Seven US chromate plants; active employees 1930–47; 193 deaths | Male oil refinery workers, 1933–38 | Respiratory system | 42 | 20.7 | Digestive system Oral region (also included in respiratory system) | 13 3 | 2.0 5.4* | Machle & Gregorius (1948) |
| Seven US chromium plants; active employees 1940–50; 5522 person-years | US male white, non-white | Respiratory system, except larynx | 10 white 16 non-white | 14.3* 80.0* | Other sites | 6 (whole cohort) | 1.0 ns | Brinton et al. (1952); Gafafer (1953) |
| Health survey, 897 workers | Boston X-ray survey | Bronchogenic/lung | 10 | 53.6 (prevalence ratio) | | | | Gafafer (1953) |
| Three US plants; men employed 1937–40, surveyed 1941–60 | Cancer mortality; US males 1950, 1953, 1958 | Respiratory (160–164) | 69 (2 maxillary sinus) | 9.4* | Digestive system | 16 | 1.5 ns | Taylor (1966); Enterline (1974) |
| 290 cases near US chromium plant | Random sample of hospital admissions | Lung | 11[a] | ∞ | | | | Baetjer (1950) |
| US chromate plant; employed one or more years 1931–37; all jobs related to exposure to soluble and insoluble chromium; lifetime exposure in months calculated | No independent comparison group | Lung | 41 | | | | | Mancuso & Hueper (1951); Mancuso (1975) |

**Table 28 (contd)**

| Study population | Reference population | Cancer of respiratory organs | | | Cancer at other sites | | | Reference |
|---|---|---|---|---|---|---|---|---|
| | | Site | Number | Estimated relative risk | Site | Number | Estimated relative risk | |
| US chromate plant; 2101 (restricted to 1803) workers initially employed three or more months 1945–74; status 1977 (88.5% complete); population working in new and/or old production sites | Baltimore City; mortality | Lung | 59 | 2.0* | Digestive system<br>Other | 13<br>14 | 0.60<br>0.40 | Hayes et al. (1979) |
| Three UK chromate factories; men employed 1949–55 | Cancer mortality, England and Wales | Lung | 12 | 3.6* | All other sites | No increase | | Bidstrup & Case (1956) |
| Same UK factories as studied by Bidstrup & Case (1956); 1948–77; 2715 males | Cancer mortality, England, Wales and Scotland | Lung | 116 | 2.4* | Other sites<br>Nasal cancer | 80<br>2 | 1.2 ns<br>7.1* | Alderson et al. (1981) |
| Two FRG chromate plants; 1140 male workers employed more than one year 1934–79 | Mortality, North Rhine Westphalen | Lung | 51 | 2.1* | Stomach | 12 | 0.94 ns | Korallus et al. (1982) |
| Tokyo chromium manufacture; 896 production workers, 1918–78 | Age-, cause-specific mortality, Japanese males | Respiratory cancers<br><br>1–10 years' exposure<br>11–20 years' exposure<br>≥21 years' exposure | 31 (6 sino-nasal)<br>5<br>9<br>17 | 9.2*<br><br>4.2*<br>7.5*<br>17.5* | Stomach | 11 | 1.0 | Satoh et al. (1981) |

**Table 28 (contd)**

| Study population | Reference population | Cancer of respiratory organs | | | Cancer at other sites | | | Reference |
|---|---|---|---|---|---|---|---|---|
| | | Site | Number | Estimated relative risk | Site | Number | Estimated relative risk | |
| 273 chromate producers in Japan; 1947–73; observed 1960–82 | Age-, cause-specific mortal-ity, Japanese males | Lung | 25 (plus 1 maxillary sinus) | 18.3* | Digestive system | 6 | 0.9 | Watanabe & Fukuchi (1984) |
| 540 Italian chromate pro-ducers employed 10 years or more, 1948–85 | Italian cause-specific death rates | Lung Highly exposed | 14 6 | 2.2* 4.2* | Larynx Pleura | 3 3 | 2.9 30* | De Marco et al. (1988) |

aIn comparison with internal reference population

*Significant at 95% level

ns Nonsignificant

**Table 29. Epidemiological studies of cancer in workers in chromate–pigment industries**

| Study population | Reference population | Cancer of respiratory organs | | | Cancer at other sites | | | Reference |
|---|---|---|---|---|---|---|---|---|
| | | Site | Number | Estimated relative risk | Site | Number | Estimated relative risk | |
| Norwegian chromium pigment production since 1948; 133 workers of whom 24 over 3 years' employment to 1972 | Cancer incidence, Norway 1955–76 | Lung | 6 (one case with <3 years' employment) | 44 / 67 (10 years' latency) | Gastrointestinal / Nasal cavity | 3 / 1 | 6.4 / – | Langård & Norseth (1975, 1979); Langård & Vigander (1983) |
| UK chromate pigment factories: A, lead & zinc chromate; B, lead & zinc chromate; C, lead chromate; followed up to 1981 | Mortality, England and Wales | Lung A (1932–54) B (1948–67) C (1946–60) | 21 11 7 | 2.2* 4.4* 1.1 ns | | | | Davies (1978, 1979, 1984a) |
| French lead and zinc chromate manufacturers; 251 males employed 6 months or more, 1958–77 | Standard death rates, northern France 1958–77 | Lung | 11 | 4.6* | | | | Haguenoer et al. (1981) |
| German and Dutch manufacturers of zinc and lead chromates; 978 workers followed up for 15 076 person-years | Local death rates, FRG and the Netherlands | Lung | 19 | 2.0* | | | | Frentzel-Beyme (1983) |

**Table 29 (contd)**

| Study population | Reference population | Cancer of respiratory organs | | | Cancer at other sites | | | Reference |
|---|---|---|---|---|---|---|---|---|
| | | Site | Number | Estimated relative risk | Site | Number | Estimated relative risk | |
| US lead and zinc chro-mate production workers employed ≥1 month 1940–69; 1181 white, 698 non-white; followed up to end of 1982 | Mortality, US whites and non-whites | Lung (30-year latency) | 24 | 1.4 ns | Stomach | 6 | 1.8 ns | Sheffet et al. (1982); Hayes et al. (1989) |
| | | <1 year exposure | 3 | 1.4** | | | | |
| | | 1–9 years' exposure | 3 | 2.0** | | | | |
| | | ≥10 years' exposure | 6 | 3.2** | | | | |

** $p$ for trend < 0.01

ns Nonsignificant

**Table 30. Epidemiological studies of cancer in workers in chromium–plating industries**

| Study population | Reference population | Cancer of respiratory organs | | | Cancer at other sites | | | Reference |
|---|---|---|---|---|---|---|---|---|
| | | Site | Number | Estimated relative risk | Site | Number | Estimated relative risk | |
| 54 UK chromium-plating plants; 1056 male platers | 1099 non-exposed males in plants and in two nonplating industries | Lung | 24 | 1.4 ns | All sites<br>Gastrointestinal<br>Other sites | 44<br>8<br>12 | 1.7*<br>1.5 ns<br>1.9 ns | Royle (1975a,b) |
| Japanese chromium platers; 952 workers with >6 months' exposure | Platers not exposed to chromium and clerical workers | Lung | 0 | – | All sites | 5 | 0.5 ns | Okubo & Tsuchiya (1977, 1979, 1987) |
| US workers in diecasting and Ni-Cr-plating plant, 1974–78 | US national mortality statistics | Lung<br>men<br>women | 28<br>10 | 1.9*<br>3.7* | Stomach<br>Larynx<br>Lymphosarcoma | 4<br>2<br>2 | 2.5 ns<br>3.3 ns<br>2.9 ns | Silverstein et al. (1981) |
| Nine plants, Parma, Italy, 116 'thick' and 62 'thin' platers; employed more than 1 year 1951–81 | Mortality, Italy | Lung | 3 | 3.3* (4.3* for 'thick' platers) | All sites | 8 | 1.9 | Franchini et al. (1983) |
| UK chromium platers; 2689 (1288 men, 1401 women) first employed 1946–75; observed 1946–83 | Mortality, England and Wales | Lung<br>men<br>women<br>Nasal cavity (men and women)<br>Larynx<br>men<br>women | 63<br>9<br>3<br><br>3<br>0 | 1.6*<br>1.1 ns<br>10*<br><br>3.0 ns<br>– | Stomach (men and women)<br>Liver<br>men<br>women | 25<br><br>4<br>0 | 1.5 ns<br><br>6.7*<br>– | Sorahan et al. (1987) |

* Significant at 95% level
ns Nonsignificant

**Table 31. Epidemiological studies of cancer in workers in ferrochromium industries**

| Study population | Reference population | Cancer of respiratory organs | | | Cancer at other sites | | | Reference |
|---|---|---|---|---|---|---|---|---|
| | | Site | Number | Estimated relative risk | Site | Number | Estimated relative risk | |
| USSR ferrochromium alloy industry; 1955–69 | Mortality, general population of municipality | Lung (men) | Not given | 4.4–6.6* by age | All sites (men) Oesophagus (men) | Not given Not given | 0.5–3.3* 2.0*–11.3* | Pokrovskaya & Shabynina (1973) |
| Swedish ferrochromium plant; ferroalloy; 1876 workers for 1 or more years 1930–75; traced by parish lists and cancer registry | County or national statistics; classification of work areas by Cr[III] and Cr[VI] | Lung All workers Maintenance workers Arc workers | 7 4 (2 mesotheliomas) 2 (1 mesothelioma) | 1.2 ns 4.0* 1.0 ns | Prostate (all workers) | 23 | 1.2 ns | Axelsson et al. (1980) |
| Norwegian ferrochromium and ferrosilicon; 1235 male workers employed 1928–65 | General population; internal comparison with unexposed | Lung (ferrochromium workers) | 10 | 1.5 ns | All sites Kidney Prostate Stomach (ferrochromium workers) | 132 5 12 7 | 0.8 ns 2.7 ns 1.5 ns 1.4 ns | Langård et al. (1980, 1989) |

*Significant at 95% level

ns, Nonsignificant

Machle and Gregorius (1948) reported high proportionate mortality from respiratory cancer among male workers at the seven chromate-producing plants in the USA: between 1930 and 1947, the annual death rate from respiratory cancer was 2.63/1000, as compared with a frequency of 0.09/1000 in a comparison group from an oil refinery in 1933-38. [The Working Group noted that the age structures of the two populations were not given.]

Brinton *et al.* (1952) and Gafafer (1953) conducted a mortality study (a US Public Health Service study) of male workers in the seven chromate manufacturing plants during 1940-50 with 5522 person-years of membership in sick-benefit associations for persons 15-74 years old, not including workers who had terminated employment with the chromate industry and those who had died more than one year after the onset of disability. Comparison was made to age- and race-specific US male mortality rates during 1940-48. Ten deaths from cancer of the respiratory system (except larynx) were observed among white employees (SMR, 1429 [95% CI, 685-2627]). Among non-white employees, 16 deaths from cancer at this site were found (SMR, 8000 [95% CI, 4573-12 991]). For the entire study group, six deaths from cancers at all other sites were observed [SMR, 95.2; 95% CI, 35-207]. [The Working Group noted that the SMR for lung cancer may have been biased, because of the exclusion of terminated and retired workers and of those who did not belong to the sick-benefit plan.] A health survey of 897 workers gave a prevalence ratio of 53.6 for bronchogenic cancer in chromate workers compared to persons who had undergone a chest X-ray survey for lung cancer (Gafafer, 1953).

Enterline (1974) reanalysed data from a study by Taylor (1966) of 1212 male workers who had been employed in three of the US plants for three months or longer for the period 1937-60. The study cohort, constructed from earnings reports in old age and survivors disability insurance records, was restricted to men born after 1889. Vital status was ascertained through 1960 by searching the death claim files of the records; death certificates were subsequently obtained for workers for whom death claims had been filed. Age-specific mortality figures for US males in the calendar years 1950, 1953 and 1958 were used as reference. A total of 69 deaths from cancers of the respiratory system (ICD codes 160-164) was observed (SMR, 943 [95% CI, 733-1193]), two of which were from maxillary sinus cancer; the author regarded this rate as greatly elevated. Furthermore, a small excess of deaths from cancer of the digestive system was observed (16 deaths; SMR, 153 [95% CI, 88-249]).

In a study of medical records from two hospitals in Baltimore, MD, USA, near a chromate-producing plant, Baetjer (1950) found that 11 (3.8%) of 290 male lung cancer patients admitted in 1925-48 had had exposure to chromates, whereas no chromate-exposed worker was found among a 'random' sample of 725 other hospital admissions. Ten of the 11 cases had worked in the local chromate production plant and one in an electrical company. Occupational history was derived only from records.

Mancuso (1975) reported on a cohort recruited from a US chromate-producing plant that had been investigated earlier (Mancuso & Hueper, 1951). In the earlier report, six lung cancer deaths were observed, giving a relative risk of 15; using hygiene data collected in 1949, cumulative exposures to soluble, insoluble and total chromium, combined with length of exposure, were computed for each worker in the cohort. The second analysis was confined to the 41 deaths from lung cancer that occurred in persons first employed between 1931 when the plant started operation and 1937 and followed through 1974, and rates were computed using direct standardization, with the entire plant population as the standard. Mortality from lung cancer was associated with cumulative exposure to insoluble chromium, to soluble chromium and to total chromium. [The Working Group noted that the three classes of exposure were highly correlated and the risks of exposure to soluble and insoluble chromium could not be distinguished.]

Hayes *et al.* (1979) studied workers at a chromate production plant in Baltimore, MD, USA, which had been partly renovated in 1950-51 and 1960 to reduce exposure to chromium dusts. The study cohort consisted of 2101 workers with more than 90 days of work experience, first employed between 1945 and 1974, and followed through July 1977; vital status was ascertained for 75% on an individual basis and for another 14% on a group basis. SMRs for 1803 hourly employees were calculated on the basis of expected values derived from the age-, race- and time-specific mortality rates for Baltimore City males. There were 404 deaths from all causes (SMR, 92). The overall SMR for cancer of the trachea, bronchus and lung (ICD code 162) was 202, based on 59 observed deaths (95% CI, 155-263). Workers hired between 1945 and 1949, before the plant was renovated, who had been employed for fewer than three years, had an SMR for lung cancer of 180 (95% CI, 110-270), based on 20 observed deaths, whereas workers with three or more years of employment hired in that period had an SMR of 300 (95% CI, 160-520), based on 13 observed deaths. For workers hired in 1950-59, when part of the plant had better environmental controls, similarly elevated risks were seen, based on 12 and nine cases for short-term and long-term employment, respectively. No case of lung cancer was detected in 1960-74 after the plant had been renovated, but, as the authors noted, the latent period is too short for an adequate assessment of risk for cancer at this site. Additional case-control analyses were performed to determine whether specific work areas were associated with lung cancer hazard. Controls who had died from causes other than cancer were matched individually by race, date of hire, age at initial employment and duration of employment to the 66 hourly or salaried employees who had died from lung cancer. A significant ($p < 0.05$) elevation in risk for lung cancer was found for employees who had worked in the 'special products' and dichromate areas, where soluble chromium[VI] compounds were produced and packaged (relative risks, 2.6 and 3.3, respectively).

On the basis of data from the previous study and the results of 555 air samples analysed in 1945-50, Braver *et al.* (1985) studied the relationship between exposure to chromium[VI] and occurrence of lung cancer. The authors reported a dose-response relationship with cumulative exposure. [The Working Group noted that the association appeared to be due predominantly to duration of exposure and not to estimated level of exposure, which did not vary substantially.]

A total of 723 chromate production workers from three factories in the UK who were interviewed and radiographed were followed up in 1949-55 by Bidstrup and Case (1956), who reported significantly higher than expected lung cancer mortality: 12 deaths [SMR, 364; 95% CI, 188-635] (based on age-adjusted rates for England and Wales). The average duration of exposure was 12.2 years; 165 (22.8%) persons had worked for more than 20 years (Bidstrup, 1951). For cancers at other sites, the observed and expected numbers of deaths did not differ significantly.

Alderson *et al.* (1981) studied 2715 chromate production workers with more than one year of work experience between 1948 and 1977 and who had undergone at least one X-ray of the lungs, 79 (2.9%) of whom were lost to follow-up, at the same three UK factories studied by Bidstrup and Case (1956). The percentage of heavy smokers was reported to be lower among the workers than among males in England and Wales [numbers not given]. During the study period, 602 deaths occurred (SMR, 135 [95% CI, 125-146]), 116 of which were from lung cancer (SMR, 242 [95% CI, 200-290]). Two deaths from nasal cancer were observed in one factory; 0.28 would have been expected for the whole cohort (SMR, 714 [95% CI, 87-2580]).

Korallus *et al.* (1982) identified 1140 workers who had been employed for one year or more at two chromate-producing plants in the Federal Republic of Germany. The study subjects were active workers and pensioners who had been hired before 1948 or workers hired thereafter. Vital status was ascertained from personnel documents and from population registries until 1979. Cause of death was determined from medical records and, in some cases, from death certificates. The SMR for respiratory cancer (ICD 8, 160-163) was 210 [95% CI, 156-276]. A total of 20 deaths from bronchial carcinomas (and one laryngeal carcinoma) was seen in one factory (SMR, 192 [95% CI, 119-294], and 30 deaths, all from bronchial carcinoma, in the second (SMR, 224 [95% CI, 151-319]). The author noted difficulties in the ascertainment of cause of death and of comparability with the standard population.

Satoh *et al.* (1981) studied 896 men who had been engaged in manufacturing chromium compounds for one or more years in a factory in the Tokyo, Japan, area between 1918 and 1975. The workers were observed from 1918 through 1978 or to death; vital status could not be ascertained for an additional 165 retired workers. The authors stated that 84% of the chromium compounds manufactured between

1934 and 1975 were hexavalent compounds and 16% trivalent compounds. The expected numbers of deaths were based on age- and cause-specific mortality rates for Japanese males. Between 1950 and 1978, 120 deaths (SMR, 90) were observed, 31 of which were from respiratory cancer [SMR, 923; 95% CI, 627-1310]; 25 of these were from lung cancer and six from sinonasal cancer. No other cancer occurred in excess. When the population was subdivided by duration of work, there were five cases of respiratory cancer in the group with one to ten years of exposure [SMR, 423; 95% CI, 138-989], nine in the group with 11-20 years' exposure [SMR, 748; 95% CI, 343-1424] and 17 in the group with more than 21 years of exposure [SMR, 1747; 95% CI, 1021-2806].

Watanabe and Fukuchi (1984) reported in an abstract a mortality study of 273 workers employed in 1947 or later at a chromate-producing factory in Japan for at least five years until 1973, previously studied by Ohsaki *et al.* (1974, 1978). The population was observed from January 1960 to December 1982. Expected numbers of deaths were based on age-, year- and cause-specific deaths rates for the Japanese male population. Sixty deaths from all causes were observed; 33 from all cancers, of which 25 were from lung cancer (SMR, 1832 [95% CI, 1190-2714]) and six from cancer of the digestive organs [SMR, 88; 95% CI, 32-192]; one cancer of the maxillary sinus was seen.

In an Italian cohort study of 981 chromate production workers employed for one year or more in 1948-85 (De Marco *et al.*, 1988), analysis was limited to the 540 workers followed up for ten years or more. Cause-specific death rates in Italy were used as a reference level. The SMR for lung cancer was 217 (14 deaths; 95% CI, 118-363), and there were three deaths each from cancers of the pleura and larynx. Among a subgroup of workers with heavy exposure to hexavalent chromium compounds (on the basis of job histories), the SMR for lung cancer was 420 (six deaths [95% CI, 154-193]).

### (b) Production of chromate pigments

#### (i) Case reports

Newman (1890) reported the first case of cancer in a 'chrome worker', which was an adenocarcinoma of the anterior half of the left nostril in a 47-year-old male worker who had had perforation of his nasal septum for 20 years; the patient had been exposed to chrome pigments. Since that time, there have been a number of case reports of lung cancer in workers involved in production of chromate pigments (Gross & Kölsch, 1943; Letterer *et al.*, 1944; Langård & Kommedal, 1975; Zober, 1979; Rivolta *et al.*, 1982).

#### (ii) Epidemiological studies

Langård and Vigander (1983) followed up 133 workers for 1953-80, who had been employed in a small Norwegian company producing chromate pigments in

1948-72, previously studied by Langård and Norseth (1975). The work force was exposed to zinc chromate from 1951; a small number of workers had also been exposed to lead chromate between 1948 and 1956. While past levels of exposure to hexavalent chromium are unknown, exposures to chromates as chromium measured in 1973 ranged from 0.01 to 1.35 mg/m³ (Langård & Norseth, 1979). One case of lung cancer occurred among 109 workers with less than three years of employment prior to 1972. Six cases of lung cancer occurred in a subpopulation of 24 workers with more than three years of work experience prior to 1972 [giving a standardized incidence ratio (SIR) of 4444 (95% CI, 1631-9674) on the basis of national incidence rates among males]. More than ten years after first exposure, the SIR was 6667 [95% CI, 2447-14 510] on the basis of national reference rates. Only 18 workers had worked at the plant for more than five years, and all six cases belonged to this subgroup. One of the cases had worked in the production of zinc chromate as well as lead chromate, while five cases had worked in the production of zinc chromate only. A previous follow-up had found one case of cancer of the nasal cavity, one of cancer of the prostate and three of cancer of the gastrointestinal tract (one cancer of the pancreas, one stomach cancer and one cancer of the large intestine) (Langård & Norseth, 1979). The three latter cases occurred in the subgroup of 24 workers employed for more than three years before 1972 [SMR, 638; 95% CI, 0.6-8.8].

Davies (1978, 1979, 1984a) studied mortality among 1002 male workers at three factories in the UK where chromate pigments were manufactured. Production of lead chromate[VI] occurred in all factories; workers in two of the factories (A and B) were additionally involved in manufacturing zinc chromate[VI] until 1964 and 1976, respectively. Small amounts of barium chromate were produced in factory A from 1942, and small amounts of strontium chromate were produced in factory B from the early 1950s to 1968. Factory A closed in 1982 and factory B in 1978. Exposure levels were classified only as high, medium or low. The 1984 report extended the follow-up from the 1930s or 1940s to the end of 1981. The expected numbers were based on calendar time period-, sex- and age-specific mortality rates for England and Wales. An excess of lung cancer appeared in two groups of workers assigned to high and medium exposure: factory A, those entering before 1955 (21 cases; SMR, 222 [95% CI, 138-340]) and factory B, those entering before 1968 (11 cases; SMR, 440 [95% CI, 220-787]). In workers with low exposure to zinc and lead chromates in factories A and B, seven lung cancer deaths were observed [SMR, 101; 95% CI, 41-208]. In factory C, where only lead chromate was produced, seven lung cancer deaths were observed [SMR, 109; 95% CI, 44-224], and the highest ratio was found for one to 29 years of follow-up of a group of 33 men among early entrants with high and medium exposure (three cases [SMR, 357; 95% CI, 74-1044]). The author indicated that moderate or heavy exposure to zinc chromate may give rise to a high risk for developing lung cancer, and that relatively mild or short-term exposure may not constitute a measurable lung cancer hazard.

Davies (1984b) also studied a subgroup of 57 workers involved in the production of lead chromate pigments from lead nitrate in the same three factories, who had been reported to the work inspectorate to have lead poisoning, mostly between 1930 and 1945. Mortality was observed through 1981, giving 1585 person-years of observation. Four deaths from lung cancer (SMR, 145 [95% CI, 40-370]) were observed. [The Working Group noted that this small sample of workers might have been highly selected.]

Haguenoer *et al.* (1981) reported deaths among a cohort of 251 workers in a factory manufacturing zinc and lead chromate pigments in France who had been employed for more than six months between 1 January 1958 and 31 December 1977. Fifty deaths occurred, the specific cause of which was known from medical records for 30. Expected numbers were derived from death certificates. Among the 30 deaths, there were 11 confirmed lung cancer deaths (SMR, 461; 95% CI, 270-790). The mean time from first employment until detection of cancer was 17 years, and the mean duration of employment among cases was 15.3 years. [The Working Group noted that cause of death was ascertained from different sources for observed and expected cases.]

Frentzel-Beyme (1983) studied mortality among men employed for more than six months in three factories in the Federal Republic of Germany and two factories in the Netherlands that produced lead and zinc chromate pigments. The total number of study participants was 1396. Regional death rates in the two countries were used to estimate expected figures. In an analysis of 978 men with exposure beginning before 1965, 117 deaths were observed [SMR, 96], of which 19 were from lung cancer [SMR, 204; 95% CI, 123-319].

Hayes *et al.* (1989) followed-up a cohort studied by Sheffet *et al.* (1982) consisting of 1879 male employees of a New Jersey (USA) lead and zinc chromate pigment production factory who had been employed for at least one month between January 1940 and December 1969; they were observed from 1940 to 1982. US age- and calendar-specific death rates for white and nonwhite men were used as reference. Vital status was ascertained for 1737 workers (92%). Airborne chromium concentrations were measured during later years, giving estimates of $> 0.5$ mg/m³ for exposed jobs and of $> 2$ mg/m³ for highly exposed jobs; the ratio of lead chromate:zinc chromate in the working atmosphere was reported to be about 9:1, and low levels of nickel may have been present. The SMR for all cancers was 93 (101 deaths; 95% CI, 76-113). Among a total of 41 lung cancer deaths (SMR, 116; 95% CI, 83-158), 24 occurred among workers exposed to chromate dusts (SMR, 143). The SMR for lung cancer among men who had not worked in chromium-exposed jobs was 92 (17 deaths; 95% CI, 53-147), and that for men who had worked for less than one year was 93 (seven deaths; 95% CI, 37-192). For those with cumulative exposure to chromate dusts of one to nine years, the SMR was 176 (nine deaths; 95% CI, 80-334), and for ten or more years, 194 (eight deaths; 95% CI, 83-383). When accounting for 30 years since first employment among men with more than ten years' exposure, the SMR rose to 321 (95% CI, 117-698), based on six cases. In jobs with exposure to chromate dusts, a nonsignificant excess of cancer of the digestive tract was found; for stomach cancer, the SMRs were 149, 185 and 214 for those with less than one, one to nine and more than ten years' exposure, respectively.

(c)   *Chromium plating*

(i)   *Case reports*

Cases of lung cancer have also been reported among chromium platers (Barbořík *et al.*, 1958; Kleisbauer *et al.*, 1972; Korallus *et al.*, 1974b,c; Michel-Briand & Simonin, 1977; Takemoto *et al.*, 1977; Sano, 1978; Zober, 1979; Brochard *et al.*, 1983; Kim *et al.*, 1985).

(ii)   *Epidemiological studies*

Royle (1975b) conducted a mortality study among past and current workers with three months or more of consecutive employment in 54 chromium-plating plants in Yorkshire, UK. The study covered 1238 chromium-plating workers (1056 men, 182 women), 142 of whom had died by 31 May 1974. A control population of 1284 manual workers (1099 men, 185 women) was drawn from non-chromium-plating departments of the largest firms and from the past and current work force of two industrial companies located in the same geographic region. The control subjects were matched individually to the platers by sex, age, date when last known to be alive and, for current workers, smoking habits. The study population represented 91% of the total exposed population and 93% of the eligible controls. Compared with the controls, chromium platers experienced a significant excess proportion of deaths from total cancer: 51/142 *versus* 24/104 in men and women combined ($p <$ 0.01). The excess was statistically significant only for individuals who had been platers for more than one year. In male chromium platers, 24 lung cancer deaths (ICD codes 162, 163) out of a total of 130 deaths were observed *versus* 13/96 among controls (nonsignificant). Cancer of the gastrointestinal tract and of 'all other sites' also occurred in excess in men, but the differences were not significant: 8/130 deaths from gastrointestinal cancers among exposed *versus* 4/96 in controls; 12/130 deaths from cancers of 'all other sites' in exposed *versus* 5/96 in controls. The smoking habits of platers and controls were similar. A higher proportion of controls had worked in asbestos processing (8.3% of controls *versus* 3.6% of platers); more platers had worked in coal mines, foundries, potteries, cotton manufacture and flax and hemp mills (Royle, 1975a). [The Working Group noted that past exposure to asbestos among the controls might have led to some underestimation of the lung cancer risk in the exposed group, and that the method of analysis used made the study difficult to interpret.]

Okubo and Tsuchiya (1977, 1979) reported results from a mortality study among 952 chromium platers in Tokyo, Japan. The cohort was constructed from records for 1970-76 of the Tokyo Health Insurance Society of the Plating Industry, and consisted of chromium platers (889 men, 63 women) who were born prior to 31 May 1937, had more than six months of work experience in chromium plating and had a work history record. Vital status was ascertained from a questionnaire sent to the management of the plating firms and, for retired workers, by contacting family registers; persons whose vital status was unknown were assumed to be alive. The expected number of deaths was derived from age-, sex- and year-specific death rates for the Tokyo general population. Twenty-one deaths from all causes were observed in chromium platers [SMR, 55; 95% CI, 34-83]. No case of lung cancer occurred, although 1.2 would have been expected in men. These results were reiterated in a 99% follow-up of a subgroup reported in an abstract (Okubo & Tsuchiya, 1987). [The Working Group questioned the completeness of assembling the cohort, the low age structure of the population and the limited period of follow-up.]

Silverstein et al. (1981) performed a proportionate mortality study in a group of hourly employees and retirees with at least ten years of service in a die-casting and nickel- and chromium-electroplating plant in the USA. The 238 subjects who had died between January 1974 and December 1978 were included in the study. Causes of death as stated on death certificates were compared with US national mortality rates. A total of 53 deaths from cancer were observed (proportionate mortality ratio (PMR), 135 [95% CI, 101-176]) among white men and 23 among white women (PMR, 127 [95% CI, 81-191]). The study revealed 28 lung cancer deaths (PMR, 191 [95% CI, 127-276]) in white men and ten among white women (PMR, 370 [95% CI, 178-681]). Smoking habits were not known. Four deaths from stomach cancer (PMR, 254 [95% CI, 69-648]), two from laryngeal cancer (PMR, 330 [95% CI, 40-1184] and two from lymphosarcoma and reticulosarcoma (PMR, 285 [95% CI, 35-1032]) occurred in white men. A case-control analysis of the lung cancer deaths, using deaths from cardiovascular disease as controls, tested the association of cancer with duration of work in different work sites, without considering possible confounders. An association was seen (odds ratio, 9.2; $p = 0.04$) for white men with more than five years' work in a department which, prior to 1971, was one of the major die-casting and plating areas in the plant. The authors noted that, although the population had been exposed primarily to chromium[VI], they had also been exposed to nickel compounds and may have been exposed to polycyclic aromatic hydrocarbons and metal fumes during die-casting.

Franchini et al. (1983) reported cancer mortality in a group of 178 Italian chromium electroplaters, 62 of whom were 'bright' (thin plating) and 116 of whom were 'hard' (thick plating) platers, and who had worked for at least one year in one of nine plants between 1951 and 1981. In 1980, exposure to chromium averaged 7 µg/m³ air as chromium trioxide near the plating baths and 3 µg/m³ in the middle of the room; measurements of urinary chromium showed that hard platers were more heavily exposed than bright platers: the median level of chromium in the urine of hard platers was 23.1 µg/g creatinine in 1974-76 and 5.7 µg/g creatinine in 1980-81. The SMR for deaths from all causes was 97 (15 deaths [95% CI, 55-163]); there were eight deaths from malignant tumours (SMR, 191; [95% CI, 82-375]) and three from lung cancer [SMR, 333; 95% CI, 69-974]. Seven of the cancer deaths occurred among hard platers [SMR, 259; 95% CI, 105-534] as did all three of the lung cancers [SMR, 429; 95% CI, 88-1252].

Sorahan *et al.* (1987) reported the mortality experience of 2689 chromium platers (1288 men, 1401 women) in the UK observed from January 1946 to December 1983 who were involved mainly in 'bright' (thin) plating of bumpers and overriders, initially reported by Waterhouse (1975). Scattered sampling of exposure had taken place before 1973, showing air concentrations of chromium trioxide up to 8.0 mg/m³, while the median values were 'nondetectable' or 'trace'; after 1973, measurements generally showed levels of chromium below 50 µg/m³. The cohort comprised workers employed in 1946-75 with more than six months' employment as a (chromium) electroplater. Death rates were compared with those of the general population of England and Wales. All members of the cohort had had at least some exposure to chromium but also some exposure to nickel chloride and nickel sulfate. A total of 213 cancer deaths (SMR, 130 [95% CI, 113-148]) and 72 lung cancer deaths (SMR, 150 [95% CI, 117-189]) were observed in men and women combined; 63 lung cancer deaths occurred in men (SMR, 158 [95% CI, 121-202]) and nine in women (SMR, 111 [95% CI, 46-261]). When the figures for each sex were combined and account was taken of time from first employment, the highest SMRs were 342 [95% CI, 182-585] after ten to 14 years and 245 [95% CI, 127-428] after 15-19 years of work at the chromium baths. Overall, three deaths (two in men, one in women) from cancer of the nose and nasal cavities occurred (SMR, 1000 [95% CI, 206-2922]); all three persons had been exposed to chromium for one to two years, while the third had also worked for 13 years plating nickel. There were 25 deaths from stomach cancer (SMR, 154 [95% CI, 100-228]), but this excess occurred only in men. Four deaths from cancer of the liver were observed in men (SMR, 667 [95% CI, 182-1707]) but none in women. In an analysis of data on first job held, the SMR for lung cancer was 199 (46 deaths [95% CI, 146-266] for men first employed as chrome bath workers and 101 (17 deaths [95% CI, 59-161]) for chromium workers who were first employed at other work sites. The authors reported that only 11% of workers had had periods of work at both the chrome baths and other chrome work. Although a significant association was found between work at chrome baths and death from lung cancer, no such association was found with work at nickel baths (Burges, 1980).

In a case-control study in Denmark of 326 cases of laryngeal cancer and 1134 controls (Olsen & Sabroe, 1984), two of the cases occurred among male chromium platers, yielding a standardized incidence odds ratio of 110 (95% CI, 30-360).

### (d) Production of ferrochromium alloys

Pokrovskaya and Shabynina (1973) studied a cohort of male and female factory workers engaged in chromium ferroalloy production between 1955 and 1969 in the USSR. Workers were reported to be exposed to chromium[VI] and chromium[III] compounds as well as benzo[a]pyrene. Death certificates were obtained from the municipal vital statistics office, and comparison was made with city mortality rates by sex and by ten-year age group. Access to complete work histories made it possible to exclude from the control cohort subjects who had been exposed to chromium in other plants. Male chromium workers aged 50-59 experienced significant [$p = 0.001$] increases in death rates from all malignancies, from lung cancer and from oesophageal cancer, as compared with deaths rates in the municipal population. The relative risk for lung cancer in men was reported to range from 4.4 in the 30-39-year age group to 6.6 ($p = 0.001$) in the 50-59-year age group. A large proportion of the cases of lung cancer among workers exposed to high concentrations of dust (cinder pit workers, metal crushers, smelter workers), including workers who were not exposed to benzo[a]pyrene in areas of furnace charge and finished products preparation. [The Working Group noted that the numbers of workers and the numbers of cancers by specific site were not reported.]

Axelsson et al. (1980) studied employees at a ferrochromium plant in Sweden producing ferrochromium alloys by furnace reduction of chromite ore, quartz, lime and coke; the study was restricted to all 1876 men employed for at least one year during the period 1 January 1930 to 31 December 1975 and alive in 1951. Records were available for all employees who had worked since 1913. Individuals were categorized according to length and place of work in the factory. Death certificates (1951-75) were obtained from the national Central Bureau of Statistics and incident cancer cases (1958-75) from a manual search of Cancer Registry files. Expected numbers of cancer deaths and incident cases were calculated assuming a 15-year latent period from onset of employment. The estimated levels of chromium metal plus chromium[III] in the work atmosphere ranged from 0 to 2.5 mg/m³, and those for chromium[VI] from 0 to 0.25 mg/m³. There were 87 cases of cancer in the period 1958-75 [SIR, 101; 95% CI, 81-125], of which seven were cancers of the trachea, bronchus, lung and pleura [SIR, 119; 95% CI, 48-245]. Among 641 arc furnace workers, who were considered as being most likely to have encountered exposure to chromium[III] and [VI], there were two cases of cancer at these sites [SIR, 95; 95%

CI, 12-344], one of which was a pleural mesothelioma. Among 326 maintenance workers, there were four cases of cancer at these sites [SIR, 400; 95% CI, 109-1024], two of which were mesotheliomas. Asbestos had been used in the factory.

Langård *et al.* (1980, 1990) studied male workers at a ferrochromium and ferro-silicon production plant in Norway, primarily to explore the hypothesis that chromium[III] might be carcinogenic to humans. Workers with one year or more of work were included. Hygiene studies in the plant in 1975 indicated the presence of chromium[III] and [VI] in the work environment; the atmosphere contained a mean of 0.01-0.29 mg/m$^3$ chromium, 11-33% of which was water-soluble chromium[VI]. The 1980 study comprised 976 workers with first employment before 1960 and alive in 1953; in the 1990 report, the cohort also included those with first employment before 1965 (to make a total of 1235 workers). In the latter report, 357 deaths from all causes were observed (SMR, 81 [95% CI, 73-90]). The SIR for all cancers was 84 (132 observed; 95% CI, 70-100); the total number of lung cancers was 17 (SIR, 88 [95% CI, 56-123]). Among the 379 ferrochromium workers, there were ten cases of lung cancer [SIR, 154; 95% CI, 74-283], 12 of the prostate [SIR, 151 [95% CI, 78-262] and five of the kidney [SIR, 273; 95% CI, 89-638]. The excess of lung cancer in ferrochromium workers was higher in the 1980 study (seven cases; SMR, 226 [95% CI, 91-466]).

### (e)    *Other industrial exposures to chromium*

In an exploratory proportionate mortality study, Tsuchiya (1965) investigated the occurrence of cancer in 1957-59 in about 200 Japanese companies with more than 1000 employees each. A total of 492 cancer deaths occurred among 1 200 000 workers during that period. The 22 lung cancer deaths that occurred among workers in industries handling chromium compounds were compared with the Japanese mortality rate for 1958 [SMR, 220; 95% CI, 138-333]. The author pointed out that because a person had handled chromium or nickel in a factory did not necessarily imply that he had been exposed to these elements. [The Working Group noted that the design of the study did not exclude selection bias, and that exposures to chromium and a variety of carcinogens were not mutually exclusive.]

Dalager *et al.* (1980) carried out a proportionate mortality study on a group of spray painters using zinc chromate primer paints in the maintenance of aircraft at two US military bases. Spray painting was carried out mainly in air-conditioned booths, but without respirators. The study cohort consisted of 977 white male workers who had spray painted for at least three months and who had terminated employment within a ten-year period prior to 31 July 1959. The relative 'frequency' of causes of death through 1977 was generated by comparing the observed number of cases with the expected relative frequency in the white US male population. There were 202 deaths among the spray painters; 50 had died of cancer (PMR, 136 [95%

CI, 101-179]), 21 of whom had respiratory cancer (ICD 160-164; PMR, 184 [95% CI, 114-282]). The proportionate cancer mortality rate for respiratory cancer was 146 (not significant).

Bertazzi *et al.* (1981) studied the causes of death in 1954-78 for 427 workers who had been employed for at least six months between 1946 and 1977 in a plant producing paints and coatings, including chromate[VI] pigments. They found 18 deaths due to cancer *versus* 9.8 expected on the basis of national rates; there were eight lung cancer deaths, giving SMRs of 227 [95% CI, 156-633] based on local rates and 334 [95% CI, 106-434] on the basis of national rates. The authors were unable to differentiate between exposures to different paints and coatings; they stated that the primary exposure was to chromate[VI] pigments but that there was low exposure to asbestos.

Cornell and Landis (1984) studied the causes of death for 851 men who had worked in 26 US nickel/chromium foundries between 1968 and 1979 and compared them with the mortality experience of US males and of a control group of foundry workers not exposed to nickel/chromium. Sixty deaths were from lung cancer *versus* 56.9 expected in the general population; a total of 103 deaths from all other neoplasms was observed with 118.0 expected. No death from nasal cancer was observed.

Stern *et al.* (1987) followed up 9365 workers from two chrome leather tanneries in Minnesota and Wisconsin, USA, from identification of the cohort in 1940 through to December 1982. Follow-up was 95% complete. By that time, 1582 deaths had occurred, giving a SMR of 89. The SMRs for cancer of the lung, trachea and bronchus (ICD 162-163) were low in both tanneries (18 deaths; SMR, 67; 95% CI, 40-106 and 42 deaths; SMR, 93; 95% CI, 67-126) in comparison with expected rates in the respective states. [The Working Group noted that exposure to chromium was low and occurred in only a small subgroup of the workers.]

Hernberg *et al.* (1983a,b) conducted a joint Danish-Finnish-Swedish case-control study among 167 living cases of cancer of the nasal or paranasal sinuses diagnosed between 1 July 1977 and 31 December 1980, who were individually matched for country, age and sex with patients with colonic or rectal cancer. Cases and controls were interviewed by telephone. Patients who had had work-related exposures during the ten years before occurrence of the illness were excluded. Sixteen patients, many of whom were included within the category 'stainless steel welding' and 'nickel', *versus* six controls reported exposure to chromium (odds ratio, 2.7; 95% CI, 1.1-6.6). Among 21 cases categorized as having been exposed to nickel and/or chromium, including the above cases, only two had been exposed to chromium only: one spray painter (chromates) and one steel worker.

In a case-control study in North Carolina and Virginia, USA, of 160 patients (93 men, 67 women) with cancers of the nasal cavity and paranasal sinuses diagnosed between 1970 and 1980, Brinton *et al.* (1984) found chromium/chromate exposure to be 5.1 times more frequent among male cases than among 290 hospital controls, based on five exposed male cases. The authors stated that the excess was associated mainly with use of chromate products in the building industry and in painting.

A hospital-based case-control study in Norway of 176 incident male lung cancer cases was performed by Kjuus *et al.* (1986). Cases were recruited between 1979 and 1983, and 176 age- and sex-matched control subjects were recruited from the same hospitals. Seven cases and six controls had been exposed to chromium and nickel compounds (welding excluded) for more than three years. The risk ratio, adjusted for smoking, was 1.4 (95% CI, 0.4-4.4).

Rafnsson and Jóhannesdóttir (1986) followed up 450 Icelandic men born between 1905 and 1945 who were licensed as masons (cement finishers). Nine deaths from cancer of the lung, trachea and bronchus (ICD 162, 163) were found (SMR, 314; 95% CI, 143-595). The eight men who had been licensed for 20 years had a SMR of 365 (95% CI, 158-720). The concentration of chromium[VI] in Icelandic cement in 1983 was 5.8-9.5 mg/kg; however, masons also work with other substances. [The Working Group noted that respiratory exposure to chromates would have been very low, suggesting that the excess may have been due to other factors.]

In an extended case-control study, Claude *et al.* (1988) further examined the possible relationship between work-related exposure and bladder cancer proposed by Claude *et al.* (1986). A total of 531 male cases were recruited from hospitals in the Federal Republic of Germany between 1977 and 1985 and were compared with sex- and age-matched controls recruited mainly from urological hospital wards. Exposure to chromium/chromate was reported for 52 cases *versus* 24 controls (odds ratio, 2.2; 95% CI, 1.4-3.5). The corresponding figures for spray painting were 49 *versus* 17 (odds ratio, 2.9; 95% CI, 1.7-4.9). Details were not given on the extent to which spray painting included exposure to chromium-containing paints. After adjustment for smoking, the rate ratio estimates for duration of exposure to chromium/chromate were (number of cases/controls in parentheses); one to nine years, 1.2 (10/8); ten to 19 years, 1.0 (9/7); 20-29 years, 2.0 (11/5); and ≥30 years, 3.0 (26/8), which gives a *p*-value for trend of 0.009. The corresponding rate ratios for spray painting were: 4.7 (13/2), 8.4 (8/1), 2.0 (14/9) and 2.4 (17/8). [The Working Group noted that the possibility of recall bias was high, since the risk ratios for 24/25 exposures exceeded unity.]

### (f) *Environmental exposure to chromium*

The possible relation between environmental exposure to chromium and mortality from lung cancer was studied by Axelsson and Rylander (1980) in a population-based study among people living close to two Swedish ferrochromium smelters. Air concentrations of chromium near the smelter were 100-400 ng/m³. The lung cancer mortality rates in the two communities where the smelters were located were 253 per million ($p < 0.05$) and 161 per million, respectively, as compared with the county rate of 194 per million during the entire period studied (1961-75).

# 4. Summary of Data Reported and Evaluation

## 4.1  Exposure data

Chromium in the form of various alloys and compounds has been in widespread commercial use for over 100 years. Early applications included chrome pigments and tanning liquors. In recent decades, chromium has also been widely used in chromium alloys and chrome plating.

Several million workers worldwide are exposed to airborne fumes, mists and dust containing chromium or its compounds. Of the occupational situations in which exposure to chromium occurs, highest exposures to chromium[VI] may occur during chromate production, welding, chrome pigment manufacture, chrome plating and spray painting; highest exposures to other forms of chromium occur during mining, ferrochromium and steel production, welding and cutting and grinding of chromium alloys.

Data on exposure levels are available for several specific industries and job categories covering several decades. In the past, exposures to chromium[VI] in excess of 1 mg/m³ were found repeatedly in some processes, including chromium plating, chromate production and certain welding operations; exposures to total chromium have been even higher. Modern control technologies have markedly reduced exposures in some processes, such as electroplating, in recent years.

Occupational exposure has been shown to give rise to elevated levels of chromium in blood, urine and some body tissues, inhalation being the main route.

Nonoccupational sources of exposure to chromium include food, air and water, but the levels are usually several orders of magnitude lower than those typically encountered in occupational situations.

## 4.2  Experimental carcinogenicity data

### Chromium[0]

Studies in rats by intratracheal, intramuscular and intrafemoral administration, in mice and rats by intrapleural and intraperitoneal administration and in mice, rats and rabbits by intravenous injections were inadequate to evaluate the carcinogenicity of *chromium metal* as a powder.

## Chromium[III]

In studies in which *chromic acetate* was administered by the oral route to mice and rats and by intrapleural and intramuscular administration to rats, the incidence of tumours was not increased. In studies in which rats were administered *chromic oxide* by intrabronchial or oral routes, no increase in the incidence of tumours was observed. In experiments by intrabronchial implantation of *chromic chloride* or *chrome tan* (a basic chromic sulfate) in rats and by intraperitoneal administration of *chromic sulfate* in mice, the incidence of tumours was not increased. Many of these studies suffered from certain limitations. *Chromite ore* has been extensively tested in rats by intrabronchial, intrapleural and intrafemoral administration; no increase in the incidence of tumours was seen.

## Chromium[VI]

*Calcium chromate* has been tested by inhalation in mice, by intratracheal administration in rats and hamsters, by intrabronchial administration and intrapleural administration in rats, by subcutaneous administration in mice, and by intramuscular administration in mice and rats. In the one study by inhalation in mice, there was an increase in the incidence of lung adenomas which was of borderline significance; in the single study by intratracheal administration and in the three studies by intrabronchial administration in rats, lung tumours were induced. No lung tumour was seen in hamsters after intratracheal instillation. Local tumours were produced in rats by intrapleural and in rats and mice by intramuscular administration of calcium chromate. *Chromium trioxide* (chromic acid) has been tested as a mist by inhalation at two dose levels in mice and as a solid by intrabronchial implantation in three studies in rats. In mice, a low incidence of lung adenocarcinomas was observed at the higher dose and of nasal papillomas at the lower dose; perforation of the nasal septum was observed at both dose levels. A few lung tumours were seen in two of the studies by intrabronchial administration in rats. *Sodium dichromate* has been tested in rats by inhalation, intratracheal, intrabronchial, intrapleural and intramuscular administration. Lung tumours, benign and malignant, were observed in the studies by inhalation and by intratracheal administration. No increase in the occurrence of local tumours was seen after intrabronchial, intrapleural or intramuscular administration. *Barium chromate* has been tested in rats by intrabronchial, intrapleural and intramuscular implantation. No increase in the occurrence of tumours was seen following intrabronchial implantation; the other studies were inadequate to allow an evaluation of the carcinogenicity of this compound. *Lead chromate* and derived pigments have been tested by intrabronchial implantation in rats without producing a significant increase in the incidence of tumours. Lead chromate and derived pigments have also been tested in rats by subcutaneous and intramuscular injection, producing malignant tumours at the site of injection and, in one study, renal carcinomas. A study by intrapleural administration to rats could not be evaluated. No increase in tumour incidence was observed when lead chromate was administered intramuscularly to mice. A single subcutaneous injection of *basic lead chromate* produced a high incidence of local sarcomas in rats. *Zinc chromates* have been tested in rats by intrabronchial implantation, producing bronchial carcinomas, by intrapleural administration, producing local tumours, and by subcutaneous and intramuscular injection, producing local sarcomas. Two samples of *strontium chromate* were tested in rats by intrabronchial implantation, producing a high incidence of bronchial carcinomas; intrapleural and intramuscular injection of strontium chromate produced local sarcomas.

**Other forms of chromium**

A range of *roasted chromite ores* (Cr[III/VI]), often described as mixed chromium dust, and other residue materials encountered in the early stages of bichromate production have been tested extensively in mice, rats, guinea-pigs and rabbits by inhalation and by intratracheal, intrabronchial, intrapleural and intramuscular administration. The results of these tests were generally negative, although a low incidence of local tumours was observed in rats following intrapleural or intramuscular implantation of roasted chromite ore. The studies were considered to suffer from certain inadequacies. *Chromium[IV] dioxide* was tested by inhalation in rats, producing a few lung lesions of questionable nature; the study had a number of limitations.

**4.3  Human carcinogenicity data**

Epidemiological studies carried out in the Federal Republic of Germany, Italy, Japan, the UK and the USA of workers in the chromate production industry have consistently shown excess risks for lung cancer. The workers in this industry may be exposed to a variety of forms of chromium, including chromium[VI] and [III] compounds.

Similarly, studies carried out in the Federal Republic of Germany, France, the Netherlands, Norway, the UK and the USA of workers in the production of chromate pigments have also consistently shown excess risks for lung cancer. Workers in this industry are exposed to chromates, not only in the pigments themselves but also from soluble chromium[VI] compounds in the raw materials used in their production. Excess risk for lung cancer has been clearly established in facilities where zinc chromate was produced, although other chromium pigments were also generally made in these plants. A small study in the UK of workers producing lead chromate pigments showed no overall excess risk for lung cancer, but a nonsignificant excess risk was seen in a subgroup of workers with lead poisoning. No data were available on risk associated with exposure to strontium chromate or to other specific chromate pigments.

In two limited reports from the UK and in a small Italian study, excesses of lung cancer were reported in workers in the chromium plating industry. In a group of persons working in die-casting and plating in the USA, similar results were seen. These findings were confirmed in a large study of chromium platers in the UK, which demonstrated an excess risk for lung cancer in platers, particularly among those with at least ten years of employment at chrome baths. Workers in this industry have been exposed to soluble chromium[VI] compounds and possibly also to nickel.

In three reports, from Norway, Sweden and the USSR, in which ferrochromium workers were studied, the overall results with regard to lung cancer were inconclusive. The major exposure in this industry is to chromium[III] compounds and to metallic chromium, although exposure to chromium[VI] may also occur.

Cases of sinonasal cancer were reported in epidemiological studies of primary chromate production workers in Japan, the UK and the USA, of chromate pigment production workers in Norway and of chromium platers in the UK, indicating a pattern of excess risk for these rare tumours.

For cancers other than of the lung and sinonasal cavity, no consistent pattern of cancer risk has been shown among workers exposed to chromium compounds.

The results of epidemiological studies of stainless-steel welders are consistent with the finding of excess mortality from lung cancer among other workers exposed to chromium[VI], but they do not contribute independently to the evaluation of chromium since welders are also exposed to other compounds. (See also the monograph on welding.)

No epidemiological study addressed the risk of cancer from exposure to metallic chromium alone.

### 4.4  Other relevant data

Inhaled chromium[VI] from welding and chrome-plating aerosols is readily absorbed from the respiratory tract. The degree of absorption depends on the extent of reduction of the hexavalent form to chromium[III], which is absorbed to a much lesser extent. The same factors apply to absorption from the gastrointestinal tract, although absorption by this route is generally much less than that from the respiratory tract.

Chromium[VI] compounds may cause adverse effects to the skin, the respiratory tract and, to a lesser degree, the kidneys in humans, while chromium[III] is less toxic.

Elevated levels of sister chromatid exchange were observed in workers exposed to chromium[VI] compounds in electroplating factories in four out of six studies.

Chromosomal aberrations were found in all three studies of exposed workers; an increased frequency of aneuploidy was reported in one of these studies. The two available studies on chromium[III] were inadequate to evaluate its cytogenetic effect in humans.

Chromates enter cells more readily than chromium[III] compounds and are reduced ultimately to chromium[III]. The reduction process and the subsequent intracellular activity of reduced chromium species are important for the mechanism of toxicity and carcinogenicity of chromium[VI]. Particulate chromium[III] compounds can also enter cells by phagocytosis.

Chromium[VI] compounds cross the placental barrier in greater amounts than chromium[III] compounds. Chromium trioxide increased fetal death rate, caused growth retardation and increased the frequency of skeletal deformities and of cleft palate in rodents. Developmental effects have also been reported in mice exposed to chromic chloride.

Chromium[VI] compounds of various solubilities in water were consistently active in numerous studies covering a wide range of tests for genetic and related effects. In particular, potassium dichromate, sodium dichromate, ammonium dichromate, potassium chromate, sodium chromate, ammonium chromate, chromium trioxide, calcium chromate, strontium chromate and zinc yellow induced a variety of effects (including DNA damage, gene mutation, sister chromatid exchange, chromosomal aberrations, cell transformation and dominant lethal mutation) in a number of targets, including animal cells *in vivo* and animal and human cells *in vitro*. Potassium chromate induced aneuploidy in insects, while chromium trioxide did not; various compounds induced gene mutation in insects. Potassium dichromate produced recombination, gene mutation and aneuploidy in fungi. All of these chromium[VI] compounds induced DNA damage and gene mutation in bacteria. Similar patterns were observed with zinc chromate, barium chromate, lead chromate and the derived pigments chromium orange, chromium yellow and molybdenum orange, which, however, often required preliminary dissolution in alkali or acids. A liquid chromium[VI] compound (chromyl chloride) and its vapours induced gene mutation in bacteria.

Although chromium[III] compounds were generally even more reactive than chromium[VI] compounds with purified DNA and isolated nuclei, 12 compounds of various solubilities (chromic chloride, chromic acetate, chromic nitrate, chromic sulfate, chromic potassium sulfate, chromium alum, neochromium, chromic hydroxide, chromic phosphate, chromic oxide, chromite ore and cupric chromite) gave positive results in only a minority of studies using cellular test systems, often under particular treatment conditions or at very high concentrations, which were generally orders of magnitude higher than those needed to obtain the same effects with chromium[VI] compounds. Some of the positive results could be ascribed to contamination with traces of chromium[VI] compounds. In particular, no DNA damage was observed in cells of animals treated *in vivo* with chromic chloride, and no micronuclei were seen in cells of animals given chromic nitrate. The chromium[III] compounds tested generally did not produce DNA damage, gene mutation, sister chromatid exchange or cell transformation in cultured animal and human cells. Chromosomal aberrations were often observed with high concentrations of chromium[III] compounds. Weak effects on gene mutation and mitotic gene conversion were observed in fungi. Negative results were obtained in the large majority of tests for DNA damage and gene mutation in bacteria. Certain complexes of chromium[III] with organic ligands, which favour the penetration of chromium[III] into cells, were reported to induce DNA damage and gene mutation in bacteria and in cultured mammalian cells.

A chromium[II] compound (chromous chloride) gave negative results in in-vitro tests with animal cells (DNA damage, chromosomal aberrations and aneuploidy). A water-insoluble chromium[0] compound (chromium carbonyl) did not induce DNA damage in bacteria.

No relevant study on the genetic and related effects of metallic chromium was available to the Working Group.

### 4.5 Evaluation[1]

There is *sufficient evidence* in humans for the carcinogenicity of chromium[VI] compounds as encountered in the chromate production, chromate pigment production and chromium plating industries.

There is *inadequate evidence* in humans for the carcinogenicity of metallic chromium and of chromium[III] compounds.

There is *sufficient evidence* in experimental animals for the carcinogenicity of calcium chromate, zinc chromates, strontium chromate and lead chromates.

There is *limited evidence* in experimental animals for the carcinogenicity of chromium trioxide (chromic acid) and sodium dichromate.

There is *inadequate evidence* in experimental animals for the carcinogenicity of metallic chromium, barium chromate and chromium[III] compounds.

The Working Group made the overall evaluation on chromium[VI] compounds on the basis of the combined results of epidemiological studies, carcinogenicity studies in experimental animals, and several types of other relevant data which support the underlying concept that chromium[VI] ions generated at critical sites in the target cells are responsible for the carcinogenic action observed.

---

[1]For definitions of the italicized terms, see Preamble, pp. 33–37

**Overall evaluation**

Chromium[VI] *is carcinogenic to humans* (Group 1).

Metallic chromium and chromium[III] compounds *are not classifiable as to their carcinogenicity to humans* (Group 3).

# 5. References

Aaseth, J., Alexander, J. & Norseth, T. (1982) Uptake of $^{51}$Cr-chromate by human erythrocytes—a role of glutathione. *Acta pharmacol. toxicol.*, *50*, 310-315

Abe, S., Ohsaki, Y., Kimura, K., Tsuneta, Y., Mikami, H. & Murao, M. (1982) Chromate lung cancer with special reference to its cell type and relation to the manufacturing process. *Cancer*, *49*, 783-787

Abell, M.T. & Carlberg, J.R. (1974) A simple reliable method for the determination of airborne hexavalent chromium. *Am. ind. Hyg. Assoc. J.*, *35*, 229-233

Ackermann, F. (1977) Method of instrumental neutron activation analysis and its application for the determination of trace metals in sediments (Ger.). *Dtsch. Gewaesserkd. Mitt.*, *21*, 53-60 [*Chem. Abstr.*, *88*, 15489g]

Adachi, S. (1987) Effects of chromium compounds on the respiratory system. Part 5. Long term inhalation of chromic acid mist in electroplating by C57BL female mice and recapitulation on our experimental studies (Jpn.). *Jpn. J. ind. Health*, *29*, 17-33

Adachi, S. & Takemoto, K. (1987) Occupational lung cancer. A comparison between humans and experimental animals (Jpn.). *Jpn. J. ind. Health*, *29*, 345-357

Adachi, S., Yoshimura, H., Katayama, H. & Takemoto, K. (1986) Effects of chromium compounds on the respiratory system. Part 4. Long term inhalation of chromic acid mist in electroplating to ICR female mice (Jpn.). *Jpn. J. ind. Health*, *28*, 283-287

Aitio, A., Järvisalo, J., Kiilunen, M., Tossavainen, A. & Vaittinen, P. (1984) Urinary excretion of chromium as an indicator of exposure to trivalent chromium sulphate in leather tanning. *Int. Arch. occup. environ. Health*, *54*, 241-249

Aitio, A., Jarvisalo, J., Kiilunen, M., Kalliomaki, P.L. & Kalliomaki, K. (1988) Chromium. In: Clarkson, T.W., Friberg, L., Nordberg, G.F. & Sager, P.R., eds, *Biological Monitoring of Toxic Metals*, New York, Plenum, pp. 369-382

Al-Badri, J.S., Sabir, S.M., Shehab, K.M., Jalil, M. & Al-Rawi, H. (1977) Determination of inorganic elements in Iraqi tobacco leaves and cigarettes by neutron activation analysis. *Iraqi J. Sci.*, *18*, 34-44

Albers, P.H., Sileo, L. & Mulhern, B.M. (1986) Effects of environmental contaminants on snapping turtles of a tidal wetland. *Arch. environ. Contam. Toxicol.*, *15*, 39-49

Alderson, M.R., Rattan, N.S. & Bidstrup, L. (1981) Health of workmen in the chromate-producing industry in Britain. *Br. J. ind. Med.*, *38*, 117-124

Alexander, J., Aaseth, J. & Norseth, T. (1982) Uptake of chromium by rat liver mitochondria. *Toxicology*, *24*, 115-122

Alwens, W. & Jonas, W. (1938) The chromate lung cancer (Ger.). *Unio int. contra cancrum, 3*, 103-118

American Chrome & Chemicals (undated a) *Product Data Sheet: Chromium Oxide Metallurgical (Cr$_2$O$_3$)*, Corpus Christi, TX

American Chrome & Chemicals (undated b) *Product Data Sheet: Accrox C (Cr$_2$O$_3$)*, Corpus Christi, TX

American Chrome & Chemicals (undated c) *Product Data Sheet: Accrox R (Cr$_2$O$_3$)*, Corpus Christi, TX

American Chrome & Chemicals (undated d) *Product Data Sheet: Accrox S (Cr$_2$O$_3$)*, Corpus Christi, TX

American Chrome & Chemicals (undated e) *Product Data Sheet: Chromic Acid (CrO$_3$)*, Corpus Christi, TX

American Chrome & Chemicals (undated f) *Product Data Sheet: Sodium Bichromate (Na$_2$Cr$_2$O$_7$.2H$_2$O)*, Corpus Christi, TX

American Chrome & Chemicals (undated g) *Product Data Sheet: Sodium Bichromate Anhydrous (Na$_2$Cr$_2$O$_7$)*, Corpus Christi, TX

American Chrome & Chemicals (undated h) *Product Data Sheet: Sodium Chromate Anhydrous (Na$_2$CrO$_4$)*, Corpus Christi, TX

American Chrome & Chemicals (undated i) *Product Data Sheet: Sodium Chromate Tetrahydrate (Na$_2$CrO$_4$.4H$_2$O)*, Corpus Christi, TX

American Conference of Governmental Industrial Hygienists (1988) *TLVs Threshold Limit Values and Biological Exposure Indices for 1988-89*, Cincinnati, OH, pp. 15-16, 24, 38

American Society for Testing and Materials (1971) *Standard Test Method for Chromium Oxide in Chrome Ores (ASTM E342-71 (Reapproved 1985))*, Philadelphia, PA, pp. 1-3

American Society for Testing and Materials (1978) *Standard Test Method for Chromic Oxide in Leather (Perchloric Acid Oxidation) (ASTM D2807-78)*, Philadelphia, PA, pp. 1-4

American Society for Testing and Materials (1981) *Standard Methods for Chemical Analysis of Chrome-containing Refractories and Chrome Ore (ASTM C572-81)*, Philadelphia, PA, pp. 1-9

American Society for Testing and Materials (1983) *Standard Methods for Chemical Analysis of Chromium and Ferrochromium (ASTM E363-83)*, Philadelphia, PA, pp. 1-6

American Society for Testing and Materials (1984a) *Standard Specification for Wrought Cobalt-Nickel-Chromium Molybdenum Alloy for Surgical Implant Applications (ASTM F562-84)*, Philadelphia, PA, pp. 1-4

American Society for Testing and Materials (1984b) *Standard Test Method for Lead and Chromium in Air Particulate Filter Samples of Lead Chromate Type Pigment Dusts by Atomic Absorption Spectroscopy (ASTM D4358-84)*, Philadelphia, PA, pp. 1-5

American Society for Testing and Materials (1985a) *Standard Test Method for Chromium in Workplace Atmospheres (Colorimetric Method) (ASTM D3586-85)*, Philadelphia, PA, pp. 1-6

American Society for Testing and Materials (1985b) *Standard Test Method for Low Concentrations of Chromium in Paint by Atomic Absorption Spectrocopy (ASTM D3718-85a)*, Philadelphia, PA, pp. 1-4

American Society for Testing and Materials (1986a) *Standard Test Method for Chromium in Water (ASTM D1687-86)*, Philadelphia, PA, pp. 1-9

American Society for Testing and Materials (1986b) *Standard Test Method for Chemical Analysis of Strontium Chromate Pigment (ASTM D1845-86)*, Philadelphia, PA, pp. 1-3

American Society for Testing and Materials (1987a) *Standard Specification for Cast Cobalt-Chromium-Molybdenum Alloy for Surgical Implant Applications (ASTM F75-87)*, Philadelphia, PA, pp. 1-2

American Society for Testing and Materials (1987b) *Standard Specification for Thermomechanically Processed Cobalt-Chromium-Molybdenum Alloy for Surgical Implant Applications (ASTM F799-87)*, Philadelphia, PA, pp. 1-3

American Society for Testing and Materials (1987c) *Standard Test Method for Analysis of Yellow, Orange, and Green Pigments Containing Lead Chromate and Chromium Oxide Green (ASTM D126-87)*, Philadelphia, PA, pp. 1-7

American Society for Testing and Materials (1988a) *Standard Specification for Wrought Cobalt-Nickel-Chromium-Molybdenum-Tungsten-Iron Alloy for Surgical Implant Applications (ASTM F563-88)*, Philadelphia, PA, pp. 1-3

American Society for Testing and Materials (1988b) *Standard Test Method for Chemical Analysis of Zinc Yellow Pigment (Zinc Chromate Yellow) (ASTM D44-88)*, Philadelphia, PA, pp. 1-5

Andersen, O. (1983) Effects of coal combustion products and metal compounds on sister chromatid exchange (SCE) in a macrophage-like cell line. *Environ. Health Perspect.*, *47*, 239-253

Angerer, J. & Schaller, K.H. (1988) *Analysen in biologischem Material* (Analysis in Biological Material), Weinheim, Deutsche Forschungsgemeinschaft, pp. 1-16

Anon. (1978) Chromic acid. *Chem. Mark. Rep.*, *213*, 9

Anon. (1979) Sodium bichromate. *Chem. Mark. Rep.*, *216*, 9

Anon. (1981) Problems of epidemiological evidence. *Environ. Health Perspect.*, *40*, 11-20

Anon. (1988a) Chemical profile: chromic acid. *Chem. Mark. Rep.*, *234*, 54

Anon. (1988b) Chemical profile: sodium bichromate. *Chem. Mark. Rep.*, *234*, 82

Arbeidsinspectie (Labour Inspection) (1986) *De Nationale MAC–Lijst 1986* (National MAC-List 1986), Voorburg, p. 10

Arbejdstilsynet (Labour Inspection) (1988) *Graensevaerdier for Stoffer og Materialer* (Limit Values for Compounds and Materials) (No 3.1.0.2), Copenhagen, p. 14

Arbetarskyddsstyrelsens (National Board of Occupational Safety and Health) (1987) *Hygieniska Gränsvärden* (Hygienic Limit Values), Stockholm, p. 28

Arlauskas, A., Baker, R.S.U., Bonin, A.M., Tandon, R.K., Crisp, P.T. & Ellis, J. (1985) Mutagenicity of metal ions in bacteria. *Environ. Res.*, *36*, 379-388

Atomergic Chemetals Corp. (1980) *Specification Sheet: Barium Chromate*, Farmingdale, NY

Axelsson, G. & Rylander, R. (1980) Environmental chromium dust and lung cancer mortality. *Environ. Res.*, *23*, 469-476

Axelsson, G., Rylander, R. & Schmidt, A. (1980) Mortality and incidence of tumours among ferrochromium workers. *Br. J. ind. Med.*, *37*, 121-127

Bacon, F.E. (1964) Chromium and chromium alloys. In: Kirk, R.E. & Othmer, D.F., eds, *Encyclopedia of Chemical Technology*, 2nd ed., Vol. 5, New York, John Wiley & Sons, pp. 453-464

Baetjer, A.M. (1950) Pulmonary carcinoma in chromate workers. II. Incidence on basis of hospital records. *Arch. ind. Hyg. occup. Med.*, 2, 505-516

Baetjer, A.M., Damron, C. & Budacz, V. (1959a) The distribution and retention of chromium in men and animals. *Arch. ind. Health*, 20, 136-150

Baetjer, A.M., Lowney, J.F., Steffee, H. & Budacz, V. (1959b) Effect of chromium on incidence of lung tumors in mice and rats. *Arch. ind. Health*, 20, 124-135

Baker, R.S.U. (1984) Evaluation of metals in in vitro assays, interpretation of data and possible mechanisms of action. *Toxicol. environ. Chem.*, 7, 191-212

Baker, R.S.U., Bonin, A.M., Arlauskas, A., Tandon, R.K., Crisp, P.T. & Ellis, J. (1984) Chromium(VI) and apparent phenotypic reversion in *Salmonella* TA100. *Mutat. Res.*, 138, 127-132

Bakke, O., Jakobsen, K. & Eik-Nes, K.B. (1984) Concentration-dependent effects of potassium dichromate on the cell cycle. *Cytometry*, 5, 482-486

Balsberg-Påhlsson, A.-M., Lithner, G. & Tyler, G. (1982) *Krom i Miljön* (Chromium in the Environment), Solna, Statens Naturvårdsverk

Baranowska-Dutkiewicz, B. (1981) Absorption of hexavalent chromium by skin in man. *Arch. Toxicol.*, 47, 47-50

Barbořík, M., Hanslian, L., Oral, L., Sehnalová, H. & Holuša, R. (1958) Carcinoma of the lungs in personnel working at electrolytic chromium plating (Czech). *Prac. Lek.*, 10, 413-417

Barceló, J., Poschenrieder, C. & Gunsé, B. (1986) Impact of chromium on the environment. II. Chromium in living organisms (Sp.). *Circ. Farm.*, 293, 31-48

Barium & Chemicals (1988a) *MSDS and Data Sheet: Calcium Chromate*, Steubenville, OH

Barium & Chemicals (1988b) *Military Specification: Barium Chromate (MIL-B-55A)*, Steubenville, OH

Barium & Chemicals (undated) *Barium, Strontium, Calcium ... and Other Chemical Products*, Steubenville, OH

Belitskaya, E.N. (1981) Physiologic and hygienic characterization of working conditions for steel smelters in open-hearth process (Russ.). *Gig. Tr.*, 24, 9-11

Belmont Metals (1989) *Typical Analysis: Electrolytic Chromium Metal*, Brooklyn, NY

Bennicelli, C., Camoirano, A., Petruzzelli, S., Zanacchi, P. & De Flora, S. (1983) High sensitivity of *Salmonella* TA102 in detecting hexavalent chromium mutagenicity and its reversal by liver and lung preparations. *Mutat. Res.*, 122, 1-5

Bertazzi, P.A., Zocchetti, C., Terzaghi, G.F., Riboldi, L., Guercilena, S. & Beretta, F. (1981) Mortality experience of paint production workers (Ital.). *Med. Lav.*, 6, 465-472

Beszedits, S. (1988) Chromium removal from industrial wastewaters. In: Nriagu, J.O. & Nieboer, E., eds, *Chromium in the Natural and Human Environments*, New York, Wiley-Interscience, pp. 231-265

Beyersmann, D. & Köster, A. (1987) On the role of trivalent chromium in chromium genotoxicity. *Toxicol. environ. Chem.*, 14, 11-22

Beyersmann, D., Köster, A., Buttner, B. & Flessel, P. (1984) Model reactions of chromium compounds with mammalian and bacterial cells. *Toxicol. environ. Chem.*, 8, 279-286

Bhargava, O.P., Bumsted, H.E., Grunder, F.I., Hunt, B.L., Manning, G.E., Riemann, R.A., Samuels, J.K., Tatone, V., Waldschmidt, S.J. & Hernandez, P. (1983) Study of an analytical method for hexavalent chromium. *Am. ind. Hyg. Assoc. J.*, 44, 433-436

Bianchi, V. & Levis, A.G. (1984) Mechanisms of chromium genotoxicity. *Toxicol. environ. Chem.*, 9, 1-25

Bianchi, V. & Levis, A.G. (1985) Metals as genotoxic agents: the model of chromium. In: Irgolic, K.J. & Martell, A.E., eds, *Environmental Organic Chemistry*, Deersfield Beach, FL, VCH Publishers, pp. 447-462

Bianchi, V. & Levis, A.G. (1987) Recent advances in chromium genotoxicity. *Toxicol. environ. Chem.*, 15, 1-24

Bianchi, V. & Levis, A.G. (1988) Genetic effects and mechanisms of action of chromium compounds. *Sci. total Environ.*, 71, 351-355

Bianchi, V., Levis, A.G. & Saggioro, D. (1979) Differential cytotoxic activity of potassium dichromate on nucleoside uptake in BHK fibroblasts. *Chem.-biol. Interact.*, 24, 137-151

Bianchi, V., Dal Toso, R., Debetto, P., Levis, A.G., Luciani, S., Majone, F. & Tamino, G. (1980) Mechanisms of chromium toxicity in mammalian cell cultures. *Toxicology*, 17, 219-224

Bianchi, V., Debetto, P., Zantedeschi, A. & Levis, A.G. (1982a) Effects of hexavalent chromium on the adenylate pool of hamster fibroblasts. *Toxicology*, 25, 19-30

Bianchi, V., Nuzzo, F., Abbondandolo, A., Bonatti, S., Capelli, E., Fiorio, R., Giulotto, E., Mazzaccaro, A., Stefanini, M., Zaccaro, L., Zantedeschi, A. & Levis, A.G. (1982b) Scintillometric determination of DNA repair in human cell lines: a critical appraisal. *Mutat. Res.*, 93, 447-463

Bianchi, V., Celotti, L., Lanfranchi, G., Majone, F., Marin, G., Montaldi, A., Sponza, G., Tamino, G., Venier, P., Zantedeschi, A. & Levis, A.G. (1983) Genetic effects of chromium compounds. *Mutat. Res.*, 117, 279-300

Bianchi, V., Zantedeschi, A., Montaldi, A. & Majone, F. (1984) Trivalent chromium is neither cytotoxic nor mutagenic in permeabilized hamster fibroblasts. *Toxicol. Lett.*, 23, 51-59

Bidstrup, P.L. (1951) Carcinoma of the lung in chromate workers. *Br. J. ind. Med.*, 8, 302-305

Bidstrup, P.L. & Case, R.A.M. (1956) Carcinoma of the lung in workmen in the bichromates-producing industry in Great Britain. *Br. J. ind. Med.*, 13, 260-264

Bigaliev, A.B. (1981) Chromosomal aberrations in a lymphocyte culture from persons in contact with chromium (Russ.). *Tsitol. Genet.*, 15, 63-68

Bigaliev, A.B., Elemesova, M.S. & Turebaev, M.N. (1977a) Evaluation of the mutagenic activity of chromium compounds (Russ.). *Gig. Tr. prof. Zabol.*, 6, 37-40

Bigaliev, A.B., Turebaev, M.N. & Elemesova, M.S. (1977b) Cytogenetic study of the in vivo mutagenic properties of chromium compounds (Russ.). In: Dubinin, N.P., ed., *Genet. Posledstviya Zagryaznenia Okruzhayushehei Sredy* (Proceedings of a Symposium), Moscow, Nauka, pp. 173-176

Bigaliev, A.B., Turebaev, M.N., Bigalieva, R.K. & Elemesova, M.S. (1977c) Cytogenetic examination of workers engaged in chrome production (Russ.). *Genetika*, *13*, 545-547

Bigaliev, A.B., Shpak, N.K. & Smagulov, A.S. (1979) Mechanisms of the cytogenetic action of chromium as an environmental pollutant. *Dokl. Biol. Sci.* (Engl. transl.), *245*, 809-810

Biggart, N.W. & Murphy, E.C., Jr (1988) Analysis of metal-induced mutations altering the expression or structure of a retroviral gene in a mammalian cell line. *Mutat. Res.*, *198*, 115-129

Bloomfield, J.J. & Blum, W. (1928) Health hazards in chromium plating. *Public Health Rep.*, *43*, 2330-2347

Bohgard, M., Jandiga, B.L. & Akselsson, K.R. (1979) An analytical procedure for determining chromium in samples of airborne dust. *Ann. occup. Hyg.*, *22*, 241-251

Bonatti, S., Meini, M. & Abbondandolo, A. (1976) Genetic effects of potassium dichromate in *Schizosaccharomyces pombe*. *Mutat. Res.*, *38*, 147-150

Bourne, H.G., Jr & Yee, H.T. (1950) Occupational cancer in a chromate plant. An environmental appraisal. *Ind. Med. Surg.*, *19*, 563-567

Bovet, P., Lob, M. & Grandjean, M. (1977) Spirometric alterations in workers in the chromium electroplating industry. *Int. Arch. occup. environ. Health*, *40*, 25-32

Bragt, P.C. & van Dura, E.A. (1983) Toxicokinetics of hexavalent chromium in the rat after intratracheal administration of chromates of different solubilities. *Ann. occup. Hyg.*, *27*, 315-322

Brakhnova, I.T. (1975) *Environmental Hazards of Metals* (translation), New York, Consultants Bureau, pp. 41-42

Brambilla, G., Sciabà, L., Carlo, P., Finollo, R., Farina, A. & Parodi, S. (1980) DNA crosslinking in mammalian cells treated with potassium dichromate (Abstract No. 394). *Proc. Am. Assoc. Cancer Res.*, *21*, 98

Brams, A., Buchet, J.P., Crutzen-Fayt, M.C., De Meester, C., Lauwerys, R. & Léonard, A. (1987) A comparative study, with 40 chemicals, of the efficiency of the *Salmonella* assay and the SOS chromotest (kit procedure). *Toxicol. Lett.*, *38*, 123-133

Braver, E.R., Infante, P. & Chu, K. (1985) An analysis of lung cancer risk from exposure to hexavalent chromium. *Teratog. Carcinog. Mutagenesis*, *5*, 365-378

Brinton, H.P., Frasier, E.S. & Koven, A.L. (1952) Morbidity and mortality experience among chromate workers. *Public Health Rep.*, *67*, 835-847

Brinton, L.A., Blot, W.J., Becker, J.A., Winn, D.M., Browder, J.P., Farmer, J.C., Jr & Fraumeni, J.F., Jr (1984) A case-control study of cancers of the nasal cavity and paranasal sinuses. *Am. J. Epidemiol.*, *119*, 896-906

British Chrome & Chemical Ltd (1988) *MSDS: Basic Chromic Sulphate (Chrometan)*, Eaglescliffe, Stockton-on-Tees

Brochard, P., Ameille, J., Brun, B., Gagnant, B. & Philbert, M. (1983) Bronchial cancer and chromium electroplating. About a new case (Fr.). *Arch. Mal. prof.*, *44*, 35-37

Bronzetti, G., Galli, A., Boccardo, P., Vellosi, R., Del Carratore, R., Sabbioni, E. & Edel, J. (1986) Genotoxicity of chromium *in vitro* on yeast: interaction with DNA. *Toxicol. environ. Chem.*, *13*, 103-111

Brune, D., Nordberg, G. & Wester, P.O. (1980) Distribution of 23 elements in the kidney, liver and lungs of workers from a smeltery and refinery in north Sweden exposed to a number of elements and of a control group. *Sci. total Environ.*, *16*, 13-35

Bryson, W.G. & Goodall, C.M. (1983) Differential toxicity and clearance kinetics of chromium (III) or (VI) in mice. *Carcinogenesis*, *4*, 1535-1539

Buckell, M. & Harvey, D.G. (1951) An environmental study of the chromate industry. *Br. J. ind. Med.*, *8*, 298-301

Bunker, V.W., Lawson, M.S., Delves, H.T. & Clayton, B.E. (1984) The uptake and excretion of chromium by the elderly. *Am. J. clin. Nutr.*, *39*, 797-802

Burges, D.C.L. (1980) Mortality study of nickel platers. In: Brown, S.S. & Sunderman, F.W., eds, *Nickel Toxicology*, London, Academic Press, pp. 15-18

Burrows, D. (1983) Adverse chromate reactions on the skin. In: Burrows, D., ed., *Chromium: Metabolism and Toxicity*, Boca Raton, FL, CRC Press, pp. 137-163

Byrne, C.J. & DeLeon, I.R. (1986) Trace metal residues in biota and sediments from Lake Pontchartrain, Louisiana. *Bull. environ. Contam. Toxicol.*, *37*, 151-158

Calder, L.M. (1988) Chromium contamination of groundwater. In: Nriagu, J.O. & Nieboer, E., eds, *Chromium in the Natural and Human Environments*, New York, Wiley Interscience, pp. 215-229

Camusso, M. & Montesissa, C. (1988) Chromium (Part 1) (Ital.). *Chim. ind. (Milan)*, *70*, 30-32

Cantoni, O. & Costa, M. (1984) Analysis of the induction of alkali sensitive sites in the DNA by chromate and other agents that induce single strand breaks. *Carcinogenesis*, *5*, 1207-1209

Carelli, G., La Bua, R., Rimatori, V., Porcelli, D. & Iannaccone, A. (1981) Interferences in the spectrophotometric s-diphenylcarbazide determination of environmental hexavalent chromium in a chromium and zinc plating plant. *Scand. J. Work Environ. Health*, *7*, 56-61

Cary, E.E. (1982) Chromium in air, soil, and natural waters. In: Langård, S., ed., *Biological and Environmental Aspects of Chromium*, Amsterdam, Elsevier, pp. 49-64

Casto, B.C., Meyers, J. & DiPaolo, J.A. (1979) Enhancement of viral transformation for evaluation of the carcinogenic or mutagenic potential of inorganic metal salts. *Cancer Res.*, *39*, 193-198

Cavalleri, A. & Minoia, C. (1985) Monitoring exposure to Cr(VI) and Cr(III) in workers by determination of chromium in urine, serum and red blood cells (Ital.). *G. ital. med. Lav.*, *7*, 35-38

Celotti, L., Furlan, D., Seccati, L. & Levis, A.G. (1987) Interactions of nitrilotriacetic acid (NTA) with Cr(VI) compounds in the induction of gene mutations in cultured mammalian cells. *Mutat. Res.*, *190*, 35-39

Chalupski, V.H. (1956) The manufacture and properties of chromium pigments. In: Udy, M.J., ed., *Chromium*, Vol. 1, New York, Reinhold, pp. 364-376

Chemical Information Services Ltd (1988) *Directory of World Chemical Producers 1989/90 Edition*, Oceanside, NY

Choi, Y.-J., Kim, Y.-W. & Cha, C.-W. (1987) A study on sister chromatid exchanges in lymphocytes in some metal plating workers (Korean). *Korea Univ. med. J.*, *24*, 249-257

Christie, N.T., Cantoni, O., Evans, R.M., Meyn, R.E. & Costa, M. (1984) Use of mammalian DNA repair-deficient mutants to assess the effects of toxic metal compounds on DNA. *Biochem. Pharmacol.*, *33*, 1661-1670

Chromium Association (1989) *World Production of Ferrochromium*, Paris

Cikrt, M. & Bencko, V. (1979) Biliary excretion and distribution of $^{51}$Cr(III) and $^{51}$Cr(VI) in rats. *J. Hyg. Epidemiol. Microbiol. Immunol.*, *23*, 241-246

Clarkson, T.W., Nordberg, G.F. & Sager, P.R. (1985) Reproductive and developmental toxicity of metals. *Scand. J. Work Environ. Health*, *11*, 145-154

Claude, J., Kunze, E., Frentzel-Beyme, R., Paczkowski, K., Schneider, J. & Schubert, H. (1986) Life-style and occupational risk factors in cancer of the lower urinary tract. *Am. J. Epidemiol.*, *124*, 578-589

Claude, J.C., Frentzel-Beyme, R.R. & Kunze, E. (1988) Occupation and risk of cancer of the lower urinary tract among men. A case-control study. *Int. J. Cancer*, *41*, 371-379

Cobalt Development Institute (1985) *Cobalt in Superalloys*, London, Strobel & Sons

Collaborative Study Group for the Micronucleus Test (1986) Sex difference in the micronucleus test. *Mutat. Res.*, *172*, 151-163

Collaborative Study Group for the Micronucleus Test (1988) Strain difference in the micronucleus test. *Mutat. Res.*, *204*, 307-316

Commission of the European Communities (1975) Council Directive of 16 June 1975 concerning the quality required of surface water intended for the abstraction of drinking water in the Member States. *Off. J. eur. Communities*, *L194*, 26-30

Connett, P.H. & Wetterhahn, K.E. (1983) Metabolism of the carcinogen chromate by cellular constitutents. *Struct. Bonding*, *54*, 93-124

Connett, P.H. & Wetterhahn, K.E. (1985) In vitro reaction of the carcinogen chromate with cellular thiols and carboxylic acids. *J. Am. chem. Soc.*, *107*, 4282-4288

Cook, W.A. (1987) *Occupational Exposure Limits — Worldwide*, Washington DC, American Industrial Hygiene Association, pp. 119, 133

Copson, R.L. (1956) Production of chromium chemicals. In: Udy, M.J., ed., *Chromium*, Vol. 1, New York, Reinhold, pp. 262-282

Corbett, T.H., Heidelberger, C. & Dove, W.F. (1970) Determination of the mutagenic activity to bacteriophage T4 of carcinogenic and noncarcinogenic compounds. *Mol. Pharmacol.*, *6*, 667-679

Cornelis, R. (1988) Analytical procedures and clinical reference materials in monitoring human exposures to trace metals with special reference to chromium, lead, and thallium. *Sci. total Environ.*, *71*, 269-283

Cornell, R.G. & Landis, J.R. (1984) Mortality patterns among nickel/chromium alloy foundry workers. In: Sunderman, F.W., Jr, ed., *Nickel in the Human Environment* (IARC Scientific Publications No. 53; IPCS Joint Symposia No. 4; CEC-EUR 916 EN), Lyon, IARC, pp. 87-93

Costa, R., Strolego, G. & Levis, A.G. (1988) Mutagenicity of lead chromate in *Drosophila melanogaster* in the presence of nitrilotriacetic acid (NTA). *Mutat. Res.*, *204*, 257-261

Cupo, D.Y. & Wetterhahn, K.E. (1984) Repair of chromate-induced DNA damage in chick embryo hepatocytes. *Carcinogenesis, 5,* 1705-1708

Cupo, D.Y. & Wetterhahn, K.E. (1985a) Binding of chromium to chromatin and DNA from liver and kidney of rats treated with sodium dichromate and chromium III chloride *in vivo. Cancer Res., 45,* 1146-1151

Cupo, D.Y. & Wetterhahn, K.E. (1985b) Modification of chromium(VI)-induced DNA damage by glutathione and cytochrome P-450 in chicken embryo hepatocytes. *Proc. natl Acad. Sci. USA, 82,* 6755-6759

Custer, T.W., Franson, J.C., Moore, J.F. & Myers, J.E. (1986) Reproductive success and heavy metal contamination in Rhode Island common terns. *Environ. Pollut. (Ser. A), 41,* 33-52

Cyprus Specialty Metals (1988) *Specification Sheets: Chromite (Chrome Ore) and Chromite, Supergray,* Malvern, PA

Dalager, N.A., Mason, T.J., Fraumeni, J.F., Jr, Hoover, R. & Payne, W.W. (1980) Cancer mortality among workers exposed to zinc chromate paints. *J. occup. Med., 22,* 25-29

Dams, R., Robbins, J.A., Rahn, K.A. & Winchester, J.W. (1970) Nondestructive neutron activation analysis of air pollution particulates. *Anal. Chem., 42,* 861-867

Danielsson, B.R.G., Hassoun, E. & Dencker, L. (1982) Embryotoxicity of chromium: distribution in pregnant mice and effects on embryonic cells *in vitro. Arch. Toxicol., 51,* 233-245

Danielsson, B.R.G., Dencker, L., Lindgren, A. & Tjälve, H. (1984) Accumulation of toxic metals in male reproduction organs. *Arch. Toxicol., Suppl. 7,* 177-180

Davies, J.M. (1978) Lung-cancer mortality of workers making chrome pigments (letter to the Editor). *Lancet, i,* 384

Davies, J.M. (1979) Lung cancer mortality of workers in chromate pigment manufacture: an epidemiological survey. *J. Oil col. chem. Assoc., 62,* 157-163

Davies, J.M. (1984a) Lung cancer mortality among workers making lead chromate and zinc chromate pigments in three English factories. *Br. J. ind. Med., 41,* 158-169

Davies, J.M. (1984b) Long term mortality study of chromate pigment workers who suffered lead poisoning. *Br. J. ind. Med., 41,* 170-178

Davis, G.K. (1956) Chromium in soils, plants, and animals. In: Udy, M.J., ed., *Chromium,* Vol. 1, New York, Reinhold, pp. 105-109

Davis, J.M.G. (1972) The fibrogenic effects of mineral dusts injected into the pleural cavity of mice. *Br. J. exp. Pathol., 53,* 190-201

De Flora, S. (1978) Metabolic deactivation of mutagens in the *Salmonella*/microsome test. *Nature, 271,* 455-456

De Flora, S. (1981a) Study of 106 organic and inorganic compounds in the *Salmonella*/microsome test. *Carcinogenesis, 2,* 283-298

De Flora, S. (1981b) A 'spiral test' applied to bacterial mutagenesis assays. *Mutat. Res., 82,* 213-227

De Flora, S. (1982) Biotransformation and interaction of chemicals as modulators of mutagenicity and carcinogenicity. In: Sugimura, T., Kondo, S. & Takebe, H., eds, *Environmental Mutagens and Carcinogens*, Tokyo, University of Tokyo Press/New York, Alan R. Liss, pp. 527-541

De Flora, S. & Boido, V. (1980) Effect of human gastric juice on the mutagenicity of chemicals. *Mutat. Res.*, 77, 307-315

De Flora, S. & Wetterhahn, K.E. (1990) Mechanisms of chromium metabolism and genotoxicity. *Life Chem. Rep.* (in press)

De Flora, S., Coppola, R., Camoirano, A., Battaglia, M.A. & Bennicelli, C. (1980) Mutagenicity and toxicity of chromyl chloride and its vapours. *Carcinogenesis*, 1, 583-587

De Flora, S., Zanacchi, P., Bennicelli, C. & Arillo, A. (1982) Influence of liver S-9 preparations from rats and rainbow trout on the activity of four mutagens. *Toxicol. Lett.*, 10, 345-349

De Flora, S., Zanacchi, P., Camoirano, A., Bennicelli, C. & Badolati, G. (1984a) Genotoxic activity and potency of 135 compounds in the Ames reversion test and in bacterial DNA-repair test. *Mutat. Res.*, 133, 161-198

De Flora, S., Camoirano, A., Zanacchi, P. & Bennicelli, C. (1984b) Mutagenicity testing with TA97 and TA102 of 30 DNA-damaging compounds, negative with other *Salmonella* strains. *Mutat. Res.*, 134, 159-165

De Flora, S., Bennicelli, C., Zanacchi, P., Camoirano, A., Morelli, A. & De Flora, A. (1984c) In vitro effects of N-acetylcysteine on the mutagenicity of direct-acting compounds and procarcinogens. *Carcinogenesis*, 5, 505-510

De Flora, S., De Renzi, G.P., Camoirano, A., Astengo, M., Basso, C., Zanacchi, P. & Bennicelli, C. (1985a) Genotoxicity assay of oil dispersants in bacteria (mutation, differential lethality, SOS DNA-repair) and yeast (mitotic crossing-over). *Mutat. Res.*, 158, 19-30

De Flora, S., Morelli, A., Basso, C., Romano, M., Serra, D. & De Flora, A. (1985b) Prominent role of DT-diaphorase as a cellular mechanism reducing chromium(VI) and reverting its mutagenicity. *Cancer Res.*, 45, 3188-3196

De Flora, S., Bennicelli, C., Camoirano, A., Serra, D., Romano, M., Rossi, G.A., Morelli, A. & De Flora, A. (1985c) In vivo effects of N-acetylcysteine on glutathione metabolism and on the biotransformation of carcinogenic and/or mutagenic compounds. *Carcinogenesis*, 6, 1735-1745

De Flora, S., Russo, P., Pala, M., Fassina, G., Zunino, A., Bennicelli, C., Zanacchi, P., Camoirano, A. & Parodi, S. (1985d) Assay of phenacetin genotoxicity using in vitro and in vivo test systems. *J. Toxicol. environ. Health*, 16, 355-377

De Flora, S., Badolati, G.S., Serra, D., Picciotto, A., Magnolia, M.R. & Savarino, V. (1987a) Circadian reduction of chromium in the gastric environment. *Mutat. Res.*, 192, 169-174

De Flora, S., Camoirano, A., Serra, D., Basso, C., Zanacchi, P. & Bennicelli, C. (1987b) DT diaphorase and the action of chemical mutagens and carcinogens. *Chem. scripta*, 27A, 151-155

De Flora, S., Camoirano, A., Romano, M., Astengo, M., Cesarone, C.F. & Millman, I. (1987c) Metabolism of mutagens and carcinogens in woodchuck liver and its relationship with hepatitis virus infection. *Cancer Res.*, 47, 4052-4058

De Flora, S., Petruzzelli, S., Camoirano, A., Bennicelli, C., Romano, M., Rindi, M., Ghelar-ducci, L. & Giuntini, C. (1987d) Pulmonary metabolism of mutagens and its relation-ship with lung cancer and smoking habits. *Cancer Res., 47,* 4740-4745

De Flora, S., Bennicelli, C., Camoirano, A., Serra, D. & Hochstein, P. (1988) Influence of DT diaphorase on the mutagenicity of organic and inorganic compounds. *Carcinogenesis, 9,* 611-617

De Flora, S., Serra, D., Camoirano, A. & Zanacchi, P. (1989a) Metabolic reduction of chro-mium, as related to its carcinogenic properties. *Biol. Trace Element Res., 21,* 179-187

De Flora, S., Camoirano, A., Serra, D. & Bennicelli, C. (1989b) Genotoxicity and metabo-lism of chromium compounds. *Toxicol. environ. Chem., 19,* 153-160

De Flora, S., Hietanen, E., Bartsch, H., Camoirano, A., Izzotti, A., Bagnasco, M. & Mill-man, I. (1989c) Enhanced metabolic activation of chemical hepatocarcinogens in wood-chucks infected with hepatitis B virus. *Carcinogenesis, 10,* 1099–1106

De Flora, S., Serra, D., Basso, C. & Zanacchi, P. (1989d) Mechanistic aspects of chromium carcinogenicity. *Arch. Toxicol., Suppl. 13,* 28-39

De Flora, S., Bagnasco, M., Serra, D. & Zanacchi, P. (1990) Genotoxicity of chromium com-pounds. A review. *Mutat. Res.* (in press)

Deknudt, G. (1982) In vivo study of the mutagenicity of heavy metals in mammals (Abstract no. 33). *Mutat. Res., 97,* 180

Delachaux (1989) *Vacuum Grade (Super Alloys); Chromium Powders; Double Degassed Bri-quettes,* Gennevilliers

De Marco, R., Bernardinelli, L. & Mangione, M.P. (1988) Death risk due to cancer of the respiratory apparatus in chromate production workers (Ital.). *Med. Lav., 79,* 368-376

Deng, C.Z., Ou, B.X., Huang, J.C., Zhuo, Z.L., Xian, H.L., Yao, M.C., Chen, M.Y., Li, Z.X., Sheng, S.Y. & Yei, Z.F. (1983) Cytogenetic effects of electroplating workers (Chin.). *Acta sci. circumst., 3,* 267-271

Deng, C.Z., Lee, H.H., Xian, H.L., Yao, M.C., Huang, J.C. & Ou, B.X. (1988) Chromosomal aberrations and sister chromatid exchanges of peripheral blood lymphocytes in Chi-nese electroplating workers: effect of nickel and chromium. *J. trace Elem. exp. Med., 1,* 57–62

Deutches Institut für Normung (German Standards Institute) (1987) *Photometric Determina-tion of Chromium (VI) using 1,5-Diphenylcarbonohydrazide (D 24) (DIN 38405),* Part 24, Berlin (West)

DiPaolo, J.A. & Casto, B.C. (1979) Quantitative studies of in vitro morphological transfor-mation of Syrian hamster cells by inorganic metal salts. *Cancer Res., 39,* 1008-1013

Dixit, M.N., Bhale, G.L. & Thomas, A. (1976) Emission spectrographic determination of trace elements in plant materials. *Indian J. pure appl. Phys., 14,* 485-487

Donaldson, R.M. & Barreras, R.F. (1966) Intestinal absorption of trace quantities of chro-mium. *J. Lab. clin. Med., 68,* 484-493

Donaldson, D.L., Smith, C.C. & Yunice, A.A. (1986) Renal excretion of chromium-51 chlo-ride in the dog. *Am. J. Physiol., 246,* F870-F878

Douglas, G.R., Bell, R.D.L., Grant, C.E., Wytsma, J.M. & Bora, K.C. (1980) Effect of lead chromate on chromosomal aberration, sister-chromatid exchange and DNA damage in mammalian cells *in vitro. Mutat. Res.*, 77, 157-163

Dry Color Manufacturers' Association (1982) *Classification and Chemical Description of the Mixed Metal Oxide Inorganic Colored Pigments*, 2nd ed., Arlington, VA

Dunkel, V.C., Pienta, R.J., Sivak, A. & Traul, K.A. (1981) Comparative neoplastic transformation responses of Balb/3T3 cells, Syrian hamster embryo cells, and Rauscher murine leukemia virus-infected Fischer 344 rat embryo cells to chemical carcinogens. *J. natl Cancer Inst.*, 67, 1303-1315

Dunkel, V.C., Zeiger, E., Brusick, D., McCoy, E., McGregor, D., Mortelmans, K., Rosenkranz, H.S. & Simmon, V.F. (1984) Reproducibility of microbial mutagenicity assays: I. Tests with *Salmonella typhimurium* and *Escherichia coli* using a standardized protocol. *Environ. Mutagenesis*, 6(Suppl. 2), 1-254

Dunstan, L.P. & Garner, E.L. (1977) Chemical preparation of biological materials for accurate chromium determination by isotope dilution mass spectrometry. *Trace Subst. environ. Health*, 11, 334-337

Dvizhkov, P.P. & Fedorova, V.I. (1967) On blastomogenic properties of chromic oxide (Russ.). *Vop. Onkol.*, 13, 57-62

Egilsson, V., Evans, I.H. & Wilkie, D. (1979) Toxic and mutagenic effects of carcinogens on the mitochondria of *Saccharomyces cerevisiae. Mol. gen. Genet.*, 174, 39-46

Eisenberg, M. & Topping, J.J. (1986) Trace metal residues in finfish from Maryland waters, 1978-1979. *J. environ. Sci. Health*, B21, 87-102

Ekholm, U., Ulfvarsson, U. & Lindberg, E. (1983) *Exposure Conditions in Swedish Chromium Plating Industry* (Swed.) (Arbete och Hälsa 1983:24), Solna, Arbetarskyddsstyrelsen

Elias, Z., Schneider, O., Aubry, F., Danière, M.C. & Poirot, O. (1983) Sister chromatid exchanges in Chinese hamster V79 cells treated with the trivalent chromium compounds chromic chloride and chromic oxide. *Carcinogenesis*, 4, 605-611

Elias, Z., Poirot, O., Schneider, O., Danière, M.C., Terzetti, F., Guedenet, J.C. & Cavelier, C. (1986) Cellular uptake, cytotoxic and mutagenic effects of insoluble chromic oxide in V79 Chinese hamster cells. *Mutat. Res.*, 169, 159-170

Elinder, C.G., Gerhardsson, L. & Oberdoerster, G. (1988) Biological monitoring of toxic metals — overview. In: Clarkson, T.W., Friberg, L., Nordberg, G.F. & Sager, P.R., eds, *Biological Monitoring of Toxic Metals*, New York, Plenum, pp. 1-71

Elkem Metals Co. (1986) *Product Data Sheet: ELCHROMER® Electrolytic Chromium*, Pittsburgh, PA

Eller, P.M., ed. (1984) *NIOSH Manual of Analytical Methods*, 3rd ed., Vols 1 and 2 (DHHS (NIOSH) Publ. No. 84-100), Washington DC, US Government Printing Office, pp. 7024-1–7024-3, 7200-1–7200-5, 7300-1–7300-5, 7600-1–7600-4, 8310-1–8310-6

Eller, P.M., ed. (1985) *NIOSH Manual of Analytical Methods*, 3rd ed., 1st Suppl. (DHHS (NIOSH) Publ. No. 84-100), Washington DC, US Government Printing Office, pp. 8005-1–8005-5

Elofsson, S.-A., Gamberale, F., Hindmarsh, T., Iregren, A., Isaksson, A., Johnsson, I., Knave, B., Lydahl, E., Mindus, P., Persson, H.E., Philipson, B., Steby, M., Struwe, G., Söderman, E., Wennberg, A. & Widén, L. (1980) Exposure to organic solvents. A cross-sectional epidemiological investigation on occupationally exposed car and industrial spray painters with special reference to the nervous system. *Scand. J. Work Environ. Health, 6*, 239-273

Enterline, P.E. (1974) Respiratory cancer among chromate workers. *J. occup. Med., 16*, 523-526

ERAMET-SLN (Entreprise de Recherches et d'Activités — Métaux — Société le Nickel) (1989) *Western World Stainless Steel Production*, Paris

Eurométaux (1986) *Usage of Nickel in Industry*, Brussels

Fabry, L. (1980) Relation between the induction of micronuclei in bone-marrow cells by chromium salts and their carcinogenic potency (Fr.). *C.R. Soc. Biol., 174*, 889-892

Fairhurst, S. & Minty, C.A. (1990) *The Toxicity of Chromium and Inorganic Chromium Compounds* (Health and Safety Executive Toxicity Review), London, Her Majesty's Stationery Office (in press)

Fan, A.M. & Harding-Barlow, I. (1987) Chromium. In: Fishbein, L., Furst, A. & Mehlman, M.A., eds, *Genotoxic and Carcinogenic Metals: Environmental and Occupational Occurrence and Exposure* (Advances in Modern Environmental Toxicology, Vol. XI), Princeton, NJ, Princeton Scientific Publishing, pp. 87-125

Farrell, R.P., Judd, R.J., Lay, P.A., Dixon, N.E., Baker, R.S.U. & Bonin, A.M. (1989) Chromium(V)-induced cleavage of DNA: are chromium(V) complexes the active carcinogens in chromium(VI)-induced cancer? *Chem. Res. Toxicol., 2*, 227-229

Filiberti, R., Ceppi, M. & Vercelli, M. (1983) Distribution in the environment and toxic and carcinogenic effects of chromium (Ital.). *Riv. med. Lav. Ig. ind., 7*, 245-259

Fishbein, L. (1976) Environmental metallic carcinogens: an overview of exposure levels. *J. Toxicol. environ. Health, 2*, 77-109

Fishbein, L. (1984) Overview of analysis of carcinogenic and/or mutagenic metals in biological and environmental samples. I. Arsenic, beryllium, cadmium, chromium and selenium. *Int. J. environ. anal. Chem., 17*, 113-170

Fitzgerald, P.R., Peterson, J. & Lue-Hing, C. (1985) Heavy metals in tissues of cattle exposed to sludge-treated pastures for eight years. *Am. J. vet. Res., 46*, 703-707

Foa, V., Riboldi, L., Patroni, M., Zocchetti, C., Sbrana, C. & Mutti, A. (1988) Effects derived from long-term low-level chromium exposure in ferro-alloy metallurgy. Study of absorption and renal function in workers. *Sci. total Environ., 71*, 389-400

Fornace, A.J., Jr (1982) Detection of DNA single-strand breaks produced during the repair of damage by DNA-protein cross-linking agents. *Cancer Res., 42*, 145-149

Fornace, A.J., Jr, Seres, D.S., Lechner, J.F. & Harris, C.C. (1981) DNA-protein cross-linking by chromium salts. *Chem.-biol. Interact., 36*, 345-354

Fradkin, A., Janoff, A., Lane, B.P. & Kuschner, M. (1975) In vitro transformation of BHK21 cells grown in the presence of calcium chromate. *Cancer Res., 35*, 1058-1063

Franchini, I., Mutti, A., Cavatorta, A., Corradi, A., Cosi, A., Olivetti, G. & Borghetti, A. (1978) Nephrotoxicity of chromium. Remarks on an experimental and epidemiological investigation. *Contrib. Nephrol.*, *10*, 98-110

Franchini, I., Magnani, F. & Mutti, A. (1983) Mortality experience among chromeplating workers. Initial findings. *Scand. J. Work Environ. Health*, *9*, 247-252

Franzen, E., Pohle, R. & Knoblich, K. (1970) Industrial hygiene studies in electroplating. III. Chromium in urine (Ger.). *Z. ges. Hyg.*, *16*, 657-661

Fregert, S. & Gruvberger, B. (1972) Chemical properties of cement. *Berufsdermatosen*, *20*, 238-245

Frentzel-Beyme, R. (1983) Lung cancer mortality of workers employed in chromate pigment factories. A multicentric European epidemiological study. *J. Cancer Res. clin. Oncol.*, *105*, 183-188

Friedman, J., Shabtai, F., Levy, L.S. & Djaldetti, M. (1987) Chromium chloride induces chromosomal aberrations in human lymphocytes *via* indirect action. *Mutat. Res.*, *191*, 207-210

Fukunaga, M., Kurachi, Y. & Mizuguchi, Y. (1982) Action of some metal ions on yeast chromosomes. *Chem. pharm. Bull.*, *30*, 3017-3019

Furst, A. (1971) Trace elements related to specific chronic diseases: cancer. In: Cannon, H.L. & Hopps, H.C., eds, *Environmental Geochemistry in Health and Disease*, Boulder, CO, Geological Society of America, pp. 109-130

Furst, A., Schlauder, M. & Sasmore, D.P. (1976) Tumorigenic activity of lead chromate. *Cancer Res.*, *36*, 1779-1783

Gafafer, W.M., ed. (1953) *Health of Workers in Chromate Producing Industry: A Study (US Public Health Service, Division of Occupational Health Publications No. 192)*, Washington DC, US Public Health Service

Gale, T.F. (1978) Embryotoxic effects of chromium trioxide in hamsters. *Environ. Res.*, *16*, 101-109

Gale, T.F. (1982) The embryotoxic response to maternal chromium trioxide exposure in different strains of hamsters. *Environ. Res.*, *29*, 196-203

Gale, T.F. & Bunch, J.D., III (1979) The effect of time of administration of chromium trioxide on the embryotoxic response in hamsters. *Teratology*, *19*, 81-86

Galli, A., Boccardo, P., Del Carratore, R., Cundari, E. & Bronzetti, G. (1985) Conditions that influence the genetic activity of potassium dichromate and chromium chloride in *Saccharomyces cerevisiae*. *Mutat. Res.*, *144*, 165-169

Gauglhofer, J. (1984) Chromium (Ger.). In: Merian, E., ed., *Metallen im Umwelt* (Metals in the Environment), Weinheim, Verlag Chemie, pp. 409-424

Gava, C., Perazzolo, L., Zentilin, L., Levis, A.G., Corain, B., Bombi, G.G., Palumbo, M. & Zatta, P. (1989a) Genotoxic potentiality and DNA binding properties of acetylacetone, maltol, and their aluminium(III) and chromium(III) neutral complexes. *Toxicol. environ. Chem.*, *22*, 149-157

Gava, C., Costa, R., Zordan, M., Venier, P., Bianchi, V. & Levis, A.G. (1989b) Induction of gene mutations in Salmonella and Drosophila by soluble Cr(VI) compounds: synergistic effects of nitrilotriacetic acid (NTA). *Toxicol. environ. Chem.* (in press)

Gentile, J.M., Hyde, K. & Schubert, J. (1981) Chromium genotoxicity as influenced by complexation and rate effects. *Toxicol. Lett.*, 7, 439-448

Gilani, S.H. & Marano, M. (1979) Chromium poisoning and chick embryogenesis. *Environ. Res.*, 19, 427-431

Glaser, U., Hochrainer, D., Klöppel, H. & Kuhnen, H. (1985) Low level chromium (VI) inhalation effects on alveolar macrophages and immune functions in Wistar rats. *Arch. Toxicol.*, 57, 250-256

Glaser, U., Hochrainer, D., Klöppel, H. & Oldiges, H. (1986) Carcinogenicity of sodium dichromate and chromium [VI/III] oxide aerosols inhaled by male Wistar rats. *Toxicology*, 42, 219-232

Gläss, E. (1955) Studies on the effect of heavy metal salts on mitosis in root tips of *Vicia faba* (Ger.). *Z. Botanik.*, 43, 359-403

Gomes, E.R. (1972) Incidence of chromium-induced lesions among electroplating workers in Brazil. *Ind. Med.*, 41, 21-25

Gómez-Arroyo, S., Altamirano, M. & Villalobos-Pietrini, R. (1981) Sister chromatid exchanges induced by some chromium compounds in human lymphocytes *in vitro*. *Mutat. Res.*, 90, 425-431

Gray, S.J. & Sterling, K. (1950) The tagging of red cells and plasma proteins with radioactive chromium. *J. clin. Invest.*, 29, 1604-1613

Green, M.H.L., Muriel, W.J. & Bridges, B.A. (1976) Use of a simplified fluctuation test to detect low levels of mutagens. *Mutat. Res.*, 38, 33-42

Gresh, J.T. (1944) Chromic acid poisoning resulting from inhalation of mist developed from five per cent chromic acid solution. II. Engineering aspects of chromic acid poisoning from anodizing operations. *J. ind. Hyg. Toxicol.*, 26, 127-130

Grogan, C.H. (1957) Experimental studies in metal carcinogenesis. VIII. On the etiological factor in chromate cancer. *Cancer*, 10, 625-638

Gross, E. & Kölsch, F. (1943) On lung cancer in the chromium pigment industry (Ger.). *Arch. Gewerbepathol. Gewerbehyg.*, 12, 164-170

Guillemin, M.P. & Berode, M. (1978) A study on the difference in chromium exposure in workers in two types of electroplating process. *Ann. occup. Hyg.*, 21, 105-112

Haguenoer, J.M., Dubois, G., Frimat, P., Cantineau, A., Lefrançois, H. & Furon, D. (1981) Mortality from bronchopulmonary cancer in a zinc- and lead-chromate producing factory (Fr.). In: *Prevention of Occupational Cancer, International Symposium* (Occupational Safety and Health Series No. 46), Geneva, International Labour Office, pp. 168-176

Haguenoer, J.M., Leveque, G. & Frimat, P. (1982) Determinations of chromium, nickel and cobalt in cement of northern France and Belgium in relation to dermatoses (Fr.). *Arch. Mal. prof.*, 43, 241-247

Haines, A.T. & Nieboer, E. (1988) Chromium hypersensitivity. In: Nriagu, J.O. & Nieboer, E., eds, *Chromium in the Natural and Human Environments*, New York, John Wiley & Sons, pp. 497-532

Hama, G., Fredrick, W., Millage, D. & Brown, H. (1954) Absolute control of chromic acid mist. Investigation of a new surface-active agent. *Am. ind. Hyg. Q.*, 15, 211-216

Hamamy, H.A., Al-Hakkak, Z.S. & Hussain, A.F. (1987) Chromosome aberrations in workers at a tannery in Iraq. *Mutat. Res.*, *189*, 395-398

Hamilton, J.W. & Wetterhahn, K.E. (1986) Chromium(VI)-induced DNA damage in chick embryo liver and blood cells *in vivo*. *Carcinogenesis*, *7*, 2085-2088

Hamilton-Koch, W., Snyder, R.D. & LaVelle, J.M. (1986) Metal-induced DNA damage and repair in human diploid fibroblasts and Chinese hamster ovary cells. *Chem.-biol. Interactions*, *59*, 17-28

Handa, B.K. (1988) Occurrence and distribution of chromium in natural waters of India. In: Nriagu, J.O. & Nieboer, E., eds, *Chromium in the Natural and Human Environments*, New York, Wiley Interscience, pp. 189-214

Hansen, K. & Stern, R.M. (1984) A survey of metal-induced mutagenicity *in vitro* and *in vivo*. *J. Am. Coll. Toxicol.*, *3*, 381-430

Hansen, K. & Stern, R.M. (1985) Welding fumes and chromium compounds in cell transformation assays. *J. appl. Toxicol.*, *5*, 306-314

Hanslian, L., Navrátil, J., Jurák, J. & Kotrle, M. (1967) The impairment of higher respiratory pathways by chromic acid aerosol (Czech.). *Prac. Lék.*, *19*, 294-298

Hartford, W.H. (1963) Chromium. In: Kolthoff, I.M. & Elving, P.J., eds, *Treatise on Analytical Chemistry*, Part II, Vol. 8, New York, John Wiley & Sons, pp. 273-377

Hartford, W.H. (1979) Chromium compounds. In: Mark, H.F., Othmer, D.F., Overberger, C.G., Seaborg, G.T. & Grayson, M., eds, *Kirk-Othmer Encyclopedia of Chemical Technology*, 3rd ed., Vol. 6, New York, John Wiley & Sons, pp. 82-120

Hartford, W.H. & Copson, R.L. (1964) Chromium compounds. In: Kirk, R.E., Othmer, D.F., Grayson, M. & Eckroth, D., eds, *Encyclopedia of Chemical Technology*, 2nd ed., Vol. 5, New York, John Wiley & Sons, pp. 485-486, 494, 499, 510

Hartwig, A. & Beyersmann, D. (1987) Enhancement of UV and chromate mutagenesis by nickel ions in the Chinese hamster HGPRT assay. *Toxicol. environ. Chem.*, *14*, 33-42

Harzdorf, A.C. (1987) Analytical chemistry of chromium species in the environment, and interpretation of results. *Int. J. environ. anal. Chem.*, *29*, 249-261

Hatch, G.G. & Anderson, T.M. (1986) Chemical enhancement of simian adenovirus SA7 transformation of hamster embryo cells: evaluation of diverse chemicals (Abstract No. OD5). In: Ramel, C., Lambert, B. & Magnusson, J., eds, *Fourth International Conference on Environmental Mutagens, Stockholm, June 24-28, 1985*, New York, Alan R. Liss, p. 34

Haworth, S., Lawlor, T., Mortelmans, K., Speck, W. & Zeiger, E. (1983) *Salmonella* mutagenicity test results for 250 chemicals. *Environ. Mutagenesis*, *5* (*Suppl. 1*), 3-142

Hayashi, M., Sofuni, T. & Ishidate, M., Jr (1982) High-sensitivity in micronucleus induction of a mouse strain (MS). *Mutat. Res.*, *105*, 253-256

Hayes, R.B. (1988) Review of occupational epidemiology of chromium chemicals and respiratory cancer. *Sci. total Environ.*, *71*, 331-339

Hayes, R.B., Lilienfeld, A.M. & Snell, L.M. (1979) Mortality in chromium chemical production workers: a prospective study. *Int. J. Epidemiol.*, *8*, 365-374

Hayes, S., Gordon, A., Sadowski, I. & Hayes, C. (1984) RK bacterial test for independently measuring chemical toxicity and mutagenicity: short-term forward selection assay. *Mutat. Res.*, *130*, 97-106

Hayes, R.B., Sheffet, A. & Spirtas, R. (1989) Cancer mortality among a cohort of chromium pigment workers. *Am. J. ind. Med.*, *16*, 127-133

Haynes, E. (1907) *Metal Alloy* (Kokomo, Ind.). Patent No. 873, 745 [Chem. Abstr., 1908, 2]

Health and Safety Executive (1987) *Occupational Exposure Limits 1987* (Guidance Note EH 4d87), London, Her Majesty's Stationery Office, p. 11

Heck, J.D. & Costa, M. (1982a) In vitro assessment of the toxicity of metal compounds. I. Mammalian cell transformation. *Biol. Trace Element Res.*, *4*, 71-82

Heck, J.D. & Costa, M. (1982b) In vitro assessment of the toxicity of metal compounds. II. Mutagenesis. *Biol. Trace Element Res.*, *4*, 319-330

Heigl, A. (1978) Polarographic determination of copper, lead, tin, cadmium, nickel, zinc, iron, cobalt and chromium in waste water (Ger.). *Chimia*, *32*, 339-344 [*Chem. Abstr.*, *90*, 76081f]

Heit, M. (1979) Variability of the concentrations of seventeen trace elements in the muscle and liver of a single striped bass, *Morone saxatilis*. *Bull. environ. Contam. Toxicol.*, *23*, 1-5

Hellquist, H., Irander, K., Edling, C. & Ödkvist, L.M. (1983) Nasal symptoms and histopathology in a group of spray painters. *Acta otolaryngol.*, *96*, 495-500

Hernberg, S., Collan, Y., Degerth, R., Englund, A., Engzell, U., Kuosma, E., Mutanen, P., Nordlinder, H., Hansen, H.S., Schultz-Larsen, K., Søgaard, H. & Westerholm, P. (1983a) Nasal cancer and occupational exposures. Preliminary report of a joint Nordic case-referent study. *Scand. J. Work Environ. Health*, *9*, 208-213

Hernberg, S., Westerholm, P., Schultz-Larsen, K., Degerth, R., Kuosma, E., Englund, A., Engzell, U., Hansen, H.S. & Mutanen, P. (1983b) Nasal and sinonasal cancer. Connection with occupational exposures in Denmark, Finland and Sweden. *Scand. J. Work Environ. Health*, *9*, 315-326

Hopkins, L.L., Jr (1965) Distribution in the rat of physiological amounts of injected $^{51}$Cr(III) with time. *Am. J. Physiol.*, *209*, 731-735

Howarth, C.L. (1956) Chromium chemicals in the textile industry. In: Udy, M.J., ed., *Chromium*, Vol. 1, New York, Reinhold, pp. 283-290

Hueper, W.C. (1955) Experimental studies in metal cancerigenesis. VII. Tissue reactions to parenterally introduced powdered metallic chromium and chromite ore. *J. natl Cancer Inst.*, *16*, 447-462

Hueper, W.C. (1958) Experimental studies in metal cancerigenesis. X. Cancerigenic effects of chromite ore roast deposited in muscle tissue and pleural cavity of rats. *Arch. ind. Health*, *18*, 284-291

Hueper, W.C. (1961) Environmental carcinogenesis and cancers. *Cancer Res.*, *21*, 842-857

Hueper, W.C. & Payne, W.W. (1959) Experimental cancers in rats produced by chromium compounds and their significance to industry and public health. *Am. ind. Hyg. Assoc. J.*, *20*, 274-280

Hueper, W.C. & Payne, W.W. (1962) Experimental studies in metal carcinogenesis. Chromium, nickel, iron, arsenic. *Arch. environ. Health*, *5*, 445-462

Huff, J.W., Sastry, K.S., Gordon, M.P. & Wacker, W.E.C. (1964) The action of metal ions on tobacco mosaic virus ribonucleic acid. *Biochemistry*, *3*, 501-506

Husgafvel-Pursiainen, K., Kalliomäki, P.-L. & Sorsa, M. (1982) A chromosome study among stainless steel welders. *J. occup. Med.*, *24*, 762-766

Hyodo, K., Suzuki, S., Furuya, N. & Meshizuka, K. (1980) An analysis of chromium, copper, and zinc in organs of a chromate workers. *Int. Arch. occup. environ. Health*, *46*, 141-150

IARC (1973) *IARC Monographs on the Evaluation of Carcinogenic Risk of Chemicals to Man*, Vol. 2, *Some Inorganic and Organometallic Compounds*, Lyon, pp. 100-125

IARC (1979) *IARC Monographs on the Evaluation of the Carcinogenic Risk of Chemicals to Humans*, Suppl. 1, *Chemicals and Industrial Processes Associated with Cancer in Humans*, IARC Monographs *Volumes 1 to 20*, Lyon, pp. 29-30

IARC (1980a) *IARC Monographs on the Evaluation of the Carcinogenic Risk of Chemicals to Humans*, Vol. 23, *Some Metals and Metallic Compounds*, Lyon, pp. 205-323

IARC (1980b) *IARC Monographs on the Evaluation of the Carcinogenic Risk of Chemicals to Humans*, Vol. 23, *Some Metals and Metallic Compounds*, Lyon, pp. 325-415

IARC (1981) *IARC Monographs on the Evaluation of the Carcinogenic Risk of Chemicals to Humans*, Vol. 25, *Wood, Leather and Some Associated Industries*, Lyon, pp. 201-247

IARC (1982) *IARC Monographs on the Evaluation of the Carcinogenic Risk of Chemicals to Humans*, Suppl. 4, *Chemicals, Industrial Processes and Industries Associated with Cancer in Humans*. IARC Monographs *Volumes 1 to 29*, Lyon, pp. 91-93

IARC (1987a) *IARC Monographs on the Evaluation of Carcinogenic Risks to Humans*, Suppl. 7, *Overall Evaluations of Carcinogenicity: An Updating of* IARC Monographs *Volumes 1 to 42*, Lyon, pp. 165-168

IARC (1987b) *IARC Monographs on the Evaluation of Carcinogenic Risks to Humans*, Suppl. 6, *Genetic and Related Effects: An Updating of Selected IARC Monographs from Volumes 1 to 42*, Lyon, pp. 165-168

IARC (1988) *Information Bulletin on the Survey of Chemicals Being Tested for Carcinogenicity*, No. 13, Lyon, pp. 34, 123, 259

IARC (1989) *IARC Monographs on the Evaluation of Carcinogenic Risks to Humans*, Vol. 47, *Some Organic Solvents, Resin Monomers and Related Compounds, Pigments and Occupational Exposures in Paint Manufacture and Painting*, Lyon, pp. 307-326

Iijima, S., Matsumoto, N. & Lu, C.-C. (1983a) Transfer of chromic chloride to embryonic mice and changes in the embryonic mouse neuroepithelium. *Toxicology*, *26*, 257-265

Iijima, S., Spindle, A. & Pedersen, R.A. (1983b) Developmental and cytogenetic effects of potassium dichromate on mouse embryos *in vitro*. *Teratology*, *27*, 109-115

Il'inykh, S.V. (1977) Method for the determination of chromium in canned food packed into cans made of chrome-plated tin (Russ.). In: *Hygienic Aspect of Defence of Health of Workers*, Moscow, Erismana Institute of Hygiene, pp. 193-194 [*Chem. Abstr.*, *89*, 88934d]

Imreh, S. & Radulescu, D. (1982) Cytogenetic effects of chromium *in vivo* and *in vitro* (Abstract No. 56). *Mutat. Res.*, *97*, 192-193

Institut National de Recherche et de Sécurité (National Institute for Research and Safety) (1986) [*Limit Values for Dangerous Substances in Work Place Air*] (ND 1609-125-86) (in French), Paris, p. 562

Ivankovic, S. & Preussmann, R. (1975) Absence of toxic and carcinogenic effects after administration of high doses of chromic oxide pigment in subacute and long-term feeding experiments in rats. *Food Cosmet. Toxicol., 13*, 347-351

Iyengar, V. & Woittiez, J. (1988) Trace elements in human clinical specimens: evaluation of literature data to identify reference values. *Clin. Chem., 34*, 474-481

Jackson, J.F. & Linskens, H.F. (1982) Metal ion induced unscheduled DNA synthesis in *Petunia* pollen. *Mol. gen. Genet., 187*, 112-115

Jacquet, P. & Draye, J.P. (1982) Toxicity of chromium salts to cultured mouse embryos. *Toxicol. Lett., 12*, 53-57

Jayjock, M.A. & Levin, L. (1984) Health hazards in a small automotive body repair shop. *Ann. occup. Hyg., 28*, 19-29

Jin, X. & Hou, D. (1984) Chemical behaviour of chromium in the environment (Chin.). *Changchun Dizhi Xueyuan Xuebao, 3*, 91-99

Johansson, A., Wiernik, A., Jarstrand, C. & Camner, P. (1986) Rabbit alveolar macrophages after inhalation of hexa- and trivalent chromium. *Environ. Res., 39*, 372-385

de Jong, G.J. & Brinkman, U.A.T. (1978) Determination of chromium (III) and chromium (VI) in sea water by atomic absorption spectrometry. *Anal. chim. Acta, 98*, 243-250

Kada, T., Hirano, K. & Shirasu, T. (1980) Screening of environmental chemical mutagens in the rec-assay system with *Bacillus subtilis*. In: de Serres, F.J. & Hollaender, A., eds, *Chemical Mutagens: Principles and Methods for Their Detection*, Vol. 6, New York, Plenum, pp. 149-173

Kalinina, L.M. & Minseitova, S.R. (1983a) Induction of mutagenic repair in cells of *Escherichia coli* under the action of potassium bichromate (translation). *Dokl. Akad. Nauk SSR, 268*, 720-722

Kalinina, L.M. & Minseitova, S.R. (1983b) Mutagenic effects and DNA-damaging action in *Escherichia coli* cells treated with potassium bichromate (translation). *Genetika, 19*, 1941-1947

Kalinina, L.M. & Minseitova, S.R. (1983c) DNA repair pathways in *Escherichia coli* K-12 cells after mutation induction by potassium dichromate (translation). *Dokl. Akad. Nauk SSR, 272*, 208-210

Kaneko, T. (1976) Chromosome damage in cultured human leukocytes induced by chromium chloride and chromium trioxide (Jpn.). *Jpn. J. ind. Health, 18*, 136-137

Kanematsu, N., Hara, M. & Kada, T. (1980) Rec assay and mutagenicity studies on metal compounds. *Mutat. Res., 77*, 109-116

Kaths, D.S. (1981) *In Vivo Cytogenetic Effect of Some Salts of the Heavy Metals Cadmium, Chromium, Mercury, and Platinum in Assays of Micronuclei and Sister Chromatid Exchange*, Thesis, Freiburg, Freiburg University

Kawanishi, S., Inoue, S. & Sano, S. (1986) Mechanism of DNA cleavage induced by sodium chromate(VI) in the presence of hydrogen peroxide. *J. biol. Chem., 261*, 5952-5958

Kelly, W.F., Ackrill, P., Day, J.P., O'Hara, M., Tye, C.T., Burton, I., Orton, C. & Harris, M. (1982) Cutaneous absorption of trivalent chromium: tissue levels and treatment by exchange transfusion. *Br. J. ind. Med.*, *39*, 397-400

Kerr, L.A. & Edwards, W.C. (1981) Chromate poisoning in livestock from oil field wastes. *Vet. hum. Toxicol.*, *23*, 401-402

Kettrup, A., zur Mühlen, T. & Angerer, J. (1985) *Luftanalysen* (Air Analysis), Weinheim, Deutsche Forschungsgemeinschaft, pp. 1-9

Kharab, P. & Singh, I. (1985) Genotoxic effects of potassium dichromate, sodium arsenite, cobalt chloride and lead nitrate in diploid yeast. *Mutat. Res.*, *155*, 117-120

Kharab, P. & Singh, I. (1987) Induction of respiratory deficiency in yeast by salts of chromium, arsenic, cobalt and lead. *Ind. J. exp. Biol.*, *25*, 141-142

Kiilunen, M., Kivistö, H., Ala-Laurila, P., Tossavainen, A. & Aitio, A. (1983) Exceptional pharmacokinetics of trivalent chromium during occupational exposure to chromium lignosulfonate dust. *Scand. J. Work Environ. Health*, *9*, 265-271

Kiilunen, M., Järvisalo, J., Mäkitie, O. & Aitio, A. (1987) Analysis, storage stability and reference values for urinary chromium and nickel. *Int. Arch. occup. environ. Health*, *59*, 43-50

Kim, S., Iwai, Y., Fujino, M., Furumoto, M., Sumino, K. & Miyasaki, K. (1985) Chromium-induced pulmonary cancer. Report of a case and a review of the literature. *Acta pathol. jpn.*, *35*, 643-654

Kishi, R., Tarumi, T., Uchino, E. & Miyake, H. (1987) Chromium content of organs of chromate workers with lung cancer. *Am. J. ind. Med.*, *11*, 67-74

Kitagawa, S., Seki, H., Kametani, F. & Sakurai, H. (1988) EPR study on the interaction of hexavalent chromium with glutathione or cysteine: production of pentavalent chromium and its stability. *Inorg. chim. Acta*, *152*, 251-255

Kjuus, H., Skjærven, R., Langård, S., Lien, J.T. & Aamodt, T. (1986) A case-referent study of lung cancer, occupational exposures and smoking. I. Comparison of title-based and occupation-based occupational information. *Scand. J. Work Environ. Health*, *12*, 193-202

Klein, F. (1985) Nickel and chromium concentrations in ambient air of work places in the iron and steel industry (Fr.). In: Brown, S.S. & Sunderman, F.W., Jr, eds, *Progress in Nickel Toxicology*, Oxford, Blackwell Scientific, pp. 195-197

Kleinfeld, M. & Rosso, A. (1965) Ulcerations of the nasal septum due to inhalation of chromic acid mist. *Ind. Med. Surg.*, *34*, 242-243

Kleisbauer, J.-P., Poirier, R., Favre, R. & Laval, P. (1972) The problem of bronchial carcinomas of occupational origin (two cases) (Fr.). *Marseille méd.*, *109*, 699-704

Knudsen, I. (1980) The mammalian spot test and its use for the testing of potential carcinogenicity of welding fume particles and hexavalent chromium. *Acta pharmacol. toxicol.*, *47*, 66-70

Koli, A.K. & Whitmore, R. (1983) Trace elements in fish from the Savannah River near Savannah River nuclear plant. *Environ. int.*, *9*, 361-362

Kolihova, D., Sychra, V. & Dudova, N. (1978) Atomic absorption spectrometric analysis of ilmenite and inorganic pigments based on titanium dioxide. III. Determination of copper, manganese, chromium and iron by atomic absorption spectrometry with electrothermic atomization (Czech.). *Chem. Listy*, 72, 1081-1087 [*Chem. Abstr.*, 90, 40259f]

Kominsky, J.R., Rinsky, R. & Stroman, R. (1978) *Goodyear Aerospace Corp.* (Health Hazard Evaluation Report No. 77-127-516), Cincinnati, OH, National Institute for Occupational Safety and Health

Koponen, M. (1985) *Applications of Some Instrumental Methods in Metal Aerosol Characterization* (Original Reports 2/1985), Kuopio, University of Kuopio

Koponen, M., Gustafsson, T., Kalliomäki, P.-L. & Pyy, L. (1981) Chromium and nickel aerosols in stainless steel manufacturing, grinding and welding. *Am. ind. Hyg. Assoc. J.*, 42, 596-601

Korallus, U., Ehrlicher, H. & Wüstefeld, E. (1974a) Trivalent chromium compounds: results of a study in occupational medicine. Part 3: Clinical study (Ger.). *Arbeitsmed. Sozialmed. Präventivmed.*, 9, 248-252

Korallus, U., Ehrlicher, H. & Wüstefeld, E. (1974b) Trivalent chromium compounds: results of a study in occupational medicine. Part 1: General; technology; preliminary study (Ger.). *Arbeitsmed. Sozialmed. Präventivmed.*, 9, 51-54

Korallus, U., Ehrlicher, H. & Wüstefeld, E. (1974c) Trivalent chromium compounds: results of study in occupational medicine. Part 2: Analysis of disease status (Ger.). *Arbeitsmed. Sozialmed. Präventivmed.*, 9, 76-79

Korallus, U., Lange, H.-J., Neiss, A., Wüstefeld, E. & Zwingers, T. (1982) Relationships between environmental hygiene control measures and mortality from bronchial cancer in the chromate producing industry (Ger.). *Arbeitsmed. Sozialmed. Präventivmed.*, 17, 159-167

Kortenkamp, A., Ozolins, Z., Beyersmann, D. & O'Brien, P. (1989) Generation of PM2 DNA breaks in the course of reduction of chromium(VI) by glutathione. *Mutat. Res.*, 216, 19-26

Koshi, K. (1979) Effects of fume particles from stainless steel welding on sister chromatid exchanges and chromosome aberrations in cultured Chinese hamster cells. *Ind. Health*, 17, 39-49

Koshi, K. & Iwasaki, K. (1983) Solubility of low-solubility chromates and their clastogenic activity in cultured cells. *Ind. Health*, 21, 57-65

Koshi, K., Yagami, T. & Nakanishi, Y. (1984) Cytogenetic analysis of peripheral blood lymphocytes from stainless steel welders. *Ind. Health*, 22, 305-318

Koshi, K., Sertia, F., Sawatari, K. & Suzuki, Y. (1987) Cytogenetic analysis of bone marrow cells and peripheral blood lymphocytes from rats exposed to chromium fumes by inhalation (Abstract No. 21). *Mutat. Res.*, 181, 365

Kramer, H.L., Steiner, J.W. & Vallely, P.J. (1983) Trace element concentrations in the liver, kidney, and muscle of Queensland cattle. *Bull. environ. Contam. Toxicol.*, 30, 588-594

Kretzschmar, J.G., Delespaul, I., De Rijck, T. & Verduyn, G. (1977) The Belgian network for the determination of heavy metals. *Atmos. Environ.*, 11, 263-271

Krishnaja, A.P. & Rege, M.S. (1982) Induction of chromosomal aberrations in fish *Boleoph-thalmus dussumieri* after exposure *in vivo* to mitomycin C and heavy metals mercury, selenium and chromium. *Mutat. Res.*, *102*, 71-82

Kroner, R.C. (1973) The occurrence of trace metals in surface waters. In: Sabadell, J.E., ed., *Proceedings of a Symposium on Traces of Heavy Metals in Water Removal Processes and Monitoring*, Springfield, VA, National Technical Information Service, pp. 311-322

Kumpulainen, J.T., Lehto, J., Koivistoinen, P., Uusitupa, M. & Vuori, E. (1983) Determinations of chromium in human milk, serum and urine by electrothermal atomic absorption spectrometry without preliminary ashing. *Sci. total Environ.*, *31*, 71-80

Kurokawa, Y., Matsushima, M., Imazawa, T., Takamura, N., Takahashi, M. & Hayashi, Y. (1985) Promoting effect of metal compounds on rat renal tumorigenesis. *J. Am. Coll. Toxicol.*, *4*, 321-330

Kuschner, M. & Laskin, S. (1971) Experimental models in environmental carcinogenesis. *Am. J. Pathol.*, *64*, 183-196

Lalor, E. (1973) Zinc and strontium chromates. In: Patton, T.C., ed., *Pigment Handbook*, Vol. 1, New York, John Wiley & Sons, pp. 847-859

Lane, B.P. & Mass, M.J. (1977) Carcinogenicity and cocarcinogenicity of chromium carbonyl in heterotopic tracheal grafts. *Cancer Res.*, *37*, 1476-1479

Lanfranchi, G., Paglialunga, S. & Levis, A.G. (1988) Mammalian cell transformation induced by chromium(VI) compounds in the presence of nitrilotriacetic acid. *J. toxicol. environ. Health*, *24*, 251-260

Langård, S. (1980) Chromium. In: Waldron, H.A., ed., *Metals in the Environment*, London, Academic Press, pp. 111-132

Langård, S. (1982) Absorption, transport and excretion of chromium in man and animals. In: Langård, S., ed., *Biological and Environmental Aspects of Chromium*, Amsterdam, Elsevier, pp. 149-169

Langård, S. & Kommedal, T.M. (1975) Bronchial carcinoma in a young man exposed to chromates (Norw.). *Tidsskr. Nor. Lægeforen.*, *95*, 819-820

Langård, S. & Norseth, T. (1975) A cohort study of bronchial carcinomas in workers producing chromate pigments. *Br. J. ind. Med.*, *32*, 62-65

Langård, S. & Norseth, T. (1979) Cancer in the gastrointestinal tract in chromate pigment workers. *Arch. Hig. Rada Toksicol.*, *30 (Suppl.)*, 301-304

Langård, S. & Vigander, T. (1983) Occurrence of lung cancer in workers producing chromium pigments. *Br. J. ind. Med.*, *40*, 71-74

Langård, S., Gundersen, N., Tsalev, D.L. & Gylseth, B. (1978) Whole blood chromium level and chromium excretion in the rat after zinc chromate inhalation. *Acta pharmacol. toxicol.*, *42*, 142-149

Langård, S., Andersen, A. & Gylseth, B. (1980) Incidence of cancer among ferrochromium and ferrosilicon workers. *Br. J. ind. Med.*, *37*, 114-120

Langård, S., Andersen, A. & Ravnestad, J. (1990) Incidence of cancer among ferrochromium and ferrosilicon workers; an extended observation period. *Br. J. ind. Med.*, *47*, 14-19

Langerwerf, J.S.A., Bakkeren, H.A. & Jongen, W.M.T. (1985) A comparison of the mutagenicity of soluble trivalent chromium compounds with that of potassium chromate. *Ecotoxicol. environ. Saf.*, *9*, 92-100

Laskin, S., Kuschner, M. & Drew, R.T. (1970) Studies in pulmonary carcinogenesis. In: Hanna, M.G., Jr, Nettesheim, P. & Gilbert, J.R., eds, *Inhalation Carcinogenesis* (US Atomic Energy Commission Symposium Series No. 18), Oak Ridge, TN, US Atomic Energy Commission, Division of Technical Information Extension, pp. 321-351

Lautner, G.M., Carver, J.C. & Konzen, R.B. (1978) Measurement of chromium(VI) and chromium (III) in stainless steel welding fumes with electron spectroscopy for chemical analysis and neutron activation analysis. *Am. ind. Hyg. Assoc. J.*, *39*, 651-660

LaVelle, J.M. (1986a) Potassium chromate potentiates frameshift mutagenesis in *E. coli* and *S. typhimurium*. *Mutat. Res.*, *171*, 1-10

LaVelle, J.M. (1986b) Chromium(VI) comutagenesis: characterization of the interaction of $K_2CrO_4$ with azide. *Environ. Mutagenesis*, *8*, 717-725

LaVelle, J.M. & Witmer, C.M. (1984) Chromium(VI) potentiates mutagenesis by sodium azide but not ethylmethanesulfonate. *Environ. Mutagenesis*, *6*, 311-320

Lee, K.P., Ulrich, C.E., Geil, R.G. & Trochimowicz, H.J. (1988) Effects of inhaled chromium dioxide dust on rats exposed for two years. *Fundam. appl. Toxicol.*, *10*, 125-145

Léonard, A. & Deknudt, G. (1981) Mutagenicity test with chromium salts in mouse (Abstract). *Mutat. Res.*, *80*, 287

Léonard, A. & Lauwerys, R.R. (1980) Carcinogenicity and mutagenicity of chromium. *Mutat. Res.*, *76*, 227-239

Letterer, E., Neidhardt, K. & Klett, H. (1944) Chromate lung cancer and chromate pneumoconioses. A clinical, patho-anatomical, and occupational hygiene study (Ger.). *Arch. Gewerbepathol. Gewerbehyg.*, *12*, 323-361

Levis, A.G. & Bianchi, V. (1982) Mutagenic and cytogenetic efects of chromium compounds. In: Langård, S., ed., *Biological and Environmental Aspects of Chromium*, Amsterdam, Elsevier, pp. 171-208

Levis, A.G. & Majone, F. (1979) Cytotoxic and clastogenic effects of soluble chromium compounds on mammalian cell cultures. *Br. J. Cancer*, *40*, 523-533

Levis, A.G. & Majone, F. (1981) Cytotoxic and clastogenic effects of soluble and insoluble compounds containing hexavalent and trivalent chromium. *Br. J. Cancer*, *44*, 219-235

Levis, A.G., Buttignol, M. & Vettorato, L. (1977) DNA synthesis inhibition in BHK fibroblasts treated *in vitro* with potassium dichromate. *Experientia*, *33*, 82-84

Levis, A.G., Bianchi, V., Tamino, G. & Pegoraro, B. (1978a) Cytotoxic effects of hexavalent and trivalent chromium on mammalian cells *in vitro*. *Br. J. Cancer*, *37*, 386-396

Levis, A.G., Buttignol, M., Bianchi, V. & Sponza, G. (1978b) Effects of potassium dichromate on nucleic acid and protein syntheses and on precursor uptake in BHK fibroblasts. *Cancer Res.*, *38*, 110-116

Levy, L.S. & Venitt, S. (1986) Carcinogenicity and mutagenicity of chromium compounds: the associaton between bronchial metaplasia and neoplasia. *Carcinogenesis*, *7*, 831-836

Levy, L.S., Martin, P.A. & Bidstrup, P.L. (1986) Investigation of the potential carcinogenicity of a range of chromium containing materials on rat lung. *Br. J. ind. Med.*, *43*, 243-256

Lewalter, J., Korallus, U., Harzdorf, C. & Weidemann, H. (1985) Chromium bond detection in isolated erythrocytes: a new principle of biological monitoring of exposure to hexavalent chromium. *Int. Arch. occup. environ. Health*, 55, 305-318

Li, M.-C., Sheng, K.-L., Ching, C.-F., Chen, C.-H., Chin, P.-K., Jung, T.-W. & Wang, H.-P. (1979) Determination of trace elements in environmental samples by proton-induced X-ray emission analysis (Chin.). *K'o Hsueh Tung Pao*, 24, 19-21 [*Chem. Abstr.*, 90, 145297v]

Lindberg, E. & Hedenstierna, G. (1983) Chrome plating: symptoms, findings in the upper airways and effects on lung function. *Arch. environ. Health*, 38, 367-374

Lindberg, E. & Vesterberg, O. (1983) Monitoring exposure to chromic acid in chrome plating by measuring chromium in urine. *Scand. J. Work Environ. Health*, 9, 333-340

Littorin, M., Högstedt, B., Strömbäck, B., Karlsson, A., Welinder, H., Mitelman, F. & Skerfving, S. (1983) No cytogenetic effects in lymphocytes of stainless steel welders. *Scand. J. Work Environ. Health*, 9, 259-264

Llagostera, M., Garrido, S., Guerrero, R. & Barbé, J. (1986) Induction of SOS genes of *Escherichia coli* by chromium compounds. *Environ. Mutagenesis*, 8, 571-577

Löfroth, G. (1978) The mutagenicity of hexavalent chromium is decreased by microsomal metabolism. *Naturwissenschaften*, 65, 207-208

Loprieno, N., Boncristiani, G., Venier, P., Montaldi, A., Majone, F., Bianchi, V., Paglialunga, S. & Levis, A.G. (1985) Increased mutagenicity of chromium compounds by nitrilotriacetic acid. *Environ. Mutagenesis*, 7, 185-200

Love, A.H.G. (1983) Chromium — biological and analytical considerations. In: Burrows, D., ed., *Chromium: Metabolism and Toxicity*, Boca Raton, FL, CRC Press, pp. 1-12

Luciani, S., Dal Toso, R., Rebellato, A.M. & Levis, A.G. (1979) Effects of chromium compounds on plasma membrane $Mg^{2+}$-ATPase activity of BHK cells. *Chem.-biol. Interact.*, 27, 59-67

Lumio, J. (1953) On the lesions in the upper airways among chromium platers (Swed.). *Nord. hyg. Tidskr.*, 5-6, 86-91

Ma, T.H., Harris, M.M., Van Anderson, A., Ahmed, I., Mohammad, K., Bare, J.L. & Lin, G. (1984) Tradescantia-micronucleus (Trad-MCN) tests on 140 health-related agents. *Mutat. Res.*, 138, 157-167

Machle, W. & Gregorius, F. (1948) Cancer of the respiratory system in the United States chromate-producing industry. *Public Health Rep.*, 63, 1114-1127

Macrae, W.D., Whiting, R.F. & Stich, H.F. (1979) Sister-chromatid exchanges induced in cultured mammalian cells by chromate. *Chem.-biol. Interactions*, 26, 281-286

Majone, F. (1977) Effects of potassium dichromate on mitosis of cultured mammalian cells. *Caryologia*, 30, 469-481

Majone, F. & Levis, A.G. (1979) Chromosomal aberrations and sister chromatid exchanges in Chinese hamster cells treated *in vitro* with hexavalent chromium compounds. *Mutat. Res.*, 67, 231-238

Majone, F. & Rensi, D. (1979) Mitotic alterations, chromosome aberrations and sister chromatid exchanges induced by hexavalent and trivalent chromium on mammalian cells *in vitro*. *Caryologia*, 32, 379-392

Majone, F., Marin, G. & Levis, A.G. (1982) Chromium-induced sister chromatid exchanges in CHO cells. *Caryologia*, *35*, 225-235

Majone, F., Montaldi, A., Ronchese, F., De Rossi, A., Chieco-Bianchi, L. & Levis, A.G. (1983) Sister chromatid exchanges induced *in vivo* and *in vitro* by chemical carcinogens in mouse lymphocytes carrying endogenized Moloney leukemia virus. *Carcinogenesis*, *4*, 33-37

Makarov-Zemlyanskii, Y.Y., Men'shikov, B.I. & Strakhov, I.P. (1978) Persulphate method for determining chromium (III) in solutions with a 'silver free' catalyst (Russ.). *Kozh.-Obuvn. Prom-st.*, *20*, 43-45 [*Chem. Abstr.*, *89*, 76343x]

Maltoni, C. (1974) Occupational carcinogenesis. *Excerpta med. int. Congr. Ser.*, *322*, 19-26

Maltoni, C. (1976) Predictive value of carcinogenesis bioassays. *Ann. N.Y. Acad. Sci.*, *271*, 431-443

Maltoni, C., Morisi, L. & Chieco, P. (1982) Experimental approach to the assessment of the carcinogenic risk of industrial inorganic pigments. *Adv. mod. environ. Toxicol.*, *2*, 77-92

Mancuso, T.F. (1975) Considerations of chromium as an industrial carcinogen. In: Hutchinson, T.C., ed., *Proceedings of the International Conference on Heavy Metals in the Environment, Toronto, 1975*, Toronto, Institute for Environmental Studies, pp. 343-356

Mancuso, T.F. & Hueper, W.C. (1951) Occupational cancer and other health hazards in a chromate plant: a medical appraisal — I. Lung cancer in chromate workers. *Ind. Med. Surg.*, *20*, 358-363

Marzin, D.R. & Phi, H.V. (1985) Study of the mutagenicity of metal derivatives with *Salmonella typhimurium* TA102. *Mutat. Res.*, *155*, 49-51

Matsui, S. (1980) Evaluation of a *Bacillus subtilis* rec-assay for the detection of mutagens which may occur in water environments. *Water Res.*, *14*, 1613-1619

Matsumoto, N., Ijima, S. & Katsunuma, H. (1976) Placental transfer of chromic chloride and its teratogenic potential in embryonic mice. *J. toxicol. Sci.*, *2*, 1-13

McGean-Rohco (1984) *Data Sheet: Speciality Chromium Chemicals*, Cleveland, OH

McGregor, D.B., Martin, R., Cattanach, P., Edwards, I., McBride, D. & Caspary, W.J. (1987) Responses of the L5178Y tk+/tk− mouse lymphoma cell forward mutation assay to coded chemicals. I: Results for nine compounds. *Environ. Mutagenesis*, *9*, 143-160

McLean, J.R., McWilliams, R.S., Kaplan, J.G. & Birnboim, H.C. (1982) Rapid detection of DNA strand breaks in human peripheral blood cells and animal organs following treatment with physical and chemical agents. *Progr. Mutat. Res.*, *3*, 137-141

Mellor, J.W. (1931) *A Comprehensive Treatise on Inorganic and Theoretical Chemistry*, Vol. 11, Chapt. 60, *Chromium*, London, Longmans, Green & Co.

Merian, E. (1984) Introduction on environmental chemistry and global cycles of arsenic, beryllium, cadmium, chromium, cobalt, nickel, selenium, and their derivatives. *Toxicol. environ. Chem.*, *8*, 9-38

Mertz, W. (1969) Chromium occurrence and function in biological systems. *Physiol. Rev.*, *49*, 163-239

Mertz, W., Roginski, E.E. & Reba, R.C. (1965) Biological activity and fate of intravenous chromium (III) in the rat. *Am. J. Physiol.*, *209*, 489-494

Meyers, J.B. (1950) Acute pulmonary complications following inhalation of chromic acid mist. *Arch. ind. Hyg. occup. Med.*, 2, 742-747

Michel-Briand, C. & Simonin, M. (1977) Bronchopulmonary carcinomas in two workers employed in the same workshop of a chrome electroplating factory (Fr.). *Arch. Mal. prof.*, 38, 1001-1013

Miller, C.A. & Costa, M. (1988) Characterization of DNA-protein complexes induced in intact cells by the carcinogen chromate. *Mol. Carcinogenesis*, 1, 125-133

Miller, C.A. & Costa, M. (1989) Immunological detection of DNA-protein complexes induced by chromate. *Carcinogenesis*, 10, 667-672

Min, B.C. (1976) A study on the concentration of heavy metals in the tributaries of Han river (Korean). *Kongjung Poken Chapchi*, 13, 337-347 [*Chem. Abstr.*, 90, 92066k]

Mineral Pigments Corp. (undated a) *Specification Sheet: Jet Milled Dark Chromium Oxide (J-5351)*, Beltsville, MD

Mineral Pigments Corp. (undated b) *Specification Sheet: Jet Milled Light Chrome Yellow (J-1222)*, Beltsville, MD

Mineral Pigments Corp. (undated c) *Specification Sheet: Jet Milled Medium Chrome Yellow (J-1238)*, Beltsville, MD

Mineral Pigments Corp. (undated d) *Specification Sheet: Jet Milled Strontium Chromate (J-1365)*, Beltsville, MD

Ministry of Health & Welfare (1978) *Drinking Water Standards*, Tokyo

Mitchell, A.J. (1969) An unsuspected hazard of chrome stripping. *Trans. Soc. occup. Med.*, 19, 128-130

Mitchell, A.D., Rudd, C.J. & Caspary, V.J. (1988) Evaluation of the L5178Y mouse lymphoma cell mutagenesis assay: intralaboratory results for sixty-three coded chemicals tested at SRI International. *Environ. mol. Mutagenesis*, 12 (Suppl. 13), 37-101

Miyaki, M., Murata, I., Osabe, M. & Ono, T. (1977) Effect of metal cations on misincorporation by *E. coli* DNA polymerases. *Biochem. biophys. Res. Commun.*, 77, 854-860

Mohn, G.R. & Ellenberger, J. (1977) The use of *Escherichia coli* K12/343/113 (λ) as a multipurpose indicator strain in various mutagenicity testing procedures. In: Kilbey, B.J., Legator, M., Nichols, W. & Ramel, C., eds, *Handbook of Mutagenicity Test Procedures*, Amsterdam, Elsevier, pp. 95-118

Molina, D. & Abell, M.T. (1987) An ion chromatographic method for insoluble chromates in paint aerosol. *Am. ind. Hyg. Assoc. J.*, 48, 830-835

Molos, J.E. (1947) Use of plastic chips in the control of chromic acid mist. *Ind. Med.*, 16, 404-405

Montaldi, A., Zentilin, L., Paglialunga, S. & Levis, A.G. (1987a) Solubilization by nitrilotriacetic acid (NTA) of genetically active Cr(VI) and Pb(II) from insoluble metal compounds. *J. Toxicol. environ. Health*, 21, 387-394

Montaldi, A., Zantilin, L., Zordan, M., Bianchi, V., Levis, A.G., Clonfero, E. & Paglialunga, S. (1987b) Chromosomal effects of heavy metals (Cd, Cr, Hg, Ni and Pb) on cultured mammalian cells in the presence of nitrilotriacetic acid (NTA). *Toxicol. environ. Chem.*, 14, 183-200

Moreton, J., Bettelley, J., Mathers, H., Nicholls, A., Perry, R.W., Ratcliffe, D.B. & Svensson, L. (1983) Investigation of techniques for the analysis of hexavalent chromium, total chromium and total nickel in welding fume: a co-operative study. *Ann. occup. Hyg.*, *37*, 137-156

Morimoto, K. & Koizumi, A. (1981) Inhibition repair of radiation-induced chromosome breaks: effects of chromium trioxide on cultured human lymphocytes. *Ind. Health*, *19*, 259-262

Morning, J.L. (1975) *Chromium* (Bulletin 667, Bureau of Mines), Washington DC, US Department of the Interior

Morning, J.L. (1978) Chromium. In: *Minerals Yearbook 1976*, Vol. 1, *Metals, Minerals and Fuels*, Washington DC, Bureau of Mines, US Government Printing Office, pp. 297-308

Morris, B.W., Griffiths, H., Hardisty, C.A. & Kemp, G.J. (1989) Increased concentrations of chromium in plasma, urine and red blood cells in a group of stainless steel welders. *At. Spectr.*, *10*, 1-3

Mukubo, K. (1978) Studies on experimental lung tumor by the chemical carcinogens and inorganic substances. III. Histopathological studies on lung tumour in rats induced by pertracheal vinyl tube infusion of 20-methylcholanthrene combined with chromium and nickel powders (Jpn.). *J. Nara med. Assoc.*, *29*, 321-340

Mutti, A., Cavatora, A., Borghi, L., Canali, M., Giaroli, C. & Franchini, I. (1979) Distribution and urinary excretion of chromium. Studies on rats after administration of single and repeated doses of potassium dichromate. *Med. Lav.*, *70*, 171-179

Mutti, A., Pedroni, C., Arfini, G., Franchini, I., Minoia, C., Micoli, G. & Baldi, C. (1984) Biological monitoring of occupational exposure to different chromium compounds at various valency states. *Int. J. environ. anal. Chem.*, *17*, 35-41

Myhr, B.C. & Caspary, W.J. (1988) Evaluation of the L5178Y mouse lymphoma cell mutagenesis assay: intralaboratory results for sixty-three coded chemicals tested at Litton Bionetics, Inc. *Environ. mol. Mutagenesis*, *12 (Suppl. 13)*, 103-194

Nagaya, T. (1986) No increase in sister-chromatid exchange frequency in lymphocytes of chromium platers. *Mutat. Res.*, *170*, 129-132

Nagaya, T., Ishikawa, N. & Hata, H. (1989) Sister chromatid exchange analysis in lymphocytes of workers exposed to hexavalent chromium. *Br. J. ind. Med.*, *46*, 48-51

Nakamura, S.-I., Oda, Y., Shimada, T., Oki, I. & Sugimoto, K. (1987) SOS-inducing activity of chemical carcinogens and mutagens in *Salmonella typhimurium* TA1535/pSK1002: examination with 151 chemicals. *Mutat. Res.*, *192*, 239-246

Nakamuro, K., Yoshikawa, K., Sayato, Y. & Kurata, H. (1978) Comparative studies of chromosomal aberration and mutagenicity of trivalent and hexavalent chromium. *Mutat. Res.*, *58*, 175-181

National Chemical Co. (undated a) *Specification Sheet: No. 10 Chromium Phosphate*, Chicago, IL

National Chemical Co. (undated b) *Specification Sheet: No. 4 Calcium Chromate*, Chicago, IL

National Chemical Co. (undated c) *Specification Sheet: No. 6 Barium Chromate*, Chicago, IL

National Chemical Co. (undated d) *Chrome Yellow Specifications*, Chicago, IL

National Chemical Co. (undated e) *Specification Sheet: Molybdate Orange Nos. 1720, 1730 and 1740*, Chicago, IL

National Chemical Co. (undated f) *Specification Sheet: No. 3 Strontium Chromate*, Chicago, IL

National Institute for Occupational Safety and Health (1973) *Occupational Exposure to Chromic Acid*, Cincinnati, OH, pp. 15-16

National Institute for Occupational Safety and Health (1975) *Occupational Exposure to Chromium VI*, Cincinnati, OH, pp. 23-24

National Institute for Occupational Safety and Health (1977) *National Occupational Hazard Survey 1972-74*, Cincinnati, OH

National Institute for Occupational Safety and Health (1984a) Method 7024. Chromium compounds as Cr. In: *NIOSH Manual of Analytical Methods*, Vol. 1, Cincinnati, OH, pp. 1-3

National Institute for Occupational Safety and Health (1984b) Method 7600. Chromium hexavalent. In: *NIOSH Manual of Analytical Methods*, Vol. 1, Cincinnati, OH, pp. 1-4

National Institute for Occupational Safety and Health (1988) NIOSH recommendations for occupational safety and health standards 1988. *Morbid. Mortal. wkly Rep.*, *37*(Suppl. 7), 9

National Oceanic and Atmospheric Administration (1987) *National Status and Trends Program for Marine Environmental Quality. Progress Report. A Summary of Selected Data on Chemical Contaminants in Tissues Collected During 1984, 1985, and 1986 (NOAA Technical Memorandum NOS OMA 38)*, Rockville, MD, National Ocean Service, US Department of Commerce, pp. 1-23, D-10–D-11, E-3

National Research Council (1974) *Chromium*, Washington DC, National Academy of Sciences

Nestmann, E.R., Matula, T.I., Douglas, G.R., Bora, K.C. & Kowbel, D.J. (1979) Detection of the mutagenic activity of lead chromate using a battery of microbial tests. *Mutat. Res.*, *66*, 357-365

Nettesheim, P., Hanna, M.G., Jr, Doherty, D.G., Newell, R.F. & Hellman, A. (1971) Effect of calcium chromate dust, influenza virus, and 100 R whole-body X radiation on lung tumor incidence in mice. *J. natl Cancer Inst.*, *47*, 1129-1144

Newbold, R.F., Amos, J. & Connell, J.R. (1979) The cytotoxic, mutagenic and clastogenic effects of chromium-containing compounds on mammalian cells in culture. *Mutat. Res.*, *67*, 55-63

Newman, D. (1890) A case of adeno-carcinoma of the left inferior turbinated body, and perforation of the nasal septum, in the person of a worker in chrome pigments. *Glasgow med. J.*, *33*, 469-470

Newton, M.F. & Lilly, L.J. (1986) Tissue-specific clastogenic effects of chromium and selenium salts *in vivo*. *Mutat. Res.*, *169*, 61-69

Ngaha, E.O. (1981) Renal effects of potassium dichromate in the rat: comparison of urinary enzyme excretion with corresponding tissue patterns. *Gen. Pharmacol.*, *12*, 497-500

Nickel Development Institute (1987a) *Design Guidelines for the Selection and Use of Stainless Steel*, Toronto

Nickel Development Institute (1987b) *Nickel Base Alloys*, Toronto

Nieboer, E. & Jusys, A.A. (1988) Biological chemistry of chromium. In: Nriagu, J.O. & Nieboer, E., eds, *Chromium in the Natural and Human Environments*, New York, John Wiley & Sons, pp. 21-79

Nieboer, E. & Shaw, S.L. (1988) Mutagenic and other genotoxic effects of chromium compounds. In: Nriagu, J.O. & Nieboer, E., eds, *Chromium in the Natural and Human Environments*, New York, John Wiley & Sons, pp. 399-441

Nieboer, E., Yassi, A., Haines, A.T. & Jusys, A.A. (1984) *Effects of Chromium Compounds on Human Health*, Toronto, Ontario Ministry of Labour

Nijs, M. & Kirsch-Volders, M. (1986) Induction of spindle inhibition and abnormal mitotic figures by Cr(II), Cr(III) and Cr(VI) ions. *Mutagenesis, 1*, 247-252

Nise, G. & Vesterberg, O. (1979) Direct determination of chromium in urine by electrothermal atomic absorption spectrometry. *Scand. J. Work Environ. Health, 5*, 404-410

Nishimura, M. & Umeda, M. (1978) Mutagenic effect of some metal compounds on cultured mammalian cells (Abstract No. 19). *Mutat. Res., 54*, 246-247

Nishio, A. & Uyeki, E.M. (1985) Inhibition of DNA synthesis by chromium compounds. *J. Toxicol. environ. Health, 15*, 237-244

Nishioka, N. (1975) Mutagenic activities of metal compounds in bacteria. *Mutat. Res., 31*, 185-189

Nishiyama, H., Yano, H., Nishiwaki, Y., Kitaya, T., Matsuyama, T., Kodama, T., Suemasu, K., Tamai, S. & Takemoto, K. (1985) Lung cancer in chromate workers — analysis of 11 cases. *Jpn. J. clin. Oncol., 15*, 489-497

Nishiyama, H., Nishiwaki, Y., Kodama, T., Matsuyama, T., Araki, T. & Takemoto, K. (1988) Lung cancer in chromate workers found by mass survey (Abstract No. 1.15). *Lung Cancer (J. int. Assoc. Study Lung Cancer), 4 (Suppl.)*

Nissing, W. (1975) Trace-element pollution of the Lower Rhine and its significance in drinking-water supply (Ger). *Ber. Arbeitsgem. Rheinwasserwerke, 32*, 83-94 [*Chem. Abstr., 88*, 176854n]

Nomiyama, H., Yotoriyama, M. & Nomiyama, K. (1980) Normal chromium levels in urine and blood of Japanese subjects determined by direct flameless atomic absorption spectrophotometry, and valency of chromium in urine after exposure to hexavalent chromium. *Am. ind. Hyg. Assoc. J., 41*, 98-102

Norseth, T. (1980) Cancer hazards caused by nickel and chromium exposure. *J. Toxicol. environ. Health, 6*, 1219-1227

Norseth, T. (1981) The carcinogenicity of chromium. *Environ. Health Perspect., 40*, 121-130

Norseth, T. (1986) The carcinogenicity of chromium and its salts. *Br. J. ind. Med., 43*, 649-651

Norseth, T., Alexander, J., Aaseth, J. & Langård, S. (1982) Biliary excretion of chromium in the rat: a role of glutathione. *Acta pharmacol. toxicol., 51*, 450-455

Nriagu, J.O. & Nieboer, E., eds (1988) *Chromium in the Natural and Human Environments*, New York, John Wiley & Sons

Oberly, T.J., Piper, C.E. & McDonald, D.S. (1982) Mutagenicity of metal salts in the L5178Y mouse lymphoma assay. *J. Toxicol. environ. Health, 9*, 367-376

O'Brien, D.M. & Hurley, D.E. (1981) *An Evaluation of Engineering Control Technology for Spray Painting* (DHSS (NIOSH) Publ. No. 81-121), Cincinnati, OH, National Institute for Occupational Safety and Health

Occidental Chemical Corp. (1987a) *Technical Bulletin: Chromic Acid*, Niagara Falls, NY

Occidental Chemical Corp. (1987b) *Technical Bulletin: Potassium Bichromate*, Niagara Falls, NY

Occidental Chemical Corp. (1987c) *Technical Bulletin: Sodium Chromate Anhydrous*, Niagara Falls, NY

Ogawa, H., Misawa, S., Morita, M., Abe, T., Kawai, K. & Nishioka, H. (1978) Sister chromatid exchanges of human lymphocytes induced by metal compounds (Jpn.). *Progr. Med. (Tokyo)*, *107*, 584-585

Ohno, H., Hanaoka, F. & Yamada, M.-A. (1982) Inducibility of sister-chromatid exchanges by heavy-metal ions. *Mutat. Res.*, *104*, 141-145

Ohsaki, Y., Abe, S., Homma, Y., Yozawa, K., Kishi, F., Murao, M., Sato, H., Date, F., Kawauchi, F., Kobayashi, T. & Fujita, I. (1974) High incidence of lung cancer in chromate workers (Jpn.). *J. Jpn. Soc. intern. Med.*, *63*, 1198-1203

Ohsaki, Y., Abe, S., Kimura, K., Tsuneta, Y., Mikami, H. & Murao, M. (1978) Lung cancer in Japanese chromate workers. *Thorax*, *33*, 372-374

Okada, S., Ohba, H. & Taniyama, M. (1981) Alterations in ribonucleic acid synthesis by chromium (III). *J. inorg. Biochem.*, *15*, 223-331

Okada, S., Suzuki, M. & Ohba, H. (1983) Enhancement of ribonucleic acid synthesis by chromium (III) in mouse liver. *J. inorg. Biochem.*, *19*, 95-103

Okada, S., Tsukada, H. & Ohba, H. (1984) Enhancement of nucleolar RNA synthesis by chromium (III) in regenerating rat liver. *J. inorg. Biochem.*, *21*, 113-124

Okubo, T. & Tsuchiya, K. (1977) An epidemiological study on lung cancer among chromium plating workers. *Keio J. Med.*, *26*, 171-177

Okubo, T. & Tsuchiya, K. (1979) Epidemiological study of chromium platers in Japan. *Biol. Trace Elem. Res.*, *1*, 35-44

Okubo, T. & Tsuchiya, K. (1987) Mortality determined in a cohort study of chromium-plating workers (Abstract). *Scand. J. Work Environ. Health*, *13*, 179

Olivier, P. & Marzin, D. (1987) Study of the genotoxic potential of 48 inorganic derivatives with the SOS chromotest. *Mutat. Res.*, *189*, 263-269

Olsen, J. & Sabroe, S. (1984) Occupational causes of laryngeal cancer. *J. Epidemiol. Community Health*, *38*, 117-121

O'Neill, I.K., Schuller, P. & Fishbein, L., eds (1986) *Environmental Carcinogens. Selected Methods of Analysis*, Vol. 8, *Some Metals: As, Be, Cd, Cr, Ni, Pb, Se, Zn* (IARC Scientific Publications No. 71), Lyon, IARC

Osaki, S., Osaki, T., Shibata, S. & Takashima, Y. (1976) Determination of hexavalent and total chromium in sea water by isotope dilution mass spectrometry (Jpn.). *Bunseki Kagaku*, *25*, 358-362 [*Chem. Abstr.*, *86*, 126960g]

Pacyna, J.M. & Nriagu, J.O. (1988) Atmospheric emissions of chromium from natural and anthropogenic sources. In: Nriagu, J.O. & Nieboer, E., eds, *Chromium in the Natural and Human Environments*, New York, John Wiley & Sons, pp. 105-123

Pagano, G., Esposito, A., Bove, P., De Angelis, M., Rota, A. & Giordano, G.G. (1983) The effects of hexavalent and trivalent chromium on fertilization and development in sea urchins. *Environ. Res., 30*, 442-452

Papp, J.F. (1983) Chromium. In: *Mineral Commodity Profiles 1983*, Washington DC, Bureau of Mines, US Department of the Interior, pp. 1-21

Papp, J.F. (1985) Chromium. In: *Bulletin 675, Mineral Facts and Problems*, Washington DC, Bureau of Mines, US Department of the Interior, pp. 1-18

Papp, J.F. (1987) Chromium. In: *1986 Bureau of Mines Minerals Yearbook*, Washington DC, Bureau of Mines, US Department of the Interior, pp. 1-20

Papp, J.F. (1988) Chromium. In: *1987 Bureau of Mines Minerals Yearbook*, Washington DC, Bureau of Mines, US Department of the Interior, pp. 1-17

Paschin, Y.V. & Kozachenko, V.I. (1981) Mutagenic activity of chromium compounds (Russ.). *Gig. Sanit., 5*, 46-49

Paschin, Y.V. & Kozachenko, V.I. (1982) The modifying effect of hexavalent chromate on the mutagenic activity of thio-TEPA. *Mutat. Res., 103*, 367-370

Paschin, Y.V. & Toropsev, S.N. (1982) Chromosome damage induced *in vivo* by heavy metal ion detected by indirect testing. *Acta biol. acad. sci. hung., 33*, 419-422

Paschin, Y.V. & Toropsev, S.N. (1983) Induction of micronuclei in mouse red cells by chromium ion (Russ.). *Bull. exp. Biol. Med., 95*, 72-74

Paschin, Y.V., Kozachenko, V.I. & Zacepilova, T.A. (1981) Complex testing of the genetic activity of the hexavalent chromium ion *in vitro* and *in vivo* (Russ.). *Tsitol. Genet., 15*, 66-69

Paschin, Y.V., Zacepilova, T.A. & Kozachenko, V.I. (1982) Induction of dominant lethal mutations in male mice by potassium dichromate. *Mutat. Res., 103*, 345-347

Paschin, Y.V., Kozachenko, V.I. & Sal'nikova, L.E. (1983) Differential mutagenic response at the HGPRT locus in V79 and CHO Chinese hamster cells after treatment with chromate. *Mutat. Res., 122*, 361-365

Patel, B., Balani, M.C. & Patel, S. (1985) Sponge 'sentinel' of heavy metals. *Sci. total Environ., 41*, 143-152

Patierno, S.R., Banh, D. & Landolph, J.R. (1988) Transformation of C3H/10T1/2 mouse embryo cells to focus formation and anchorage independence by insoluble lead chromate but not soluble calcium chromate: relationship to mutagenesis and internalization of lead chromate particles. *Cancer Res., 48*, 5280-5288

Payne, W.W. (1960a) Production of cancers in mice and rats by chromium compounds. *Arch. ind. Health, 21*, 530-535

Payne, W.W. (1960b) The role of roasted chromite ore in the production of cancer. *Arch. environ. Health, 1*, 20-26

Pedersen, N.B. (1982) The effects of chromium on the skin. In: Langård, S., ed., *Biological and Environmental Aspects of Chromium*, Amsterdam, Elsevier, pp. 249-277

Pedersen, P., Thomsen, E. & Stern, R.M. (1983) Detection by replica plating of false revertant colonies induced in the *Salmonella*-mammalian microsome assay by hexavalent chromium. *Environ. Health Perspect., 51*, 227-230

Pedersen, B., Thomsen, E. & Stern, R.M. (1987) Some problems in sampling, analysis and evaluation of welding fumes containing Cr(VI). *Ann. occup. Hyg.*, 31, 325-338

Pelkonen, L. & Fräki, J. (1983) Prevalence of dichromate sensitivity. *Contact Derm.*, 9, 190-194

Perone, V.B., Moffitt, A.E., Jr, Possick, P.A., Key, M.M., Danzinger, S.J. & Gellin, G.A. (1974) The chromium, cobalt, and nickel contents of American cement and their relationship to cement dermatitis. *Am. ind. Hyg. Assoc. J.*, 35, 301-306

Petrilli, F.L. & De Flora, S. (1977) Toxicity and mutagenicity of hexavalent chromium on *Salmonella typhimurium*. *Appl. environ. Microbiol.*, 33, 805-809

Petrilli, F.L. & De Flora, S. (1978a) Oxidation of inactive trivalent chromium to the mutagenic hexavalent form. *Mutat. Res.*, 58, 167-173

Petrilli, F.L. & De Flora, S. (1978b) Metabolic deactivation of hexavalent chromium mutagenicity. *Mutat. Res.*, 54, 139-147

Petrilli, F.L. & De Flora, S. (1980) Mutagenicity of chromium compounds. In: *Chromium Symposium 80. Focus of a Standard*, Pittsburg, PA, Industrial Health Foundation, pp. 76-99

Petrilli, F.L. & De Flora, S. (1982) Interpretations on chromium mutagenicity and carcinogenicity. In: Sorsa, M. & Vainio, H., eds, *Mutagens in Our Environment*, New York, Alan R. Liss, pp. 453-464

Petrilli, F.L., De Renzi, G.P. & De Flora, S. (1980) Interaction between polycyclic aromatic hydrocarbons, crude oil and oil dispersants in the *Salmonella* mutagenesis assay. *Carcinogenesis*, 1, 51-56

Petrilli, F.L., Camoirano, A., Bennicelli, C., Zanacchi, P., Astengo, M. & De Flora, S. (1985) Specificity and inducibility of the metabolic reduction of chromium(VI) mutagenicity by subcellular fractions of rat tissues. *Cancer Res.*, 45, 3179-3187

Petrilli, F.L., Zanacchi, P., Camoirano, A., Astengo, M., Basso, C. & De Flora, S. (1986a) Selective genotoxicity of chromium compounds. In: Serrone, D., ed., *Chromium Symposium 1986. An Update*, Pittsburg, PA, Industrial Health Foundation, pp. 100-111

Petrilli, F.L., Bennicelli, C., Serra, D., Romano, M., De Flora, A. & De Flora, S. (1986b) Metabolic reduction and detoxification of hexavalent chromium. In: Serrone, D., ed., *Chromium Symposium 1986. An Update*, Pittsburg, PA, Industrial Health Foundation, pp. 112-130

Petrilli, F.L., Rossi, G.A., Camoirano, A., Romano, M., Serra, D., Bennicelli, C., De Flora, A. & De Flora, S. (1986c) Metabolic reduction of chromium by alveolar macrophages and its relationships to cigarette smoke. *J. clin. Invest.*, 77, 1917-1924

Petruzzelli, S., De Flora, S., Bagnasco, M., Hietanen, E., Camus, A.-M., Saracci, R., Izzotti, A., Bartsch, H. & Giuntini, C. (1989) Carcinogen metabolism studies in human bronchial and lung parenchymal tissues. *Am. Rev. respir. Dis.*, 140, 417-422

Pfeil, E. (1935) Lung tumors as occupational disease in chromate plants (Ger.). *Dtsch. med. Wochenschr.*, 61, 1197-1200

Pokrovskaya, L.V. & Shabynina, N.K. (1973) Carcinogenous hazards in the production of chromium ferroalloys (Russ.). *Gig. Tr. prof. Zabol.*, 10, 23-26

Pokrovskaya, L., Tushnakova, N., Gorodnova, N. & Andreeva, T. (1976) Dust factor and occupational disease of workers at open-cast mining of chromium-ore (Russ.). In: Domin, S., Kaznelson, B. & Zislin, D., eds, *Occupational Diseases of Dust Etiology*, Vol. 3, Moscow, Medizina, pp. 38-43

Polak, L. (1983) Immunology of chromium. In: Burrows, D., ed., *Chromium: Metabolism and Toxicology*, Boca Raton, FL, CRC Press, pp. 51-123

Polak, L., Turk, J.L. & Frey, J.R. (1973) Studies on contact hypersensitivity to chromium compounds. *Progr. Allergy*, *17*, 145-226

Poschenrieder, C., Barceló, J. & Gunsé, B. (1986) The impact of chromium in the environment. I. Natural and anthropogenic presence of chromium in the environment (Sp.). *Circ. Farm.*, *290*, 23-38

Price-Jones, M.J., Gubbings, G. & Chamberlain, M. (1980) The genetic effects of crocidolite asbestos: comparison of chromosome abnormalities and sister-chromatid exchanges. *Mutat. Res.*, *79*, 331-336

Princi, F., Miller, L.H., Davis, A. & Cholak, J. (1962) Pulmonary disease of ferrochromium workers. *J. occup. Med.*, *4*, 301-310

Raffetto, G., Parodi, S., Parodi, C., De Ferrari, M., Troiano, R. & Brambilla, G. (1977) Direct interaction with cellular targets as the mechanism for chromium carcinogenesis. *Tumori*, *63*, 503-512

Rafnsson, V. & Jóhannesdóttir, S.G. (1986) Mortality among masons in Iceland. *Br. J. ind. Med.*, *43*, 522-525

Rainaldi, G., Colella, C.M., Piras, A. & Mariani, T. (1982) Thioguanine resistance, ouabain resistance and sister chromatid exchanges in V79/AP4 Chinese hamster cells treated with potassium dichromate. *Chem.-biol. Interact.*, *42*, 45-51

Raithel, H.J., Ebner, G., Schaller, K.H., Schellmann, B. & Valentin, H. (1987) Problems in establishing norm values for nickel and chromium concentrations in human pulmonary tissue. *Am. J. ind. Med.*, *12*, 55-70

Rasmuson, A. (1985) Mutagenic effects of some water-soluble metal compounds in a somatic eye-color test system in *Drosophila melanogaster*. *Mutat. Res.*, *157*, 157-162

Rasmussen, L. (1977) Epiphytic bryophytes as indicators of the changes in the background levels of airborne metals from 1951-75. *Environ. Pollut.*, *14*, 37-45

Retnev, V.M. (1960) On the effect produced by chromium compounds contained in cement dust on the development of bronchial asthma (Russ.). *Gig. Tr. prof. Zabol.*, *7*, 29-33

Reuzel, P.G.J., Beems, R.B., De Raat, W.K. & Lohman, P.H.M. (1986) Carcinogenicity and in vitro genotoxicity of the particulate fraction of two stainless steel welding fumes. *Excerpta med. int. Congr. Ser.*, *676*, 329-332

Riley, E.C. & Goldman, F.H. (1937) Control of chromic acid mists from plating tanks. *Public Health Rep.*, *52*, 172-174

Rivedal, E. & Sanner, T. (1981) Metal salts as promoters of in vitro morphological transformation of hamster embryo cells initiated by benzo[a]pyrene. *Cancer Res.*, *41*, 2950-2953

Rivolta, G., Tomasini, M. & Colombi, A. (1982) Case study of lung cancer due to chromates diagnosed through cytologic examination of the sputum without X-ray evidence (Ital.). *Med. Lav.*, *73*, 40-44

Robison, S.H., Cantoni, O. & Costa, M. (1982) Strand breakage and decreased molecular weight of DNA induced by specific metal compounds. *Carcinogenesis*, *3*, 657-662

Robison, S.H., Cantoni, O. & Costa, M. (1984) Analysis of metal-induced DNA lesions and DNA-repair replication in mammalian cells. *Mutat. Res.*, *131*, 173-181

Rodriguez-Arnaiz, R. & Molina Martinez, R.F. (1986) Genetic effects of potassium dichromate and chromium trioxide in *Drosophila melanogaster*. *Cytologia*, *51*, 421-425

Roe, F.J.C. & Carter, R.L. (1969) Chromium carcinogenesis: calcium chromate as a potent carcinogen for the subcutaneous tissues of the rat. *Br. J. Cancer*, *23*, 172-176

Rogers, S.J., Pagano, D.A. & Zeiger, E. (1987) Mutagenicity of CrIII and CrVI compounds in the presence of mannitol, dithiothreitol and anaerobiosis (Abstract No. 237). *Environ. Mutagenesis*, *9* (Suppl. 8), 91

Rosensteel, R.E. (1974) *Harris Structural Steel Company (Health Hazard Evaluation Report No. 73-99-108)*, Cincinnati, OH, National Institute for Occupational Safety and Health

Roskill Information Services (1974) *Chromium: World Survey of Production, Consumption and Prices*, 2nd ed., London, pp. 8, 80-93

Rossi, S.C. & Wetterhahn, K.E. (1989) Chromium[V] is produced upon reduction of chromate by mitochondrial electron transport chain complexes. *Carcinogenesis*, *10*, 913-920

Rossman, T.G. & Molina, M. (1986) The genetic toxicology of metal compounds: II. Enhancement of ultraviolet light-induced mutagenesis in *Escherichia coli* WP2. *Environ. Mutagenesis*, *8*, 263-271

Rossman, T.G., Molina, M. & Meyer, L.W. (1984) The genetic toxicology of metal compounds: I. Induction of λ prophage in *E. coli* WP2$_s$(λ). *Environ. Mutagenesis*, *6*, 59-69

Rössner, P., Bencko, V. & Šrám, R.J. (1981) Combined action of chromium and nickel on mouse and hamster fibroblast cell lines. *J. Hyg. Epidemiol. Microbiol.*, *25*, 252-258

Royle, H. (1975a) Toxicity of chromic acid in the chromium plating industry (2). *Environ. Res.*, *10*, 141-163

Royle, H. (1975b) Toxicity of chromic acid in the chromium plating industry (1). *Environ. Res.*, *10*, 39-53

Rudnykh, A.A. & Saichenko, S.Pl (1985) Reparative DNA synthesis in the lymphocytes of rats exposed to potassium dichromate and manganese chloride *in vivo* (Russ.). *Tsitol. Genet.*, *19*, 391-392

Ruiz-Rubio, M., Alejandre-Durán, E. & Pueyo, C. (1985) Oxidative mutagens specific for A.T base pairs induced forward mutations to L-arabinose resistance in *Salmonella typhimurium*. *Mutat. Res.*, *147*, 153-163

Ryberg, D. & Alexander, J. (1984) Inhibitory action of hexavalent chromium (Cr(VI)) on the mitochondrial respiration and a possible coupling to the reduction of Cr(VI). *Biochem. Pharmacol.*, *33*, 2461-2466

Sadiq, M., Zaidi, T.H., Hoda, A.-U. & Mian, A.A. (1982) Heavy metal concentrations in shrimp, crab, and sediment obtained from AD-Damman sewage outfall area. *Bull. environ. Contam. Toxicol.*, *29*, 313-319

Salmon, L., Atkins, D.H.F., Fischer, E.M.R. & Law, D.V. (1977) Retrospective analysis of air samples in the UK 1957-1974. *J. radioanal. Chem.*, *37*, 867-880

Sanderson, C.J. (1976) The uptake and retention of chromium by cells. *Transplantation, 21,* 526-529

Saner, G., Yüzbasiyan, V. & Çigdem, S. (1984) Hair chromium concentration and chromium excretion in tannery workers. *Br. J. ind. Med., 41,* 263-266

Sano, T. (1978) Pathology of chromium lesions (Jpn.). *Rodo no Kagaku, 33,* 4-14

Sarto, F., Levis, A.G. & Paulon, C. (1980) Clastogenic activity of hexavalent and trivalent chromium in cultured human lymphocytes. *Caryologia, 33,* 239-250

Sarto, F., Cominato, I., Bianchi, V. & Levis, A.G. (1982) Increased incidence of chromosomal aberrations and sister chromatid exchanges in workers exposed to chromic acid ($CrO_3$) in electroplating factories. *Carcinogenesis, 3,* 1011-1016

Sasaki, I. (1985) Inorganic pigments. In: Japan Chemical Week, ed., *Japan Chemical Annual 1985,* Tokyo, The Chemical Daily Co. Ltd, p. 78

Sasaki, I. (1986) Inorganic pigments. In: Japan Chemical Week, ed., *Japan Chemical Annual 1986,* Tokyo, The Chemical Daily Co. Ltd, p. 78

Sasaki, I. (1987) Inorganic pigments. In: Japan Chemical Week, ed., *Japan Chemical Annual 1987/1988,* Tokyo, The Chemical Daily Co. Ltd, p. 88

Satoh, K., Fukuda, Y., Torii, K. & Katsuno, N. (1981) Epidemiological study of workers engaged in the manufacture of chromium compounds. *J. occup. Med., 23,* 835-838

Sax, I.R. & Lewis, R.J., Sr (1987) *Hawley's Condensed Chemical Dictionary,* 11th ed., New York, Van Nostrand-Reinhold, pp. 66, 118, 278-281, 953-954, 1057-1058, 1098

Sayato, Y. & Nakamuro, K. (1980) Chromium as an inorganic pollutant (Jpn.). *Kagaku no Ryoiki Zokan, 126,* 111-117

Schaaper, R.M., Koplitz, R.M., Tkeshelashvili, L.K. & Loeb, L.A. (1987) Metal-induced lethality and mutagenesis: possible role of apurinic intermediates. *Mutat. Res., 177,* 179-188

Schaller, K.-H., Essing, H.-G., Valentin, H. & Schäcke, G. (1972) Quantitative chromium determination in urine by flameless atomic absorption spectrometry (Ger.). *Z. klin. Chem. klin. Biochem., 10,* 434-437

Schiek, R.C. (1973) Lead chromate pigments. Chrome yellow and chrome orange. In: Patton, T.C., ed., *Pigment Handbook,* Vol. 1, New York, John Wiley & Sons, pp. 357-363

Schroeder, H.A., Balassa, J.J. & Vinton, W.H., Jr (1964) Chromium, lead, cadmium, nickel and titanium in mice: effect on mortality, tumors and tissue levels. *J. Nutr., 83,* 239-250

Schroeder, H.A., Balassa, J.J. & Vinton, W.H., Jr (1965) Chromium, cadmium and lead in rats: effects on lifespan, tumors and tissue levels. *J. Nutr., 86,* 51-66

Sen, P. & Costa, M. (1986) Incidence and localization of sister chromatid exchanges induced by nickel and chromium compounds. *Carcinogenesis, 7,* 1527-1533

Sen, P., Conway, K. & Costa, M. (1987) Comparison of the localization of chromosome damage induced by calcium chromate and nickel compounds. *Cancer Res., 47,* 2142-2147

Sequi, P. (1980) Behaviour of chromium and mercury in soil (Ital.). In: Frigerio, A., ed., *Rischi Tossic. Inquin. Met.: Cromo Mercurio [Conv. Naz.],* Milan, DST Publishers, pp. 27-50

Sharma, B.K., Singhal, P.C. & Chugh, K.S. (1978) Intravascular haemolysis and acute renal failure following potassium dichromate poisoning. *Postgrad. med. J., 54,* 414-415

Sheehy, J.W., Mortimer, V.D, Jones, J.H. & Spottswood, S.E. (1984) *Control Technology Assessment: Metal Plating and Cleaning Operations* (NIOSH Technical Report), Cincinnati, OH, National Institute for Occupational Safety and Health

Sheffet, A., Thind, I., Miller, A.M. & Louria, D.B. (1982) Cancer mortality in a pigment plant utilizing lead and zinc chromates. *Arch. environ. Health, 37*, 44-52

Shimkin, M.B. & Leiter, J. (1940) Induced pulmonary tumors in mice. III. The role of chronic irritation in the production of pulmonary tumors in strain A mice. *J. natl Cancer Inst., 1*, 241-254

Shimkin, M.B., Stoner, G.D. & Theiss, J.C. (1977) Lung tumor response in mice to metals and metal salts. *Adv. exp. Med. Biol., 91*, 85-91

Sibley, S.F. (1976) Cobalt. In: *Mineral Facts and Problems*, Washington DC, Bureau of Mines, US Government Printing Office, pp. 269-280

Silverstein, M., Mirer, F., Kotelchuck, D., Silverstein, B. & Bennett, M. (1981) Mortality among workers in a die-casting and electroplating plant. *Scand. J. Work Environ. Health, 7 (Suppl. 4)*, 156-165

Sina, J.F., Bean, C.L., Dysart, G.R., Taylor, V.I. & Bradley, M.O. (1983) Evaluation of the alkaline elution/rat hepatocyte assay as a predictor of carcinogenic/mutagenic potential. *Mutat. Res., 113*, 357-391

Singh, I. (1983) Induction of reverse mutation and mitotic gene conversion by some metal compounds in *Saccharomyces cerevisiae*. *Mutat. Res., 117*, 149-152

Sirover, M.A. & Loeb, L.A. (1976) Infidelity of DNA synthesis *in vitro*: screening for potential metal mutagens or carcinogens. *Science, 194*, 1434-1436

Slavin, W. (1981) Determination of chromium in the environment and in the work place. *Atmos. Spectrosc., 2*, 8-12

Smith, D.E., Slade, M.D., Spencer, O.K., Roberts, W.L. & Ruckman, J.H. (1976) Metal concentrations in air particulate in the Four Corners area. *Utah Acad. Proc., 53*, 75-83

Snow, E.T. & Xu, L.-S. (1989) Effects of chromium(III) on DNA replication *in vitro*. *Biol. Trace Element Res., 21*, 61-72

Snyder, R.D. (1988) Role of active oxygen species in metal-induced DNA strand breakage in human diploid fibroblasts. *Mutat. Res., 193*, 237-246

Sokolowska, D.M. & Jongen, W.M.F. (1984) Heavy metals and *Salmonella typhimurium*: mutagenicity and interaction with model compounds (Abstract No. I.1.7). *Mutat. Res., 130*, 168

Sontag, G., Kerschbaumer, M. & Kainz, G. (1977) Determination of toxic heavy metals in effluent Austrian medicinal and table water (Ger.). *Z. Wasser Abwasser Forsch., 10*, 166-169 [*Chem. Abstr., 88*, 110183m]

Sora, S., Agostoni Carbone, M.L., Pacciarini, M. & Magni, G.E. (1986) Disomic and diploid meiotic products induced in *Saccharomyces cerevisiae* by the salts of 27 elements. *Mutagenesis, 1*, 21-28

Sorahan, T., Burges, D.C.L. & Waterhouse, J.A.H. (1987) A mortality study of nickel/chromium platers. *Br. J. ind. Med., 44*, 250-258

Sponza, G. & Levis, A.G. (1980) Effects of potassium dichromate, mitomycin C and methyl-methane-sulphonate on the in vitro synthesis of poly dT catalyzed by DNA-polymerase α from calf thymus with poly dA.(dT)$_n$ (Abstract). In: *Atti Associazione Genetica Italiana*, Vol. 26, Sassari, Poddighe, pp. 303-305

Steffee, C.H. & Baetjer, A.M. (1965) Histopathologic effects of chromate chemicals. Report of studies in rabbits, guinea pigs, rats and mice. *Arch. environ. Health, 11*, 66-75

Steinhoff, D., Gad, S.C., Hatfield, K. & Mohr, U. (1986) Carcinogenicity study with sodium dichromate in rats. *Exp. Pathol., 30*, 129-141

Stella, M., Montaldi, A., Rossi, R., Rossi, G. & Levis, A.G. (1982) Clastogenic effects of chromium on human lymphocytes *in vitro* and *in vivo*. *Mutat. Res., 101*, 151-164

Stern, R.M. (1982) Chromium compounds: production and occupational exposure. In: Langård, S., ed., *Biological and Environmental Aspects of Chromium*, Amsterdam, Elsevier, pp. 5-47

Stern, R.M., Thomsen, E. & Furst, A. (1984) Cr(VI) and other metallic mutagens in fly ash and welding fumes. *Toxicol. environ. Chem., 8*, 95-108

Stern, F.B., Beaumont, J.J., Halperin, W.E., Murthy, L.I., Hills, B.W. & Fajen, J.M. (1987) Mortality of chrome leather tannery workers and chemical exposures in tanneries. *Scand. J. Work Environ. Health, 13*, 108-117

Stoner, G.D., Shimkin, M.B., Troxell, M.C., Thompson, T.L. & Terry, L.S. (1976) Test for carcinogenicity of metallic compounds by the pulmonary tumor response in strain A mice. *Cancer Res., 36*, 1744-1747

Stowe, H.D., Braselton, W.E., Kaneene, J.B. & Slanker, M. (1985) Multielement assays of bovine tissue specimens by inductively coupled argon plasma emission spectroscopy. *Am. J. vet. Res., 46*, 561-565

Sugiyama, M., Patierno, S.R., Cantoni, O. & Costa, M. (1986a) Characterization of DNA lesions induced by CaCrO$_4$ in synchronous and asynchronous cultured mammalian cells. *Mol. Pharmacol., 29*, 606-613

Sugiyama, M., Wang, X.-W. & Costa, M. (1986b) Comparison of DNA lesions and cytotoxicity induced by calcium chromate in human, mouse and hamster cell lines. *Cancer Res., 46*, 4547-4551

Sugiyama, M., Ando, A., Foruno, A., Furlong, N.B., Hidaka, T. & Ogura, R. (1987) Effects of vitamin E, vitamin B$_2$ and selenite on DNA single strand breaks induced by sodium chromate(VI). *Cancer Lett., 38*, 1-7

Sugiyama, M., Costa, M., Nakagawa, T., Hidaka, T. & Ogura, R. (1988) Stimulation of polyadenosine diphosphoribose synthesis by DNA lesions induced by sodium chromate in Chinese hamster V-79 cells. *Cancer Res., 48*, 1100-1104

Sullivan, C.P., Donachie, M.J., Jr & Morral, F.R. (1970) *Cobalt-base Superalloys 1970*, Brussels, Centre d'information du Cobalt, pp. 1-4, 38-44

Sunderman, F.W., Jr (1976) A review of the carcinogenicities of nickel, chromium and arsenic compounds in man and animals. *Prev. Med., 5*, 279-294

Sunderman, F.W., Jr (1984) Recent advances in metal carcinogenesis. *Ann. clin. Lab. Sci., 14*, 93-122

Sunderman, F.W., Jr (1986) Carcinogenicity and mutagenicity of some metals and their compounds. In: O'Neill, I.K., Schuller, P. & Fishbein, L., eds, *Environmental Carcinogens: Selected Methods of Analysis*, Vol. 8, *Some Metals: As, Be, Cd, Cr, Ni, Pb, Se, Zn* (IARC Scientific Publications No. 71), Lyon, IARC, pp. 17-43

Sunderman, F.W., Jr, Lau, T.J. & Cralley, L.J. (1974) Inhibitory effect of manganese upon muscle tumorigenesis by nickel subsulfide. *Cancer Res., 34*, 92-95

Sunderman, F.W., Jr, McCully, K.S., Taubman, S.B., Allpass, P.R., Reid, M.C. & Rinehimer, L.A. (1980) Manganese inhibition of sarcoma induction by benzo[a]pyrene in rats. *Carcinogenesis, 1*, 613-620

Suzuki, Y. (1988) Reduction of hexavalent chromium by ascorbic acid in rat lung lavage fluid. *Arch. Toxicol., 62*, 116-122

Suzuki, Y., Homma, K., Minami, M. & Yoshikawa, H. (1984) Distribution of chromium in rats exposed to hexavalent chromium and trivalent chromium aerosols. *Ind. Health, 22*, 261-277

Takahashi, W., Pfenninger, K. & Wong, L. (1983) Urinary arsenic, chromium, and copper levels in workers exposed to arsenic-based wood preservatives. *Arch. environ. Health, 38*, 209-214

Takemoto, K., Kawai, H. & Yoshimura, H. (1977) Studies on the relation of chromium and pulmonary disease. II. Chromium contamination of lung cancer (Jpn.). In: *Proceedings of the 50th Annual Meeting of the Japan Association of Industrial Health*, Tokyo, Japan Association of Industrial Health, pp. 368-369

Tamaro, M., Banfi, E., Venturini, S. & Monti-Bragadin, C. (1975) Hexavalent chromium compounds are mutagenic for bacteria (Ital.). In: *Proceedings of the 17th National Congress of the Italian Society of Microbiology*, Padua, Società Italiana di Microbiologia, pp. 411-415

Tamino, G. & Peretta, L. (1980) Variations of DNA physico-chemical parameters in its interactions with mutagenic and/or carcinogenic compounds. In: Borsellino, A., Omodeo, P., Strom, R., Vecli, A. & Wamke, E., eds, *Developments in Biophysical Research*, New York, Plenum, pp. 335-346

Tamino, G., Peretta, L. & Levis, A.G. (1981) Effects of trivalent and hexavalent chromium on physico-chemical properties of mammalian cell nucleic acids and synthetic polynucleotides. *Chem.-biol. Interactions, 37*, 309-319

Tandon, S.K., Mathur, A.K. & Gaur, J.S. (1977) Urinary excretion of chromium and nickel among electroplaters and pigment industry workers. *Int. Arch. occup. environ. Health, 40*, 71-76

Taylor, F.H. (1966) The relationship of mortality and duration of employment as reflected by a cohort of chromate workers. *Am. J. public Health, 56*, 218-229

Teleky, L. (1936) Cancer in chromium workers (Ger.). *Dtsch. med. Wochenschr., 62*, 1353

Teraoka, H. (1987) Distribution of 24 elements in the internal organs of normal males and the metallic workers in Japan. *Arch. environ. Health, 36*, 155-165

Thomsen, E. & Stern, R.M. (1979) A simple analytical technique for the determination of hexavalent chromium in welding fumes and other complex matrices. *Scand. J. Work Environ. Health, 5*, 386-403

Tkeshelashvili, L.K., Shearman, C.W., Zakour, R.A., Koplitz, R.M. & Loeb, L.A. (1980) Effects of arsenic, selenium and chromium on the fidelity of DNA synthesis. *Cancer Res.*, *40*, 2455-2460

Torgrimsen, T. (1982) Analysis of chromium. In: Langård, S., ed., *Biological and Environmental Aspects of Chromium*, Amsterdam, Elsevier, pp. 65-99

Tossavainen, A. (1976) Metal fumes in foundries. *Scand. J. Work Environ. Health*, *2* (Suppl. 1), 42-49

Traul, K.A., Takayama, K., Kachevsky, V., Hink, R.J. & Wolff, J.S. (1981) A rapid in vitro assay for carcinogenicity of chemical substances in mammalian cells utilizing an attachment-independence endpoint. *J. appl. Toxicol.*, *1*, 190-195

Triebig, G., Zschiesche, W., Schaller, K.H., Weltle, D. & Valentin, H. (1987) Studies on the nephrotoxicity of heavy metals in iron and steel industries. In: Foá, V., Emmett, E.A., Maroni, M. & Colombi, A., eds, *Occupational and Environmental Chemical Hazards. Cellular and Biochemical Indices for Monitoring Toxicity*, Chichester, Ellis Horwood, pp. 334-338

Tsapakos, M.J. & Wetterhahn, K.E. (1983) The interaction of chromium with nucleic acids. *Chem.-biol. Interactions*, *46*, 265-277

Tsapakos, M.J., Hampton, T.H. & Jennette, K.W. (1981) The carcinogen chromate induces DNA cross-links in rat liver and kidney. *J. biol. Chem.*, *256*, 3623-3626

Tsapakos, M.J., Hampton, T.H. & Wetterhahn, K.E. (1983a) Chromium(VI)-induced DNA lesions and chromium distribution in rat kidney, liver and lung. *Cancer Res.*, *43*, 5662-5667

Tsapakos, M.J., Hampton, T.H., Sinclair, P.R., Sinclair, J.F., Bement, W.J. & Wetterhahn, K.E. (1983b) The carcinogen chromate causes DNA damage and inhibits drug-mediated induction of porphyrin accumulation and glucuronidation in chick embryo hepatocytes. *Carcinogenesis*, *4*, 959-966

Tso, W.-W. & Fung, W.-P. (1981) Mutagenicity of metallic cations. *Toxicol. Lett.*, *8*, 195-200

Tsuchiya, K. (1965) The relation of occupation to cancer, especially cancer of the lung. *Cancer*, *18*, 136-144

Tsuda, H. & Kato, K. (1977) Chromosomal aberrations and morphological transformation in hamster embryonic cells treated with potassium dichromate in vitro. *Mutat. Res.*, *46*, 87-94

Tsuneta, Y. (1982) Investigations of the pathogenesis of lung cancer observed among chromate factory workers (Jpn.). *Hokkaido J. med. Sci.*, *57*, 175-187

Työsuojeluhallitus (National Finnish Board of Occupational Safety and Health) (1987) *HTP-Azvot 1987* (TLV-Values 1987) (Safety Bull. 25), Helsinki, p. 19

Udy, M.C. (1956) The physical and chemical properties of compounds of chromium. In: Udy, M.J., ed., *Chromium*, Vol. 1, New York, Reinhold, pp. 164-165, 206

Ulitzur, S. & Barak, M. (1988) Detection of genotoxicity of metallic compounds by the bacterial bioluminescence test. *J. Biolumin. Chemilumin.*, *2*, 95-99

Umeda, M. & Nishimura, M. (1979) Inducibility of chromosomal aberrations by metal compounds in cultured mammalian cells. *Mutat. Res.*, *67*, 221-229

US Department of Commerce (1978) *US Imports for Consumption and General Imports* (FT 246/Annual 1977), Washington DC, Bureau of the Census, US Government Printing Office, pp. 231-233, 247, 293

US Environmental Protection Agency (1977) *Environmental Monitoring Near Industrial Sites, Chromium* (US NTIS PB-271 881), Washington DC

US Environmental Protection Agency (1978) *Reviews of the Environmental Effects of Pollutants. III. Chromium* (US EPA 600/1-78-023), Washington DC

US Environmental Protection Agency (1979) Facilities engaged in leather tanning and finishing; effluent limitations guidelines, pretreatment standards, and new source performance standards. *Fed. Regist.*, *44*, 38746-38776

US Environmental Protection Agency (1983) *Methods for the Chemical Analysis of Water and Wastes* (US EPA-600/4-79-020), Cincinnati, OH, Environmental Monitoring and Support Laboratory

US Environmental Protection Agency (1984) *Health Assessment Document for Chromium, Final Report* (US EPA-600/8-83-014F), Research Triangle Park, NC, Environmental Criteria and Assessment Office

US Environmental Protection Agency (1986) *Test Methods for Evaluating Solid Waste*, Vol. 1A, *Laboratory Manual Physical/Chemical Methods* (SW-846), 3rd ed., Washington DC, Office of Solid Waste and Emergency Response

US Environmental Protection Agency (1988) Maximum contaminant levels for inorganic chemicals. *US Code fed. Regul.*, *Title 40*, Part 141.11, p. 530

US Occupational Safety and Health Administration (1987) Air contaminants. *US Code fed. Regul.*, *Title 29*, Part 1910.1000, pp. 676-682

Uyeki, E.M. & Nishio, A. (1983) Antiproliferative and genotoxic effects of chromium on cultured mammalian cells. *J. Toxicol. environ. Health*, *11*, 227-235

Van Bemst, A., Beaufils, B., Hewett, P.J. & Stern, R.M. (1983) Interlaboratory calibration of a standardized analytical method for hexavalent and total chromium in welding fumes. *Weld. World*, *21*, 10-15

Vandenbalck, J.L. & Patriarche, G.J. (1987) Electrochemical micro-determinations of thallium(I) and chromium (VI) ions using DPASV and DP polarography. *Sci. total Environ.*, *60*, 97-104

Vandervort, R. & Cromer, J. (1975) *Peabody Galion Corp.* (Health Hazard Evaluation/Toxicity Determination Report NIOSH-TR-73-47-172), Cincinnati, OH, National Institute for Occupational Safety and Health

Venier, P., Montaldi, A., Majone, F., Bianchi, V. & Levis, A.G. (1982) Cytotoxic, mutagenic and clastogenic effects of industrial chromium compounds. *Carcinogenesis*, *3*, 1331-1338

Venier, P., Montaldi, A., Busi, L., Gava, C., Zentilin, L., Tecchio, G., Bianchi, V. & Levis, A.G. (1985a) Genetic effects of chromium tannins. *Carcinogenesis*, *6*, 1327-1335

Venier, P., Montaldi, A., Gava, G., Zentilin, L., Tecchio, G., Bianchi, V., Paglialunga, S. & Levis, A.G. (1985b) Effects of nitrilotriacetic acid on the induction of gene mutations and sister-chromatid exchanges by insoluble chromium compounds. *Mutat. Res.*, *156*, 219-228

Venier, P., Gava, C., Zordan, M., Bianchi, V., Levis, A.G., De Flora, S., Bennicelli, C. & Camoirano, A. (1987) Interactions of chromium with nitrilotriacetic acid (NTA) in the induction of genetic effects in bacteria. *Toxicol. environ. Chem.*, *14*, 201-218

Venier, P., Montini, R., Zordan, M., Clonfero, E., Paleologo, M. & Levis, A.G. (1989) Induction of SOS response in *Escherichia coli* strain PQ37 by 16 chemical compounds and human urine extracts. *Mutagenesis*, *4*, 51-57

Venitt, S. (1986) Genetic toxicology in chromium and nickel compounds. In: Stern, R.M., Berlin, A., Fletcher, A.C. & Järvisalo, J., eds, *Health Hazards and Biological Effects of Welding Fumes and Gases*, Amsterdam, Excerpta Medica, pp. 249-266

Venitt, S. & Bosworth, D. (1983) The development of anaerobic methods for bacterial mutation assays: aerobic and anaerobic fluctuation test of human faecal extracts and reference mutagens. *Carcinogenesis*, *4*, 339-345

Venitt, S. & Levy, S.L. (1974) Mutagenicity of chromates in bacteria and its relevance to chromate carcinogenesis. *Nature*, *250*, 493-495

Verschoor, M.A., Bragt, P.C., Herber, R.F.M., Zielhuis, R.L. & Zwennis, W.C.M. (1988) Renal function of chrome-plating workers and welders. *Int. Arch. occup. environ. Health*, *60*, 67-70

Versieck, J., Hoste, J., Barbier, F., Steyaert, H., De Rudder, J. & Michels, H. (1978) Determination of chromium and cobalt in human serum by neutron activation analysis. *Clin. Chem.*, *24*, 303-308

Vieux, B., Garland, J., Warren, G. & Rogers, S. (1986) Mutagenic mechanisms of substitutionally inert metal complexes of PtII, PtIV, CrIII and potassium dichromate (Abstract No. PM 30). In: Ramel, C., Lambert, B. & Magnusson, J., eds, *Proceedings of the Fourth International Conference on Environmental Mutagens, Stockholm, June 24-28 1985*, New York, Alan R. Liss, p. 262

Vigliani, E.C. & Zurlo, N. (1955) Experiences of the 'Clinica del Lavoro' with some MAKs of industrial toxins (Ger.). *Arch. Gewerbepathol. Gewerbehyg.*, *13*, 528-534

Vos, G., Hovens, J.P.C. & Hagel, P. (1986) Chromium, nickel, copper, zinc, arsenic, selenium, cadmium, mercury and lead in Dutch fishery products 1977-1984. *Sci. total Environ.*, *52*, 25-40

Wacker, W.E.C. & Vallee, B.L. (1959) Nucleic acids and metals. I. Chromium, manganese, nickel, iron and other metals in ribonucleic acid from diverse biological sources. *J. biol. Chem.*, *234*, 3257-3262

Wahlberg, J.E. & Skog, E. (1963) The percutaneous absorption of sodium chromate ($^{51}$Cr) in the guinea-pig. *Acta dermatovenerol.*, *43*, 102-108

van der Wal, J.F. (1985) Exposure of welders to fumes, Cr, Ni, Cu and gases in Dutch industries. *Ann. occup. Hyg.*, *29*, 377-389

Wallach, S. & Verch, R.L. (1984) Placental transport of chromium. *J. Am. Coll. Nutr.*, *3*, 69-74

Wapner, K.L., Morris, D.M. & Black, J. (1986) Release of corrosion products by F-75 cobalt base alloy in the rat. II: Morbidity apparently associated with chromium release *in vivo*: a 120-day rat study. *J. biomed. Mat. Res.*, *20*, 219-233

Warner, J.S. (1984) Occupational exposure to airborne nickel in producing and using primary nickel products. In: Sunderman, F.W., Jr, ed., *Nickel in the Human Environment* (IARC Scientific Publications No. 53), Lyon, IARC, pp. 419-437

Warren, G., Schultz, P., Bancroft, D., Bennett, K., Abbott, E.H. & Rogers, S. (1981) Mutagenicity of a series of hexacoordinate chromium(III) compounds. *Mutat. Res., 90,* 111-118

Watanabe, S. & Fukuchi, Y. (1984) Cancer mortality of chromate-producing workers. In: Eustace, I.E., ed., *XXI International Congress on Occupational Health, 9-14 September, 1984, Dublin, Ireland,* London, Permanent Commission and International Association on Occupational Health, p. 442

Watanabe, M., Takayama, Y.-I., Koike, M. & Yamamoto, M. (1985) In vivo clastogenicity of lead chromate in mice. *Tohoku J. exp. Med., 146,* 373-374

Waterhouse, J.A.H. (1975) Cancer among chromium platers (Abstract). *Br. J. Cancer, 32,* 262

Watling, H.R. & Watling, R.J. (1982) Metal concentrations in oysters from the southern African coast. *Bull. environ. Contam. Toxicol., 28,* 460-466

Wayne Pigment Corp. (1985a) *MSDS: Molybdate Orange Light 64,* Milwaukee, WI

Wayne Pigment Corp. (1985b) *MSDS: Molybdate Orange Dark 664,* Milwaukee, WI

Weast, R.C., ed. (1985) *CRC Handbook of Chemistry and Physics,* 66th ed., Boca Raton, FL, CRC Press, pp. B-70, B-75, B-82, B-88—B-89, B-106, B-127, B-142, B-147, B-159

Wedrychowski, A., Schmidt, W.N. & Hnilica, L.S. (1986a) DNA-protein crosslinking by heavy metals in Novikoff hepatoma. *Arch. Biochem. Biophys., 251,* 397-402

Wedrychowski, A., Schmidt, W.N., Ward, W.S. & Hnilica, L.S. (1986b) Cross-linking of cytokeratins to DNA *in vivo* by chromium salt and *cis*-diamminedichloroplatinum(II). *Biochemistry, 25,* 1-9

Westbrook, J.H. (1979) Chromium and chromium alloys. In: Mark, H.F., Othmer, D.F., Overberger, C.G., Seaborg, G.T. & Grayson, M., eds, *Kirk-Othmer Encyclopedia of Chemical Technology,* 3rd ed., Vol. 6, New York, John Wiley & Sons, pp. 54-82

Wetterhahn-Jennette, K. (1981) The role of metals in carcinogenicity: biochemistry and metabolism. *Environ. Health Perspect., 40,* 233-252

Whiting, R.F., Stich, H.F. & Koropatnick, D.J. (1979) DNA damage and DNA repair in cultured human cells exposed to chromate. *Chem.-biol. Interactions, 26,* 267-280

Whitney, R.G. & Risby, T.H. (1975) *Selected Methods in the Determination of First Row Transition Metals in Natural Fresh Water,* University Park, PA, Pennsylvania University Press

Wiegand, H.J., Ottenwälder, H. & Bolt, H.M. (1984a) Disposition of intratracheally administered chromium(III) and chromium(VI) in rabbits. *Toxicol. Lett., 22,* 273-276

Wiegand, H.J., Ottenwälder, H. & Bolt, H.M. (1984b) The reduction of chromium (VI) to chromium (III) by glutathione: an intracellular redox pathway in the metabolism of the carcinogen chromate. *Toxicology, 33,* 341-348

Wild, D. (1978) Cytogenetic effects in the mouse of 17 chemical mutagens and carcinogens evaluated by the micronucleus test. *Mutat. Res., 56,* 319-327

Windholz, M., ed. (1983) *The Merck Index,* 10th ed., Rahway, NJ, Merck & Co., pp. 76-77, 140, 229, 315-319, 777, 1100, 1233-1234, 1267, 1456-1457

Wong, M.H., Choy, C.K., Lau, W.M. & Cheung, Y.H. (1981) Heavy-metal contamination of the Pacific oysters (*Crassostrea gigas*) cultured in Deep Bay, Hong Kong. *Environ. Res.*, 25, 302-309

World Health Organization (1970) *European Standards for Drinking Water*, 2nd ed., Geneva, p. 33

World Health Organization (1988) *Chromium* (Environmental Health Criteria 61), Geneva, International Programme on Chemical Safety

Yagi, T. & Nishioka, H. (1977) DNA damage and its degradation by metal compounds. *Sci. Eng. Rev. Doshisha Univ.*, 18, 1-8

Yamamoto, A., Wada, O. & Ono, T. (1981) A low-molecular-weight, chromium-binding substance in mammals. *Toxicol. appl. Pharmacol.*, 59, 515-523

Yassi, A. & Nieboer, E. (1988) Carcinogenicity of chromium compounds. In: Nriagu, J.O. & Nieboer, E., eds, *Chromium in the Natural and Human Environments*, New York, John Wiley & Sons, pp. 443-495

Yasuda, Y. (1980) Abnormalities in mouse sperm and sterility after injection of potassium bichromate (Abstract). *Teratology*, 22, 13A

Yunusova, K.K. & Pavlovskaya, G.S. (1975) The effect of the chromium plating regimen on the protective properties of chromine (Russ.). *Zashch. Met.*, 11, 248-250 [*Chem. Abstr.*, 83, 123027k]

Zakour, R.A. & Glickman, B.W. (1984) Metal-induced mutagenesis in the *lacI* gene of *Escherichia coli*. *Mutat. Res.*, 126, 9-18

Zey, J.N. & Aw, T.-C. (1984) *American Transportation Corp.* (*Health Hazard Evaluation Report No. 82-025-1413*), Cincinnati, OH, National Institute for Occupational Safety and Health

Zhang, X., Jixun, D. & Tsungci, F. (1984) The mutagenic effect of hexavalent chromium and antimutagenic effect of cysteine detected by the Tradescantia-micronucleus technique (Chin.). *Zhandong Haiyang Xueyan Xuebao*, 14, 81-83

Zimmering, S. (1983) The *mei-9$^a$* test for chromosome loss in *Drosophila*: a review of assays of 21 chemicals for chromosome breakage. *Environ. Mutagenesis*, 5, 907-921

Zober, A. (1979) On the problems of evaluating bronchial carcinoma after exposure to chromium compounds (Ger.). *Int. Arch. occup. environ. Health*, 43, 107-121

# NICKEL AND NICKEL COMPOUNDS

Nickel and nickel compounds were considered by previous IARC Working Groups, in 1972, 1975, 1979, 1982 and 1987 (IARC, 1973, 1976, 1979, 1982, 1987). Since that time, new data have become available, and these are included in the present monograph and have been taken into consideration in the evaluation.

## 1. Chemical and Physical Data

The list of nickel alloys and compounds given in Table 1 is not exhaustive, nor does it necessarily reflect the commercial importance of the various nickel-containing substances, but it is indicative of the range of nickel alloys and compounds available, including some compounds that are important commercially and those that have been tested in biological systems. A number of intermediary compounds occur in refineries which cannot be characterized and are not listed.

### 1.1 Synonyms, trade names and molecular formulae of nickel and selected nickel-containing compounds

**Table 1. Synonyms (Chemical Abstracts Service names are given in bold), trade names and atomic or molecular formulae or compositions of nickel, nickel alloys and selected nickel compounds**

| Chemical name | Chem. Abstr. Serv. Reg. Number[a] | Synonyms and trade names | Formula | Oxidation state[b] |
|---|---|---|---|---|
| **Metallic nickel and nickel alloys** | | | | |
| **Nickel** | 7440-02-0 (8049-31-8; 17375-04-1; 39303-46-3; 53527-81-4; 112084-17-0) | C.I. 77775; N1; Ni 233; Ni 270; Nickel 270; Nickel element; NP 2 | Ni | 0 |

## Table 1 (contd)

| Chemical name | Chem. Abstr. Serv. Reg. Number[a] | Synonyms and trade names | Formula | Oxidation state[b] |
|---|---|---|---|---|
| Ferronickel | 11133-76-9 (11148-37-1; 12604-55-6) | **Iron alloy (base), Fe,Ni;** nickel alloy (non-base), Fe, Ni | Fe, Ni | 0 |
| Nickel aluminium alloys | 61431-86-5 37187-84-1 | **Raney nickel;** Raney alloy | NiAl | 0 |
| Nickel-containing steels[c] | 12681-83-3 | **Iron alloy (base);** 21-6-9; 21-6-9 alloy; Alloy 21-6-9; **AMS 5656C;** Armco 21-6-9; ASTM XM10; 21-6-9 austenitic steel; Nitronic 40; Nitronic 40 stainless steel; Pyromet 538; 21-6-9 Stainless steel; Stainless steel 21-6-9; 21-6-9 steel; Steel 21-6-9 | Fe 60-69, Cr 18-21, Mn 8-10, Ni 5-7, Si 0-1, N 0.2-0.4, C 0-0.1, P 0-0.1 | 0 |
| High nickel alloys[c] | 12605-70-8 | **ASTM B344-60Ni,** 16 Cr; Chromel C; 06Kh15N60; Kh15N60N; Nichrome; NiCr 60/15; PNKh; Tophet C | Ni 57-62, Fe 22-28, Cr 14-18, Si 0.8-1.6, Mn 0-1, C 0-0.2 | 0 |
| | 11121-96-3 | AFNOR ZFeNC45-36; AISI 332; Alloy 800; **ASTM B163-800;** DIN 1.4876; IN 800; Incoloy alloy 800; JIS NCF 800; NCF Steel; NCF 800 HTB; Pyromet 800; Sanicro 31; Thermax 4876; TIG N800 | Fe 39-47, Ni 30-35; Cr 19-23, Mn 0-1.5, Si 0-1; Cu 0-0.8; Al 0-0.6; Ti 0-0.6; C 0-0.1 | 0 |
| | 12675-92-2 | **Haynes alloy No. 188** | Ni(Co) | 0 |
| | 11105-19-4 | Alloy 400; ASTM B127; ASTM B164-A; H3261; Monel alloy 400; Monel (NiCu30Fe) | Ni 63-70; Cu 25-37, Fe 0-2.5, Mn 0-2, Si 0-0.5, C 0-0.3 | 0 |
| **Nickel oxides and hydroxides** | | | | |
| Nickel hydroxide (amorphous | 12054-48-7 11113-74-9) | Nickel dihydroxide; nickel (II) hydroxide; nickel (2+) hydroxide; **nickel hydroxide (Ni(OH)$_2$);** nickelous hydroxide | Ni(OH)$_2$ | +2 |
| Nickel monoxide | 1313-99-1 11099-02-8 | Black nickel oxide[d]; green nickel oxide; mononickel oxide; nickel monooxide; nickelous oxide; **nickel oxide (NiO);** nickel (II) oxide; nickel (2+) oxide | NiO | +2 |
| | 34492-97-2 | **Bunsenite (NiO)** | | |
| Nickel trioxide | 1314-06-3 (34875-54-2) | Black nickel oxide[d]; dinickel trioxide; nickelic oxide; nickel oxide; nickel (III) oxide; **nickel oxide (Ni$_2$O$_3$);** nickel peroxide; nickel sesquioxide | Ni$_2$O$_3$ | +3 |
| **Nickel sulfides** | | | | |
| Nickel disulfide | 12035-51-7 | **Nickel sulfide (NiS$_2$)** | NiS$_2$ | +4 |
| | 12035-50-6 | **Vaesite (NiS$_2$)** | NiS$_2$ | +4 |

## Table 1 (contd)

| Chemical name | Chem. Abstr. Serv. Reg. Number[a] | Synonyms and trade names | Formula | Oxidation state[b] |
|---|---|---|---|---|
| Nickel sulfide (amorphous | 16812-54-7 (1344-49-6) 11113-75-0) | Mononickel monosulfide; nickel monosulfide; nickel monosulfide (NiS); nickelous sulfide; nickel (II) sulfide; nickel (2+) sulfide; nickel sulfide (NiS) | NiS | +2 |
| | 1314-04-1 (61026-96-8) | Millerite (NiS) | NiS | +2 |
| Nickel sub-sulfide | 12035-72-2 | Nickel sesquisulfide; nickel subsulfide ($Ni_3S_2$); nickel sulfide ($Ni_3S_2$); trinickel disulfide | $Ni_3S_2$ | NS |
| | 12035-71-1 | Heazlewoodite ($Ni_3S_2$); Khizlevudite | | |
| Pentlandite | 53809-86-2 | Pentlandite ($Fe_9Ni_9S_{16}$) | $Fe_9Ni_9S_{16}$ | NS |
| | 12174-14-0 | Pentlandite | $(Fe_{0.4-0.6}Ni_{0.4-0.6})_9S_8$ | NS |
| Nickel salts | | | | |
| Nickel carbonate | 3333-67-3 | Carbonic acid, nickel (2+) salt (1:1); nickel carbonate (1:1); nickel (II) carbonate; nickel (2+) carbonate; nickel carbonate ($NiCO_3$); nickel (2+) carbonate ($NiCO_3$); nickel monocarbonate; nickelous carbonate | $NiCO_3$ | +2 |
| Basic nickel carbonates | 12607-70-4 (63091-15-6) | Carbonic acid, nickel salt, basic; nickel carbonate hydroxide ($Ni_3(CO_3)(OH)_4$); nickel, (carbonato(2-)) tetrahydroxytri- | $NiCO_3.2Ni(OH)_2$ | +2 |
| | 12122-15-5 | Nickel bis(carbonato(2-))hexahydroxypenta-; nickel hydroxycarbonate | $2NiCO_3.3Ni(OH)_2$ | +2 |
| Nickel acetate | 373-02-4 (17593-69-0) | Acetic acid, nickel (2+) salt; nickel (II) acetate; nickel (2+) acetate; nickel diacetate; nickelous acetate | $Ni(OCOCH_3)_2$ | +2 |
| Nickel acetate tetrahydrate | 6018-89-9 | Acetic acid, nickel (+2) salt, tetrahydrate | $Ni(OCOCH_3)_2.4H_2O$ | +2 |
| Nickel ammonium sulfates | 15699-18-0 | Ammonium nickel sulfate $((NH_4)_2Ni(SO_4)_2)$; nickel ammonium sulfate $(Ni(NH_4)_2(SO_4)_2)$; sulfuric acid, ammonium nickel (2+) salt (2:2:1) | $Ni(NH_4)_2(SO_4)_2$ | +2 |
| Nickel ammonium sulfate hexahydrate | 25749-08-0 | Ammonium nickel sulfate $((NH_4)_2Ni_2(SO_4)_3)$; sulfuric acid, ammonium nickel (2+) salt (3:2:2) | $Ni_2(NH_4)_2(SO_4)_3$ | +2 |

**Table 1 (contd)**

| Chemical name | Chem. Abstr. Serv. Reg. Number[a] | Synonyms and trade names | Formula | Oxi-dation state[b] |
|---|---|---|---|---|
| | 7785-20-8 (51287-85-5, 55526-16-4) | Ammonium nickel (2+) sulfate hexahydrate; ammonium nickel sulfate ((NH$_4$)$_2$Ni(SO$_4$)$_2$); diammonium nickel disulfate hexahydrate; diammonium nickel (2+) disulfate hexahydrate; diammonium nickel (II) disulfate hexahydrate; nickel ammonium sulfate (Ni(NH$_4$)$_2$(SO$_4$)$_2$) hexahydrate; nickel diammonium disulfate hexahydrate; **sulfuric acid, ammonium nickel (2+) salt (2:2:1), hexahydrate** | Ni(NH$_4$)$_2$(SO$_4$)$_2$. 6H$_2$O | +2 |
| Nickel chromate | 14721-18-7 | **Chromium nickel oxide (NiCrO$_4$); nickel chromate (NiCrO$_4$); nickel chromium oxide (NiCrO$_4$)** | NiCrO$_4$ | +2 |
| Nickel chloride | 7718-54-9 (37211-05-5) | Nickel (II) chloride; nickel (2+) chloride; **nickel chloride (NiCl$_2$);** nickel dichloride; nickel dichloride (NiCl$_2$); nickelous chloride | NiCl$_2$ | +2 |
| Nickel chloride hexahydrate | 7791-20-0 | **Nickel chloride (NiCl$_2$) hexahydrate** | NiCl$_2$.6H$_2$O | +2 |
| Nickel nitrate hexahydrate | 13478-00-7 | Nickel (2+) bis(nitrate)hexahydrate; nickel dinitrate hexahydrate; nickel (II) nitrate hexahydrate; nickel nitrate (Ni(NO$_3$)$_2$) hexahydrate; nickelous nitrate hexahydrate; **nitric acid, nickel (2+) salt, hexahydrate** | Ni(NO$_3$)$_2$.6H$_2$O | +2 |
| Nickel sulfate | 7786-81-4 | Nickel monosulfate; nickelous sulfate; nickel sulfate (1:1); nickel (II) sulfate; nickel (2+) sulfate; nickel (2+) sulfate (1:1); nickel sulfate (NiSO$_4$); **sulfuric acid, nickel (2+) salt (1:1)** | NiSO$_4$ | +2 |
| Nickel sulfate hexahydrate | 10101-97-0 | **Sulfuric acid, nickel (2+) salt (1:1), hexahydrate** | NiSO$_4$.6H$_2$O | +2 |
| Nickel sulfate heptahydrate | 10101-98-1 | **Sulfuric acid, nickel (2+) salt (1:1), heptahydrate** | NiSO$_4$.7H$_2$O | +2 |
| **Other nickel compounds** | | | | |
| Nickel carbonyl | 13463-39-3 (13005-31-7, 14875-95-7, 36252-60-5, 42126-46-5, 71327-12-3) | **Nickel carbonyl (Ni(CO)$_4$), (T-4)-;** nickel tetracarbonyl; tetracarbonylnickel; tetracarbonylnickel (0) | Ni(CO)$_4$ | 0 |

## Table 1 (contd)

| Chemical name | Chem. Abstr. Serv. Reg. Number[a] | Synonyms and trade names | Formula | Oxidation state[b] |
|---|---|---|---|---|
| Nickel antimonide | 12035-52-8 (73482-18-5) | **Antimony compound with nickel (1:1);** nickel antimonide (NiSb); nickel compound with antimony (1:1); nickel monoantimonide | NiSb | NS |
| | 12125-61-0 | **Breithauptite (SbNi)** | NiSb | NS |
| Nickel arsenides | 27016-75-7 (12068-59-6 24440-79-7) | **Nickel arsenide (NiAs)** | NiAs | NS |
| | 1303-13-5 (23292-74-2) | Nickeline; **nickeline (NiAs)**; nicolite | NiAs | NS |
| | 12256-33-6 | **Nickel arsenide ($Ni_{11}As_8$); nickel arsenide** tetragonal | $Ni_{11}As_8$ | NS |
| | 12044-65-4 | **Maucherite ($Ni_{11}As_8$); Placodine; Temiskamite** | $Ni_{11}As_8$ | NS |
| | 12255-80-0 | **Nickel arsenide ($Ni_5As_2$); nickel arsenide** hexagonal | $Ni_5As_2$ | NS |
| Nickel selenide | 1314-05-2 | Nickel monoselenide; **nickel selenide (NiSe)** | NiSe | NS |
| | 12201-85-3 | Maekinenite; **Makinenite (NiSe)** | NiSe | NS |
| Nickel subselenide | 12137-13-2 | **Nickel selenide ($Ni_3Se_2$)** | $Ni_3Se_2$ | NS |
| Nickel sulfarsenide | 12255-10-6 | **Nickel arsenide sulfide (NiAsS)** | NiAsS | NS |
| | 12255-11-7 | **Gersdorffite (NiAsS)** | NiAsS | NS |
| Nickel telluride | 12142-88-0 | Nickel monotelluride; **nickel telluride (NiTe)** | NiTe | NS |
| | 24270-51-7 | **Imgreite (NiTe)** | NiTe | NS |
| Nickel titanate | 12035-39-1 | Nickel titanate(IV); nickel titanate ($NiTiO_3$); **nickel titanium oxide ($NiTiO_3$);** nickel titanium trioxide | $NiTiO_3$ | +2 |
| Chrome iron nickel black spinel | 71631-15-7 | CI 77504; **CI Pigment Black 30;** DCMA-13-50-9; nickel iron chromite black spinel | $(Ni,Fe)(CrFe)_2O_4$ | NS |

**Table 1 (contd)**

| Chemical name | Chem. Abstr. Serv. Reg. Number[a] | Synonyms and trade names | Formula | Oxidation state[b] |
|---|---|---|---|---|
| Nickel ferrite brown spinel | 68187-10-0 | CI Pigment Brown 34; DCMA-13-35-7 | NiFe$_2$O$_4$ | NS |
| Nickelocene | 1271-28-9 (51269-44-4) | Bis($\eta$5-2,4-cyclopentadien-1-yl)nickel; di-$\pi$-cyclopentadienylnickel; dicyclopentadienylnickel; nickel, bis($\eta$5-2,4-cyclopentadien-1-yl)-; nickel, di-$\pi$-cyclopentadienyl- | $\pi$-(C$_5$H$_5$)$_2$Ni | +2 |

[a]Replaced CAS Registry numbers are given in parentheses.

[b]NS, not specified; mixed formal oxidation states of nickel and/or complex coordination in the solid form

[c]Chemical Abstracts Service Registry lists hundreds of these compounds; some typical examples are given.

[d]In commercial usage, 'black nickel oxide' usually refers to the low-temperature crystalline form of nickel monoxide, but nickel trioxide (Ni$_2$O$_3$), an unstable oxide of nickel, may also be called 'black nickel oxide'.

## 1.2 Chemical and physical properties of the pure substance

Known physical properties of some of the nickel compounds considered in this monograph are given in Table 2. Data on solubility refer to saturated solutions of the compound in water or other specified solvents. Nickel compounds are sometimes classed as soluble or insoluble in water; such a classification can be useful in technical applications of the various compounds but may not be relevant to determining their biological activity. Water-soluble nickel compounds include nickel chloride (642 g/l at 20°C) and nickel sulfate (293 g/l at 20°C), while nickel monosulfide (3.6 mg/l at 18°C) and nickel carbonate (93 mg/l at 25°C) are classed as insoluble (Weast, 1986). Compounds with solubilities towards the middle of this range are not easily classified in this way. Different forms of nominally the same nickel compound can have very different solubilities in a given solvent, and particle size, hydration and crystallinity can markedly affect the rate of dissolution. For example, anhydrous nickel sulfate and the hexahydrate are similarly soluble in unbuffered water (Grandjean, 1986), but the hexahydrate dissolves several orders of magnitude faster than the anhydrate.

**Table 2. Physical properties of nickel and nickel compounds[a]**

| Chemical name | Atomic/molecular weight | Melting-point (°C) | Boiling-point (°C) | Typical physical description | Solubility |
|---|---|---|---|---|---|
| **Metallic nickel and nickel alloys** | | | | | |
| Nickel | 58.69 | 1455 | 2730 | Lustrous white, hard ferromagnetic metal[b] or grey powder | Soluble in dilute nitric acid; slightly soluble in hydrochloric and sulfuric acids; insoluble in cold or hot water |
| Ferronickel alloy | – | – | – | Grey solid[c] | Combined properties of metallic iron and nickel, ammonia and alkali hydroxides |
| **Nickel oxides and hydroxides** | | | | | |
| Nickel hydroxide | 92.70 | 230 | – | Green crystals or amorphous solid | Nearly insoluble (0.13 g/l)[d] in cold water; soluble in acid, ammonium hydroxide |
| Nickel monoxide | 74.69 | 1984 | – | Grey, black or green[c] powder | Insoluble in water (0.0011 g/l at 20°C); soluble in acid, ammonium hydroxide[d] |
| **Nickel sulfides** | | | | | |
| Nickel disulfide | 122.81 | Decomposes at 400[d] | – | Black crystals[c] or powder | Insoluble in water[d] |
| **Nickel sulfide** | | | | | |
| Amorphous | 90.75 | 797 | – | Black crystals or powder | Nearly insoluble (0.0036 g/l, β-form)[d] in water at 18°C; soluble in aqua regia, nitric acid, potassium hydrosulfide; slightly soluble in acids |
| α–form | 90.75 | – | – | – | |
| β–form | 90.75 | – | – | Dark-green crystals[c] | |
| Nickel subsulfide (α–form) | 240.19 | 790 | – | Lustrous pale-yellowish or bronze metallic crystals | Insoluble in cold water; soluble in nitric acid |

# Table 2 (contd)

| Chemical name | Atomic/molecular weight | Melting-point (°C) | Boiling-point (°C) | Typical physical description | Solubility |
|---|---|---|---|---|---|
| **Nickel salts** | | | | | |
| Nickel acetate | 176.78 | Decomposes | 16.6 | Dull-green crystals | Soluble in water (166 g/l at 20°C)[d]; insoluble in ethanol |
| Nickel acetate tetrahydrate | 248.84 | Decomposes | 16 | Dull-green crystals | Soluble in water (160 g/l at 20°C)[d]; soluble in dilute ethanol |
| **Nickel ammonium sulfates** | | | | | |
| Hexahydrate | 394.94 | - | - | - | Soluble in water (104 g/l at 20°C)[d] |
| Anhydrous | 286.88 | Decomposes[e] | - | Green crystals[e] | Soluble in water (300 g/l at 20°C)[d]; less soluble in ammonium sulfate solution; insoluble in ethanol[e] |
| Nickel carbonate | 118.70 | Decomposes | - | Light-green crystals | Nearly insoluble (0.093 g/l) in water at 25°C; insoluble in hot water, soluble in acids |
| Nickel hydroxycarbonate | 587.67 | Decomposes | - | Light-green crystals or brown powder[e] or wet green paste | Insoluble in cold water; decomposes in hot water; soluble in acids |
| **Nickel chlorides** | | | | | |
| Anhydrous | 129.60 | 1001 | Sublimes at 973 | Yellow deliquescent scales | Soluble in water at 20°C (642 g/l) and at 100°C (876 g/l); soluble in ethanol, ammonium hydroxide; insoluble in nitric acid |
| Hexahydrate | 237.70 | - | - | Green deliquescent crystals | Soluble in water (2540 g/l at 20°C)[d]; very soluble in ethanol |
| Nickel chromate | 174.71 | - | - | Black crystals | Insoluble in water |

**Table 2 (contd)**

| Chemical name | Atomic/molecular weight | Melting-point (°C) | Boiling-point (°C) | Typical physical description | Solubility |
|---|---|---|---|---|---|
| Nickel nitrate hexa-hydrate | 290.79 | 56.7 | Decom-poses at 136.7 | Green deliquescent crystals | Soluble in water (2385 g/l at 0°C), am-monium hydroxide and ethanol |
| **Nickel sulfates** | | | | | |
| Anhydrous | 154.75 | Decom-poses at 848 | – | Pale–green to yellow crystals | Soluble in water (293 g/l at 20°C); insol-uble in ethanol and diethyl ether[d,e] |
| Hexahydrate | 262.84 | 53.3 | – | Blue or emerald–green crystals[e] | Soluble in water (625 g/l at 0°C); solu-ble in ethanol[d] |
| Heptahydrate | 280.85 | 99 | – | Green crystals | Soluble in water (756 g/l at 20°C); solu-ble in ethanol[d] |
| **Other nickel compounds** | | | | | |
| Nickel antimonide | 180.44 | 1158 | Decom-poses at 1400 | Light–copper to mauve crystals[c] | Insoluble in water[d] |
| Nickel arsenides NiAs | 133.61 | 968 | – | Grey crystals[c] | Insoluble in hot or cold water, soluble in aqua regia |
| Ni₁₁As₈ | 1244.96 | 1000 | – | Platinum–grey crystals | Insoluble in water[d] |
| Ni₅As₂ | 443.39 | 993 | – | Grey crystals[c] | Insoluble in water[d] |
| Nickel carbonyl | 170.73 | –25 | 43 | Colourless to yellow liquid | Nearly insoluble (0.18 g/l) in water at 9.8°C; soluble in aqua regia, ethanol, diethyl ether, benzene, nitric acid; insol-uble in dilute acids or dilute alkali |

**Table 2 (contd)**

| Chemical name | Atomic/ molecular weight | Melting–point (°C) | Boiling–point (°C) | Typical physical description | Solubility |
|---|---|---|---|---|---|
| Nickelocene | 188.88 | 171–173[e] | – | Dark–green crystals[e] | Soluble in most organic solvents; insoluble in water; decomposes in acetone, ethanol, diethyl ether |
| Nickel selenide (NiSe) | 137.65 | Red heat | – | White or grey crystals | Insoluble in water and hydrochloric acid; soluble in aqua regia, nitric acid |
| Nickel subselenide (Ni$_3$Se$_2$) | 333.99 | – | – | Green crystals[c] | Insoluble in water[d] |
| Nickel telluride | 186.29 | Decomposes at 600–900[d] | – | Grey crystals[c] | Insoluble in water; soluble in nitric acid, aqua regia, bromine water[d] |
| Nickel titanate | 154.57 | Decomposes at 1000 | – | Yellow crystals[c] | Insoluble in water[d] |

[a]From Weast (1986), unless otherwise specified; –, depending on composition
[b]From Windholz (1983)
[c]From Sunderman (1984)
[d]From Grandjean (1986)
[e]From Sax & Lewis (1987)

## 1.3  Technical products and impurities

This section does not include nickel-containing intermediates and by-products specific to nickel production and use, which are considered in section 2.

### (a)  Metallic nickel and nickel alloys

*Ferronickel* contains 20-50% nickel (Sibley, 1985). Other components include carbon (1.5-1.8%), sulfur (<0.3%), cobalt (<2%), silicon (1.8-4%), chromium (1.2-1.8%) and iron (balance of alloy). It is delivered as ingots or granules (ERAMET-SLN, 1986).

Pure unwrought *nickel* is available commercially in the form of cathodes, powder, briquets, pellets, rondelles, ingots and shot. Its chemical composition is >99% nickel, with carbon, copper, iron, sulfur and oxygen as impurities (Sibley, 1985). Metallic nickel undergoes surface oxidation in air; oxidation of finely divided nickel powder can result in the conversion of a large fraction of the metal to oxide upon prolonged storage (Cotton & Wilkinson, 1988).

*Nickel-aluminium alloy* (for the production of Raney nickel) is available as European Pharmacopoeia grade with the following typical analysis: nickel, 48-52%; aluminium, 48-52%; and chloride, 0.001% (Riedel-de Haën, 1986).

*Nickel alloys* can be categorized as nickel-chromium, nickel-chromium-cobalt, iron-nickel-chromium and copper-nickel alloys. Typical analyses are given in Table 3. Austenitic steels are the major group of *nickel-containing steels*. Typical compositions are given in Table 4.

### (b)  Nickel oxides and hydroxides

The temperature of formation of *nickel oxide* (up to 1045°C) determines the colour of the crystal (jet-black to apple green), the crystalline surface area and the nickel [III] content (<0.03-0.81% by weight). The temperature of formation may also affect the crystalline structure and the incidence of defects within it (Sunderman *et al.*, 1987; Benson *et al.*, 1988a).

*Nickel monoxides* are available commercially in different forms as laboratory reagents and as industrial products. Laboratory reagents are either green powder (Aldrich Chemical Co., Inc., 1988) or black powders; industrial products are either black powders, coarse particles (Sinter 75) or grey sintered rondelles (INCO, 1988; Queensland Nickel Sales Pty Ltd, 1989). Sinter 75 (76% Ni) contains about 22% oxygen and small amounts of copper (0.75%), iron (0.3%), sulfur (0.006%) and cobalt (1.0%) (Sibley, 1985). Sintered rondels (≥85% Ni) are formed by partially reducing a cylindrical pressing of granular nickel oxide to nickel metal. The degree of reduction achieved determines the nickel content of the finished rondel (Queensland Nickel Sales Pty Ltd, 1989).

Table 3. Elemental analyses of representative nickel alloys (weight %)[a]

| Alloy | Ni | Cu | Cr | Co | Fe | Mo | W | Ta | Nb | Al | Ti | Mn | Si | C | Zr |
|---|---|---|---|---|---|---|---|---|---|---|---|---|---|---|---|
| **Nickel–chromium** | | | | | | | | | | | | | | | |
| Cast alloy 625 | 63.0 | – | 21.6 | – | 2.0 | 8.7 | – | – | 3.9 | 0.2 | 0.2 | 0.06 | 0.20 | 0.20 | – |
| Hastelloy alloy X | 47.0 | – | 22.0 | 1.5 | 18.5 | 9.0 | 0.6 | – | – | – | – | 0.50 | 0.50 | 0.10 | – |
| Inconel alloy 617 | 54.0 | – | 22.0 | 12.5 | – | 9.0 | – | – | – | 1.0 | – | – | – | 0.07 | – |
| **Nickel–chromium–cobalt** | | | | | | | | | | | | | | | |
| Haynes Alloy 1002 | 16.0 | – | 22.0 | Bal | 1.5 | – | 7.0 | 3.8 | – | 0.3 | 0.2 | 0.70 | 0.40 | 0.60 | 0.30 |
| Haynes Alloy No. 188 | 22.0 | – | 22.0 | 39.0 | 3.0 max | – | 14.0 | – | – | – | – | 1.25 max | 0.40 | 0.10 | – |
| **Nickel–iron–chromium** | | | | | | | | | | | | | | | |
| Haynes Alloy 556 | 20.0 | – | 22.0 | 20.0 | 29.0 | 3.0 | 2.5 | 0.9 | 0.1 | 0.3 | – | 1.50 | 0.40 | 0.10 | – |
| Incoloy Alloy 800[b] | 32.5 | – | 21.0 | – | 46.0 | – | – | – | – | 0.4 | 0.4 | 0.80 | 0.50 | 0.05 | – |
| **Nickel–copper** | | | | | | | | | | | | | | | |
| Monel alloy 400[b] | 66.5 | 31.5 | – | – | 1.3 | – | – | – | – | – | – | 1.0 | 0.25 | 0.15 | – |
| Monel alloy K–500[b] | 65.0 | 29.5 | – | – | 1.0 | – | – | – | – | 2.8 | 0.5 | 0.6 | 0.15 | 0.15 | – |

[a]From Nickel Development Institute (1987a); Bal, balance
[b]From Tien & Howson (1981)

**Table 4. Typical composition of nickel-containing steels (weight %)[a]**

| Grade | Cr | Ni | Mn | Mo | C | Si | S | P | Fe |
|---|---|---|---|---|---|---|---|---|---|
| AISI-201 | 16-18 | 3.5-5.5 | 5.5-7.5 | - | 0.15 | 1.0 | 0.03 | 0.06 | Balance |
| AISI-302 | 17-19 | 8.0-10.0 | 2.0 | - | 0.15 | 1.0 | 0.03 | 0.045 | Balance |
| AISI-304 | 18-20 | 8.0-10.5 | 2.0 | - | 0.08 | 1.0 | 0.03 | 0.045 | Balance |
| AISI-316 | 16-18 | 10-14 | 2.0 | 2-3 | 0.08 | 1.0 | 0.03 | 0.045 | Balance |

[a]From Nickel Development Institute (1987b); AISI, American Iron and Steel Institute

*Nickel hydroxide* is commercially available at 97% purity (Aldrich Chemical Co., Inc., 1988).

### (c)  Nickel sulfides

*Nickel sulfide* exists in three forms: the high-temperature, hexagonal crystal form, in which each nickel atom is octahedrally coordinated to six sulfur atoms; the low-temperature, rhombohedral form (which occurs naturally as millerite), in which each nickel atom is coordinated to two other nickel atoms and five sulfur atoms (Grice & Ferguson, 1974); and amorphous nickel sulfide. Amorphous nickel sulfide is gradually converted to nickel hydroxy sulfide on contact with air (Cotton & Wilkinson, 1988). Grice and Ferguson (1974) referred to the rhombohedral (millerite) form as β-nickel sulfide and the high-temperature hexagonal form as α-nickel sulfide. Different nomenclatures have been used by other authors (Abbracchio *et al.*, 1981; Grandjean, 1986). The term β-nickel sulfide is used to denote the rhombohedral millerite form throughout this monograph.

*Nickel subsulfide* exists in two forms: α-nickel subsulfide, the low-temperature, rhombohedral form (heazlewoodite), in which nickel atoms exist in distorted tetrahedral coordination and the sulfur atoms form an almost cubic body-centred sublattice, with six equidistant nickel neighbours; and β-nickel subsulfide, the high-temperature form (Sunderman & Maenza, 1976).

An examination of the surface of crystalline and amorphous nickel sulfide particles revealed that crystalline particles have a net negative surface charge, while the surface charge of amorphous nickel sulfide appears to be positive. X-Ray photoelectron spectroscopy analysis of amorphous and crystalline nickel sulfide showed that the outermost surface of the two compounds differed with respect to the Ni/S ratio and the sulfur oxidation state (Abbracchio *et al.*, 1981).

Nickel sulfides are intermediates in nickel smelting and refining which can be isolated as crude mattes for further processing but are not significant materials of commerce. Most nickel subsulfide is produced as an intermediate in many nickel refining processes (Boldt & Queneau, 1967).

(d)   *Nickel salts*

*Nickel acetate* is available as the tetrahydrate at a purity of > 97% (Mallinckrodt, Inc., 1987).

*Nickel ammonium sulfate* hexahydrate is available as analytical reagent-grade crystals at a purity of 99.0% min or at a grade for nickel plating (purity, 99-100%; Riedel-de-Haën, 1986).

*Nickel carbonate* is available mainly as hydroxycarbonates, such as basic nickel carbonate. Laboratory reagent grades may contain 47.5% or 45% nickel; industrial grades, as green powders or wet pastes, contain approximately 45% nickel (INCO, 1981-82; Pharmacie Centrale, 1988).

*Nickel chloride* is available as the hexahydrate as a laboratory reagent of > 99% purity and as industrial products with about 24.7% nickel. It is also available in industrial quantities as an aqueous solution (ERAMET-SLN, 1985).

*Nickel nitrate* is available as the hexahydrate at > 99% purity and as crystals and flakes (J.T. Baker, 1988).

*Nickel sulfate* is available as the heptahydrate at > 99% purity and as the hexahydrate at 99% purity (Aldrich Chemical Co., Inc., 1988).

(e)   *Other nickel compounds*

*Nickelocene* is available in solid form at > 90% purity or as an 8-10% solution in toluene (American Tokyo Kasei, 1988).

# 2.  Production, Use, Occurrence and Analysis

## 2.1  Production

Nickel was first isolated in 1751 by a Swedish chemist, Cronstedt, from an arsenosulfide ore (Considine, 1974).

(a)   *Metallic nickel and nickel alloys*

Table 5 gives world mine production of nickel by region. Table 6 shows world nickel plant production, including refined nickel, ferronickel and nickel recycled from scrap (Chamberlain, 1988).

Various combinations of pyrometallurgical, hydrometallurgical and vapometallurgical operations are used in the nickel producing industry (Boldt & Queneau, 1967; Evans *et al.*, 1979; Tien & Howsen, 1981; Tyroler & Landolt, 1988). The description that follows is a generalized discussion of some of the more common smelting and refining processes.

**Table 5. World mine production of nickel, by region (thousand tonnes)[a]**

| Region | 1982 | 1983 | 1984 | 1985 | 1986 |
|---|---|---|---|---|---|
| Albania | 6.0 | 7.2 | 9.2 | 9.6 | 9.7 |
| Australia | 87.7 | 76.6 | 77.1 | 85.8 | 69.9 |
| Botswana | 17.8 | 18.2 | 18.6 | 19.6 | 20.0 |
| Brazil | 14.5 | 15.6 | 23.6 | 20.3 | 23.1 |
| Burma | 0.02 | 0.02 | 0.02 | 0.02 | 0.02 |
| Canada | 88.7 | 128.1 | 174.2 | 170.0 | 181.0 |
| China | 12.0 | 13.0 | 14.0 | 25.1 | 25.5 |
| Colombia | 1.8 | 17.5 | 21.9 | 15.5 | 22.1 |
| Cuba | 36.2 | 37.7 | 31.8 | 32.4 | 32.7 |
| Dominican Republic | 5.4 | 19.6 | 24.0 | 25.4 | 22.1 |
| Finland | 6.3 | 5.3 | 6.9 | 7.9 | 6.5 |
| France (New Caledonia) | 60.2 | 46.2 | 58.3 | 73.0 | 65.1 |
| German Democratic Republic | 2.5 | 2.2 | 2.0 | 1.6 | 1.5 |
| Greece | 5.0 | 16.8 | 16.7 | 18.7 | 17.5 |
| Indonesia | 46.0 | 49.4 | 47.6 | 40.6 | 43.9 |
| Morocco | 0.13 | -- | -- | -- | -- |
| Norway | 0.39 | 0.36 | 0.33 | 0.44 | 0.40 |
| Philippines | 19.7 | 13.9 | 13.6 | 28.2 | 13.6 |
| Poland | 2.1 | 2.1 | 2.1 | 2.0 | 2.0 |
| South Africa | 22.0 | 20.5 | 25.1 | 25.1 | 25.1 |
| USA | 2.9 | -- | 13.2 | 5.6 | 1.1 |
| USSR | 165.1 | 170.0 | 174.2 | 180.0 | 186.0 |
| Yugoslavia | 4.0 | 3.0 | 4.0 | 5.0 | 5.0 |
| Zimbabwe | 15.8 | 12.0 | 12.2 | 11.1 | 11.0 |
| Total | 622.24 | 675.28 | 770.65 | 802.96 | 784.82 |

[a]From Chamberlain (1988)

**Table 6. World production of processed nickel by region (thousands of tonnes)[a]**

| Region | 1982 | 1983 | 1984 | 1985 | 1986 |
|---|---|---|---|---|---|
| Australia | 45.9 | 41.8 | 38.7 | 40.9 | 41.9 |
| Brazil | 3.5 | 8.3 | 9.2 | 13.3 | 13.5 |
| Canada | 58.6 | 87.2 | 104.0 | 100.0 | 115.0 |
| China | 12.0 | 13.0 | 14.0 | 22.5 | 22.5 |
| Colombia | 1.3 | 13.1 | 17.1 | 11.8 | 18.6 |
| Cuba | 9.0 | 9.3 | 8.5 | 8.5 | 7.7 |
| Czechoslovakia | 1.5 | 3.0 | 4.5 | 4.5 | 4.5 |
| Dominican Republic | 5.3 | 21.2 | 24.2 | 25.8 | 22.0 |

**Table 6 (contd)**

| Region | 1982 | 1983 | 1984 | 1985 | 1986 |
|---|---|---|---|---|---|
| Finland | 12.6 | 14.8 | 15.3 | 15.7 | 16.0 |
| France | 7.4 | 4.9 | 5.2 | 7.1 | 10.0 |
| France (New Caledonia) | 28.0 | 21.7 | 29.2 | 36.1 | 33.0 |
| German Democratic Republic | 3.0 | 3.0 | 3.0 | 3.0 | 3.0 |
| Germany, Federal Republic of | 1.2 | 1.2 | 1.0 | 0.7 | - |
| Greece | 4.5 | 12.9 | 15.8 | 16.0 | 12.0 |
| Indonesia | 5.0 | 4.9 | 4.8 | 4.8 | 5.0 |
| Japan | 90.6 | 82.2 | 89.3 | 92.7 | 88.8 |
| Norway | 25.8 | 28.6 | 35.6 | 37.5 | 38.2 |
| Philippines | 11.2 | 6.1 | 3.5 | 17.0 | 2.1 |
| Poland | 2.1 | 2.1 | 2.1 | 2.1 | 2.1 |
| South Africa | 14.4 | 17.0 | 20.5 | 20.0 | 20.0 |
| UK | 7.4 | 23.2 | 23.3 | 17.8 | 31.0 |
| USA | 40.8 | 30.3 | 40.8 | 33.0 | 1.5 |
| USSR | 180.0 | 185.1 | 191.4 | 198.0 | 215.0 |
| Yugoslavia | 1.5 | 1.5 | 2.0 | 3.0 | 3.0 |
| Zimbabwe | 13.3 | 10.2 | 10.3 | 9.4 | 9.8 |
| Total | 585.9 | 646.6 | 713.3 | 741.2 | 736.2 |

ªFrom Chamberlain (1988)

Nickel is produced from two kinds of ore: sulfide and silicate-oxide. The latter occurs in tropical regions, such as New Caledonia, and in regions that used to be tropical, such as Oregon (USA). Both types of ore generally contain no more than 3% nickel (Warner, 1984). Mining is practised by open pit and underground methods for sulfide ores and by open pit for silicate-oxide ores. Sulfide ores are extracted by flotation and magnetic separation into concentrates containing nickel and various amounts of copper and other metals, such as cobalt, precious metals and iron. Silicate-oxide ores are extracted by chemical means.

The extractive metallurgy of sulfide nickel ores (see Fig. 1) is practised in a large variety of processes. Most of these processes begin with oxidation of iron and sulfur at high temperatures in multiple hearth roasters or in fluid bed roasters, or, in the early days, in linear calciners or on travelling grate sinter machines ('sintering'). The roaster calcine is smelted in reverberatory or electric furnaces to remove rock and oxidized iron as a slag, leaving a ferrous nickel (copper) matte. In modern processes, both operations — roasting and smelting — are combined in a single operation called 'flash smelting'. The furnace matte is upgraded by oxidizing and slagging most of the remaining iron in converters. If the converter matte or 'Bessemer matte' contains copper, the matte can be separated into nickel subsulfide, copper sulfide

## Fig. 1. Extraction and refining of nickel and its compounds from sulfides ores[a]

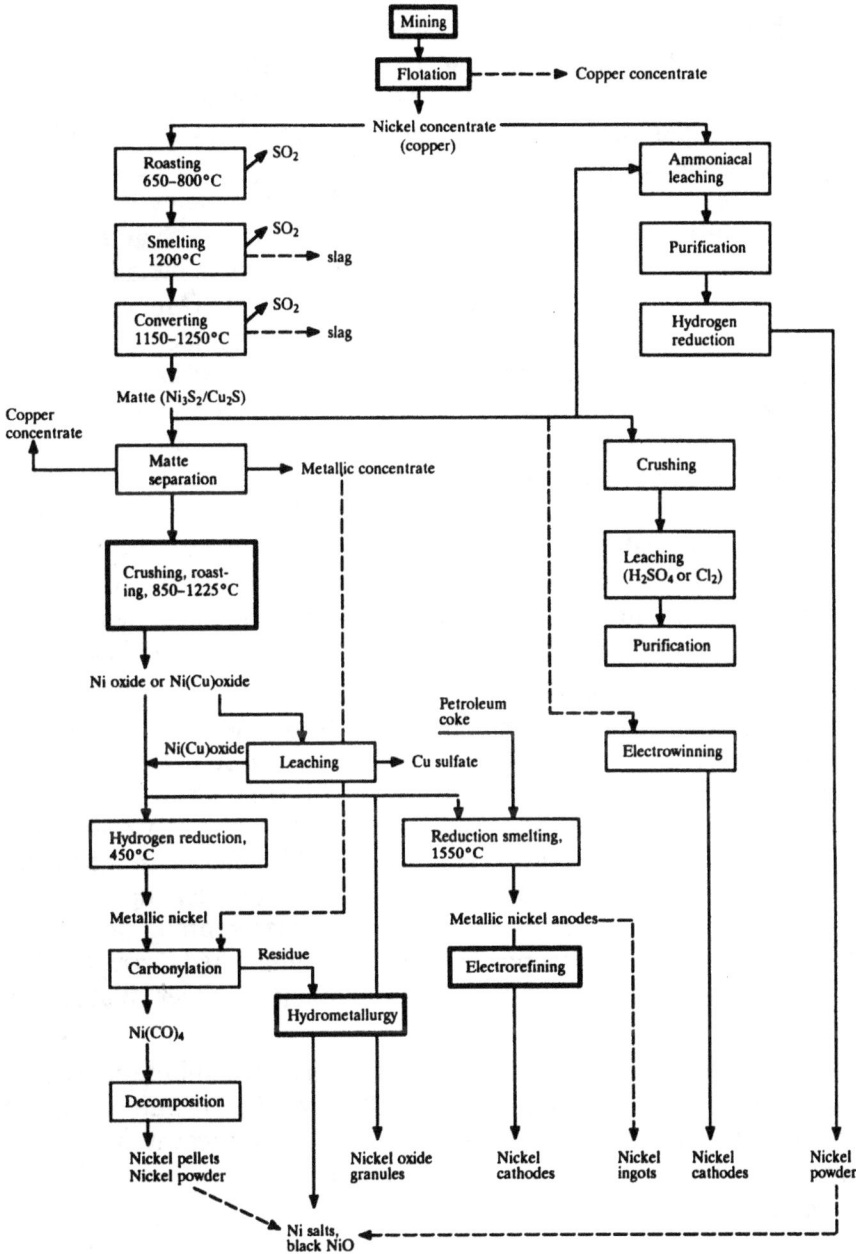

[a]Modified from Mastromatteo (1986)

and metallic concentrates by a slow cooling process followed by magnetic concentration and froth flotation.

The high-grade nickel subsulfide concentrate is then refined by various processes. Most of them begin with roasting of the concentrate to a crude nickel oxide. When the copper content is low, this crude oxide is directly saleable ('Sinter 75'). In older processes, copper was leached directly from the crude oxide with sulfuric acid (as in Clydach, Wales) or by an acidic anolyte from copper electrowinning (as in Kristiansand, Norway). Refining can be pursued after reducing the crude nickel oxide to metal either in a rotary kiln or in an electric furnace with addition of a carbonaceous reductant. In the first case, the crude particulate metallic nickel is refined by the atmospheric pressure nickel-carbonyl process (Mond carbonyl process) which allows a clear-cut separation of nickel from other metals. Nickel is then produced either as nickel powder or as nickel pellets. The carbonylation residue is further processed to recover precious metals and some nickel and cobalt salts. In the second case, the molten crude nickel is cast into anodes which are 'electrorefined'. The anolyte is purified outside the electrolytic cell by removal of the main impurities, which are iron, arsenic, copper and cobalt. These impurities are generally extracted as filter cakes containing significant amounts of nickel, warranting recycling upstream in the process. Nickel is then produced in the form of electrolytic cathodes or small 'rounds'. This electrorefining process, which was used in Kristiansand, Norway, and Port Colborne, Ontario, is no longer practised there.

The Bessemer nickel (copper) matte can also be refined without roasting, either by a combination of hydrometallurgy and electrolysis ('electrowinning') or by hydrometallurgy alone. There are three types of nickel 'electrowinning' processes: (i) directly from matte cast into (soluble) anodes; (ii) from nickel sulfate solutions obtained by leaching matte with a very low sulfur content; and (iii) from nickel chloride solutions obtained by leaching matte with chloride solution in the presence of chlorine gas. In the three cases, the solutions obtained by dissolving the matte must be purified before plating pure nickel, as for the electrorefining process. In the chloride-electrowinning process, purification is accomplished through solvent extraction methods using tributylphosphate and aliphatic amines diluted in petroleum extracts.

Complete hydrometallurgy can be practised directly on sulfide concentrates or on Bessemer matte by ammonia leaching in sulfate medium in autoclaves. The solution is purified by precipitation of sulfides, and nickel is recovered as metal powder by hydrogen precipitation in autoclaves. The nickel powder can be further sintered into briquettes.

Silicate-oxide ores ('garnierites'/'laterites') are processed either by pyrometallurgy or by hydrometallurgy (Fig. 2). Pyrometallurgy consists of drying, calcining in rotary kilns, then reduction/smelting in electric furnaces. The crude ferronickel

**Fig. 2. Extraction and refining of nickel and its compounds from silicate-oxide (laterite) ores**[a]

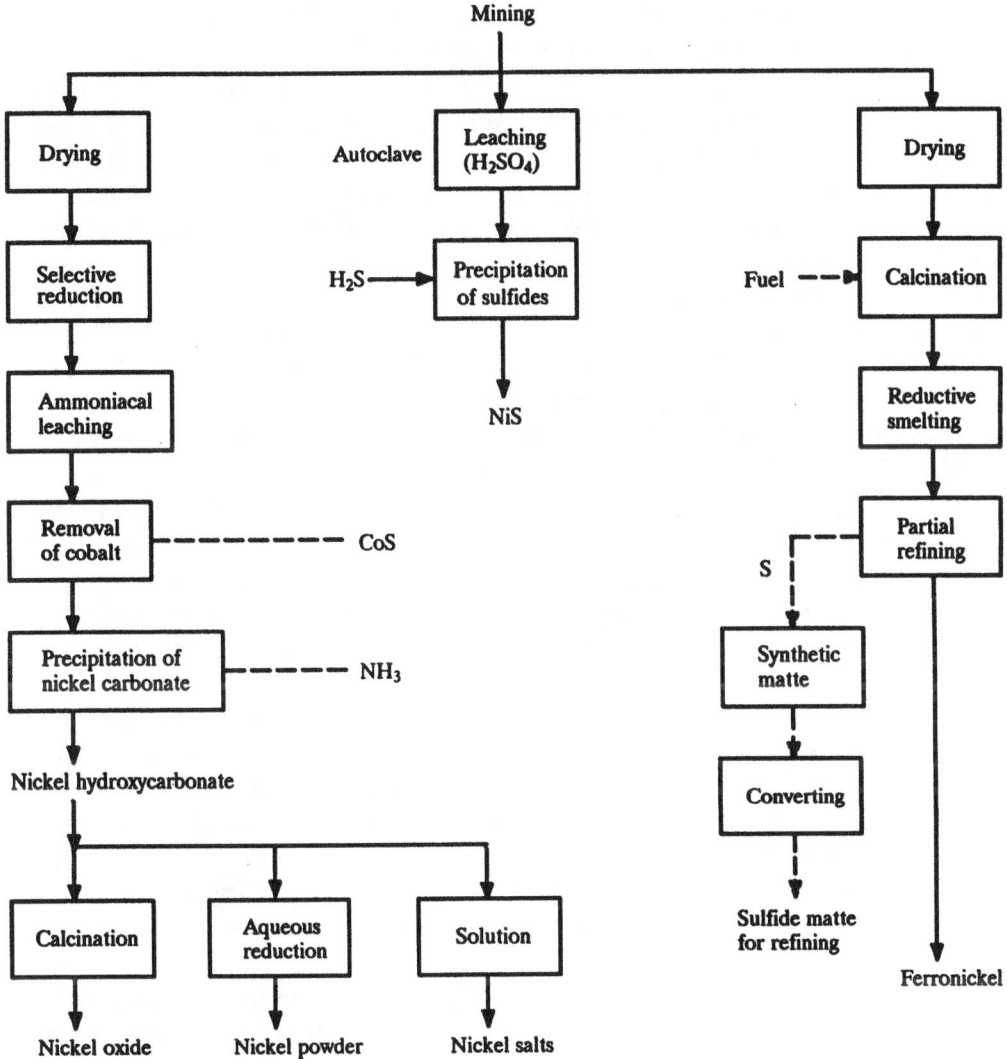

[a]Modified from Mastromatteo (1986)

obtained (containing 20-40% Ni) is partially refined by thermic processes (in ladles) before being cast into ingots or granulated in water. With pyrometallurgy, nickel matte can be produced from silicate-oxide ore either by smelting the ore in the presence of calcium sulfate in a blast furnace (old process) or in an electric furnace, or by direct injection of molten sulfur into molten ferronickel.

Hydrometallurgy of silicate-oxide ores, preferentially poor in silica and magnesia, is practised by ammoniacal leaching or by sulfuric acid leaching. Ammoniacal leaching is used for ore that is selectively reduced in rotary kilns by a mixture of hydrogen and carbon monoxide. Cobalt, the main dissolved impurity, is removed from solution by precipitation as cobalt monosulfide (containing nickel monosulfide). This by-product is further refined to separate and refine nickel and cobalt. The purified nickel stream is then transformed into the hydroxycarbonate by ammonia distillation. The hydroxycarbonate is then dried, calcined and partially reduced to a saleable nickel oxide sinter. Sulfuric acid leaching is conducted under pressure in autoclaves. Nickel and cobalt are extracted from the process liquor by precipitation with hydrogen sulfide, and the mixed nickel-cobalt (10:1) sulfide is further refined in one of the processes described above.

Nickel is obtained not only by recovery from nickel ores but also by recycling process or consumer scrap. Nickel scrap is generated in forming and shaping operations in fabricating plants where nickel-containing materials are used and is also recovered from obsolete consumer goods containing nickel. Small amounts of nickel are also produced as a coproduct of copper and platinum metal refining (Sibley, 1985).

*Nickel-containing steels* (stainless steels and others) are produced by melting cast iron and adding ferronickel and/or pure nickel or steel scraps in large electric furnaces. The melt is transferred to a refining vessel to adjust the carbon content and impurity levels and is then cast into ingots or continuously into casting shapes. Defects in cast steel are repaired by cutting or scarfing or by chipping or grinding. The desired shapes are produced by a variety of operations, including grinding, polishing and pickling (Warner, 1984). Production volumes of stainless-steel are given in Table 7.

The technology for the production of *nickel alloys* is very similar to that used for steel production, except that melting and decarburizing units are generally smaller, and greater use is made of vacuum melting and remelting (Warner, 1984). In western Europe, it was estimated that 15% of nickel consumption was in nonferrous nickel alloys (Eurométaux, 1986).

**Table 7. Stainless-steel[a] production (in thousands of tonnes) in selected regions[b]**

| Region | 1987 | 1988 |
|---|---|---|
| Austria | 54 | 67 |
| Belgium | 182 | 254 |
| Finland | 189 | 206 |
| France | 720 | 784 |
| Germany, Federal Republic of | 957 | 1186 |
| Italy | 550 | 623 |
| Spain | 327 | 426 |
| Sweden | 457 | 482 |
| United Kingdom | 393 | 427 |
| Yugoslavia | 30 | 30 |
| Total Europe | 3859 | 4485 |
| USA | 1840 | 1995 |
| Japan | 2722 | 3161 |
| Other countries | 787 | 798 |
| Total | 9208 | 10 439 |

[a]Stainless steels with and without nickel
[b]ERAMET-SLN (1989a)

### (b)   Nickel oxides and hydroxides

*Nickel oxide sinter* (a coarse, somewhat impure form of nickel monoxide) is manufactured by roasting a semipure nickel subsulfide at or above 1000°C or by decomposing nickel hydroxycarbonate. The sinters produced commercially contain either 76% nickel or, in partially reduced form, 90% nickel. Nickel oxide sinter is produced in Australia, Canada and Cuba (Sibley, 1985).

*Green nickel oxide*, a finely divided, relatively pure form of nickel monoxide, is produced by firing a mixture of nickel powder and water in air at 1000°C (Antonsen, 1981). Nickel monoxide is currently produced by two companies in the USA, six in Japan, two in the UK and one in the Federal Republic of Germany (Chemical Information Services Ltd, 1988).

*Black nickel oxide*, a finely divided, pure nickel monoxide, is produced by calcination of nickel hydroxycarbonate or nickel nitrate at 600°C (Antonsen, 1981). It is produced by one company each in Argentina, Brazil, Canada, Japan, Mexico, the UK and the USA (Chemical Information Services Ltd, 1988).

*Nickel hydroxide* is prepared by (1) treating a nickel sulfate solution with sodium hydroxide to yield a gelatinous nickel hydroxide which forms a fine precipitate when neutralized, (2) electrodeposition at an inert cathode using metallic nickel as the anode and nickel nitrate as the electrolyte, or (3) extraction with hot alcohol of the gelatinous precipitate formed by nickel nitrate solution and potassium hydroxide (Antonsen, 1981). Nickel hydroxide is currently produced by four companies in Japan, three in the USA and one each in the Federal Republic of Germany and the UK (Chemical Information Services Ltd, 1988).

### (c)  Nickel sulfides

Purified *nickel sulfide* can be prepared by (i) fusion of nickel powder with molten sulfur or (ii) precipitation using hydrogen sulfide treatment of a buffered solution of a nickel[II] salt (Antonsen, 1981).

*Nickel subsulfide* can be made by the direct fusion of nickel with sulfur. Impure nickel subsulfide is produced during the processing of furnace matte.

Nickel sulfide and nickel subsulfide are formed in large quantities as intermediates in the processing of sulfidic and silicate-oxide ores and are traded and transported in bulk quantities for further processing. No data on production volumes are available for any of the nickel sulfides.

### (d)  Nickel salts

*Nickel acetate* is produced by heating nickel hydroxide with acetic acid in the presence of metallic nickel (Sax & Lewis, 1987). This salt is currently produced by six companies in the USA, three each in Argentina, Brazil, Italy, Japan and the UK, two each in the Federal Republic of Germany and Mexico, and one each in Australia and Spain (Chemical Information Services Ltd, 1988).

An impure basic *nickel carbonate* (roughly $2NiCO_3.3Ni(OH)_2.4H_2O$) is obtained as a precipitate when sodium carbonate is added to a solution of a nickel salt. A pure nickel carbonate is prepared by oxidation of nickel powder in ammonia and carbon dioxide (Antonsen, 1981). Nickel carbonate is currently produced by six companies each in the USA and Japan, three each in India and the Federal Republic of Germany, two each in Argentina, France, Italy, Mexico and the UK, and one each in Belgium, Brazil, Canada, Spain and Switzerland (Chemical Information Services Ltd, 1988). Finland and Japan produce the largest volumes of nickel carbonate (ERAMET-SLN, 1989b).

*Nickel ammonium sulfate* is prepared by reacting nickel sulfate with ammonium sulfate and crystallizing the salt from a water solution (Antonsen, 1981; Sax & Lewis, 1987). Nickel ammonium sulfate (particular form unknown) is currently produced by three companies in the UK, two in the USA and one in Japan (Chemical Information Services, Ltd, 1988).

*Nickel chloride* (hexahydrate) is prepared by the reaction of nickel powder or nickel oxide with hot aqueous hydrochloric acid (Antonsen, 1981). It is currently produced by eight companies in the USA, six in India, four each in the Federal Republic of Germany, Japan and the UK, three in Mexico, two each in Brazil, France and Italy and one each in Spain, Switzerland and Taiwan (Chemical Information Services Ltd, 1988). The countries or regions that produce the largest volumes are: Czechoslovakia, Federal Republic of Germany, France, Japan, Taiwan, UK, USA and USSR (ERAMET-SLN, 1989b).

*Nickel nitrate* (anhydrous) can be prepared by the reaction of fuming nitric acid and nickel nitrate hexahydrate. The hexahydrate is prepared by reaction of dilute nitric acid and nickel carbonate (Antonsen, 1981). Nickel nitrate hexahydrate is manufactured on a commercial basis by three methods: (1) slowly adding nickel powder to a stirred mixture of nitric acid and water; (2) a two-tank reactor system, one with solid nickel and one with nitric acid and water; and (3) adding nitric acid to a mixture of black nickel oxide powder and hot water (Antonsen, 1981). Nickel nitrate is currently produced by six companies in the USA, four each in Brazil, Japan and the UK, two each in the Federal Republic of Germany, France, India, Italy and Spain and one each in Argentina, Australia, Belgium, Mexico and Switzerland (Chemical Information Services Ltd, 1988).

*Nickel sulfate* hexahydrate is made by adding nickel powder or black nickel oxide to hot dilute sulfuric acid or by the reaction of nickel carbonate and dilute sulfuric acid. Large-scale manufacture of the anhydrous form may be achieved by gas-phase reaction of nickel carbonyl with sulfur dioxide and oxygen at 100°C or in a closed-loop reactor that recovers the solid product in sulfuric acid (Antonsen, 1981).

Nickel sulfate hexa- and heptahydrates are currently produced by nine companies each in Japan and the USA, six in India, four each in Argentina, the Federal Republic of Germany, Mexico and the UK, three in Canada, two each in Austria, Belgium, Brazil and Italy, and one each in Australia, Czechoslovakia, Finland, the German Democratic Republic, Spain, Sweden, Switzerland, Taiwan and the USSR (Chemical Information Services Ltd, 1988). The countries or regions that produce nickel sulfate in the largest volumes are: Belgium, Czechoslovakia, the Federal Republic of Germany, Finland, Japan, Taiwan, the UK, the USA and the USSR (ERAMET-SLN, 1989b).

(e)   *Other nickel compounds*

*Nickel carbonyl* can be prepared by the Mond carbonyl process, described above for nickel. Two commercial processes are used to manufacture nickel carbonyl. In the UK, the pure compound is produced by an atmospheric method in which carbon monoxide is passed over freshly reduced nickel. In Canada, high-pressure carbon monoxide is used in the formation of iron and nickel carbonyl, which are separated by distillation. In the USA, nickel carbonyl was prepared commercially by the reaction of carbon monoxide with nickel sulfate solution (Antonsen, 1981). Nickel carbonyl is currently produced by two companies each in the Federal Republic of Germany and the USA and by one in Japan (Chemical Information Services, Ltd., 1988).

*Nickelocene* is formed by the reaction of nickel halides with sodium cyclopentadienide (Antonsen, 1981). It is currently produced by two companies in the USA (Chemical Information Services Ltd, 1988).

*Nickel selenide* (particular form unknown) is produced by one company each in Japan and the USA, *nickel titanate* by one company each in the UK and the USA and *potassium nickelocyanate* by one company each in India and the USA (Chemical Information Services Ltd, 1988).

## 2.2  Use

Uncharacterized alloys of nickel have been used in tools and weapons since 1200 AD or earlier (Considine, 1974; Tien & Howsen, 1981). In fact, the principal use of nickel has always been in its metallic form combined with other metals and nonmetals as alloys. Nickel alloys are typically characterized by their strength, hardness and resistance to corrosion (Tien & Howsen, 1981). The principal current uses of nickel are in the production of stainless and heat-resistant steels, nonferrous alloys and superalloys. Other major uses of nickel and nickel salts are in electroplating, in catalysts, in the manufacture of alkaline (nickel-cadmium) batteries, in coins, in welding products (coated electrodes, filter wire) and in certain pigments and electronic products (Antonsen, 1981; Tien & Howsen, 1981; Mastromatteo, 1986). Nickel imparts strength and corrosion resistance over a wide range of temperatures and pressures (Sibley, 1985; Chamberlain, 1988).

Worldwide demand for nickel in 1983 was 685 000 tonnes (Sibley, 1985). US consumption of nickel ranged from approximately 93 000 to 122 000 tonnes over the period 1982-86 (Chamberlain, 1988). Table 8 shows the US consumption pattern by end-use for 1983. In 1978, 44% was used in stainless steels and alloy steels, 33% in nonferrous and high-temperature alloys, 17% in electroplating and the remaining 6% primarily as catalysts, in ceramics, in magnets and as salts (Tien & Howson, 1981). In western Europe, it was estimated that, in 1982, 50% of the nickel was used in stainless steels, 10% in alloy steel, 15% in nonferrous alloys, 10% in foundry alloys, 10% in plating and 5% in other applications, such as catalysts and batteries (Eurométaux, 1986).

**Table 8. US consumption pattern of nickel in 1983 (%)[a]**

| Use | Consumption (%) |
|---|---|
| Transportation | |
|    Aircraft | 10.3 |
|    Motor vehicles and equipment | 10.2 |
|    Ship and boat building and repairs | 4.3 |
| Chemicals | 15.6 |
| Petroleum | 8.2 |
| Fabricated metal products | 8.8 |
| Electrical | 10.7 |
| Household appliances | 7.9 |
| Machinery | 7.2 |
| Construction | 9.7 |
| Other | 7.1 |

[a]From Sibley (1985)

(a)   *Metallic nickel and nickel alloys*

*Pure nickel metal* is used to prepare nickel alloys (including steels). It is used as such for plating, electroforming, coinage, electrical components, tanks, catalysts, battery plates, sintered components, magnets and welding rods (Eurométaux, 1986).

*Ferronickel* is used to prepare steels. Stainless and heat-resistant steels accounted for 93% of its end use in 1986 (Chamberlain, 1988).

*Nickel-containing steels* with low nickel content (<5% Ni) are used for construction and tool fabrication. Stainless steels are used for general engineering equipment, chemical equipment, domestic applications, hospital equipment, food processing, architectural panels and fasteners, pollution control equipment, cryogenic uses, automotive parts and engine components.

*Nickel*-copper *alloys* are used for coinage, in industrial piping and valves, marine components, condenser tubes, heat exchangers, architectural trim, thermocouples, desalination plants, ship propellers, etc. Nickel-chromium alloys are used in many high-temperature applications, such as furnaces, jet engine parts and reaction vessels. Molybdenum-containing nickel alloys are notable for their corrosion resistance and thermal stability, as are the nickel-iron-chromium alloys, and are used in nuclear and fossil-fuel steam generators, food-processing equipment and chemical-processing and heat-treating equipment. The majority of permanent magnets are made from nickel-cast iron alloys (Mastromatteo, 1986). The other groups of nickel alloys are used according to their specific properties for acid-resistant equipment, heating elements for furnaces, low-expansion alloys, cryogenic uses, storage of liquefied gases, high magnetic-permeability alloys and surgical implant prostheses.

### (b)   Nickel oxides and hydroxides

The *nickel oxide sinters* are used in the manufacture of alloys, steels and stainless steels (Antonsen, 1981).

*Green nickel oxide* is used to make nickel catalysts and in the ceramics industry. In specialty ceramics, it is added to frit compositions used for porcelain enamelling of steel; in the manufacture of magnetic nickel-zinc ferrites used in electric motors, antennas and television tube yokes; and as a colourant in glass and ceramic stains used in ceramic tiles, dishes, pottery and sanitary ware (Antonsen, 1981).

*Black nickel oxide* is used in the manufacture of nickel salts and specialty ceramics. It is also used to enhance the activity of three-way catalysts containing rhodium, platinum and palladium used in automobile exhaust control. Like green nickel oxide, black nickel oxide is also used for nickel catalyst manufacture and in the ceramic industry (Antonsen, 1981).

The major use of *nickel hydroxide* is in the manufacture of nickel-cadmium batteries. It is also used as a catalyst intermediate (Antonsen, 1981).

### (c)   Nickel sulfides

*Nickel sulfide* is used as a catalyst in petrochemical hydrogenation when high concentrations of sulfur are present in the distillates. The major use of nickel monosulfide is as an intermediate in the hydrometallurgical processing of silicate-oxide nickel ores.

### (d)   Nickel salts

*Nickel acetate* is used as a catalyst intermediate, as an intermediate in the formation of other nickel compounds, as a dye mordant, as a sealer for anodized aluminium and in nickel electroplating (Antonsen, 1981).

*Nickel carbonate* is used in the manufacture of nickel catalysts, in the preparation of coloured glass, in the manufacture of nickel pigments, in the production of nickel oxide and nickel powder, as a neutralizing compound in nickel electroplating solutions, and in the preparation of specialty nickel compounds (Antonsen, 1981).

*Nickel ammonium sulfate* has limited use as a dye mordant and is used in metal-finishing compositions and as an electrolyte for electroplating (Sax & Lewis, 1987).

*Nickel chloride* is used as an intermediate in the manufacture of nickel catalysts and to absorb ammonia in industrial gas masks. The hexahydrate is used in nickel electroplating (Antonsen, 1981) and hydrometallurgy (Warner, 1984).

*Nickel nitrate* hexahydrate is used as an intermediate in the manufacture of nickel catalysts, especially sulfur-sensitive catalysts, and as an intermediate in loading active mass in nickel-cadmium batteries of the sintered-plate type (Antonsen, 1981).

*Nickel sulfate* hexahydrate is used as an electrolyte primarily for nickel electroplating and also for nickel electrorefining. It is also used in 'electro-less' nickel plating, as a nickel strike solution for replacement coatings or for nickel flashing on steel that is to be porcelain-enamelled, as an intermediate in the manufacture of other nickel chemicals, such as nickel ammonium sulfate, and as a catalyst intermediate (Antonsen, 1981).

### (e)   Other nickel compounds

The primary use for *nickel carbonyl* is as an intermediate in the Mond carbonyl-refining process to produce highly pure nickel. Other uses of nickel carbonyl are in chemical synthesis as a catalyst, as a reactant in carbonylation reactions such as the synthesis of acrylic and methacrylic esters from acetylene and alcohols, in the vapour plating of nickel, and in the fabrication of nickel and nickel alloy components and shapes (Antonsen, 1981; Sax & Lewis, 1987).

*Nickelocene* is used as a catalyst and complexing agent and *nickel titanate* as a pigment (Sax & Lewis, 1987).

No information was available on the use of *nickel selenides* or *potassium nickelocyanate*.

## 2.3   Occurrence

### (a)   Natural occurrence

Nickel is widely distributed in nature, forming about 0.008% of the earth's crust (0.01% in igneous rocks). It ranks twenty-fourth among the elements in order of abundance (Grandjean, 1984), just above copper, lead and zinc (Mastromatteo, 1986). The core of the earth contains about 8.5% nickel; meteorites have been found to contain 5-50% (National Research Council, 1975). Nickel is also an important constituent of deep–sea nodules, typically comprising about 1.5% (Mastromatteo, 1986). Nickel–containing ores are listed in Table 9.

Laterites are formed by the long-term weathering of igneous rocks which are rich in magnesia and iron and contain about 0.25% nickel. Leaching by acidified groundwater over a long period removes the iron and magnesia, leaving a nickel-enriched residue with nickel contents up to 2.5%. Nickel is found as mixed nickel/iron oxide and as nickel magnesium silicate (garnierite) (Grandjean, 1986; Mastromatteo, 1986). Laterite deposits have been mined in many regions of the world, including New Caledonia, Cuba, the Dominican Republic, Indonesia, the USSR, Greece, Colombia, the Philippines, Guatemala and the USA (Mastromatteo, 1986).

**Table 9. Nickel-containing minerals**[a]

| Name | Chemical composition |
|------|---------------------|
| Breithauptite | NiSb |
| Niccolite | NiAs |
| Zaratite | $NiCO_3 2Ni(OH)_2.4H_2O$ |
| Bunsenite | NiO |
| Morenosite | $NiSO_4.7H_2O$ |
| Millerite | NiS |
| Vaesite | $NiS_2$ |
| Polydomite | $Ni_3S_4$ |
| Heazlewoodite | $Ni_3S_2$ |
| Pentlandite | $(Ni,Fe)_9S_8$ |
| Pyrrhotite, nickeliferous | $(Fe,Ni)_{1-x}S$[b] |
| Garnierite | $(Ni, Mg) SiO_3.nH_2O$ |

[a]From Grandjean (1986)
[b]From Warner (1984); Grandjean (1986)

Nickel and sulfur combine in a wide range of stoichiometric ratios. Nickel monosulfide (millerite), nickel subsulfide (heazlewoodite), nickel disulfide (vaesite) and $Ni_3S_4$ (polydymite) are found in mineral form in nature (Considine, 1974). Sulfide nickel ores contain a mixture of metal sulfides, principally pentlandite, chalcopyrite ($CuFeS_2$) and nickeliferous pyrrhotite in varying proportions. The major nickel mineral is pentlandite. While pentlandite may contain about 35% of nickel by weight, the nickel content of pyrrhotite is usually 1% or less, and the sulfide ore available for nickel production generally contains only 1-2% nickel (Grandjean, 1986). A large deposit of pentlandite is located in Sudbury, Ontario, Canada.

Other nickel ores include the nickel-arsenicals and the nickel-antimonials, but these are of much less commercial importance (Mastromatteo, 1986).

### (b) Occupational exposures

Occupational exposure to nickel may occur by skin contact or by inhalation of dusts, fumes or mists containing nickel or by inhalation of gaseous nickel carbonyl. Nickel-containing dusts may also be ingested by nickel workers (Grandjean, 1984). The National Institute for Occupational Safety and Health (1977a) published a list of occupations with potential exposure to nickel (Table 10); it has estimated that about 1.5 million workers in the USA are exposed to nickel and nickel compounds (National Institute for Occupational Safety and Health, 1977b).

**Table 10. Occupations with potential exposure to nickel[a]**

| | |
|---|---|
| Battery makers, storage | Mould makers |
| Catalyst workers | Nickel miners |
| Cemented carbide makers | Nickel refiners |
| Ceramic makers | Nickel smelters |
| Chemists | Nickel workers |
| Disinfectant makers | Oil hydrogenators |
| Dyers | Organic chemical synthesizers |
| Electroplaters | Paint makers |
| Enamellers | Penpoint makers |
| Gas-mask makers | Petroleum refinery workers |
| Ink makers | Spark-plug makers |
| Jewellers | Stainless-steel makers |
| Magnet makers | Textile dyers |
| Metallizers | Vacuum tube makers |
| Mond process workers | Varnish makers |
| Nickel-alloy makers | Welders |

[a]Adapted from National Institute for Occupational Safety and Health (1977b)

Occupational exposure to nickel is evaluated by monitoring air and blood serum, plasma or urine. (For recent reviews on this subject, see Rigaut, 1983; Grandjean, 1984; Nieboer *et al.*, 1984a; Warner, 1984; Grandjean, 1986; Sunderman *et al.*, 1986a). Tables 11-13 summarize exposure to nickel as measured by air and biological monitoring in various industries and occupations. The biological indicator levels are influenced by the chemical and physical properties of the nickel compound studied and by the time of sampling. It should be noted that the nickel compounds, the timing of collection of biological samples (normally at the end of a shift) and the analytical methods used differ from study to study, and elevated levels of nickel in biological fluids and tissue samples (Table 11) are mentioned only as indications of uptake of nickel, and may not correlate directly to exposure levels (Angerer *et al.*, 1989). (See also section 3.3(*b*) and the monographs on chromium and chromium compounds, and on welding.)

Table 11. Occupational exposure to nickel in the nickel producing industry

| Industry and activity (country) [year, when available] | No. of workers | Air (µg/m³) Mean ±SD | Range | Urine (µg/l) Mean ±SD | Range | Serum (µg/l) (mean ±SD) | Reference |
|---|---|---|---|---|---|---|---|
| Mines, Ontario (Canada) [1976] | | 20 | 6-40 | | | | Rigaut (1983) |
| Mines, Oregon (USA) [1981] | | 30 | | | | | Rigaut (1983) |
| Mines, New Caledonia [1982] | | 20 | 6-40 | | | | Rigaut (1983) |
| Smelter, producing ferronickel and matte, New Caledonia | | 5-76[a] | 2-274[b] | <10 (86% of samples) <br> <20 (98% of samples) | | | Warner (1984) |
| Laterite mining and smelting, Oregon (USA)[b] | | | | | | | Warner (1984) |
| Ore handling | 3 | 52 | 5-145 | | | | |
| Drying | 4 | 17 | 9-21 | | | | |
| Calcining | 4 | 90 | 37-146 | | | | |
| Skull drilling | 8 | 16 | 4-43 | | | | |
| Ferrosilicon manufacturing | 15 | 32 | 4-214 | | | | |
| Mixing | 17 | 6 | 4-7 | | | | |
| Refining | 10 | 11 | 4-34 | | | | |
| Handling of finished products | 6 | 5 | 4-9 | | | | |
| Maintenance | 9 | 39 | 7-168 | | | | |
| Miscellaneous | 3 | 193 | 8-420 | | | | |
| Refinery, Clydach (Wales, UK) Kiln | | | | | | | Morgan & Rouge (1984) |
| Before shut-down[c] | | 310 (26 samples) | 10-5000 | 24±24 (67 samples) | | 8.9±5.9 (37 samples) | |
| On return to work[c] | | | | 14±7 (20 samples) | | 3.0±2.0 (20 samples) | |

**Table 11 (contd)**

| Industry and activity (country) [year, when available] | No. of workers | Air (µg/m³) Mean ±SD | Range | Urine (µg/l) Mean ±SD | Range | Serum (µg/l) (mean ±SD) | Reference |
|---|---|---|---|---|---|---|---|
| Refinery, Clydach (Wales, UK) | | | | | | | |
| Kiln (contd) | | | | | | | |
| One month later | | 190 (30 samples) | 10–2890 | 22±10 (14 samples) | | 5.5±2.0 (16 samples) | |
| New powder plant | | 310 (20 samples) | 90–1530 | | | | |
| Before shut–down[c] | | | | 37±30 (48 samples) | | 7.2±4.8 (25 samples) | |
| On return to work[c] | | | | 13±12 (17 samples) | | 4.0±2.3 (17 samples) | |
| One month later | | 500 (22 samples) | 50–1810 | 31±13 (16 samples) | | 7.6±3.5 (15 samples) | |
| Old powder plant | | 1460 (5 samples) | 80–5000 | 33±13 (12 samples) | | 9.0±3.7 (6 samples) | |
| Wet–treatment (A)[d] | | 1540 (8 samples) | 220–4180 | 39±28 (15 samples) | | 7.4±5.1 (7 samples) | |
| Wet–treatment (B)[e] | | 90 (17 samples) | 30–150 | 34±24 (36 samples) | | 3.4±1.9 (13 samples) | |
| Refinery, Kristiansand (Norway)[b] | | | | | | | Høgetveit et al. (1978) |
| Roasting–smelting | 24 | 860±1200 | | 65±58 | | 7.2±2.8 | |
| Electrolytic department | 90 | 230±420 | | 129±106 | | 11.9±8.0 | |
| Other processes | 13 | 420±490 | | 45±27 | | 6.4±1.9 | |

Table 11 (contd)

| Industry and activity (country) [year, when available] | No. of workers | Air (μg/m³) Mean ±SD | Range | Urine (μg/l) Mean ±SD | Range | Serum (μg/l) (mean ±SD) | Reference |
|---|---|---|---|---|---|---|---|
| Refinery, Kristiansand (Norway) | | | | | | | Torjussen & Andersen (1979) |
| Roasting-smelting | 97 | | | 34±35 | | 5.2±2.7 | |
| Electrolysis | 144 | | | 73±85 | | 8.1±6.0 | |
| Other processes | 77 | | | 22±18 | | 4.3±2.2 | |
| Electrolytic refinery (USA) | 15 | 489 | 20–2200 | 222 | 8.6–813 | | Bernacki et al. (1978a) |
| | | | | 124 (μg/g creatinine) | 6.1–287 | | |
| Electrolytic refinery (FRG) | | 50 | | 14.8 (μg/g creatinine) | 2.5–63 | | Raithel (1987) |
| Electrolytic refinery (Czechoslovakia) | | 600 | 86–1265 | 264 | 125–450 | | Rigaut (1983) |
| Hydrometallurgical refinery (Canada) | | | | | | | Warner (1984) |
| Acid leaching of matte | | 99 | 5–1630 | | | | |
| Purification of nickel electrolyte: | | | | | | | |
| Tube filterman | 12 | 144 | 13–316 | | | | |
| | 12f | 129 | 11–316 | | | | |
| Filter pressman | 16 | 209 | 61–535 | | | | |
| | 16f | 152 | 31–246 | | | | |
| Filter-press area | 11 | 242 | 64–508 | | | | |
| | 11f | 221 | 52–466 | | | | |

**Table 11 (contd)**

| Industry and activity (country) [year, when available] | No. of workers | Air (µg/m³) Mean ±SD | Range | Urine (µg/l) Mean ±SD | Range | Serum (µg/l) (mean ±SD) | Reference |
|---|---|---|---|---|---|---|---|
| Hydrometallurgical refinery (Canada) (contd) | | | | | | | |
| Purification of nickel electrolyte[a]: | | | | | | | |
| Cementation of copper on nickel in Pachuca tanks | 39 / 39[f] | 168 / 38 | 48–644 / 1–133 | | | | |
| Removal of iron slimes with a tube filter | 56 / 56[f] | 200 / 85 | 27–653 / 3–433 | | | | |
| Oxidizing cobalt with chlorine | 47 / 47[f] | 183 / 66 | 30–672 / 1–267 | | | | |
| General operations in a tank house using insoluble anodes | 96[a] / 45[b] | 336 / 185 | 40–1100 / 80–400 | | | | |
| Tankhouse using nickel matte anodes: | | | | | | | |
| General area | 11[a] / 11[a,f] | 48 / 29 | 14–223 / 5–210 | | | | |
| Tankman | 15[b] / 15[b,f] | 48 / 30 | 18–88 / 12–71 | | | | |
| Anode scrapman | 11[b] / 11[b,f] | 179 / 52 | 43–422 / 1–236 | | | | |

[a]Area air sampling
[b]Personal air sampling
[c]Specimens obtained before and after six months' closure of refinery operations
[d]Short exposures to high levels of insoluble nickel compounds
[e]Chronic exposures to soluble nickel sulfate
[f]Soluble nickel

**Table 12. Occupational exposure in industries using primary nickel products**

| Industry and activity (country) | No. of workers | Air (µg/m³) | | Urine (µg/l) | | Reference |
|---|---|---|---|---|---|---|
| | | Mean | Range | Mean | Range | |
| Stainless-steel production | | | | | | Warner (1984) |
| Electric furnace shop | 8[a] | 36 | 9–65 | | | |
| Argon–oxygen decarburization | 5 | 35 | 13–58 | | | |
| Continuous casting | 2 | 14 | 11–15 | | | |
| Grinding/polishing (machine) | 6 | 134 | 75–189 | | | |
| Grinding/chipping (hand tool) | 2 | 39 | 23–48 | | | |
| Welding, cutting and scarfing[b] | 5 | 111[c] | 13–188[c] | | | |
| Heat treating | 1 | 54[d] | <1–104[d] | | | |
| Rolling and forging | 6 | 49 | <11–72 | | | |
| Other operations (maintenance, pickling) | 5 | 58 | 10–107 | | | |
| High nickel alloy production (FRG) (a few persons exposed to nickel powder) | 59 | 300[e] | | 2.6 | 0.5–52 | Raithel (1987) |
| High nickel alloy production[f] | | | | | | Warner (1984) |
| Weighing and melting | 369 | 83[f] | 1–4400 | | | |
| Hot working | 153 | 111 | 1–4200 | | | |
| Cold working | 504 | 64 | 1–2300 | | | |
| Grinding | 96 | 298 | 1–2300 | | | |
| Pickling and cleaning | 18 | 8 | 1–15 | | | |
| Maintenance | 392 | 58 | 1–73 | | | |
| Production of wrought nickel and alloys via metal powder foundries | 226 | 1500[f] | 1–60000 | | | Warner (1984) |

**Table 12 (contd)**

| Industry and activity (country) | No. of workers | Air (µg/m³) Mean | Range | Urine (µg/l) Mean | Range | Reference |
|---|---|---|---|---|---|---|
| Six jobbing foundries processing alloys containing 0–60% nickel, averaging 10–15% nickel: | | | | | | Scholz & Holcomb (1980) |
| Melting | 15 | 21 | <5–62 | | | |
| Casting | 7 | 14 | <4–35 | | | |
| Cleaning room: | | | | | | |
| Cutting and gouging | 11 | 233 | 7–900 | | | |
| Welding | 14 | 94 | 20–560 | | | |
| Hand grinding | 24 | 94 | <5–440 | | | |
| Swing grinding | 3 | 19 | 13–30 | | | |
| Jobbing foundry processing carbon, alloy and stainless steel containing 0–10% nickel: | | | | | | Warner (1984) |
| Melting and casting | 16 | 13 | ND$^e$–70 | | | |
| Cleaning room: | | | | | | |
| Air arc gouging | 7 | 310 | 40–710 | | | |
| Welding | 34 | 67 | 10–170 | | | |
| Three low alloy (0–2% nickel) iron and steel foundries | | | | | | Warner (1984) |
| Melting and casting | 16 | 13 | 4–32 | | | |
| Cleaning room (grinding, air arc gouging, welding) | 18 | 54 | 7–156 | | | |
| Steel foundry (Finland) (steel cutters) | 4 | 518 | 145–1100 | 39 | 18–77 | Aitio et al. (1985) |
| Production of soluble nickel salts (Wales, UK)$^f$ | 66 | 500 | 10–20 000 | (68) 65$^h$ | 10–200$^h$ | Morgan & Rouge (1979) |
| | 60 | 450 | <10–12 070 | (60) 49$^h$ | <10–210$^h$ | |

**Table 12 (contd)**

| Industry and activity (country) | No. of workers | Air (μg/m³) | | Urine (μg/l) | | Reference |
|---|---|---|---|---|---|---|
| | | Mean | Range | Mean | Range | |
| Production of nickel salts from nickel or nickel oxide: | | | | | | Warner (1984) |
| Nickel sulfate | 12 | 117[f] | 9–590 | | | |
| Nickel chloride | 10 | 196[f,i] | 20–485[i] | | | |
| Nickel acetate/nitrate | 6 | 155[f] | 38–525 | | | |

[a]Companies reporting exposures
[b]Samples taken outside protective hood
[c]Excludes one suspiciously high measurement (1460 μg Ni/m³)
[d]Excludes one suspiciously high measurement (500 μg Ni/m³)
[e]The median nickel concentration in workroom air was 300 μg/m³; values that exceeded 500 μg/m³ were found at 2 of 8 measuring stations
[f]Mainly from personal sampling
[g]Not detected
[h]Corrected to 1.6 g/l creatinine
[i]Excludes one suspiciously high value (2780 μg Ni/m³)

**Table 13. Occupational exposure in industries using nickel in special applications**

| Industry and activity (country) | No. of workers | Air ($\mu g/m^3$) Mean | Air Range | Urine ($\mu g/l$) Mean ± SD | Urine Range | Serum ($\mu g/l$) Mean | Serum Range | Reference |
|---|---|---|---|---|---|---|---|---|
| Ni/Cd–battery production with nickel and nickel hydroxide; assembly and welding of plates | 36 | 378[a,b] | 20–1910[a,b] | | | | | Warner (1984) |
| Ni/Cd–battery production (FRG) | 51 | | | 4.0[c] | 1.9–10.9 | | | Raithel (1987) |
| Ni/Cd or Ni/Zn–battery production (USA) | 6 | | | 11.7±7.5 10.2 | 3.4–25 7.2–23 ($\mu g/g$ creatinine) | | | Bernacki et al. (1978a) |
| Ni/H$_2$–battery production | 7 | | | 32.2±40.4 | 2.8–103 | | | Adamsson et al. (1980) |
| Ni/Cd–battery production | | | 12–33 | | 24–27 ($\mu g/g$ creatinine) | | | |
| Ni-catalyst production (Netherlands) | 73 | | <200–5870 | 64 ($\mu g/g$ creatinine) | 9–300 | 8 | 2–41 | Zwennis & Franssen (1983) |
| Ni-catalyst production from nickel sulfate (USA) | 7 5 | 150[a] 370[d] | 10–600[a] 190–530[d] | | | | | Warner (1984) |
| Ni-catalyst use; coal gasification workers (USA) | 9 | | | 4.2 3.2 | 0.4–7.9 0.1–5.8 ($\mu g/g$ creatinine) | | | Bernacki et al. (1978a) |
| Electroplating Sulfate bath, 45°C | | | | | | | | |
| Area 1 sample | 16 | <6 | <5–<8 | | | | | Warner (1984) |
| Area 2 samples | 3 | <4 | <2–<7 | | | | | |
| Personal samples | 6 | <11 | <7–<16 | | | | | |

**Table 13 (contd)**

| Industry and activity (country) | No. of workers | Air (µg/m³) Mean | Air (µg/m³) Range | Urine (µg/l) Mean ± SD | Urine (µg/l) Range | Serum (µg/l) Mean | Serum (µg/l) Range | Reference |
|---|---|---|---|---|---|---|---|---|
| Electroplating (contd) | | | | | | | | |
| Sulfate bath, 70°C | | | | | | | | |
| Area samples | 6 | <3 | <2-<3 | | | | | |
| Sulfamate bath, 45–55°C | | | | | | | | |
| Area 1 sample | 9 | <4 | <4 | | | | | |
| Area 2 samples | 6 | <4 | <4 | | | | | |
| Electroplating (Finland) | | 90 | 20–170 | 53.5 | 12–109 | 6.1 | 1.2–14.1 | Tossavainen et al. (1980) |
| Electroplating (Finland) | | – | 30–160 | – | 25–120 | – | 3–14 | Tola et al. (1979) |
| Electroplating (USA) | | 9.3[a] | 0.5–21.2 | 48 | 5–262 | | | Bernacki et al. (1980) |
| Electroplating (USA) | 21 | | | 30.4 (21.0) | 3.6–85 2.4–62 µg/g creatinine) | | | Bernacki et al. (1978a) |
| Electroplating (India) | 12 | | | 12.2 | 11–26 | | | Tandon et al. (1977) |
| Electroplating (FRG) | | 10 (soluble anode) 110 (insoluble anode) 7 (insoluble anode and wetting agent) | | | 1.7–3.6 | | | Gross (1987) |
| Exposed persons in the hollow glass industry (FRG) | 9 | | 3–3800 | 11.9 (946 samples) | 3.6–42.1[e] | 1.6 | 0.75–3.25[e] (288 samples) | Raithel (1987) |
| Flame sprayer | | | 3–600 | 25.3 (114 samples) | 8.5–81.5 | 1.95 | 0.75–3.25 (40 samples) | |

**Table 13 (contd)**

| Industry and activity (country) | No. of workers | Air (µg/m³) Mean | Air Range | Urine (µg/l) Mean ± SD | Urine Range | Serum (µg/l) Mean | Serum Range | Reference |
|---|---|---|---|---|---|---|---|---|
| Grinder, polisher | | | 18–3800 | 7.4 (406 samples) | 2.9–24.3 | 0.9 | 0.75–2.05 (140 samples) | Gross (1987) |
| Mixed mechanical work and flame spraying | | | 300–410 | 17.5 (394 samples) | 4.9–53.9 | 1.65 | 0.75–4.10 (108 samples) | Gross (1987) |
| Plasma spraying (FRG) | 6 | 200 | | | 3.4–12.5 | | | Gross (1987) |
| Spark eroding (FRG) | 6 | <10 | | | 0.7–2.1 | | | Gross (1987) |
| Flame spraying (USA) | 5 | 2.4 | <1–6.5 | 17.2 (16.0 | 1.4–26 1.4–54 µg/g creatinine | | | Bernacki et al. (1978a) |
| Plasma cutting (FRG) | 17 | | <100 | | 1.1–6.5 | | | Gross (1987) |
| Painting | | | | | | | | |
| Spray painting in a construction shipyard (USA) | 13 | | | 3.2 | <0.5–9.2 | 4.4 | <0.5–17.2 | Grandjean et al. (1980) |
| Painting in repair shipyard (USA) | 18 | | | | | 5.9 | <0.5–13 | Grandjean et al. (1980) |
| Manufacturing paints (USA) | 10 | | | 15.3±11.1 | 6–39 | | | Tandon et al. (1977) |
| Buffing, polishing, grinding | | | | | | | | |
| Buffers and polishers (aircraft engine factory) (USA) | 7 | 26 | <1–129 | 4.1 (2.4 | 0.5–9.5 0.5–4.7 µg/g creatinine | | | Bernacki et al. (1978a) |
| Grinders (abrasive wheel grinding of aircraft parts) (USA) | 9 | 1.6 | <1–9.5 | 5.4 (3.5 | 2.1–8.8 1.7–6.1 µg/g creatinine | | | Bernacki et al. (1978a) |

**Table 13 (contd)**

| Industry and activity (country) | No. of workers | Air (µg/m³) | | Urine (µg/l) | | Serum (µg/l) | | Reference |
|---|---|---|---|---|---|---|---|---|
| | | Mean | Range | Mean ± SD | Range | Mean | Range | |
| Polisher, grinder (FRG) | 15 | 140 | | | 0.7-9.9 | | | Gross (1987) |
| Polisher, grinder (stainless steel) (FRG) | 46 | 350[c] | 10-10 000[f] | 28 | (12) 3-7[f] | | | Heidermanns et al. (1983) |
| Miscellaneous exposure | | | | | | | | |
| Bench mechanics (assembling, fittings and finishing aircraft parts made of Ni-alloys) (USA) | 8 | 52 | <1-252 | 12.2 (7.2 | 1.4-41 0.7-20 µg/g creatinine) | | | Bernacki et al. (1978a) |
| Riggers/carpenters (construction shipyard) (USA) | 16 | | | 3.7 | 1.1-13.5 | 3.3 | 1.1-13.5 | Grandjean et al. (1980) |
| Riggers/carpenters (repair shipyard) (USA) | 11 | | | | | 3.6 | <0.5-7.4 | Grandjean et al. (1980) |
| Shipfitters/pipefitters (construction shipyard) (USA) | 6 | | | 4.9 | 3.7-7.1 | 4.1 | 1.5-6.8 | Grandjean et al. (1980) |
| Shipfitters/pipefitters (repair shipyard) (USA) | 15 | | | | | 9.1 | 0.5-3.8 | Grandjean et al. (1980) |

[a]Personal air sampling

[b]Excludes three suspiciously high values (5320; 18 300; 53 300 µg/m³)

[c]Median

[d]Area air monitoring

[e]68th percentile range

[f]90th percentile range

### (i)  Nickel mining and ore comminution

On the basis of personal gravimetric sampling among Canadian underground miners of nickel, the time-weighted average concentration of total airborne nickel was about 25 μg/m³ and that of respirable nickel, < 5 μg/m³ (see Table 11; Warner, 1984). Ore miners may also be exposed to radon, oil mist, diesel exhausts and asbestos (see IARC, 1977, 1988a, 1989).

### (ii)  Nickel roasting, calcining, smelting and refining

The nickel content of air samples from a Sudbury (Canada) smelter seldom exceeded 0.5 mg/m³ but could be as high as 1 mg/m³. The average concentrations of airborne nickel were higher in the roaster areas (0.048 mg/m³) than in the converter areas (0.033 mg/m³), because the handling of fine solids is a greater source of dust than the handling of molten phases. Thus, work-place air may contain roaster feed and product, which include various nickel-containing minerals and solid solutions of nickel in iron oxides. Nickel-bearing dusts from converters contain mainly nickel subsulfide (Warner, 1984). Arsenic, silica, copper, cobalt and other metal compounds may also occur in work-place air.

Emissions from the high-temperature ore calcining and smelting furnaces used to produce ferronickel from lateritic ores would contain nickel predominantly in the form of silicate oxides and iron-nickel mixed/complex oxides of the ferrite or spinel type. The nickel content of these dusts can range from 1 to 10% (International Committee on Nickel Carcinogenesis in Man, 1990).

Average concentrations of airborne nickel in refining operations can be considerably higher than those encountered in mining and smelting because of the higher nickel content of the materials being handled in the refining process (Table 11). The nickel species that may be present in various refining operations include nickel subsulfide, nickel monoxide, nickel-copper oxides, nickel-iron oxides, metallic nickel, pure and alloyed, nickel sulfate, nickel chloride and nickel carbonate. Other possible exposures would be to hydrogen sulfide, ammonia, chlorine, sulfur dioxide, arsenic and polycyclic aromatic hydrocarbons (Warner, 1984; International Committee on Nickel Carcinogenesis in Man, 1990).

A recent attempt has been made, in conjunction with a large epidemiological study (International Committee on Nickel Carcinogenesis in Man, 1990), to estimate past exposures in various nickel refineries using different processes. Exposure estimates were made first for total airborne nickel, based either on historical measurements (after 1950) or on extrapolation of recent measurements. In all cases, further estimates were made of nickel species (metallic, oxidic, sulfidic and soluble), as defined in the report, on the basis of knowledge of the processes and rough estimates of the ratio of the various species generated in each process.

Prior to the widespread use of personal samplers, high-volume samplers were used to take area samples; however, in many instances, neither personal gravimetric nor high-volume samples were available, and konimeter readings were the only available means of assessing the level of airborne dust. No measurement of the actual concentration of nickel, and especially nickel species, in work places exists for any refining operation prior to 1950. More recently, measurements have been made of total dust and, in some cases, total nickel content of dust or mist in refinery work-place air. Conversion of high-volume sampler and konimeter measurements to concentrations comparable to personal gravimetric sampler measurements introduces another uncertainty in the environmental estimates. The main reason for this uncertainty is that it is impossible to derive unique conversion factors to interrelate measurements from the three devices; different particle size distributions give rise to different conversion factors. Information concerning particle size in airborne dusts was seldom available in the work places under study (International Committee on Nickel Carcinogenesis in Man, 1990).

Estimates of nickel exposure were further divided into four categories representing different nickel species: (i) metallic nickel, (ii) oxidic nickel [undefined, but generally understood to include nickel oxide combined with various other metal oxides, such as iron, cobalt and copper oxides], (iii) sulfidic nickel (including nickel subsulfide) and (iv) soluble nickel, defined as consisting 'primarily of nickel sulfate and nickel chloride but may in some estimates include the less soluble nickel carbonate and nickel hydroxide'. No actual measurement of specific nickel species in work-place air was available upon which to base exposure estimates. As a result, the estimates are necessarily very approximate. This is clear, for example, from the estimates for linear calciners at the Clydach refinery (Wales, UK), which gave total nickel concentrations of 10-100 mg/m³, with 0-5% soluble nickel. Because of the inherent error in the processes of measurement and speciation and the uncertainty associated with extrapolating estimates from recent periods to earlier periods, the estimated concentrations of nickel species in work places in this study (International Committee on Nickel Carcinogenesis in Man, 1990) must be interpreted as broad ranges indicating only estimates of the order of magnitude of the actual exposures.

### (iii) *Production of stainless steel and nickel alloys*

While some stainless steels contain up to 25-30% nickel, nearly half of that produced contains only 8-10% nickel. Nickel oxide sinter is used as raw material for stainless and alloy steelmaking in some plants, and oxidized nickel may be found in the fumes from many melting/casting and arc/torch operations in the melting trades. The nickel concentrations in air in the stainless and alloy producing industries were given in Table 12. Occupational exposure in alloy steel making should generally be lower than those observed for comparable operations with stainless steel. The normal range of nickel in alloy steels is 0.3-5% but the nickel content can be as high as 18% for certain high-strength steels. The production of 'high nickel' alloys consumes about 80% of the nickel used for nonferrous applications. The technology is very similar to that used for stainless steel production except that melting and decarburizing units are generally smaller and greater use is made of vacuum melting and remelting. Since these alloys contain more nickel than stainless and alloy steels, the concentrations of nickel in workroom air are generally higher than for comparable operations with stainless and alloy steels (Warner, 1984).

### (iv)   *Steel foundries*

In foundries, shapes are cast from a wide variety of nickel-containing materials. Melts ranging in size from 0.5 to 45 tonnes are prepared in electric arc or induction furnaces and cast into moulds made of sand, metal or ceramic. The castings are further processed by chipping and grinding and may be repaired by air arc gouging and welding. Foundry operations can thus be divided roughly into melting/casting and cleaning room operations. Typical levels of airborne nickel in steel foundries were presented in Table 12 (Warner, 1984). Health hazards in foundry operations include exposure to silica and metal fumes and to degradation products from moulds and cores, such as carbon monoxide, formaldehyde and polycyclic aromatic hydrocarbons (see IARC, 1984).

### (v)   *Production of nickel-containing batteries*

The principal commercial product in nickel-containing batteries is the electrochemical couple nickel/cadmium. Other couples that have been used include nickel/iron, nickel/hydrogen and nickel/zinc. In nickel-cadmium batteries, the positive electrode is primarily nickel hydroxide, contained in porous plates. The positive material is made from a slurry of nickel hydroxide, cobalt sulfate and sodium hydroxide, dried and ground with graphite flake. Sintered nickel plates impregnated with the slurry may also be used. The nickel/hydrogen system requires a noble metal catalyst and operates at high pressures, requiring a steel pressure vessel. Nickel/iron batteries can be produced using nickel foil (Malcolm, 1983).

The concentrations of nickel in air and in biological samples from workers in the nickel-cadmium battery industry were summarized in Table 13. Workers in such plants are also exposed to cadmium.

### (vi)   *Production and use of nickel catalysts*

Metallic nickel is used as a catalyst, often alloyed with copper, cobalt or iron, for hydrogenation and reforming processes and for the methane conversion and Fischer-Tropsch reactions. Mixed, nickel-containing oxides are used as partial oxidation catalysts and as hydrodesulfuration catalysts (cobalt nickel molybdate) (Gentry *et al.*, 1983). Occupational exposure occurs typically in the production of catalysts from metallic nickel powder and nickel salts such as nickel sulfate (Warner, 1984), but coal gasification process workers who use Raney nickel as a hydrogenation catalyst have also been reported to be exposed to nickel (Bernacki *et al.*, 1978a). Exposure levels are generally higher in catalyst production than during the use of catalysts (see Table 13).

### (vii)  *Nickel plating*

Metal plating is an operation whereby a metal, commonly nickel, is deposited on a substrate for protection or decoration purposes. Nickel plating can be performed by electrolytic processes (electroplating) or 'electroless' processes (chemical plating), with aqueous solutions (the 'baths'). During electroplating, nickel is taken out of the solution and deposited on the substrate, which acts as the cathode. Either soluble anodes, made from metallic nickel feed, or insoluble anodes, in which the nickel is introduced as the hydroxycarbonate, are used. The baths contain a mixture of nickel sulfate and/or chloride or, less often, sulfamate. In electroless processes, a hypophosphite medium is used, the nickel feed being nickel sulfate.

The electrolyte contains soluble nickel salts, such as nickel fluoborate, nickel sulfate and nickel sulfamate (Warner, 1984). Nickel plating can be performed with a soluble (metallic nickel) or insoluble anode. The principal source of air contamination in electroplating operations is release of the bath electrolyte into the air. Electroplaters are exposed to readily absorbed soluble nickel salts by inhalation, which subsequently causes high levels in urine (Tola *et al.*, 1979; see Table 13).

### (viii)  *Welding*

Welding produces particulate fumes that have a chemical composition reflecting the elemental content of the consumable used. For each couple of process/material of application, there is a wide range of concentrations of elements present in the fume. Nickel and chromium are found in significant concentrations in fumes from welding by manual metal arc, metal inert gas and tungsten inert gas processes on stainless and alloy steels. Typical ranges of total fume and nickel, as found in the breathing zone of welders, are presented in Table 14. Certain special process applications not listed can also produce high nickel and chromium concentrations, and manual metal arc and metal inert gas welding of nickel in confined spaces produce significantly higher concentrations of total fume and elemental constituents. Exposure to welding fumes that contain nickel and chromium can lead to elevated levels of these elements in tissues, blood and urine (see monograph on welding for details).

### (ix)  *Thermal spraying of nickel*

Thermal spraying of nickel is usually performed by flame spraying or plasma spraying (Gross, 1987). For flame spraying, nickel in wire form is fed to a gun

**Table 14. Total fume and nickel concentrations found in the breathing zone of welders**[a]

| Process[b] | Total fume[c] (mg/m³) | Ni (μg/m³) |
|---|---|---|
| MMA/SS | 4-10 | 10-1000 |
| MIG/SS | 2-5 | 30-500 |
| TIG/SS | 2-6 | 10-40 |

[a]Compiled from Table 4 of monograph on welding
[b]MMA, manual metal arc; SS, stainless steel; MIG, metal inert gas; TIG, tungsten inert gas
[c]50-90% range

fuelled by a combustible gas such as acetylene, propane or natural gas. The wire is melted in the oxygen-fuel flame, atomized with compressed air, and propelled from the torch at velocities up to 120 m/s. The material bonds to the workpiece by a combination of mechanical interlocking of the molten particles and a cementation of partially oxidized material.

The material can also be sprayed in powder form, the fuel gases being either acetylene or hydrogen and oxygen. The powder is aspirated by an air stream, and the molten particles are deposited on the workpiece with high efficiency. For plasma spraying, an electric arc is established in the controlled atmosphere of a special nozzle. Argon is passed through the arc, where it ionizes to form a plasma that continues through the nozzle and recombines to create temperatures as high as 16 700°C. Powder is melted in the stream and released from the gun at a velocity of approximately 10 m/s (Burgess, 1981; Pfeiffer & Willert, 1986).

Workers who construct or repair nickel-armoured moulds in hollow-glass and ceramics factories use flame spraying with metallic powder (70-98% Ni) and are exposed to nickel dusts (as metallic and oxidic nickel) and fumes. After the moulds have been polished with grinding discs, abrasives and emery paper, they are installed in glass-making machines. Exposure levels in various types of thermal spraying, cutting and eroding were shown in Table 13.

### (x)   Production and use of paints

Some pigments for paints (e.g., nickel flake) and colours for enamels (e.g., nickel oxide) contain nickel. Exposure to nickel can occur when spraying techniques are used and when the paints are manufactured (Tandon *et al.*, 1977; Mathur & Tandon, 1981). Paint and pigment workers have slightly higher concentrations of nickel in plasma and urine than controls (see Table 13). Sandblasters may be exposed to dusts from old paints containing nickel and, additionally, to nickel-containing abrasive materials (Stettler *et al.*, 1982).

### (xi)  *Grinding, polishing and buffing of nickel-containing metals*

Grinding, polishing and buffing involve controlled use of bonded abrasives for metal finishing operations; in many cases the three operations are conducted in sequence (for review, see Burgess, 1981). Grinding includes cutting operations in foundries for removal of gates, sprues and risers, rough grinding of forgings and castings, facing off of welded assemblies and grinding out major surface imperfections. Grinding is done with wheels made of selected abrasives in bonding structural matrices. The commonly used abrasives are aluminium oxide and silicon carbide. The wheel components normally make up only a small fraction of the total airborne particulates released during grinding, and the bulk of the particles arise from the workpiece. Polishing techniques are used to remove workpiece surface imperfections such as tool marks, and this may remove as much as 0.1 mm of stock from a workpiece. In buffing, little metal is removed from the workpiece, and the process merely provides a high lustre surface by smearing any surface roughness with a high weight abrasive; e.g., ferric oxide and chromium oxide are used for soft metals, aluminium oxide for harder metals. Sources of airborne contaminants from grinding, polishing and buffing have been identified (Burgess, 1981; König *et al.*, 1985). Grinding, polishing and buffing cause exposures to metallic nickel and to nickel-containing alloys and steels (see Table 13).

### (xii)  *Miscellaneous exposure to nickel*

A group of employees exposed to metallic nickel dust was identified among employees of the Oak Ridge Gaseous Diffusion Plant in the USA. In one department, finely-divided, highly pure, nickel powder was used to manufacture 'barrier', a special porous medium employed in the isotope enrichment of uranium by gaseous diffusion. The metallic powder was not oxidized during processing. Routine air sampling was performed at the plant from 1948 to 1963, during which time 3044 air samples were collected in seven areas of the barrier plant and analysed for nickel content. The median nickel concentration was 0.13 mg/m$^3$ (range, <0.1-566 mg/m$^3$), but the authors acknowledged that the median exposures were probably underestimated (Godbold & Tompkins, 1979). Other determinations of nickel in miscellaneous industries and activities were presented in Table 13.

### (c)  *Air*

Nickel enters the atmosphere from natural sources (e.g., volcanic emissions and windblown dusts produced by weathering of rocks and soils), from combustion of fossil fuels in stationary and mobile power sources, from emissions from nickel mining and refining operations, from the use of metals in industrial processes and from incineration of wastes (Sunderman, 1986a; US Environmental Protection Agency, 1986). The estimated global emission rates are given in Table 15. The predominant forms of nickel in the ambient air appear to be nickel sulfate and complex oxides of nickel with other metals (US Environmental Protection Agency, 1986).

Table 15. Emission of nickel into the global atmosphere[a]

| Source | Emission rate ($10^6$ kg/year) |
|---|---|
| Natural | |
| Wind-blown dusts | 4.8 |
| Volcanoes | 2.5 |
| Vegetation | 0.8 |
| Forest fires | 0.2 |
| Meteoric dusts | 0.2 |
| Sea spray | 0.009 |
| Total | 8.5 |
| Anthropogenic[b] | |
| Residual and fuel oil combustion | 27 |
| Nickel mining and refining | 7.2 |
| Waste incineration | 5.1 |
| Steel production | 1.2 |
| Industrial applications | 1.0 |
| Gasoline and diesel fuel combustion | 0.9 |
| Coal combustion | 0.7 |
| Total | 43.1 |

[a]From Bennett (1984)
[b]Emissions during the mid-1970s

Nickel concentrations in the atmosphere at remote locations were about 1 ng/m³ (Grandjean, 1984). Ambient levels of nickel in air ranged from 5 to 35 ng/m³ at rural and urban sites (Bennett, 1984). Surveys have indicated wide variations but no overall trend. In the USA, atmospheric nickel concentrations averaged 6 ng/m³ in nonurban areas and 17 ng/m³ (in summer) and 25 ng/m³ (in winter) in urban areas (National Research Council, 1975). Salmon *et al.* (1978) reported nickel concentrations in 1957-74 at a semirural site in England to range from 10 to 50 ng/m³ (mean, 19 ng/m³). Nickel concentrations at seven sites in the UK ranged, with one exception, from <2 to 4.8 ng/kg [<2.5 to 5.9 ng/m³] (Cawse, 1978). Annual averages in four Belgian cities were 9-60 ng/m³ during 1972-77 (Kretzschmar *et al.*, 1980). Diffuse sources (traffic, home heating, distant sources) generally predominated.

High levels of nickel in air (110-180 ng/m³) were recorded in heavily industrialized areas and larger cities (Bennett, 1984).

Local airborne concentrations of nickel are high around locations where nickel is mined (e.g., 580 ng/m³ in Ontario, Canada) (McNeely et al., 1972). The average atmospheric nickel concentration near a nickel refinery in West Virginia (USA) was 1200 ng/m³, compared to 40 ng/m³ at six sampling stations not contiguous to the nickel plant. The highest concentration on a single day was about 2000 ng/m³ near a large nickel production facility (Grandjean, 1984).

Average exposure to nickel by inhalation has been estimated to be 0.4 µg/day (range, 0.2-1.0 µg/day) for urban dwellers and 0.2 µg/day (range, 0.1-0.4 µg/day) for rural dwellers (Bennett, 1984).

### (d)  Tobacco smoke

Cigarette smoking can cause a daily absorption of nickel of 1 µg/pack due to the nickel content of tobacco (Grandjean, 1984). Sunderman and Sunderman (1961) and Szadkowski et al. (1969) found average nickel contents of 2.2 and 2.3 µg/ cigarette, respectively, with a range of 1.1-3.1. The latter authors also showed that 10-20% of the nickel in cigarettes is released in mainstream smoke; most of the nickel was in the gaseous phase. The nickel content of mainstream smoke ranges from 0.005 to 0.08 µg/cigarette (Klus & Kuhn, 1982). It is not yet known in what form nickel occurs in mainstream smoke (US Environmental Protection Agency, 1986); it has been speculated that it may be present as nickel carbonyl (Grandjean, 1984), but, if so, it must occur at concentrations of < 0.1 ppm (Alexander et al., 1983). Pipe tobacco, cigars and snuff have been reported to contain nickel at levels of the same magnitude (2-3 µg/g tobacco) (National Research Council, 1975).

### (e)  Water and beverages

Nickel enters groundwater and surface water by dissolution of rocks and soils, from biological cycles, from atmospheric fallout, and especially from industrial processes and waste disposal, and occurs usually as nickel ion in the aquatic environment. Most nickel compounds are relatively soluble in water at pH values less than 6.5, whereas nickel exists predominantly as nickel hydroxides at pH values exceeding 6.7. Therefore, acid rain has a pronounced tendency to mobilize nickel from soil and to increase nickel concentrations in groundwater.

The nickel content of groundwater is normally below 20 µg/l (US Environmental Protection Agency, 1986), and the levels appear to be similar in raw, treated and distributed municipal water. In US drinking-water, 97% of all samples (n = 2503) contained ≤20 µg/l, while about 90% had ≤10 µg/l (National Research Council, 1975). Unusually high levels were found in groundwater polluted with soluble nickel compounds from a nickel-plating facility (up to 2500 µg/l) and in water from 12 wells (median, 180 µg/l) (Grandjean, 1984). The median level in Canadian ground-water was < 2 µg/l, but high levels were reported in Ontario (Méranger et al., 1981). In municipal tap-water near large open-pit nickel mines, the average nickel concentration was about 200 µg/l, while that in a control area had an average level of about 1 µg/l (McNeely et al., 1972).

Nickel concentrations in drinking-water in European countries were reported to range in general from 2-13 µg/l (mean, 6 µg/l) (Amavis et al., 1976). Other studies have suggested low background levels in drinking-water, e.g., in Finland an average of about 1 µg/l (Punsar et al., 1975) and in Italy mostly below 10 µg/l. In the German Democratic Republic, drinking-water from groundwater showed an average level of 10 µg/l nickel, slightly below the amount present in surface water (Grandjean, 1984). In the Federal Republic of Germany, the mean concentration of nickel in drinking-water was 9 µg/l, with a maximal value of 34 µg/l (Scheller et al., 1988).

The nickel concentration in seawater ranges from 0.1 to 0.5 µg/l, whereas the average level in surface waters is 15-20 µg/l. Freshly fallen arctic snow was reported to contain 0.02 µg/kg, a level that represents 5–10% of those in annual condensed layers (Mart, 1983).

Nickel concentrations of 100 µg/l have been found in wine; average levels of about 30 µg/l were measured in beer and levels of a few micrograms per litre in mineral water (Grandjean, 1984). In the Federal Republic of Germany, however, the mean concentration of nickel in mineral waters was 10 µg/l, with a maximal value of 31 µg/l (Scheller et al., 1988).

(f)    Soil

The nickel content of soil may vary widely, depending on mineral composition: a normal range of nickel in cultivated soils is 5-500 µg/g, with a typical level of 50 µg/g (National Research Council, 1975). In an extensive survey of soils in England and Wales, nickel concentrations were generally 4-80 µg/g (median, 26 µg/g; maximum, 228 µg/g) (Archer, 1980). Farm soils from different parts of the world contained 3-1000 µg/g. Nickel may be added to agricultural soils by application of sewage sludge (National Research Council, 1975).

The nickel content of coal was 4-24 µg/g, whereas crude oils (especially those from Angola, Colombia and California) contained up to 100 µg/g (Tissot & Weltle, 1984; World Health Organization, 1990).

### (g)  Food

Nickel levels in various foods have been summarized recently (Grandjean, 1984; Smart & Sherlock, 1987; Scheller *et al.*, 1988; Grandjean *et al.*, 1989). Table 16 gives the results of analyses for nickel in various foodstuffs in Denmark; the mean level of nickel in meat, fruit and vegetables was ≤0.2 mg/kg fresh weight. This result was confirmed by analysis of hundreds of food samples from Denmark, the Federal Republic of Germany and the UK (Nielsen & Flyvholm, 1984; Veien & Andersen, 1986; Smart & Sherlock, 1987; Scheller *et al.*, 1988): the nickel content of most samples was < 0.5 mg/kg. The nickel concentration in nuts was up to 3 mg/kg (Veien & Andersen, 1986) and that in cocoa up to 10 mg/kg (Nielsen & Flyvholm, 1984). The nickel content of wholemeal flour and bread was significantly higher than that of more refined products due to the high nickel content of wheat germ (Smart & Sherlock, 1987). High nickel levels in flour may also originate from contamination during milling. In addition, fats can contain nickel, probably owing to the use of nickel catalysts in commercial hydrogenation. Margarine normally contains less than 0.2 mg/kg, but levels up to 6 mg/kg have been found (Grandjean, 1984).

**Table 16. Nickel content (mg/kg) in foods in the average Danish diet**[a]

| Food | No. of samples | Range | Mean |
|------|----------------|-------|------|
| Milk products | | | |
|   Full milk | 63 | BDL[b]-0.13 | 0.02 |
|   Yogurt | 3 | 0.004-0.03 | 0.01 |
|   Cream | 3 | 0.01-0.04 | 0.03 |
|   Cheese | 25 | 0.02-0.34 | 0.10 |
| Meat, fish, eggs | | | |
|   Beef | 32 | 0.01-0.03 | 0.02 |
|   Pork | 20 | < 0.02-0.02 | 0.02 |
|   Chicken | 9 | 0.02-0.24 | 0.11 |
|   Lamb | 12 | < 0.02-0.02 | 0.02 |
|   Liver, kidney | 108 | 0-0.94 | 0.11 |
|   Fish | 658 | 0.005-0.303 | 0.04 |
|   Egg | 30 | 0.01-0.35 | 0.05 |
| Roots and vegetables | | | |
|   Potatoes | 45 | BDL-0.44 | 0.14 |
|   Carrots | 17 | < 0.01-0.16 | 0.04 |
|   Celery root | 8 | 0.04-0.1 | 0.06 |
|   Beetroot | 7 | 0.01-0.3 | 0.12 |
|   Cabbage | 31 | 0.01-0.63 | 0.17 |
|   Cauliflower | 5 | 0.03-1.0 | 0.3 |

**Table 16 (contd)**

| Food | No. of samples | Range | Mean |
|------|----------------|-------|------|
| Roots and vegetables (contd) | | | |
| Kale | 2 | 0.15-0.24 | 0.20 |
| Lettuce | 21 | BDL-1.4 | 0.36 |
| Spinach | 15 | 0.02-2.99 | 0.52 |
| Asparagus | 1 | - | 0.42 |
| Cucumber | 8 | 0.01-0.11 | 0.04 |
| Tomatoes | 21 | 0.01-0.25 | 0.07 |
| Peas | 24 | 0.13-0.8 | 0.42 |
| Fruits | | | |
| Apples | 11 | BDL-0.03 | 0.01 |
| Pears | 10 | 0.07-0.42 | 0.14 |
| Plums | 10 | 0.03-0.20 | 0.12 |
| Currants | 13 | 0.01-0.2 | 0.06 |
| Strawberries | 9 | 0.03-0.08 | 0.05 |
| Rhubarb | 10 | 0.01-0.22 | 0.13 |
| Grapes | 4 | 0.01-0.04 | 0.02 |
| Raisins | 3 | 0.02-0.04 | 0.03 |
| Citrus fruits | 3 | 0.01-0.04 | 0.03 |
| Bananas | 4 | 0.01-0.03 | 0.02 |
| Canned fruits | 65 | 0.02-1.36 | 0.31 |
| Juice | 11 | 0.01-0.17 | 0.04 |
| Meal, grain and bread | | | |
| Wheat flour | 32 | 0.03-0.3 | 0.13 |
| Rye flour | 15 | 0.03-0.3 | 0.1 |
| Oatmeal | 18 | 0.80-4.7 | 1.76 |
| Rice | 16 | 0.08-0.45 | 0.21 |
| Other | | | |
| Butter | 4 | 0.03-0.2 | 0.1 |
| Margarine | 13 | 0.2-2.5 | 0.34 |
| Sugar | 22 | 0.01-0.09 | 0.05 |

[a]From Grandjean et al. (1989)
[b]BDL, below detection limit [not specified]

Stainless-steel kitchen utensils have been shown to release nickel into acid solutions, especially during boiling (Christensen & Möller, 1978). The amount of nickel liberated depends on the composition of the utensil, the pH of the food and the length of contact. The average contribution of kitchen utensils to the oral intake of nickel is unknown, but they could augment alimentary exposure by as much as 1 mg/day (Grandjean et al., 1989).

A study of hospital diets in the USA showed that the general diet contained 160 μg/day, and special diets varied by less than 40% from this level (Myron *et al.*, 1978). A recent study (Nielsen & Flyvholm, 1984) suggested a daily intake of 150 μg in the average Danish diet. Knutti and Zimmerli (1985) found dietary intakes in Switzerland of 73 ± 9 μg in a restaurant, 83 ± 9 μg in a hospital, 141 + 33 μg in a vegetarian restaurant and 142 ± 20 μg in a military canteen. The mean nickel intake in the UK in 1981-84 was 140-150 μg/day (Smart & Sherlock, 1987).

### (h)  Humans tissues and secretions

The estimated average body burden of nickel in adults is 0.5 mg/70 kg (7.4 μg/ kg bw). In post-mortem tissue samples from adults with no occupational or iatrogenic exposure to nickel compounds, the highest nickel concentrations were found in lung, bone, thyroid and adrenals, followed by kidney, heart, liver, brain, spleen and pancreas in diminishing order (Seemann *et al.*, 1985; Sunderman, 1986b; Raithel, 1987; Raithel *et al.*, 1987; Rezuke *et al.*, 1987; Kollmeier *et al.*, 1988; Raithel *et al.*, 1988). Reference values for nickel concentrations in autopsy tissues from nonexposed persons are listed in Table 17.

The mean nickel concentration in lung tissues from 39 nickel refinery workers autopsied during 1978-84 was 150 (1-1344) μg/g dry weight. Workers employed in the roasting and smelting department had an average nickel concentration of 333 (7-1344) μg/g, and those who had worked in the electrolysis department had an average nickel concentration of 34 (1-216) μg/g dry weight. Lung tissue from 16 persons who were not connected with the refinery contained an average level of 0.76 (0.39-1.70) μg/g dry weight (Andersen & Svenes, 1989).

The concentrations of nickel in body fluids have diminished substantially over the past ten years as a consequence of improved analytical techniques, including better procedures to minimize nickel contamination during collection and assay. Concentrations of nickel in human body fluids and faeces are given in Table 18 (see also Sunderman, 1986b; Sunderman *et al.*, 1986a).

### (i)  Iatrogenic exposures

Potential iatrogenic sources of exposure to nickel are dialysis treatment, leaching of nickel from nickel-containing alloys used as prostheses and implants and contaminated intravenous medications (for review, see Grandjean, 1984; Sunderman *et al.*, 1986a).

**Table 17. Concentrations of nickel in human autopsy tissues**

| Tissue | No. of subjects | Nickel concentration | | | | Reference |
|--------|-----------------|----------------------|---|---|---|-----------|
| | | ng/g wet weight | | ng/g dry weight | | |
| | | Mean±SD | Range | Mean±SD | Range | |
| Lung | 4 | 16 ± 8 | 8-24 | 86 ± 56 | 33-146 | Rezuke et al. (1987) |
| | 8 | 119 ± 50 | 48-221 | - | - | |
| | 9 | - | - | 132 ± 99 | 50-290 | |
| | 41 | 7 ± 10 | < 1-70 | - | - | |
| | 9 | 18 ± 12 | 7-46 | 173 ± 94 | 71-371 | |
| | 15 | - | - | 180 ± 105 | 43-361 | Seemann et al. (1985) |
| | 70 | 137 ± 187 | - | 754 ± 1010 | - | Kollmeier et al. (1988) |
| | 30 | 20-40[a] | 8-120[a] | 107-195[a] | 42-600[a] | Raithel et al. (1988) |
| | 16 | - | - | 760 ± 390 | 390-1700 | Andersen & Svenes (1989) |
| Kidney | 8 | 11 ± 4 | 7-15 | - | - | Rezuke et al. (1987) |
| | 6 | - | - | 125 ± 54 | 50-120 | |
| | 36 | 14 ± 27 | < 1-165 | - | - | |
| | 10 | 9 ± 6 | 3-25 | 62 ± 43 | 19-171 | |
| | 18 | - | - | 34 ± 22 | < 5-84 | Seemann et al. (1985) |
| Liver | 4 | 9 ± 3 | 5-13 | 32 ± 12 | 21-48 | Rezuke et al. (1987) |
| | 8 | 8 ± 2 | 6-11 | - | - | |
| | 10 | 10 ± 7 | 8-21 | 50 ± 31 | 11-102 | |
| | 23 | - | - | 18 ± 21 | < 5-86 | Seemann et al. (1985) |
| Heart | 4 | 6 ± 2 | 4-8 | 23 ± 6 | 16-30 | Rezuke et al. (1987) |
| | 8 | 7 ± 2 | 4-9 | - | - | |
| | 9 | 8 ± 5 | 1-14 | 54 ± 40 | 10-110 | |
| Spleen | 22 | - | - | 23 ± 20 | < 5-85 | Seemann et al. (1985) |
| | 10 | 7 ± 5 | 1-15 | 37 ± 31 | 9-95 | Rezuke et al. (1987) |

[a]Range of median values and 68th percentile of range on the basis of 600 lung specimens from 30 autopsies

**Table 18. Nickel concentrations in specimens from healthy, unexposed adults**[a]

| Specimen | Mean ± SD | Range | Units |
|---|---|---|---|
| Whole blood | 0.34 ± 0.28 | <0.05-1.05 | μg/l |
| Serum | 0.28 ± 0.24 | <0.05-1.08 | μg/l |
| Urine (spot collection) | 2.0 ± 1.5 | 0.5-6.1 | μg/l |
| | 2.0 ± 1.5 | 0.4-6.0 | μg/g creatinine |
| | 2.8 ± 1.9 | 0.5-8.8 | μg/l[b] |
| Urine (24-h collection) | 2.2 ± 1.2 | 0.7-5.2 | μg/l |
| | 2.6 ± 1.4 | 0.5-6.4 | μg/day |
| Faeces (3-day collection) | 14.2 ± 2.7 | 10.8-18.7 | μg/g (dry weight) |
| | 258 ± 126 | 80-540 | μg/day |

[a]From Sunderman *et al.* (1986a)
[b]Factored to specific gravity = 1.024

Hypernickelaemia has been observed in patients with chronic renal disease who are maintained by extracorporeal haemodialysis or peritoneal dialysis (Table 19; Linden *et al.*, 1984; Drazniowsky *et al.*, 1985; Hopfer *et al.*, 1985; Savory *et al.*, 1985; Wills *et al.*, 1985). In one severe incident, water from a nickel-plated stainless-steel water-heater contaminated the dialysate to approximately 250 μg/l, resulting in plasma nickel levels of 3000 μg/l and acute nickel toxicity (Webster *et al.*, 1980). Even during normal operation, the average intravenous uptake of nickel may be 100 μg per dialysis (Sunderman, 1983a).

Nickel-containing alloys may be implanted in patients as joint prostheses, plates and screws for fractured bones, surgical clips and steel sutures (Grandjean, 1984). Corrosion of these prostheses and implants can result in accumulation of alloy-specific metals in the surrounding soft tissues and in release of nickel to the extracellular fluid (Sunderman *et al.*, 1986a, 1989a).

High concentrations of nickel have been reported in human albumin solutions prepared by six manufacturers for intravenous infusion. In three lots that contained 50 g/l albumin, the average nickel concentration was 33 μg/l (range, 11-17 μg/l); in nine lots that contained 250 g/l albumin, the average nickel concentration was 83 μg/l (range, 26-222 μg/l) (Leach & Sunderman, 1985). Meglumine diatrizoate ('Renografin-76'), an X-ray contrast medium, tends to be contaminated with nickel. Seven lots of this preparation (containing 760 g/l diatrizoate) contained

**Table 19. Nickel concentrations in dialysis fluids and in serum specimens from patients with chronic renal disease (CRD)[a]**

| Region and patients | No. of subjects | Ni conc. in dialysis fluid (μg/l) | Serum Ni concentration (μg/l) | |
|---|---|---|---|---|
| | | | Pre-dialysis | Post-dialysis |
| **USA** | | | | |
| Healthy controls | 30 | | 0.3 ± 0.2 | |
| Non-dialysed CRD patients | 7 | | 0.6 ± 0.3 | |
| CRD patients on haemodialysis | | | | |
| Hospital A | 40 | 0.82 | 6.2 ± 1.8 | 7.2 ± 2.2 |
| Hospital B | 9 | 0.40-0.42 | 3.9 ± 2.0 | 5.2 ± 2.5 |
| Hospital C | 10 | 0.68 | 3.0 ± 1.3 | 3.7 ± 1.3 |
| **USA** | | | | |
| Healthy controls | 50 | | 0.4 ± 0.2 | |
| CRD patients on haemodialysis | 28 | | 3.7 ± 1.5 | |
| **UK and Hong Kong** | | | | |
| Healthy controls | 71 | | 1.0 (<0.6-3.0) | |
| Non-dialysed CRD patients | 31 | | 1.6 (<0.6-3.6) | |
| CRD patients on haemodialysis | | | | |
| Hospital A | 25 | 2-3 | 8.6 (0.6-16.6) | 8.8 (3.0-21.4) |
| Hospital B | 16 | | 2.9 (1.8-4.0) | 3.4 (2.2-5.4) |
| CRD patients on peritoneal dialysis | 13 | 2-3 | 8.6 (5.4-11.4) | |

[a]From Sunderman *et al.* (1986a)

nickel at 144 ± 44 μg/l. Serum nickel concentrations in 11 patients who received intra-arterial injections of 'Renografin-76' (164 ± 10 ml per patient [giving 19.1 ± 4.0 μg Ni per patient]) for coronary arteriography increased from a pre-injection level of 1.33 μg/l (range, 0.11-5.53 μg/l) to 2.95 μg/l (range, 1.5-7.19 μg/l) 15 min post-injection. Serum levels remained significantly elevated for 4 h and returned to baseline levels only 24 h post-injection (Leach & Sunderman, 1987).

*(j)  Regulatory status and guidelines*

Occupational exposure limits for nickel in various forms are given in Table 20.

**Table 20. Occupational exposure limits for airborne nickel in various forms**[a]

| Country or region | Year | Nickel species | Concentration (mg/m³) | Interpretation[b] |
|---|---|---|---|---|
| Belgium | 1987 | Nickel metal and insoluble nickel compounds (as Ni) | 0.1 | TWA |
| | | Nickel carbonyl (as Ni) | 0.35 | TWA |
| Brazil | 1987 | Nickel carbonyl (as Ni) | 0.28 | TWA |
| Chile | 1987 | Soluble nickel compounds (as Ni) | 0.08 | TWA |
| China | 1987 | Nickel carbonyl (as Ni) | 0.001 | TWA |
| Denmark | 1988 | Nickel metal | 0.5 | TWA |
| | | Nickel carbonyl | 0.007 | TWA |
| | | Soluble nickel compounds (as Ni) | 0.1 | TWA |
| | | Insoluble nickel compounds (as Ni) | 1 | TWA |
| Finland | 1987 | Nickel metal | 1 | TWA |
| | | Nickel carbonyl | 0.007 | TWA |
| | | Soluble nickel compounds (as Ni) | 0.1 | TWA |
| France | 1986 | Nickel sulfide (as Ni) | 1 | TWA |
| German Democratic Republic | 1987 | Nickel compounds (as Ni) | 0.25 | TWA |
| | | Nickel carbonyl (as Ni) | 0.01 | TWA |
| | | Nickel compounds (as Ni) | 0.5 | STEL |
| | | Nickel carbonyl (as Ni) | 0.03 | STEL |
| Hungary | 1987 | Nickel compounds (as Ni) | 0.005 | TWA/STEL |
| | | Nickel carbonyl (as Ni) | 0.007 | TWA/STEL |
| India | 1987 | Nickel carbonyl (as Ni) | 0.35 | TWA |
| Indonesia | 1987 | Nickel metal and insoluble nickel compounds (as Ni) | 1 | TWA |
| | | Nickel carbonyl (as Ni) | 0.007 | TWA |
| Italy | 1987 | Nickel carbonyl (as Ni) | 0.007 | TWA |
| Japan | 1987 | Nickel | 1 | TWA |
| | | Nickel carbonyl (as Ni) | 0.007 | TWA |
| Mexico | 1987 | Nickel metal and insoluble nickel compounds (as Ni) | 1 | TWA |
| | | Soluble nickel compounds (as Ni) | 0.1 | TWA |
| | | Nickel carbonyl (as Ni) | 0.35 | TWA |

**Table 20 (contd)**

| Country or region | Year | Nickel species | Concentration (mg/m³) | Interpretation[b] |
|---|---|---|---|---|
| Netherlands | 1986 | Nickel | 1 | TWA |
| | | Soluble nickel compounds (as Ni) | 0.1 | TWA |
| | | Nickel carbonyl (as Ni) | 0.35 | TWA |
| Poland | 1987 | Nickel carbonyl (as Ni) | 0.007 | TWA |
| Romania | 1987 | Nickel carbonyl (as Ni) | 0.002 | TWA |
| | | Nickel carbonyl (as Ni) | 0.005 | Ceiling |
| Sweden | 1987 | Nickel metal | 0.5 | TWA |
| | | Nickel carbonyl | 0.007 | TWA |
| | | Nickel subsulfide | 0.01 | TWA |
| | | Other nickel compounds (as Ni) | 0.1 | TWA |
| Switzerland | 1987 | Nickel metal and insoluble nickel compounds (as Ni) | 0.5 | TWA |
| | | Soluble nickel compounds (as Ni) | 0.05 | TWA |
| Taiwan | 1987 | Nickel carbonyl (as Ni) | 0.35 | TWA |
| UK | 1987 | Nickel and insoluble nickel compounds (as Ni) | 1 | TWA |
| | | Soluble nickel compounds (as Ni) | 0.1 | TWA |
| | | Soluble nickel compounds (as Ni) | 0.3 | STEL (10 min) |
| | | Insoluble nickel compounds (as Ni) | 3 | STEL (10 min) |
| | | Nickel carbonyl (as Ni) | 0.35 | TWA |
| USA | | | | |
| ACGIH | 1988 | Nickel metal; nickel sulfide roasting, fume and dust (as Ni) | 1 | TWA |
| | | Soluble compounds (as Ni) | 0.1 | TWA |
| | | Nickel carbonyl | 0.35 | TWA |
| NIOSH | 1988 | Nickel, inorganic compounds (as Ni) | 0.015 | TWA |
| | | Nickel carbonyl | 0.007 | TWA |
| OSHA | 1987 | Metallic nickel | 1 | TWA |
| | | Nickel carbonyl | 0.007 | TWA |
| | | Soluble nickel compounds (as Ni) | 0.1 | TWA |

**Table 20 (contd)**

| Country or region | Year | Nickel species | Concentration (mg/m³) | Interpretation[b] |
|---|---|---|---|---|
| USSR | 1987 | Nickel metal and insoluble nickel compounds (as Ni) | 0.5 | MAC |
| | | Nickel carbonyl (as Ni) | 0.0005 | MAC |
| | | Nickel monoxide, oxide, sulfide | 0.5 | MAC |

[a]From Arbeidsinspectie, 1986; Institut National de Recherche et de Sécurité, 1986; National Institute for Occupational Safety and Health (NIOSH), 1988; Arbetarskyddsstyrelsens, 1987; Cook, 1987; Health and Safety Executive, 1987; Työsuojeluhallitus, 1987; US Occupational Safety and Health Administration (OSHA), 1987; American Conference of Governmental Industrial Hygienists (ACGIH), 1988; Arbejdstilsynet, 1988

[b]TWA, time-weighted average; STEL, short-term exposure limit; MAC, maximum allowable concentration

## 2.4 Analysis

Typical methods for the analysis of nickel in air, water, food and biological materials are summarized in Table 21. A method has been developed for classifying nickel in airborne dust samples into four species — 'water-soluble', 'sulfidic', 'metallic' and 'oxidic' — on the basis of a sequential leaching procedure (Blakeley & Zatka, 1985; Zatka, 1987, 1988; Zatka et al., undated).

Atomic absorption spectrometry and differential pulse anodic stripping voltammetry (DPASV) are the most common methods for analysis of nickel in environmental and biological media. Air samples are collected on cellulose ester membrane filters, wet digested with nitric acid—perchloric acid and analysed by electrothermal atomic absorption spectrometry (EAAS) or inductively coupled argon plasma emission spectrometry (ICP) (National Institute for Occupational Safety and Health, 1984; Kettrup et al., 1985). The National Institute for Occupational Safety and Health (1977b, 1981) has recommended standard procedures for personal air sampling and analysis of nickel. The routine procedure does not permit identification of individual nickel compounds.

Assessment of individual nickel compounds, especially as components of complex mixtures, necessitates procedures such as X-ray diffraction and would not be feasible for routine monitoring. Sampling and analytical methods used to monitor air, water and soil have been summarized (US Environmental Protection Agency, 1986).

Nickel concentrations in blood, serum or urine are used as biological indicators of exposure to or body burden of nickel. Biological monitoring as a part of biomedical surveillance has been evaluated in several reviews (Aitio, 1984; Norseth,

**Table 21. Methods for the analysis of nickel**

| Sample matrix | Sample preparation | Assay procedure[a] | Sensitivity/detection limit | Reference |
|---|---|---|---|---|
| Air | Collect on cellulose ester membrane filter; digest with nitric acid and perchloric acid | AAS | – | National Institute for Occupational Safety and Health (1981) |
|  | Collect on cellulose acetate membrane filter; digest with nitric acid and hydrochloric acid | AAS | 1 µg absolute; 10 µg/m³ (sample volume, 0.1 m³) | Hauptverband der gewerblichen Berufsgenossenschaften (1981) |
|  | Collect on cellulose ester membrane filter; digest with nitric acid and perchloric acid | ICP | 1.5 µg/sample | National Institute for Occupational Safety and Health (1984) |
|  | Collect on cellulose ester membrane filter; digest with nitric acid | AAS | 20 ng/m³ (sample volume, 1.5 m³) | Kettrup et al. (1985) |
| Water | Chelate; extract with ammonium pyrrolidine dithiocarbamate: methyl isobutyl ketone | AAS | 0.04 µg/l | McNeely et al. (1972) |
|  | Filter; irradiate with ultraviolet | DPASV (dimethylglyoxime-sensitized) | 1 ng/l | Pihlar et al. (1981) |
|  | Chelate; extract with ammonium pyrrolidine dithiocarbamate: methyl isobutyl ketone | EAAS | 0.2 µg/l | Sunderman (1986b) |
| Food | Digest with acid | AAS | – | Evans et al. (1978) |
|  | Wet digest with nitric acid, hydrogen peroxide and sulfuric acid | DPASV (dimethylglyoxime-sensitized) | 1 ng/l digestion solution | Pihlar et al. (1981) |
|  | Dry ash | DPASV (dimethylglyoxime-sensitized) | 5 ng/sample | Meyer & Neeb (1985) |
|  | Dry ash, chelate with sodium(ditrifluoroethyl)dithiocarbamate | Chelate–GC | 100 ng/sample | Meyer & Neeb (1985) |
| Blood | Wet digest with nitric acid, hydrogen peroxide and sulfuric acid | DPASV (dimethylglyoxime-sensitized) | 1 ng/l digestion solution | Pihlar et al. (1981) |

**Table 21 (contd)**

| Sample matrix | Sample preparation | Assay procedure[a] | Sensitivity/detection limit | Reference |
|---|---|---|---|---|
| Serum/whole blood | Digest with nitric acid; heat | EAAS (Zeeman) | 0.05 μg/l serum<br>0.1 μg/l whole blood | Sunderman et al. (1984a) |
| Body fluids/ tissues | Digest with nitric acid, perchloric acid and sulfuric acid; chelate; extract with ammonium pyrrolidine dithiocarbamate: methyl isobutyl ketone | EAAS | 0.2 μg/l body fluids<br>0.4 μg/kg tissues | Sunderman (1986b) |
| Tissues | Homogenize; digest with nitric acid, perchloric acid and sulfuric acid | EAAS (Zeeman) | 0.01 μg/g dry wt | Sunderman et al. (1985a) |
|  | Digest with nitric acid and sulfuric acid | EAAS (Zeeman) | 0.8 μg/g wet wt | Raithel et al. (1987) |
| Serum/urine | Digest with nitric acid, perchloric acid and sulfuric acid; chelate; extract with ammonium pyrrolidine dithiocarbamate: methyl isobutyl ketone | EAAS | - | Brown et al. (1981) |
| Urine | Chelate; extract with ammonium pyrrolidine dithiocarbamate: methyl isobutyl ketone | EAAS | 0.5 μg/l | Schaller & Zober (1982) |
|  | Digest with nitric acid, perchloric acid and sulfuric acid | DPASV | 1 μg/l | Schramel et al. (1985) |
|  | Chelate; extract with hexamethylene ammonium: hexamethylene dithiocarbamate: diisopropylketone | AAS | 0.2 μg/l | Angerer & Schaller (1985) |
|  | Dilute with nitric acid | EAAS (Zeeman) | 0.5 μg/l | Sunderman et al. (1986b) |
|  | Dilute directly with nitric acid | EAAS | 1.2 μg/l | Kiilunen et al. (1987) |

[a]AAS, flameless atomic absorption spectrometry; ICP, inductively coupled argon plasma spectrometry; DPASV, differential pulse anodic stripping voltammetry; EAAS, electrothermal atomic absorption spectrometry; GC, gas chromatography

1984; Sunderman *et al.*, 1986a). Choice of specimen, sampling strategies, specimen collection, transport, storage and contamination control are of fundamental importance for an adequate monitoring programme (Sunderman *et al.*, 1986a). As discussed in recent reviews (Stoeppler, 1980; Schaller *et al.*, 1982; Stoeppler, 1984a,b; Sunderman *et al.*, 1986a, 1988a), EAAS and DPASV are practical, reliable techniques that furnish the requisite sensitivity for measurements of nickel concentrations in biological samples. The detection limits for determination of nickel by EAAS with Zeeman background correction are approximately 0.45 µg/l for urine, 0.1 µg/l for whole blood, 0.05 µg/l for serum or plasma, and 10 ng/g (dry wet) for tissues, foods and faeces (Andersen *et al.*, 1986; Sunderman *et al.*, 1986a,b; Kiilunen *et al.*, 1987; Angerer & Heinrich-Ramm, 1988). An EAAS procedure for the determination of nickel in serum and urine, which was developed on the basis of collaborative interlaboratory trials involving clinical biochemists in 13 countries, has been accepted as a reference method by the International Union of Pure and Applied Chemists (Brown *et al.*, 1981). This procedure, with additional applications for analysis of nickel in biological matrices, water and intravenous fluids, has also been accepted as a reference method by the IARC (Sunderman, 1986b). A new working method based on EAAS and Zeeman background correction for the analysis of nickel in serum, whole blood, tissues, urine and faeces has been recommended (Sunderman *et al.*, 1986a,b, 1988a). Sample preparation depends on the specimen and involves acid digestion for tissue and faeces, protein precipitation with nitric acid and heat for serum and whole blood, and simple acidification for urine.

Greater sensitivity can be achieved with DPASV analysis using a dimethylglyoxime-sensitized mercury electrode; this method has been reported to have a detection limit of 1 ng/l for determination of nickel in biological media (Flora & Nieboer, 1980; Pihlar *et al.*, 1981; Ostapczuk *et al.*, 1983). However, DPASV techniques are generally more cumbersome and time consuming than EAAS procedures. Isotope dilution mass spectrometry provides the requisite sensitivity, specificity and precision for determination of nickel (Fassett *et al.*, 1985) but has not yet been used to analyse nickel in biological samples.

Nickel carbonyl has been measured in air and exhaled breath by gas chromatography and chemiluminescence (Sunderman *et al.*, 1968; Stedman *et al.*, 1979).

# 3. Biological Data Relevant to the Evaluation of Carcinogenic Risk to Humans

## 3.1 Carcinogenicity studies in animals[1]

Experimental studies on animals exposed to nickel and various nickel compounds were reviewed previously in the *IARC Monographs* (IARC, 1976, 1987). Recent reviews on the biological and carcinogenic properties of nickel have been compiled by Fairhurst and Illing (1987), Kasprzak (1987) and Sunderman (1989), among others. In addition, a detailed document on the health effects of nickel has been prepared for the Ontario (Canada) Ministry of Labour (Odense University, 1986). A comprehensive technical report on nickel, emphasizing mutagenicity and carcinogenicity, was published by the European Chemical Industry Ecology and Toxicology Centre (1989).

### (a) Metallic nickel and nickel alloys

#### (i) Inhalation

*Mouse*: A group of 20 female C57Bl mice, two months of age, was exposed by inhalation to 15 mg/m³ metallic nickel powder ( > 99% pure; particle diameter, ≤4 µm) for 6 h per day on four or five days per week for 21 months. All mice had died by the end of the experiment. No lung tumour was observed. No control group was available (Hueper, 1958). [The Working Group noted the short duration of treatment.]

*Rat*: Groups of 50 male and 50 female Wistar rats and 60 female Bethesda black rats, two to three months of age, were exposed by inhalation to 15 mg/m³ metallic nickel powder ( > 99% pure nickel; particle diameter, ≤4 µm) for 6 h per day on four or five days per week for 21 months and observed up to 84 weeks. Histological examination of the lungs of 50 rats showed numerous multicentric, adenomatoid alveolar lesions and bronchial proliferations that were considered by the author as benign neoplasms. No specific control was included in the study (Hueper, 1958).

---

[1]The Working Group was aware of studies in progress of the carcinogenicity of nickel, nickel acetate tetrahydrate, nickel alloys, nickel–aluminium alloys, nickel chloride hexahydrate, nickel oxide, nickel sulfide and nickel sulfate hexa– and heptahydrate in experimental animals by intraperitoneal, subcutaneous, inhalation and intratracheal administration (IARC, 1988b).

In a further experiment with Bethesda black rats, exposure to metallic nickel powder (99.95% nickel; particle diameter, 1-3 μm) was combined with 20-35 ppm (50-90 mg/m³) sulfur dioxide as a mucosal irritant; powdered chalk was added to prevent clumping. Exposure was for 5-6 h per day [nickel concentration unspecified]. Forty-six of 120 rats lived for longer than 18 months. No lung tumour was observed, but many rats developed squamous metaplasia and peribronchial adenomatoses (Hueper & Payne, 1962).

*Guinea-pig.* A group of 32 male and 10 female strain 13 guinea-pigs, about three months of age, was exposed by inhalation to 15 mg/m³ metallic nickel powder (>99% pure nickel) for 6 h per day on four or five days per week for 21 months. Mortality was high: only 23 animals survived to 12 months and all animals had died by 21 months. Almost all animals developed adenomatoid alveolar lesions and terminal bronchiolar proliferations. No such lesion was observed in nine controls. One treated guinea-pig had an anaplastic intra-alveolar carcinoma, and another had an apparent adenocarcinoma metastasis in an adrenal node, although the primary tumour was not identified (Hueper, 1958).

### (ii) *Intratracheal instillation*

*Rat.* Two groups of female Wistar rats [number unspecified], 11 weeks of age, received either ten weekly intratracheal instillations of 0.9 mg metallic nickel powder [purity unspecified] or 20 weekly injections of 0.3 mg metallic nickel powder in 0.3 ml saline (total doses, 9 and 6 mg, respectively) and were observed for almost 2.5 years. Lung tumour incidence in the two groups was 8/32 (seven carcinomas, one mixed) and 10/39 (nine carcinomas, one adenoma), respectively; no lung tumour developed in 40 saline-treated controls maintained for up to 124 weeks. Pathological classification of the tumours in the two groups combined revealed one adenoma, four adenocarcinomas, 12 squamous-cell carcinomas and one mixed tumour. Average time to observation of the tumours was 120 weeks, the first tumour being observed after 98 weeks (Pott *et al.*, 1987).

*Hamster.* In a study reported in an abstract, groups of 100 Syrian golden hamsters received either a single intratracheal instillation of 10, 20 or 40 mg of metallic nickel powder (particle diameter, 3-8 μm) or of one of two nickel alloy powders (particle diameter, 0.5-2.5 μm; alloy I: 26.8% nickel, 16.2% chromium, 39.2% iron, 0.04% cobalt; alloy II: 66.5% nickel, 12.8% chromium, 6.5% iron, 0.2% cobalt) or four intratracheal instillations of 20 mg of one of the substances every six months (total dose, 80 mg). In the groups receiving single instillations of alloy II, the incidence of malignant intrathoracic tumours was reported as 1, 8 and 12%, respectively, suggesting a dose-response relationship. In the group receiving multiple instillations of alloy II, 10% of the animals developed intrathoracic malignant neoplasms, diagnosed as fibrosarcomas, mesotheliomas and rhabdomyosarcomas. Metallic nickel induced comparable numbers and types of intrathoracic neoplasms, but no tumour was observed in animals treated with alloy I or in control animals (Ivankovic et al., 1987).

A group of approximately 60 male and female Syrian golden hamsters (strain Cpb-ShGa 51), ten to 12 weeks of age, received 12 intratracheal instillations of 0.8 mg metallic nickel powder (99.9% nickel; mass median diameter, 3.1 μm) in 0.15 ml saline at two-week intervals (total dose, 9.6 mg). Additional groups were treated similarly with 12 intratracheal instillations of 3 mg pentlandite (containing 34.3% nickel; total dose, 36 mg), 3 or 9 mg chromium/nickel stainless-steel dust (containing 6.79% nickel; total doses, 36 and 108 mg) or 9 mg chromium stainless-steel dust (containing 0.5% nickel; total dose, 108 mg). The median lifespan was 90-130 weeks in the different groups. Two lung tumours were observed: an adenocarcinoma in the group that received nickel powder and an adenoma in the pentlandite-treated group. No lung tumour was observed in vehicle-treated controls or in the groups treated with stainless-steels (Muhle et al., 1990). [The Working Group noted that no lung tumour was observed in the positive control group.]

### (iii)  *Intrapleural administration*

*Rat*: A group of 25 female Osborne-Mendel rats, six months of age, received injections of a 12.5% suspension of metallic nickel powder in 0.05 ml lanolin into the right pleural cavity [6.25 mg nickel powder] once a month for five months. A group of 70 rats received injections of lanolin only. The experiment was terminated after 16 months. Four of the 12 treated rats that were examined had developed round-cell and spindle-cell sarcomas at the site of injection; no control animal developed a local tumour [$p < 0.01$] (Hueper, 1952).

A group of five male and five female Fischer 344 rats, 14 weeks of age, received injections of 5 mg metallic nickel powder suspended in 0.2 ml saline into the pleura (total dose, 25 mg) once a month for five months. Two rats developed mesotheliomas within slightly over 100 days; no tumour occurred in 20 controls (Furst et al., 1973). [The Working Group noted the limited reporting of the experiment.]

### (iv)  *Subcutaneous administration*

*Rat*: Groups of five male and five female Wistar rats, four to six weeks of age, received four subcutaneous implants of pellets (approximately 2×2 mm) of metallic nickel or nickel-gallium alloy (60% nickel) used for dental prostheses and were observed for 27 months. Local sarcomas were noted in 5/10 rats that received the metallic nickel and in 9/10 rats that received the nickel-gallium alloy. No local tumour occurred in ten groups of rats that received similar implants of other dental materials (Mitchell et al., 1960).

### (v) Intramuscular administration

*Rat*: A group of ten female hooded rats, two to three months of age, received a single intramuscular injection of 28.3 mg pure metallic nickel powder in 0.4 ml fowl serum into the right thigh. All animals developed rhabdomyosarcomas at the injection site within 41 weeks. Historical controls injected with fowl serum alone did not develop local tumours (Heath & Daniel, 1964).

Groups of 25 male and 25 female Fischer 344 rats [age unspecified] received five monthly intramuscular injections of 5 mg metallic nickel powder in 0.2 ml trioctanoin. Fibrosarcomas occurred in 38 treated animals but in none of a group of 25 male and 25 female controls given trioctanoin alone (Furst & Schlauder, 1971).

Two groups of ten male Fischer 344 rats, three months of age, received a single intramuscular injection of metallic nickel powder (3.6 or 14.4 mg/rat) in 0.5 ml penicillin G procaine. Surviving rats were killed 24 months after the injection. Sarcomas at the injection site were found in 0/10 and 2/9 treated rats, respectively, as compared with 0/20 vehicle controls (Sunderman & Maenza, 1976). [The Working Group noted the small number of animals used.]

Groups of 20 WAG rats [sex and age unspecified] received a single intramuscular injection of 20 mg metallic nickel powder in an oil vehicle [type unspecified]. A group of 56 control rats received 0.3 ml of the vehicle alone. Local sarcomas developed in 17/20 treated and 0/56 control rats (Berry *et al.*, 1984). [The Working Group noted the inadequate reporting of tumour induction.]

Groups of 20 or 16 male Fischer 344 rats, two to three months of age, received a single intramuscular injection of 14 mg metallic nickel powder (99.5% pure) or 14 mg (as nickel) of a ferronickel alloy ($NiFe_{1.6}$) in 0.3-0.5 ml penicillin G vehicle into the right thigh. Of the 20 rats receiving nickel powder, 13 developed tumours at the site of injection (mainly rhabdomyosarcomas), with an average latency of 34 weeks. No local tumour developed in the 16 rats given the ferronickel alloy, in 44 controls given penicillin G or in 40 controls given glycerol (Sunderman, 1984).

Groups of 40 male inbred WAG rats, 10-15 weeks of age, received a single intramuscular injection of 20 mg metallic nickel in paraffin oil. One group also received intramuscular injections of interferon at $5 \times 10^4$ U/rat twice a week beginning in the tenth week after nickel treatment. Rhabdomyosarcomas occurred in 14/30 and 5/10 rats in the two groups, respectively. Metallic nickel depressed natural killer cell activity. Prospective analysis of individual natural killer cell responses indicated that a persistent depression was restricted to rats that subsequently developed a tumour (Judde *et al.*, 1987).

*Hamster*: Furst and Schlauder (1971) compared the tumour response in Syrian hamsters with that of Fischer 344 rats (see above) to metallic nickel powder. Groups of 25 male and 25 female hamsters, three to four weeks old, received five monthly intramuscular injections of 5 mg nickel powder in 0.2 ml trioctanoin. Two fibrosarcomas occurred in males. No local tumour occurred in 25 male and 25 female controls injected with trioctanoin alone.

### (vi) *Intraperitoneal administration*

*Rat*: As reported in an abstract, a group of male and female Fischer rats [numbers unspecified], weighing 80-100 g, received intraperitoneal injections of 5 mg metallic nickel powder in 0.3 ml corn oil twice a month for eight months. A control group received injections of corn oil only. In the treated group, 30-50% of rats were reported to have developed intraperitoneal tumours (Furst & Cassetta, 1973).

A group of 50 female Wistar rats, 12 weeks of age, received ten weekly intraperitoneal injections of 7.5 mg metallic nickel powder [purity unspecified] (total dose, 75 mg). Abdominal tumours (sarcomas, mesotheliomas or carcinomas) developed in 46/48 (95.8%) rats at an average tumour latency of approximately eight months. Concurrent controls were not reported, but, in non-concurrent groups of saline controls, abdominal tumours were found in 0-6% of animals (Pott *et al.*, 1987).

Groups of female Wistar rats, 18 weeks of age, received single or repeated intraperitoneal injections of metallic nickel powder (100% nickel) or of one of three nickel alloys in 1 ml saline once or twice a week. All animals were sacrificed 30 months after the first injection. The incidences of local sarcomas and mesotheliomas in the peritoneal cavity are shown in Table 22. A dose-response trend was apparent for metallic nickel, and the tumour responses to the nickel alloys increased with the proportion of nickel present and the dose (Pott *et al.*, 1989, 1990). [The Working Group noted that the results at 30 months were available as an extended abstract only.]

### (vii) *Intravenous administration*

*Mouse*: A group of 25 male C57Bl mice, six weeks old, received two intravenous injections of 0.05 ml of a 0.005% suspension of metallic nickel powder in 2.5% gelatin into the tail vein. Nineteen animals survived more than 52 weeks, and six survived over 60 weeks. No tumour was observed. No control group was used (Hueper, 1955). [The Working Group noted the short period of observation.]

*Rat*: A group of 25 Wistar rats [sex unspecified], 24 weeks of age, received intravenous injections of 0.5 ml/kg bw metallic nickel powder as a 0.5% suspension in saline into the saphenous vein once a week for six weeks. Seven rats developed sarcomas in the groin region along the injection route [probably from seepage at the time of treatment]. No control group was used (Hueper, 1955).

**Table 22. Tumour responses of rats to intraperitoneal injection of nickel and nickel alloys**[a]

| Compound | Total dose (mg, as Ni) | Schedule | Mesotheliomas at two years | Sarcomas at two years | Local tumours at 30 months[b] |
|---|---|---|---|---|---|
| Metallic nickel | 6 | Single injection | 3 | 0 | 4/34 |
| | 12 | 2 × 6 mg | 3 | 2 | 5/34 |
| | 25 | 25 × 1 mg | 16 | 9 | 25/35 |
| Alloy (50% Ni) | 50 | Single injection | 1 | 7 | 8/35 |
| | 150 | 3 × 50 mg | 2 | 8 | 13/35 |
| Alloy (29% Ni)[c] | 50 | Single injection | 0 | 0 | 2/33 |
| | 100 | 2 × 50 mg | 0 | 1 | 1/36 |
| Alloy (66% Ni)[d] | 50 | Single injection | 0 | 11 | 12/35 |
| | 150 | 3 × 50 mg | 4 | 20 | 22/33 |
| Saline | | 3 × 1 ml | 0 | 1 | 1/33 |
| | | 50 × 1 ml | 0 | 0 | 0/34 |

[a]From Pott *et al.* (1989, 1990)
[b]Results not given separately for mesotheliomas and sarcomas
[c]Before milling: 32% Ni, 21% Cr, 0.8% Mn, 55% Fe
[d]Before milling: 74% Ni, 16% Cr, 7% Fe

### (viii) *Intrarenal administration*

*Rat*: A group of 20 female Sprague-Dawley rats, weighing 120-140 g, received an injection of 5 mg metallic nickel in 0.05 ml glycerine into each pole of the right kidney. No renal carcinoma or erythrogenic response developed within the 12-month period of observation (Jasmin & Riopelle, 1976).

Groups of male Fischer 344 rats, approximately two months of age, received an intrarenal injection of 7 mg metallic nickel powder or of a ferronickel alloy ($NiFe_{1.6}$; 7 mg Ni per rat) in 0.1 or 0.2 ml saline solution into each pole of the right kidney. The study was terminated after two years; the median survival time was 100 weeks in the two treated groups compared with 91 weeks in controls. Renal cancers occurred in 0/18 and 1/14 rats, respectively, compared with 0/46 saline-treated controls. The tumour was a nephroblastoma which was observed at 25 weeks (Sunderman *et al.*, 1984b).

### (ix) *Implantation of ear-tags*

*Rat*: In a study carried out to assess the carcinogenicity of cadmium chloride, 168 male Wistar rats, six weeks of age, received identification ear-tags fabricated of nickel-copper alloy (65% Ni, 32% Cu, 1% Fe, 1% Mn). A total of 14 tumours, mostly osteosarcomas, developed within 104 weeks at the site of implantation. The authors implicated nickel in the alloy as the probably causative agent and apparent local microbial infection as a contributory factor (Waalkes *et al.*, 1987).

### (x) *Other routes of administration*

*Rat*: In groups of 20 WAG rats [sex and age unspecified] *subperiosteal injection* of 20 mg metallic nickel powder resulted in local tumours in 11/20 rats; *intramedullary injection* of 20 mg metallic nickel resulted in local tumours in 9/20 rats (Berry *et al.*, 1984). [The Working Group noted the absence of controls and the inadequate reporting of tumour induction.]

### (xi) *Administration with known carcinogens*

*Rat*: Four groups of female Wistar rats [initial numbers unspecified], four to six weeks old, received intratracheal instillations of 1 or 5 mg 20-methylcholanthrene (MC) alone or with 10 mg metallic nickel powder (99.5% nickel). A fifth group received 10 mg metallic nickel powder only. At 12 weeks, squamous-cell carcinomas had developed as follows: 5 mg MC, 2/7; 5 mg MC plus Ni, 3/5; 1 mg MC, 0/8; 1 mg MC plus Ni, 0/7; metallic Ni alone, 0/7. Pretumorous lesions were more marked and the amount of epithelial metaplasia enhanced in groups receiving the combined treatment or MC only (Mukubo, 1978). [The Working Group noted the small number of animals used and the short duration of observation.]

### (b) *Nickel oxides and hydroxides*

The compounds considered under this heading include a variety of substances of nominally similar composition, which, however, may vary considerably due to differences in production methods. These differences were not generally defined in the studies described below, beyond the relatively recent designation of green and black nickel oxide.

### (i) *Inhalation*

*Rat*: Groups of six or eight male Wistar rats, two months of age, were exposed by inhalation to 0.6 or 8.0 mg/m³ nickel monoxide (green) particles (median aerodynamic diameter, 1.2 µm) for 6 h per day on five days per week for one month, after which they were maintained with no further exposure for an additional 20 months. Histopathological examination revealed one adenocarcinoma and one adenomatous lesion of the lung in the low-exposure rats and one adenomatosis in the high-exposure group. Bronchial glandular hyperplasia was seen in five and six rats in the low- and high-dose groups, respectively; a malignant histiocytoma that emanated from the paranasal region was noted in the upper respiratory tract of one rat [group unspecified]. None of the five control rats developed these lesions, although both control and exposed animals exhibited some squamous metaplasia (Horie *et al.*, 1985). [The Working Group noted the small number of animals used and the short exposure period.]

Groups of 40 and 20 male Wistar rats, five weeks of age, were exposed by inhalation to 60 and 200 $\mu g/m^3$ nickel as nickel monoxide aerosol (particle size, $<0.3$ $\mu m$) continuously for 18 months, followed by an observation period of one year under normal atmospheric conditions. At 24 months, 80% of animals in the treatment group had died, and at termination of the study (30 months) 62.5% of controls had died. No carcinogenic effect was observed (Glaser et al., 1986). [The Working Group noted that the toxic effects, particularly alveolar proteinosis, were severe, that the survival of the animals was too short for carcinogenicity to be evaluated fully, and that nickel oxide aerosols were generated by atomization of aqueous nickel acetate solutions.]

Hamster: A group of 51 male Syrian golden hamsters, two months of age, was exposed by inhalation to a mean aerosol concentration of 53.2 $mg/m^3$ nickel monoxide (mean particle diameter, 0.3 $\mu m$) for 7 h per day on five days per week for life. Another group of 51 males was exposed to nickel monoxide plus cigarette smoke. Two control groups of 51 animals were exposed to smoke and sham dust or to sham smoke and sham dust. Massive pneumoconiosis with lung consolidation developed in the nickel monoxide-exposed animals but did not affect their lifespan. Mean lifespan was $19.6 \pm 1.6$ months for animals exposed to smoke and nickel monoxide, $16.1 \pm 1.1$ for sham-exposed nickel oxide-treated animals and $19.6 \pm 1.4$ and $15.3 \pm 1.3$ months for the respective controls. No significant increase in the incidence of respiratory tumours or any evidence of cocarcinogenic interaction with cigarette smoke was noted for nickel monoxide. One osteosarcoma occurred in the nickel monoxide-treated group and one osteosarcoma and one rhabdomyosarcoma in the muscle of the thorax were seen in the group given nickel monoxide plus cigarette smoke (Wehner et al., 1975, 1979).

### (ii) Intratracheal instillation

Rat: Groups of female Wistar rats [numbers unspecified], 11 weeks of age, received ten weekly intratracheal instillations of 5 or 15 mg nickel as nickel monoxide (99.99% pure) in 0.3 ml saline to give total doses of 50 and 150 mg nickel, respectively. A control group of 40 rats received injections of saline only and were observed for 124 weeks. Lung tumour incidence in the two treated groups was 10/37 (27%) and 12/38 (31.6%), respectively; the tumours in the two groups consisted of four adenocarcinomas, two mixed tumours and 16 squamous-cell carcinomas. No lung tumour occurred in controls (Pott et al., 1987).

Hamster: In an experiment designed to study the effects of particulates on the carcinogenesis of N-nitrosodiethylamine, groups of 25 male and 25 female hamsters [strain unspecified], five weeks old, received intratracheal instillations of 0.2 ml of a suspension of 2 g nickel monoxide (particle size, 0.5-1.0 $\mu m$) in 100 ml 0.5% w/v gelatin/saline once a week for 30 weeks. A group of 50 controls received injections of carbon dust in the vehicle. Only three hamsters in each group survived beyond 48 weeks. One respiratory tract tumour [unspecified] was found in the 47 nickel monoxide-treated animals that were necropsied and four in controls. A high incidence of respiratory-tract tumours was observed in animals treated with N-nitrosodiethylamine alone (Farrell & Davis, 1974). [The Working Group noted the poor survival of treated and control animals.]

### (iii) *Intrapleural administration*

*Rat*: A group of 32 male Wistar rats, three months of age, received a single intrapleural injection of 10 mg nickel monoxide in 0.4 ml saline suspension. A positive control group of 32 rats received a 10 mg injection of crocidolite, and a negative control group of 32 rats received saline alone. After 30 months, 31/32 rats in the nickel monoxide-treated group had developed injection-site tumours (mostly rhabdomyosarcomas). Median survival time was 224 days. Nine of 32 rats in the crocidolite-treated group had local tumours, but none of the saline controls developed local sarcomas (Skaug *et al.*, 1985).

### (iv) *Intramuscular administration*

*Mouse*: Two groups of 50 Swiss and 52 C3H mice, equally divided by sex, two to three months of age, received single intramuscular injections of 5 mg nickel monoxide in penicillin G procaine into each thigh muscle and were observed for up to 476 days. Local sarcomas (mainly fibrosarcomas) occurred in 33 Swiss and 23 C3H mice. No control was reported (Gilman, 1962).

*Rat*: A group of 32 Wistar rats [sex unspecified], two to three months of age, received single intramuscular injections of 20 mg nickel monoxide powder into each thigh muscle and were observed for up to 595 days. Twenty-one rats developed a total of 26 tumours at the site of injection; 80% of the tumours were rhabdomyosarcomas, and the average latent period was 302 days. No control was reported (Gilman, 1962).

Groups of 20 Fischer rats [sex and age unspecified] received single intramuscular injections at two sites of either nickel hydroxide or nickel monoxide [dose unspecified] in aqueous penicillin G procaine. Local sarcomas developed in 15/20 (19 tumours at 40 sites) and 2/20 rats, respectively. Concurrent vehicle controls were not used. Seventeen of 20 animals given nickel subsulfide [dose unspecified] as positive controls developed local sarcomas. No tumour developed at the injection sites in two other groups of rats in the same experimental series injected intramuscularly with either nickel sulfate or nickel sulfide [presumed to be amorphous] (Gilman, 1966).

Ten male and ten female Wistar rats, weighing 150-170 g, received an intramuscular injection of 3 mg nickel trioxide powder. No control group was reported. No neoplasm developed at the injection site (Sosiński, 1975).

A group of 15 male Fischer 344 rats, two months of age, received a single intramuscular injection of nickel at 14 mg/rat as nickel monoxide (bunsenite, green-grey (Sunderman, 1984); 99.9% pure; particle diameter, <2 μm) in 0.3 ml of a 1:1 v/v glycerol:water vehicle into the right thigh and were observed for 104 weeks. Fourteen animals developed local sarcomas (mostly rhabdomyosarcomas) with a median tumour latency of 49 weeks and a median survival time of 58 weeks; metastases occurred in 4/14 rats. None of 40 control rats injected with vehicle alone developed tumours at the site of injection; 25/40 control rats were still alive at termination of the experiment (Sunderman & McCully, 1983).

Groups of 20 male Wistar rats, weighing 200-220 g, received a single intramuscular injection of 120 μmol [7.1 mg] nickel as one of three nickel hydroxide preparations — an air-dried gel, crystalline industrial nickel hydroxide and a freshly prepared colloidal nickel hydroxide — in 0.1 ml distilled water. A positive control group was treated with 120 μmol [7.1 mg] nickel as nickel subsulfide (see also p. 337) and a negative control group was treated with sodium sulfate. Seven rats treated with the colloidal preparation and one treated with the gel died from haematuria one to two weeks after the treatment. Six ulcerating, tumour-like growths developed between five and six months after treatment in the crystalline-treated group, but these regressed and were not included in tabulations. Local tumours occurred in 5/19 rats (four rhabdomyosarcomas, one fibrosarcoma) given the dried gel, 3/20 (all rhabdomyosarcomas) given the crystalline compound, 0/13 given the colloidal preparation, 16/20 positive controls and 0/20 negative controls (Kasprzak et al., 1983). [See also pp. 360-361.]

In the study by Berry et al. (1984) described on p. 321, no tumour was induced by 20 mg nickel monoxide by either the intramuscular or subperiosteal route in groups of 20 rats.

In the study by Judde et al. (1987) described on p. 321, no tumour was induced by 20 mg nickel trioxide in ten rats.

### (v) Intraperitoneal administration

Rat: A group of 50 female Wistar rats, 12 weeks of age, received two intraperitoneal injections of 500 mg nickel as nickel monoxide (99.99% pure); 46/47 of the animals developed abdominal tumours (sarcomas, mesotheliomas or carcinomas) with an average tumour latency of 31 months. Concurrent controls were not reported but, in other groups of saline controls, the incidence of abdominal tumours ranged from 0 to 6% (Pott et al., 1987).

In a study described earlier (p. 322), single injections of 25 and 100 mg nickel as nickel monoxide induced local sarcomas and mesotheliomas in the peritoneal cavity in 12/34 and 15/36 female Wistar rats, respectively, after 30 months (Pott et al.,

1989, 1990). [The Working Group noted that the results at 30 months were available as an extended abstract only.]

### (vi) *Intrarenal administration*

*Rat*: A group of 12 male Fischer 344 rats, two months of age, received an injection of nickel monoxide (green; 7 mg/rat nickel) in 0.1 or 0.2 ml saline into each pole of the right kidney and were observed for two years. No renal carcinoma was observed (Sunderman *et al.*, 1984b; see also p. 323).

### (vii) *Intracerebral injection*

*Rat*: A group of ten male and ten female Wistar rats, weighing 150-170 g, received an intracerebral injection of 3 mg nickel trioxide powder into the cerebral cortex. No control group was reported. Cerebral sarcomas [gliomas] were observed in two rats that were killed at 14 and 21 months, respectively, and a meningioma was found in one rat that was killed at 21 months (Sosiński, 1975).

### (c) *Nickel sulfides*

The experiments described below refer primarily to α-nickel subsulfide and to other crystalline forms of nickel sulfide, except where specifically stated that an amorphous form was tested.

### (i) *Inhalation*

*Rat*: A group of 122 male and 104 female Fischer 344 rats [age unspecified] was exposed by inhalation to 0.97 mg/m$^3$ nickel subsulfide (particle diameter, < 1.5 μm) for 6 h per day on five days per week for 78 weeks. The remaining rats were observed for another 30 weeks, by which time survival was less than 5%. Survival of a group of 241 control rats exposed to filtered room air was 31% at 108 weeks. A significant increase in the incidence of benign and malignant lung tumours was observed compared to controls. Among treated rats, 14 malignant (ten adenocarcinomas, three squamous-cell carcinomas, one fibrosarcoma) and 15 benign lung tumour-bearing animals were identified; one adenocarcinoma and one adenoma developed among controls. The earliest tumour appeared at 76 weeks, and the average tumour latency was approximately two years. An elevated incidence of hyperplastic and metaplastic lung lesions was also noted among nickel subsulfide-treated rats (Ottolenghi *et al.*, 1974).

### (ii) *Intratracheal instillation*

*Mouse*: Groups of 20 male B6C3F1 mice, eight weeks of age, received intratracheal instillations of 0.024, 0.056, 0.156, 0.412 or 1.1 mg/kg bw nickel subsulfide (particle size, < 2 μm) in saline once a week for four weeks and were observed for up to 27 months, at which time about 50% of the animals had died. Lung tumours occurred in all groups; no significant difference from controls and no dose-response relationship was observed. No damage to the respiratory tract that was attributable to treatment was seen (Fisher et al., 1986). [The Working Group noted the low doses used.]

Rat: Groups of 47, 45 and 40 female Wistar rats, 11 weeks of age, received intratracheal instillations of 0.063, 0.125 or 0.25 mg/animal nickel subsulfide in 0.3 ml saline (total doses, 0.94, 1.88 and 3.75 mg/animal) once a week for 15 weeks. At 120 weeks, 50% of the animals were still alive; the experiment was terminated at 132 weeks. The incidences of malignant lung tumours were 7/47, 13/45 and 12/40 in the low-, medium- and high-dose groups; 12 adenocarcinomas, 15 squamous-cell carcinomas and five mixed tumours occurred in the lungs of treated animals. No lung tumour occurred in 40 controls given 20 intratracheal injections of 0.3 ml saline (Pott et al., 1987).

Hamster: In the study reported on p. 320 (Muhle et al., 1990), no lung tumour was seen in 62 animals given 12 doses of 0.1 mg α-nickel subsulfide by intratracheal instillation. [The Working Group noted the low total dose given.]

### (iii) Intrapleural administration

Rat: A group of 32 male Wistar rats, three months of age, received a single intrapleural injection of 10 mg nickel subsulfide in 0.4 ml saline. Average survival was 177 days. Local malignant tumours (mainly rhabdomyosarcomas) developed in 28/32 animals but in none of 32 saline-injected controls (Skaug et al., 1985)

### (iv) Topical administration

Hamster: Groups of male golden Syrian hamsters of the LVG/LAK strain, two to three months of age, were painted on the mucosa of the buccal pouches with 1 or 2 mg α-nickel subsulfide in 0.1 ml glycerol three times a week for 18 weeks (six to seven animals; total doses, 54 and 108 mg nickel subsulfide) or with 5 or 10 mg three times a week for 36 weeks (13-15 animals; total doses, 540 and 1080 mg nickel subsulfide), and were observed for more than 19 months. Two control groups received applications of glycerol. No tumour developed in the buccal pouch, oral cavity or intestinal tract in the treated or control groups. Squamous-cell carcinomas of the buccal pouch developed in all four hamsters that received applications of 1 mg dimethylbenz[a]anthracene in glycerol three times a week for 18 weeks (Sunderman, 1983b).

### (v) Intramuscular administration

Mouse: Groups of 45 Swiss and 18 C3H mice, approximately equally divided by sex, two to three months of age, received single intramuscular injections of 5 mg nickel subsulfide into both or only one thigh muscle. Local tumours (mainly sarcomas) developed in 27 and nine mice, respectively. No control was reported (Gilman, 1962).

Three groups of ten female and one group of ten male NMRI mice, six weeks of age, received an injection of 10 mg labelled nickel subsulfide into the left thigh muscle, or of 5 mg into the interscapular subcutaneous tissue, in 0.1 ml olive oil:streptocillin (3:1). Two mice from each group were killed two months after injection for whole-body autoradiography; no tumour was seen at this stage. The remaining animals were autopsied at 14 months, when local sarcomas were seen in 7/8 and 4/8 females that received subcutaneous injections and in 4/8 males and 4/8 females that received intramuscular injections. Metastases to the lung, liver and regional lymph nodes occurred in approximately half of the 19 tumour-bearing mice. No control group was used (Oskarsson *et al.*, 1979).

Groups of four male and six female DBA/2 and five male and five female C57Bl6 mice, two to three months of age, received a single intramuscular injection of 2.5 mg α-nickel subsulfide in 0.1-0.5 ml penicillin G procaine solution into one thigh muscle. Local sarcomas developed in six DBA/2 ($p < 0.01$) and in five C57Bl6 ($p < 0.05$) mice, with median latent periods of 13 and 14 months, respectively. None of nine control mice of each strain injected with penicillin G alone developed a sarcoma (Sunderman, 1983b).

*Rat*: A group of 32 male and female Wistar rats, two to three months of age, received a single intramuscular injection of 20 mg nickel subsulfide into one or both thigh muscles. After an average of 21 weeks, 25/28 rats had developed 36 local tumours. Vehicle controls were not available, but two further groups of 30 rats each injected with ferrous sulfide did not develop tumours at the site of injection after 627 days (Gilman, 1962).

Groups of ten male and ten female Fischer rats, five months of age, were administered nickel subsulfide either by an intramuscular injection of 10 mg powder (particle size, 2-4 μm), by implantation of an intact 11-mm disc (500 mg), by implantation of 3-5-mm disc fragments or by implantation of 10 mg powder in a 0.45-μm porosity millipore diffusion chamber. Local tumours (mostly rhabdomysarcomas) developed in 71-95% of rats, which demonstrated diffusion of soluble nickel from the chambers. The mean tumour latency for the last group was 305 days, almost twice that for the other three groups. Among 19 controls given 38 implants of empty diffusion chambers, one tumour developed after 460 days. The authors considered that the experiment demonstrated that the induction of neoplasms by nickel subsulfide is a chemical rather than a physical (foreign-body) reaction and that phagocytosis is not essential for nickel tumorigenesis (Gilman & Herchen, 1963).

Groups of 15 Fischer rats received implants of nickel subsulfide discs (250 mg) or 8 × 1-mm discs of ferric oxide (control) in opposite sides of the gluteal musculature. The nickel subsulfide discs were removed in a geometric sequence at two, four, eight... up to 256 days after implantation, and average tumour incidence after 256 days was 66%. The critical exposure (tissue contact) period necessary for nickel subsulfide to induce malignant transformation was 32-64 days (Herchen & Gilman, 1964).

Groups of 15 male and 15 female hooded and 15 male and 12 female NIH (Bethesda) black rats, two to three months of age, received injections of 10 mg nickel subsulfide in penicillin G procaine into each gastrocnemius muscle. NIH Black rats were less susceptible to local tumour induction (14/23 rats) than hooded rats (28/28). Massive phagocytic invasion of the nickel injection site occurred in the NIH black rats (Daniel, 1966).

Groups of 20 male and 20 female Fischer 344 rats, five weeks of age, received a single subcutaneous injection of 10 or 3.3 mg nickel subsulfide in 0.25 ml saline. Two further groups received single intramuscular injections of 10 or 3.3 mg nickel subsulfide. A group of 60 male and 60 female control rats received injections of 0.25 ml saline twice a week for 52 weeks, and a further control group received no treatment. At 18 months, the groups injected subcutaneously with nickel subsulfide had tumour incidences of 90 and 95%, and the groups injected intramuscularly had tumour incidences of 85% and 97%. Most tumours in both groups were rhabdomyosarcomas. No local tumour occurred in controls (Mason, 1972).

Groups of ten male Fischer 344 rats, three months of age, received intramuscular injections of amorphous nickel sulfide and α-nickel subsulfide in 0.5 ml penicillin G procaine suspension at two comparable dose levels (about 5 and 20 mg/rat), to provide 60 and 240 µg Ni per rat. A further group received injections of nickel ferrosulfide matte (85 and 340 µg atom of nickel per rat). Sarcomas at the injection site developed in 8/10 and 9/9 of the low- and high-dose nickel subsulfide-treated groups and in 1/10 and 8/10 of the low- and high-dose nickel ferrosulfide matte-treated groups, respectively. No local sarcoma developed in the groups given nickel sulfide, among control rats given penicillin G procaine suspension alone or in two control groups treated with metallic iron powder (Sunderman & Maenza, 1976).

Groups of 63 male and female inbred Fischer and 20 male and female hooded rats, ten to 14 weeks old, received an intramuscular injection of 10 mg nickel subsulfide in penicillin G procaine. Tumour-bearing rats were autopsied 30 days after detection of the tumour. Tumours occurred in 59/63 Fischer and 11/20 hooded rats; 81.9% of tumours in hooded rats metastasized, compared to 25.4% in Fischer rats. Metastatic lesions were observed in the heart, pleura, liver and adrenal glands, as well as in lungs and lymph nodes of nine hooded rats. Of the primary tumours, 67% were rhabdomyosarcomas (Yamashiro et al., 1980).

Groups of 30 male Fischer 344 rats, approximately two months of age, received a single intramuscular injection of 0.6, 1.2, 2.5 or 5 mg nickel subsulfide. Local sarcomas were recorded in 7/30, 23/30, 28/30 and 29/30 of the animals, respectively [$p < 0.01$], indicating a dose-related increase in incidence. No such tumour developed in 60 untreated controls (Sunderman *et al.*, 1976). In an extension of this study, a total of 383 animals received injections of 0.63-20 mg $\alpha$-nickel subsulfide. Sarcoma incidence at 62 weeks after treatment ranged from 24% at the lowest dose level to 100% at the highest dose level. Of the 336 sarcomas induced, 161 were rhabdomyosarcomas, 91 undifferentiated sarcomas, 72 fibrosarcomas, nine liposarcomas, two neurofibrosarcomas and one a haemangiosarcoma. Metastasis was seen in 137 of the 336 tumour-bearing animals (Sunderman, 1981).

In a study on the relationship between physical and chemical properties and carcinogenic activities of 18 nickel compounds at a standard 14-mg intramuscular dose of nickel under comparable experimental conditions in male Fischer 344 rats (see p. 321), five nickel sulfides were among the compounds tested. Three of these ($\alpha$-nickel subsulfide, crystalline $\beta$-nickel sulfide and nickel ferrosulfide matte) induced local sarcomas in 100% of animals (9/9, 14/14 and 15/15). Metastases developed in 56, 71 and 67%, respectively, of the tumour-bearing rats. Nickel disulfide induced local tumours in 86% (12/14) animals and amorphous nickel sulfide in 12% (3/25). Median latent periods were 30 weeks for nickel subsulfide, 40 weeks for crystalline nickel sulfide, 36 weeks for nickel disulfide, 41 weeks for amorphous nickel sulfide, but only 16 weeks for nickel ferrosulfide. Median survival times were 39, 48, 47, 71 and 32 weeks, respectively (Sunderman, 1984).

In the study by Berry *et al.* (1984) described on p. 321, tumours developed in 10/20 rats given 5 mg nickel subsulfide intramuscularly, in 0/20 treated subperiosteally and in 10/20 given intrafemoral injections.

In the study by Judde *et al.* (1987) described on p. 321, a single intramuscular injection of 5 mg nickel subsulfide induced tumours in 2/100 rats.

[The Working Group was aware of several other studies in which nickel subsulfide was used as a positive control or as a model for the induction of rhabdomyosarcomas.]

*Hamster.* Groups of 15 or 17 male Syrian hamsters, two to three months of age, received a single intramuscular injection of 5 or 10 mg nickel subsulfide in 0.02-0.5 ml sterile saline. Of the 15 animals receiving the 5-mg dose, four developed local sarcomas, with a median latent period of ten months. At the 10-mg dose, 12/17 hamsters had local tumours, with a mean latency of 11 months [$p < 0.01$, trend test]. No tumour occurred among 14 controls injected with saline alone (Sunderman, 1983a).

*Rabbit*: Six-month-old white rabbits [sex and number unspecified] received intramuscular implants of agar-agar blocks containing approximately 80 mg nickel subsulfide powder. Sixteen rabbits with local tumours (rhabdomyosarcomas) were examined. Tumours were first observed about four to six months after implantation as small growths, which usually ceased active progression for up to 80 weeks then grew rapidly over the next four or five weeks (Hildebrand & Biserte, 1979a,b). [The Working Group noted the limited reporting of the study.]

Four male New Zealand albino rabbits, two months old, received bilateral intramuscular injections of 25 mg α-nickel subsulfide (50 mg/rabbit) in 0.1-0.5 ml penicillin G procaine suspension. All animals died between 16 and 72 months. No local tumour was found on autopsy (Sunderman, 1983a). [The Working Group noted the short observation period.]

### (vi) *Intraperitoneal administration*

*Rat*: Of a group of 37 Fischer rats [sex and age unspecified] that received a single intraperitoneal injection of nickel subsulfide [dose unspecified], nine developed tumours, eight of which were rhabdomyosarcomas and one a mesothelioma (Gilman, 1966). [The Working Group noted the limited reporting of the study.]

A group of 50 female Wistar rats, 12 weeks of age, received a single intraperitoneal injection of 25 mg nickel subsulfide. Abdominal tumours (sarcomas, mesotheliomas and carcinomas) occurred in 27/42 animals, with an average latent period of eight months (Pott *et al.*, 1987).

In a study described above (p. 322), three doses of nickel subsulfide were injected into the peritoneal cavities of groups of female Wistar rats. Local tumours were observed at 30 months in 20/36 animals that received 6 mg (as Ni) as a single injection, in 23/35 receiving 12 mg (as Ni) as two 6-mg injections and in 25/34 given 25 mg (as Ni) as 25 1-mg injections. The tumours were mesotheliomas or sarcomas of the abdominal cavity (Pott *et al.*, 1989, 1990). [The Working Group noted that the results at 30 months were available as an extended abstract only.]

### (vii) *Intrarenal administration*

*Rat*: Groups of 16 and 24 female Sprague-Dawley rats, weighing 120-140 g, received a single injection of 5 mg nickel subsulfide in 0.05 ml glycerine or 0.5 ml saline into each pole of the right kidney. Renal-cell carcinomas occurred in 7/16 and 11/24 animals compared with 0/16 in animals given 0.5 ml glycerine (Jasmin & Riopelle, 1976).

In a second experiment (Jasmin & Riopelle, 1976), the activity of other nickel compounds and divalent metals was investigated under identical experimental conditions using glycerine as the vehicle; all rats were autopsied after 12 months' exposure. In one group of 18 rats, nickel sulfide [probably amorphous] exhibited no renal tumorigenic activity. [The Working Group noted that it was not stated whether crystalline or amorphous nickel sulfide was used.]

Groups of male and female Wistar Lewis, NIH black, Fischer 344 and Long-Evans rats, eight weeks of age, received an intrarenal injection of 5 mg α-nickel subsulfide. The incidence of malignant renal tumours 100 weeks after exposure was 7/11 in Wistar Lewis, 6/12 in NIH black, 9/32 in Fischer and 0/12 in Long-Evans rats. Groups of 11-24 male Fischer rats were given an intrarenal injection of 0.6, 1.2, 2.5, 5 or 10 mg nickel subsulfide; no tumour was seen with 0.6, 1.2 or 2.5 mg, but responses of 5/18 and 18/24 were obtained with 5 mg and 10 mg, showing a dose-response effect. All tumours were malignant, but the authors could not establish whether the tumours were of epithelial or mesenchymal origin; 70% had distant metastases (Sunderman *et al.*, 1979a).

Groups of male Fischer 344 rats [initial number unspecified], approximately eight weeks old, received an intrarenal injection of 7 mg nickel as one of several sulfides in 0.1 or 0.2 ml saline or in glycerol:distilled water (1:1, v/v) in each pole of the right kidney and were observed for two years after treatment. The incidence of renal cancer was significantly elevated in treated groups: nickel disulfide, 2/10 (fibrosarcomas); crystalline β-nickel sulfide, 8/14 (three fibrosarcomas, three other sarcomas, one renal-cell carcinoma, one carcinosarcoma); and α-nickel subsulfide, 4/15 (mesangial-cell sarcomas). Renal cancers occurred in 1/12 (sarcoma) rats treated with nickel ferrosulfide and in 0/15 rats treated with amorphous nickel sulfide. No local tumour developed in vehicle controls (Sunderman *et al.*, 1984b).

### (viii) *Intratesticular administration*

*Rat*: A group of 19 male Fischer 344 rats, eight weeks of age, received an injection of 10 mg α-nickel subsulfide in 0.3 ml saline into the centre of the right testis and were observed for 20 months, at which time all the animals had died. A control group of 18 rats received an injection of 0.3 ml saline only, and a further two groups of four rats each received injections of either 10 mg metallic iron powder in saline or 2 mg zinc[II] as zinc chloride in distilled water. Of the nickel subsulfide-treated rats, 16/19 developed sarcomas in the treated testis, ten of which were fibrosarcomas, three malignant fibrous histiocytomas and three rhabdomyosarcomas. Four of the rats had distant metastases. No tumour occurred in the other groups (Damjanov *et al.*, 1978).

### (ix) *Intraocular administration*

*Rat*: A group of 14 male and one female Fischer 344 rats, four weeks of age, received an injection of 0.5 mg α-nickel subsulfide in 20 μl saline into the vitreous cavity of the right eye under anaesthetic. Eleven male controls were similarly injected with saline alone. The experiment was terminated at 40-42 weeks after treatment, when 11 control and one surviving treated rats were killed. Between 26 and 36 weeks after injection, 14/15 rats developed ocular tumours. Five of the tumorous eyes contained multiple neoplasms, and 22 distinct ocular tumours were identified as 11 melanomas, four retinoblastomas, three gliomas, one phakocarcinoma [lens capsular tumour] and three unclassified malignant tumours. No tumour developed in either the controls or in the uninjected, left eyes of treated rats. It was postulated that the very high incidence (93%) and short latent periods may have been due in part to the relative isolation of the vitreous bodies from the systemic circulation (blood-retina barrier), which would result in a high concentration of nickel[II]. The authors also pointed out that nickel particles within the vitreous body were relatively sequestered from phagocytosis. The visibility of developing tumours within the chamber permits their very early recognition (Albert *et al.*, 1980; Sunderman, 1983b).

*Salamander*. A group of eight lentectomized Japanese common newts received a single injection of 40-100 μg nickel subsulfide into the vitreous chamber of the eye under anaesthetic. Seven newts developed ocular melanoma-like tumours within nine months, while no tumour occurred in six controls injected with 2-3 μl sterile 0.6% saline or eye-dropper oil after lens extirpation. The lens regenerated in each of the control eyes. The site of tumour origin could not be determined, although it was suggested to be the iris, which showed numerous aberrant proliferating cells at three months (Okamoto, 1987).

### (x) *Transplacental administration*

*Rat*: A group of eight pregnant female Fischer 344 rats, 120-150 days of age, received an intramuscular injection of 20 mg α-nickel subsulfide in 0.2 ml procaine penicillin G suspension on day 6 of gestation, allowing for gradual dissolution of the nickel subsulfide throughout the remainder of the pregnancy. A group of controls received an injection of vehicle only. No difference in the incidence of benign or malignant tumours was seen between the 50 pups born to treated dams and 53 control pups observed for 26 months (Sunderman *et al.*, 1981). [The Working Group noted that only one dose was used, which was not toxic to the fetuses.]

### (xi) *Implantation into subcutaneously implanted tracheal grafts*

*Rat*: Groups of 30 and 32 female Fischer 344 rats, ten weeks of age, received five gelatin pellets containing 1 or 3 mg nickel subsulfide in heterotopic tracheal transplants inserted under the dorsal skin. At the lower dose level, tumours developed in 9/60 tracheas (six carcinomas and three sarcomas); at the higher dose level, tumours developed in 45/64 tracheas (one carcinoma and 44 sarcomas). No tumour developed in 20 control transplanted tracheas. The high dose resulted in necrosis of the epithelium and thus favoured the development of sarcomas (Yarita & Nettesheim, 1978).

(xii)  *Intramuscular, subcutaneous or intra-articular injection or injection into retroperitoneal fat*

*Rat*: In a study designed to determine the types of sarcoma that develop from various mesenchymal tissue components, groups of 20 male Fischer 344 rats, seven to eight weeks of age, received injections of 5 mg nickel subsulfide either intramuscularly, subcutaneously, into the intra-articular space or into retroperitoneal fat. Control groups of ten rats each were injected with 0.5 ml aqueous procaine penicillin G vehicle. The incidences and types of sarcoma that developed in the experimental groups were: intramuscular, 19/20 (all rhabdomyosarcomas); subcutaneous, 18/19 (ten malignant fibrous histiocytomas, five rhabdomyosarcomas, three fibrosarcomas or unclassified); intra-articular, 16/19 (eight rhabdomyosarcomas, three malignant fibrous histiocytomas, five fibrosarcomas or unclassified); and retroperitoneal fat, 9/20 (five malignant fibrous histiocytomas, three rhabdomyosarcomas, one fibrosarcoma or unclassified). Controls did not develop tumours (Shibata *et al.*, 1989).

(xiii)  *Administration with known carcinogens*

*Rat*: Groups of 30 male Fischer rats, eight to nine weeks of age, received intramuscular injections in both thighs of either 10 mg nickel subsulfide, 10 mg benzo[a]pyrene or 20 mg nickel subsulfide plus 10 mg benzo[a]pyrene in penicillin G procaine suspension, or vehicle alone. All treated rats developed sarcomas; rhabdomyosarcomas occurred in 24/30 given 10 mg nickel subsulfide, 4/30 given benzo[a]pyrene and 28/30 given 20 mg nickel subsulfide plus benzo[a]pyrene. No sarcoma occurred in controls (Maenza *et al.*, 1971).

Groups of 13, 13 and 12 male Wistar rats, weighing approximately 200 g, received single intratracheal injections of 5 mg nickel subsulfide, 2 mg benzo[a]pyrene or 5 mg nickel subsulfide plus 2 mg benzo[a]pyrene and were observed for 15 months. One rat from each group developed a tumour, consisting of one hepatoma, one retroperitoneal tumour and one squamous-cell carcinoma of the lung, respectively. Significant differences were seen in the incidence of preneoplastic lesions (peribronchial adenomatoid proliferation and bronchial squamous metaplasia), the occurrence decreasing in the order: nickel subsulfide plus benzo[a]pyrene > benzo[a]pyrene > nickel subsulfide (Kasprzak *et al.*, 1973).

(*d*)  *Nickel salts*

(i)  *Intramuscular administration*

*Rat*: A group of 32 male and female Wistar rats, two to three months of age, received an injection of 5 mg nickel sulfate hexahydrate in one or both thigh muscles (54 injected sites). Thirteen rats survived until the end of the experiment at 603 days.

No local tumour was found at the site of injection. No vehicle control was used (Gilman, 1962).

In a study reported as an abstract, sheep fat pellets, each containing 7 mg of either nickel sulfate, nickel chloride, nickel acetate, anhydrous nickel acetate, nickel carbonate or nickel ammonium sulfate, were given as three intramuscular implants [interval unspecified] into groups of 35 Bethesda black [NIH black] rats. Animals were observed for 18 months. Six tumours developed in the nickel carbonate group; single tumours developed in the nickel acetate and nickel sulfate groups. No tumour developed in any of the other groups or in 35 controls (Payne, 1964).

In a study comparing the in-vitro solubility and carcinogenicity of several nickel compounds, nickel fluoride and nickel sulfate were suspended in penicillin G procaine and injected intramuscularly [dose unspecified] into groups of 20 Fischer rats [sex and age unspecified]. The incidence of local sarcomas was 3/18 (17%; 3/36 sites) with nickel fluoride and 0/20 with nickel sulfate. Seventeen of 20 (85%) rats given nickel subsulfide as a positive control developed local sarcomas. No tumour developed in 20 rats injected with nickel sulfide [presumed to be amorphous] (Gilman, 1966). [The Working Group noted that no concurrent vehicle control was used and that the length of observation was not specified.]

A group of 20 male Wistar rats, weighing 200-220 g, received 15 intramuscular injections of 20 µl of a 0.2 M solution of nickel sulfate (4.4 µmol [0.26 mg]/injection of nickel; total dose, 66 µmol [4 mg]/rat nickel) every other day during one month. Further groups of 20 male rats received injections of nickel subsulfide (total dose, 40 µmol [7.1 mg nickel]; positive control) or sodium sulfate (15 injections of 20 µl of a 0.2 M solution; negative control). Nickel subsulfide induced local tumours in 16/20 rats; no tumour developed in nickel sulfate- or sodium sulfate-treated rats (Kasprzak et al., 1983).

One local sarcoma was found in 16 male Fischer 344 rats, two to three months old, given an intramuscular injection of nickel chromate into the right thigh as 14 mg/rat nickel. Ten rats survived two years (Sunderman, 1984).

### (ii) Intraperitoneal administration

Mouse: In a screening assay for lung adenomas in strain A mice, groups of ten male and ten female Strong strain A mice, six to eight weeks old, received intraperitoneal injections of nickel acetate in 0.85% physiological saline (total doses, 72, 180 and 360 mg/kg bw) three times a week for 24 weeks and were observed for 30 weeks, at which time all survivors were autopsied. Further groups of mice received a single intraperitoneal injection of 20 mg urethane (positive control), 24 injections of saline only or remained untreated. The incidences of lung tumours were: saline control, 37% (0.42 tumours/animal); untreated control, 31% (0.28 tumours/animal); positive control, 100% (21.6 tumours/animal); 72 mg nickel acetate, 44% (0.67 tumours/

animal); 180 mg nickel acetate, 50% (0.71 tumours/animal); and 360 mg nickel ace-tate, 63% (1.26 tumours/animal). The difference in response between the group giv-en 360 mg nickel acetate and the negative control group was significant ($p < 0.01$). Five adenocarcinomas of the lung were observed in the nickel-treated mice com-pared to none in controls (Stoner *et al.*, 1976).

In the same type of screening assay, 30 male and female Strong strain A mice, six to eight weeks of age, received intraperitoneal injections of 10.7 mg/kg bw nickel acetate tetrahydrate (maximal tolerated dose; 0.04 mmol [2.4 mg]/kg bw nickel) three times a week for 24 weeks. A control group received injections of 0.9% saline under the same schedule. Animals were autopsied 30 weeks after the first injection. Of the nickel-treated group, 24/30 animals survived to 30 weeks and had an average of 1.50 lung adenomas/animal, whereas 25/30 controls had an average of 0.32 lung adenoma/animal ($p < 0.05$) (Poirier *et al.*, 1984).

*Rat*: In a study described earlier (p. 322), groups of female Wistar rats were given repeated intraperitoneal injections of 1 mg of each of four soluble nickel salts. The dose schedule and tumour responses at 30 months are shown in Table 23. The tumours were either mesotheliomas or sarcomas (tumours of the uterus were not included) (Pott *et al.*, 1989, 1990). [The Working Group noted that administration of nickel sulfate and nickel chloride by intramuscular injection has not been shown to induce tumours in rats. They suggest that in this instance the repeated small intra-peritoneal doses permitted repeated exposure of potential target cells. Repeated intramuscular injections would result in nickel coming into contact with different cells at each injection. The Group also noted that the results at 30 months were reported only as an extended abstract.]

### (iii) *Administration with known carcinogens*

*Rat*: Groups of 12 rats [strain, sex and age unspecified] received a single sub-cutaneous injection of 9 mg/ml dinitrosopiperazine in aqueous Tween 80. The fol-lowing day, one group received topical insertion into the nasopharynx of 0.02 ml of a 0.5% solution of nickel sulfate in 4% aqueous gelatin once a week for seven weeks. A further group was held for six days and then administered 1 ml of aqueous 1% nickel sulfate solution in the drinking-water for six weeks. Additional groups of 12 rats received treatment with dinitrosopiperazine, nickel sulfate solution or nickel sulfate in gelatin only. Survival at 371 days was lower in the group treated with dini-tropiperazine plus nickel sulfate solution in the drinking-water than in the group given the nitrosamine or the nickel sulfate solution alone. Two nasopharyngeal tu-mours (one squamous-cell carcinoma, one fibrosarcoma) occurred in the group treated with dinitropiperazine plus nickel sulfate in drinking-water and two (one papilloma, one early carcinoma) in the group treated with dinitropiperazine plus

**Table 23. Tumour responses of rats to intraperitoneal injection of soluble nickel salts[a]**

| Compound | Total dose (mg, as Ni) | Schedule | Incidence of abdominal tumours |
|---|---|---|---|
| Nickel chloride.6H$_2$O | 50 | 50 × 1 mg | 4/32 [$p < 0.05$] |
| Nickel sulfate.7H$_2$O | 50 | 50 × 1 mg | 6/30 [$p < 0.05$] |
| Nickel acetate.4H$_2$O | 25 | 25 × 1 mg | 3/35 |
|  | 50 | 50 × 1 mg | 5/31 [$p < 0.05$ for trend] |
| Nickel carbonate | 25 | 25 × 1 mg | 1/35 |
| Nickel hydroxide.2H$_2$O | 50 | 50 × 1 mg | 3/33 |
| Saline |  | 3 × 1 ml | 1/33 |
|  |  | 50 × 1 ml | 0/34 |

[a]From Pott *et al.* (1989, 1990)

insertion of nickel sulfate in gelatin. No tumour occurred in the other groups. The authors concluded that 'probably nickel has a promoting action in the induction of nasopharyngeal carcinoma in rats following dinitrosopiperazine initiation' (Ou *et al.*, 1980). [The Working Group noted the small number of animals used and the poor survival.]

As reported in an abstract, in an extension of the study by Ou *et al.* (1980), five of 22 rats given an initiating injection of dinitrosopiperazine developed carcinomas following oral administration of nickel sulfate in gelatin. Two of the carcinomas were of the nasopharynx, two of the nasal cavity and one of the hard palate. No tumour developed in rats [numbers unspecified] treated with dinitrosopiperazine plus aqueous nickel sulfate, with nickel sulfate in gelatin alone or with dinitrosopiperazine alone (Liu *et al.*, 1983). [The Working Group noted the small number of animals used and the poor survival.]

As reported in an abstract, a group of 13 female rats [strain and age unspecified] received a single subcutaneous injection of 9 mg dinitrosopiperazine on day 18 of gestation. Pups of treated dams were fed 0.05 ml of 0.05% nickel sulfate beginning at four weeks of age every day for one month. The dose of nickel sulfate was increased by 0.1 ml per month for a further five months, by which time 5/21 pups had developed carcinomas of the nasal cavity. In a group of untreated pups of treated dams, 3/11 rats developed tumours (one nasopharyngeal squamous-cell carcinoma, one neurofibrosarcoma of the peritoneal cavity and one granulosa-thecal-cell carcinoma of the ovary). Groups given nickel sulfate and untreated control groups of seven pups each did not develop tumours. None of the pregnant rats that had been injected with dinitrosopiperazine alone developed tumours (Ou *et al.*, 1983).

Groups of 15 male Fischer 344 rats, seven weeks old, were administered 500 mg/l N-nitrosoethylhydroxyethylamine (NEHEA) in the drinking-water for two weeks. Thereafter, rats received drinking-water alone or drinking-water containing 600 mg/l nickel chloride hexahydrate for 25 weeks, when the study was terminated. The incidence of renal-cell tumours in the group receiving NEHEA and nickel chloride (8/15) was significantly higher ($p < 0.05$) than that in controls given NEHEA alone (2/15) or nickel chloride alone (0/15) (Kurokawa *et al.*, 1985). Nickel chloride did not show promoting activity in livers of Fischer 344 rats after initiation with N-nitrosodiethylamine, in gastric tissue of Wistar rats after initiation with N-methyl-N'-nitro-N-nitrosoguanidine, in the pancreas of Syrian golden hamsters following initiation with N-nitrosobis(2-oxypropyl)amine or in skin of SENCAR mice initiated with 7,12-dimethylbenz[a]anthracene. The authors concluded that nickel chloride is a promoter in renal carcinogenesis in rats (Hayashi *et al.*, 1984; Kurokawa *et al.*, 1985).

### (e)   Other nickel compounds

#### (i)  Inhalation

*Rat*: Groups of 64 or 32 male Wistar rats, weighing 200-250 g, were exposed by inhalation for 30 min to 30 or 60 mg/m³ nickel carbonyl vapourized from a solution in 50:50 ethanol:diethyl ether, respectively, three times a week for 52 weeks. Another group of 80 rats was exposed once to 250 mg/m³ nickel carbonyl. All treated animals had died by 30 months. One lung carcinoma appeared in each of the first two groups, and two pulmonary carcinomas developed in the last group. No pulmonary tumour occurred among 41 vehicle-treated control rats (Sunderman *et al.*, 1957, 1959). A further group of 285 rats was exposed for 30 min to 600 mg/m³ nickel carbonyl; 214 died from acute toxicity. One lung adenocarcinoma was observed in the remaining 71 animals. Similar exposure to nickel carbonyl followed by intraperitoneal injection of sodium diethyl dithiocarbamate, an antidote, resulted in survival of all 60 treated rats and the development of a single anaplastic lung carcinoma. Minimal time to observation of lung tumours in these groups was in excess of 24 months. No lung carcinoma was observed in a group of 32 controls (Sunderman & Donnelly, 1965).

A group of five non-inbred rats [sex and age unspecified] was exposed by inhalation to 70 mg/m³ nickel refinery dust (containing 11.3% metallic nickel, 58.3% nickel sulfide [identity unspecified], 1.7% nickel monoxide and 0.2% water-soluble nickel [composition of sample unclear]) for 5 h per day on five days per week for six months. Seventeen months after the start of treatment, one of five rats developed a squamous-cell carcinoma of the lung. No tumour developed among 47 untreated controls (Saknyn & Blokhin, 1978). [The Working Group noted the small number of animals used.]

*Hamster*: Groups of 102 male Syrian golden outbred LAK:LVG hamsters, two months old, were exposed by inhalation to concentrations of 17 or 70 mg/m³ nickel-enriched fly ash from the addition of nickel acetate to pulverized coal before combustion (nickel content, 6%) for 6 h per day on five days per week for 20 months. Further groups were exposed to 70 mg/m³ fly ash containing 0.3% nickel, or were sham-exposed. Five animals from each group were autopsied at four-month intervals up to 16 months, and all survivors were sacrificed at 20 months. No significant difference in mortality rate or body weight was observed between the groups. There were 14, 16, 16 and seven benign and malignant tumours in the sham-exposed, fly ash, low-dose and high-dose nickel-enriched fly ash groups, respectively. The only two malignant pulmonary neoplasms (one adenocarcinoma, one mesothelioma) occurred in the group receiving fly ash enriched with the high dose of nickel (Wehner *et al.*, 1981, 1984).

### (ii) *Intratracheal instillation*

*Rat*: A group of 26 white non-inbred rats [sex and age unspecified] received a single intratracheal instillation of 20-40 mg aerosol dust (64.7% nickel monoxide (black), 0.13% nickel sulfide, 0.18% metallic nickel) in 0.6 ml saline. One squamous-cell carcinoma of the lung had developed by 17 months. No tumour developed among a group of 47 controls (Saknyn & Blokhin, 1978). [The Working Group noted that it was not stated whether the controls were untreated or received the vehicle alone.]

### (iii) *Intramuscular administration*

*Mouse*: A group of 40 female Swiss mice, two to three months of age, received an intramuscular injection in each thigh of 10 mg of a nickel refinery dust (57% nickel subsulfide, 20% nickel sulfate hexahydrate, 6.3% nickel monoxide) suspended in penicillin G procaine. Of the 36 mice that survived more than 90 days, 20 developed a total of 23 local sarcomas, with an average latent period of 46 weeks. No tumour occurred among 48 control mice injected with the vehicle alone (Gilman & Ruckerbauer, 1962).

*Rat*: A group of 35 male and female hooded rats, two to three months of age, received an intramuscular injection in each thigh of 20 mg of a nickel refinery dust (57% nickel subsulfide, 20% nickel sulfate hexahydrate, 6.3% nickel oxide) suspended in penicillin G procaine. Of the 27 rats that survived more than 90 days, 19 developed local sarcomas. Another group of 31 male and female rats received injections of the same refinery dust after repeated washing in distilled water; 20/28 of the rats that survived more than 90 days developed local tumours at one or other of the injection sites. No tumour occurred among 30 control rats injected with the vehicle alone (Gilman & Ruckerbauer, 1962).

Groups of 25 male and 25 female Fischer 344 rats [age unspecified] received 12 intramuscular injections of 12 or 25 mg nickelocene in trioctanoin. Tumour incidences were 18/50 and 21/50, respectively. No local tumour occurred in a group of 25 male and 25 female controls (Furst & Schlauder, 1971).

Groups of 15-30 male Fischer 344 rats, approximately eight weeks old, received a single intramuscular injection of 14 mg nickel as one of four nickel arsenides, nickel antimonide, nickel telluride, nickel sinter matte ($Ni_4FeS_4$; positive control), nickel titanate or ferronickel alloy ($NiFe_{1.6}$; negative controls) in 0.3 ml glycerol:water (1:1; v/v) into the exterior thigh. The compounds were > 99.9% pure and were ground down to a median particle size of < 2 μm. Rats that died within two months of the injection were excluded from the experiment; remaining animals were observed for two years. Median survival ranged from 32 weeks (positive controls) to over 100 weeks (negative controls). The incidences of local tumours in the groups were: nickel sinter matte, 15/15; nickel sulfarsenide, 14/16; nickel arsenide hexagonal, 17/20; nickel antimonide, 17/29; nickel telluride, 14/26; and nickel arsenide tetragonal, 8/16. No tumour was observed in the groups treated with nickel arsenide, ferronickel alloy or nickel titanate nor in a vehicle control group. Median latency for tumour induction ranged from 16 weeks (positive controls) to 33 weeks (nickel arsenide tetragonal-treated group). The incidence of tumours induced by the test compounds was significantly greater than that in the vehicle control group ($p < 0.001$); 67% of all the sarcomas were rhabdomyosarcomas, 11% fibrosarcomas, 15% osteosarcomas and 5% undifferentiated sarcomas. Metastases occurred in 57% of tumour-bearing rats (Sunderman & McCully, 1983).

In a continuation of these tests, nickel selenide, nickel subselenide and nickel monoxide (positive control; see p. 327) were tested using the same experimental techniques. Nickel selenide and nickel subselenide induced significant increases in the incidence of local tumours (8/16 and 21/23, respectively; $p < 0.001$); the positive control group had 14/15 tumours. Metastases occurred in 38 and 86%, respectively, of tumour-bearing rats in the selenium-treated groups and in 29% of positive controls. Approximately 50% of the tumours were rhabdomyosarcomas (Sunderman, 1984).

*Hamster.* Groups of 25 male and 25 female hamsters, three to four weeks old, received eight monthly injections of 5 mg nickelocene in 0.2 ml trioctanoin into the right thigh. No tumour was induced. A group of survivors from another test [age unspecified] received a single intramuscular injection of 25 mg nickelocene in trioctanoin; fibrosarcomas occurred in 1/13 females and 3/16 males. No tumour occurred in 25 male or 25 female vehicle controls (Furst & Schlauder, 1971).

### (iv) *Intraperitoneal administration*

*Rat*: Groups of 16 and 23 non-inbred albino rats [sex and age unspecified] received a single intraperitoneal injection of 90-150 mg of one of two refinery dusts: the first contained 11.3% metallic nickel, 58.3% nickel sulfide, 1.7% nickel monoxide and 0.2% water-soluble nickel; the second contained 2.9% metallic nickel, 26.8% nickel sulfide, 6.8% nickel monoxide and 0.07% water-soluble nickel. Each was given in 1.5 ml physiological saline. Three local sarcomas developed within six to 15 months in animal treated with the first dust, and three local sarcomas developed within nine to 11 months in animals treated with the second dust. No tumour was observed in 47 control rats (Saknyn & Blokhin, 1978). [The Working Group noted that it was not specified whether control rats were untreated or were treated with the vehicle.]

### (v) *Intravenous administration*

*Rat*: A group of 61 male and 60 female Sprague-Dawley rats, eight to nine weeks of age, received six injections of 9 mg/kg bw nickel carbonyl (as Ni) at two- to four-week intervals and were observed for life. Nineteen animals developed malignancies, six of which were undifferentiated sarcomas and three, fibrosarcomas at various sites; the other tumours were single carcinomas of the liver, kidney and mammary gland, one haemangioendothelioma, one undifferentiated leukaemia and five pulmonary lymphomas. Two pulmonary lymphomas developed in 15 male and 32 female sham-injected controls. The difference in total tumour incidence was significant ($p < 0.05$) (Lau *et al.*, 1972).

### (vi) *Intrarenal administration*

Groups of male fischer rats [initial number unspecified], approximately eight weeks old, received intrarenal injections of 7 mg nickel as one of several nickel compounds in 0.1 or 0.2 ml saline solution or in glycerol:distilled water (1:1, v/v) in each pole of the right kidney and were observed for two years after treatment. The incidence of renal cancer was significantly elevated in the groups treated with nickel sulfarsenide (3/15 sarcomas) but not in those treated with nickel arsenide (1/20 renal-cell carcinoma), nickel selenide (1/12 sarcoma), nickel subselenide (2/23 sarcomas), nickel telluride (0/19), nickel subarsenides (tetragonal and hexagonal; 0/15 and 0/17), nickel antimonide (0/20) or nickel titanate (0/19). No local tumour developed in vehicle controls (Sunderman *et al.*, 1984b).

The experiments described in section 3.1 are summarized in Table 24.

**Table 24. Summary of studies used to evaluate the carcinogenicity to experimental animals of metallic nickel and nickel compounds**

| Compound | Route | Species (No. at start) | Tumour incidence (no. of animals with tumours/effective number) | Reference |
|---|---|---|---|---|
| **Metallic nickel powder and nickel alloys** | | | | |
| Cr/Ni stainless steel | Intratracheal | Hamster (60) | 36 mg, no local tumour<br>108 mg, no local tumour | Muhle et al. (1990) |
| Metallic nickel powder | Inhalation | Mouse (20) | No lung tumour | Hueper (1958) |
| Metallic nickel powder | Inhalation | Rat (160) | Benign lung neoplasms | Hueper (1958) |
| Metallic nickel powder (plus sulfur dioxide) | Inhalation | Rat (120) | 0/46 lung tumour | Hueper & Payne (1962) |
| Metallic nickel powder | Inhalation | Guinea-pig (42) | 1/23 intra-alveolar carcinoma, 1/23 metastasis of adenocarcinoma | Hueper (1958) |
| Metallic nickel powder | Intratracheal | Rat (80) | $10 \times 0.9$ mg, 8/32 lung tumours [$p < 0.05$]<br>$20 \times 0.3$ mg, 10/39 lung tumours [$p < 0.05$]<br>Controls, 0/40 lung tumour | Pott et al. (1987) |
| Metallic nickel powder | Intratracheal | Hamster (100 per group) | 10 mg, 1% local tumours<br>20 mg, 8% local tumours<br>40 mg, 12% local tumours<br>$4 \times 20$ mg, 10% local tumours | Ivankovic et al. (1987) |
| Metallic nickel powder | Intratracheal | Hamster (60) | 1/56 lung tumour | Muhle et al. (1990) |
| Metallic nickel powder | Intrapleural | Rat (25) | 4/12 local sarcomas vs 0/70 in controls [$p < 0.01$] | Hueper (1952) |
| Metallic nickel powder | Intrapleural | Rat (10) | 2/10 mesotheliomas vs 0/20 in controls | Furst et al. (1973) |
| Metallic nickel powder | Subcutaneous | Rat (10) | 5/10 local tumours | Mitchell et al. (1960) |
| Metallic nickel powder | Intramuscular | Rat (10) | 10/10 local tumours vs 0 in controls | Heath & Daniel (1964) |

**Table 24 (contd)**

| Compound | Route | Species (No. at start) | Tumour incidence (no. of animals with tumours/effective number) | Reference |
|---|---|---|---|---|
| Metallic nickel powder | Intramuscular | Rat (50) | 38/50 local tumours vs 0 in controls | Furst & Schlauder (1971) |
| Metallic nickel powder | Intramuscular | Rat (20) | 3.6 mg, 0/10 local tumours 14.4 mg, 2/9 local tumours Controls, 0/20 local tumour | Sunderman & Maenza (1976) |
| Metallic nickel powder | Intramuscular | Rat (20) | 17/20 local tumours vs 0/56 in controls | Berry et al. (1984) |
| Metallic nickel powder | Intramuscular | Rat (20) | 13/20 local tumours vs 0/44 in controls | Sunderman (1984) |
| Metallic nickel powder | Intramuscular | Rat (40) | 14/30 local tumours vs 0/60 in controls | Judde et al. (1987) |
| Metallic nickel powder | Intramuscular | Hamster (50) | 2/50 local tumours vs 0/50 in controls | Furst & Schlauder (1971) |
| Metallic nickel powder | Intraperitoneal | Rat | 30–50% local tumours vs none in controls | Furst & Cassetta (1973) |
| Metallic nickel powder | Intraperitoneal | Rat (50) | 46/48 abdominal tumours | Pott et al. (1987) |
| Metallic nickel powder | Intraperitoneal | Rat | 6 mg, 4/34 local tumours 2×6 mg, 5/34 local tumours 25×1 mg, 25/35 local tumours | Pott et al. (1990) |
| Metallic nickel powder | Intravenous | Mouse (25) | No tumour | Hueper (1955) |
| Metallic nickel powder | Intravenous | Rat (25) | 7/25 local tumours | Hueper (1955) |
| Metallic nickel powder | Intrarenal | Rat (20) | No local tumour | Jasmin & Riopelle (1976) |
| Metallic nickel powder | Intrarenal | Rat | No local tumour | Sunderman et al. (1984b) |
| Metallic nickel powder | Subperiosteal | Rat (20) | 11/20 local tumours | Berry et al. (1984) |
| Metallic nickel powder | Intrafemoral | Rat (20) | 9/20 local tumours | Berry et al. (1984) |

**Table 24 (contd)**

| Compound | Route | Species (No. at start) | Tumour incidence (no. of animals with tumours/effective number) | Reference |
|---|---|---|---|---|
| Nickel alloy: 26.8%, Ni, 16.2% Cr, 39.2% Fe, 0.04% Co | Intratracheal | Hamster (100 per group) | 10 mg, no local tumour<br>20 mg, no local tumour<br>40 mg, no local tumour<br>4×20 mg, no local tumour | Ivankovic et al. (1987) |
| Nickel alloy: 66.5%, Ni, 12.8% Cr, 6.5% Fe, 0.2% Co | Intratracheal | Hamster (100 per group) | 10 mg, 1% local tumours<br>20 mg, 8% local tumours<br>40 mg, 12% local tumours<br>4×20 mg, 10% local tumours | Ivankovic et al. (1987) |
| Nickel-gallium alloy (60% Ni) | Subcutaneous | Rat (10) | 9/10 local tumours | Mitchell et al. (1960) |
| Nickel-iron alloy (NiFe$_{1.6}$) | Intramuscular | Rat (16) | 0/16 local tumours | Sunderman (1984) |
| Nickel-iron alloy (NiFe$_{1.6}$) | Intrarenal | Rat | 1/14 renal cancers vs 0/46 controls | Sunderman et al. (1984b) |
| Nickel alloy (50% Ni) | Intraperitoneal | Rat | 50 mg, 8/35 local tumours<br>3×50 mg, 13/35 local tumours | Pott et al. (1989, 1990) |
| Nickel alloy (29% Ni) | Intraperitoneal | Rat | 50 mg, 2/33 local tumours<br>2×50 mg, 1/36 local tumours | Pott et al. (1989, 1990) |
| Nickel alloy (66% Ni) | Intraperitoneal | Rat | 50 mg, 12/35 local tumours<br>3×50 mg, 22/33 local tumours | Pott et al. (1989, 1990) |
| Pentlandite | Intratracheal | Hamster (60) | 1/60 local tumour | Muhle et al. (1990) |
| **Nickel oxides and hydroxides** | | | | |
| Nickel monoxide (green) | Inhalation | Rat (6, 8) | 8 mg/m³, 1/8 lung tumour<br>0.6 mg/m³, 0/6 lung tumour | Horie et al. (1985) |
| Nickel monoxide | Inhalation | Rat (40, 20) | 0.06 mg/m³, no tumour<br>0.2 mg/m³, no tumour | Glaser et al. (1986) |
| Nickel monoxide | Inhalation | Hamster (51) | 1/51 osteosarcoma | Wehner et al. (1975, 1979) |

**Table 24 (contd)**

| Compound | Route | Species (No. at start) | Tumour incidence (no. of animals with tumours/effective number) | Reference |
|---|---|---|---|---|
| Nickel monoxide | Intrapleural | Rat (32) | 31/32 local tumours *vs* 0/32 in controls | Skaug *et al.* (1985) |
| Nickel monoxide | Intratracheal | Rat | 10×5 mg, 10/37 lung tumours 10×15 mg, 12/38 lung tumours controls, 0/40 | Pott *et al.* (1987) |
| Nickel monoxide | Intratracheal | Hamster (50) | 1/49 lung tumours *vs* 4/50 in controls | Farrell & Davis (1974) |
| Nickel monoxide | Intramuscular | Mouse (50, 52) | 33/50 and 23/52 local tumours | Gilman (1962) |
| Nickel monoxide | Intramuscular | Rat (32) | 21/32 local tumorus | Gilman (1962) |
| Nickel monoxide | Intramuscular | Rat (20) | 2/20 local tumours | Gilman (1966) |
| Nickel monoxide | Intramuscular | Rat (20) | No local tumour | Sosiński (1975) |
| Nickel monoxide | Intramuscular | Rat (15) | 14/15 local tumours | Sunderman & McCully (1983) |
| Nickel monoxide | Intramuscular | Rat (20) | 0/20 local tumour | Berry *et al.* (1984) |
| Nickel monoxide | Subperiosteal | Rat (20) | 0/20 local tumour | Berry *et al.* (1984) |
| Nickel monoxide | Intraperitoneal | Rat (50) | 46/47 local tumours | Pott *et al.* (1987) |
| Nickel monoxide | Intraperitoneal | Rat | 25 mg, 12/34 local tumours 100 mg, 15/36 local tumours | Pott *et al.* (1989, 1990) |
| Nickel monoxide (green) | Intrarenal | Rat (12) | 0/12 local tumour | Sunderman *et al.* (1984b) |
| Nickel hydroxide | Intramuscular | Rat | 15/20 local tumours | Gilman (1966) |
| Nickel hydroxide | Intramuscular | Rat (3 x 20) | Dried gel: 5/19 local tumours Crystalline: 3/20 local tumours Colloidal: 0/13 local tumour | Kasprzak *et al.* (1983) |
| Nickel trioxide | Intramuscular | Rat (10) | 0/10 local tumour | Judde *et al.* (1987) |
| Nickel trioxide | Intracerebral | Rat (20) | 3/20 local tumours | Sosiński (1975) |

**Table 24 (contd)**

| Compound | Route | Species (No. at start) | Tumour incidence (no. of animals with tumours/effective number) | Reference |
|---|---|---|---|---|
| **Nickel sulfides** | | | | |
| Nickel disulfide | Intramuscular | Rat | 12/14 local tumours | Sunderman (1984) |
| Nickel disulfide | Intrarenal | Rat | 2/10 local tumours | Sunderman et al. (1984b) |
| Nickel sulfide (amorphous) | Intramuscular | Rat (10 per group) | 5.6 mg, no local tumour 22.4 mg, no local tumour | Sunderman & Maenza (1976) |
| β–Nickel sulfide | Intramuscular | Rat | 14/14 local tumours | Sunderman (1984) |
| Nickel sulfide (amorphous) | Intramuscular | Rat | 3/25 local tumours | Sunderman (1984) |
| Nickel sulfide | Intrarenal | Rat (18) | 0/18 local tumour | Jasmin & Riopelle (1976) |
| β–Nickel sulfide | Intrarenal | Rat | 8/14 local tumours | Sunderman et al. (1984b) |
| Nickel sulfide (amorphous) | Intrarenal | Rat | 0/15 local tumour | Sunderman et al. (1984b) |
| Nickel subsulfide | Inhalation | Rat (226) | 14/208 malignant lung tumours; 15/208 benign lung tumours | Ottolenghi et al. (1974) |
| Nickel subsulfide | Intratracheal | Mouse (100) | No increase in lung tumours | Fisher et al. (1986) |
| Nickel subsulfide | Intratracheal | Rat | 0.94 mg: 7/47 lung tumours 1.88 mg: 13/45 lung tumours 3.75 mg: 12/40 lung tumours | Pott et al. (1987) |
| α–Nickel subsulfide | Intratracheal | Hamster (62) | 0/62 lung tumour | Muhle et al. (1990) |
| Nickel subsulfide | Intrapleural | Rat (32) | 28/32 local tumours | Skaug et al. (1985) |
| Nickel subsulfide | Subcutaneous | Mouse (20) | 5 mg, 4/8 local tumours 10 mg, 7/8 local tumours | Oskarsson et al. (1979) |
| Nickel subsulfide | Subcutaneous | Rat (40 per group) | 3.3 mg, 37/39 local tumours 10 mg, 37/40 local tumours | Mason (1972) |
| Nickel subsulfide | Subcutaneous | Rat (20) | 18/19 local tumours | Shibata et al. (1989) |

**Table 24 (contd)**

| Compound | Route | Species (No. at start) | Tumour incidence (no. of animals with tumours/effective number) | Reference |
|---|---|---|---|---|
| Nickel subsulfide | Intramuscular | Mouse (45, 18) | Swiss, 27/45 local tumours C3H, 9/18 local tumours | Gilman (1962) |
| Nickel subsulfide | Intramuscular | Mice (20) | 5 mg, 4/8 local tumours 10 mg, 4/8 local tumours | Oskarsson et al. (1979) |
| Nickel subsulfide | Intramuscular | Mouse (10, 10) | C57Bl6, 5/10 local tumours DBA/2, 6/10 local tumours | Sunderman (1983b) |
| Nickel subsulfide | Intramuscular | Rat (32) | 25/28 local tumours | Gilman (1962) |
| Nickel subsulfide | Intramuscular | Rat (20) | 10 mg powder, 19/20 local tumours 500 mg fragments, 5/7 local tumours 500 mg discs, 14/17 local tumours 10 mg diffusion chamber, 14/17 local tumours controls, 1/19 local tumour | Gilman & Herchen (1963) |
| Nickel subsulfide (disc) | Intramuscular | Rat (groups of 15) | 4/10 local tumours with removal of disc after 64 days 7/10 local tumours with removal of disc after 128 days 10/10 local tumours with removal of disc after 206 days | Herchen & Gilman (1964) |
| Nickel subsulfide | Intramuscular | Rat (30, 27) | NIH black, 28/28 local tumours Hooded, 14/23 local tumours | Daniel (1966) |
| Nickel subsulfide | Intramuscular | Rat (40 per group) | 3.3 mg, 38/39 local tumours 10 mg, 34/40 local tumours | Mason (1972) |
| Nickel subsulfide | Intramuscular | Rat (10 per group) | 5 mg, 8/20 local tumours 20 mg, 9/9 local tumours | Sunderman & Maenza (1976) |
| Nickel subsulfide | Intramuscular | Rat (63,20) | Fischer, 59/63 local tumours Hooded, 11/20 local tumours | Yamashiro et al. (1980) |

**Table 24 (contd)**

| Compound | Route | Species (No. at start) | Tumour incidence (no. of animals with tumours/effective number) | Reference |
|---|---|---|---|---|
| Nickel subsulfide | Intramuscular | Rats (groups of 30) | 0.6 mg, 7/30 local tumours<br>1.2 mg, 23/30 local tumours<br>2.5 mg, 28/30 local tumours<br>5 mg, 29/30 local tumours | Sunderman et al. (1976) |
| Nickel subsulfide | Intramuscular | Rat | 0.63 mg, 7/29 local tumours<br>20 mg, 9/9 local tumours | Sunderman (1981) |
| α–Nickel subsulfide | Intramuscular | Rat | 9/9 local tumours | Sunderman (1984) |
| Nickel subsulfide | Intramuscular | Rat (20) | 10/20 local tumours | Berry et al. (1984) |
| Nickel subsulfide | Intramuscular | Rat (100) | 2/100 local tumours | Judde et al. (1987) |
| Nickel subsulfide | Intramuscular | Hamster (15, 17) | 5 mg, 4/15 local tumours<br>10 mg, 12/17 local tumours<br>controls, 0/14 local tumour | Sunderman (1983a) |
| Nickel subsulfide | Intramuscular | Rabbit | 16 local tumours | Hildebrand & Biserte (1979a,b) |
| α–Nickel subsulfide | Intramuscular | Rabbit (4) | 0/4 local tumour | Sunderman (1983a) |
| Nickel subsulfide | Intramuscular | Rat (20) | 19/20 local tumours | Shibata et al. (1989) |
| α–Nickel subsulfide | Topical | Hamster (6–7, 13–15) | 54 mg total, 0/6 local tumour;<br>108 mg total, 0/7 local tumour;<br>540 mg total, 0/15 local tumour;<br>1080 mg total, 0/13 local tumour | Sunderman (1983b) |
| Nickel subsulfide | Intraperitoneal | Rat (37) | 9/37 local tumours | Gilman (1966) |
| Nickel subsulfide | Intraperitoneal | Rat (50) | 27/42 local tumours | Pott et al. (1987) |
| Nickel subsulfide | Intraperitoneal | Rat | 6 mg, 20/36 local tumours<br>12 mg, 23/35 local tumours<br>25 mg, 25/34 local tumours | Pott et al. (1989, 1990) |

**Table 24 (contd)**

| Compound | Route | Species (No. at start) | Tumour incidence (no. of animals with tumours/effective number) | Reference |
|---|---|---|---|---|
| Nickel subsulfide | Subperiosteal | Rat (20) | 0/20 local tumour | Berry et al. (1984) |
| Nickel subsulfide | Intrafemoral | Rat (20) | 10/20 local tumours | Berry et al. (1984) |
| Nickel subsulfide | Intrarenal | Rat (16/24) | In glycerin, 7/16 local tumours In saline, 11/24 local tumours | Jasmin & Riopelle (1976) |
| α-Nickel subsulfide | Intrarenal | Rat (11–32) | Wistar Lewis, 7/11 local tumours NIH black, 6/12 local tumours Fischer 344, 9/32 local tumours Long–Evans, 0/12 local tumour | Sunderman et al. (1979a) |
| Nickel subsulfide | Intratesticular | Rat (19) | 16/19 local tumours | Damjanov et al. (1978) |
| Nickel subsulfide | Intraocular | Rat (15) | 14/15 local tumours | Albert et al. (1980); Sunderman (1983b) |
| Nickel subsulfide | Intraocular | Salamander (8) | 7/8 local tumours | Okamoto (1987) |
| Nickel subsulfide | Transplacental | Rat (8) | No difference in tumour incidence | Sunderman et al. (1981) |
| Nickel subsulfide | Pellet implantation into subcutaneous implanted tracheal grafts | Rat (60, 64) | 5 mg, 9/60 local tumours 15 mg, 45/64 local tumours | Yarita & Nettesheim (1978) |
| Nickel subsulfide | Intra-articular | Rat (20) | 16/19 local tumours | Shibata et al. (1989) |
| Nickel subsulfide | Intra-fat | Rat (20) | 9/20 local tumours | Shibata et al. (1989) |
| Nickel ferrosulfide | Intramuscular | Rat | 15/15 local tumours | Sunderman (1984) |
| Nickel ferrosulfide | Intrarenal | Rat | 1/12 local tumour | Sunderman et al. (1984b) |

**Table 24 (contd)**

| Compound | Route | Species (No. at start) | Tumour incidence (no. of animals with tumours/effective number) | Reference |
|---|---|---|---|---|
| **Nickel salts** | | | | |
| Basic nickel carbonate tetrahydrate | Intraperitoneal | Rat | 25 mg, 1/35 lung tumours vs 1/33 in controls; 50 mg, 3/33 lung tumours vs 1/33 in controls | Pott et al. (1989, 1990) |
| Nickel acetate | Intramuscular | Rat (35) | 1/35 local tumour | Payne (1964) |
| Nickel acetate | Intraperitoneal | Mouse (3 x 20) | 72 mg, 8/18 lung tumours; 180 mg, 7/14 lung tumours; 360 mg, 12/19 lung tumours | Stoner et al. (1976) |
| Nickel acetate tetrahydrate | Intraperitoneal | Mouse (30) | 1.50 lung tumours/animal Controls, 0.32 lung tumours/animal | Poirier et al. (1984) |
| Nickel acetate tetrahydrate | Intraperitoneal | Rat | 25 mg, 3/35 lung tumours vs 1/33 in controls; 50 mg, 5/31 lung tumours vs 1/33 in controls | Pott et al. (1989, 1990) |
| Nickel ammonium sulfate | Intramuscular | Rat (35) | 0/35 local tumour | Payne (1964) |
| Nickel carbonate | Intramuscular | Rat (35) | 6/35 local tumours | Payne (1964) |
| Nickel chloride | Intramuscular | Rat (35) | 0/35 local tumour | Payne (1964) |
| Nickel chloride hexahydrate | Intraperitoneal | Rat | 4/32 lung tumours vs 1/33 in controls | Pott et al. (1989, 1990) |
| Nickel chromate | Intramuscular | Rat (16) | 1/16 local tumour | Sunderman (1984) |
| Nickel fluoride | Intramuscular | Rat (20) | 3/18 local tumours | Gilman (1966) |
| Nickel sulfate | Intramuscular | Rat (35) | 1/35 local tumour | Payne (1964) |
| Nickel sulfate | Intramuscular | Rat (20) | 0/20 local tumour | Gilman (1966) |
| Nickel sulfate | Intramuscular | Rat (20) | 0/20 local tumour | Kasprzak et al. (1983) |
| Nickel sulfate hexahydrate | Intramuscular | Rat (32) | 0/32 local tumour | Gilman (1962) |

**Table 24 (contd)**

| Compound | Route | Species (No. at start) | Tumour incidence (no. of animals with tumours/effective number) | Reference |
|---|---|---|---|---|
| Nickel sulfate heptahydrate | Intraperitoneal | Rat | 6/30 lung tumours vs 1/33 in controls | Pott et al. (1989, 1990) |
| **Other nickel compounds** | | | | |
| Ferronickel alloy | Intramuscular | Rat | No local tumour | Sunderman & McCully (1983) |
| Nickel antimonide | Intramuscular | Rat | 17/29 vs 0/40 control ($p < 0.05$) | Sunderman & McCully (1983) |
| Nickel antimonide | Intrarenal | Rat | 0/20 local tumour | Sunderman et al. (1984b) |
| Nickel arsenide | Intramuscular | Rat | No local tumour | Sunderman & McCully (1983) |
| Nickel arsenide | Intrarenal | Rat | 1/20 local tumour | Sunderman et al. (1984b) |
| Nickel arsenide hexagonal | Intramuscular | Rat | 17/20 vs 0/40 controls ($p < 0.05$) | Sunderman & McCully (1983) |
| Nickel arsenide hexagonal | Intrarenal | Rat | 0/17 local tumour | Sunderman et al. (1984b) |
| Nickel arsenide tetragonal | Intramuscular | Rat | 8/16 vs 0/40 control ($p < 0.05$) | Sunderman & McCully (1983) |
| Nickel arsenide tetragonal | Intrarenal | Rat | 0/15 local tumour | Sunderman et al. (1984b) |
| Nickel carbonyl | Inhalation | Rat (64, 32, 80) | 30 mg/m³ for 32 weeks: 1/64 pulmonary tumour 60 mg/m³ for 32 weeks: 1/32 pulmonary tumour 250 mg/m³ once: 1/80 pulmonary tumour | Sunderman et al. (1957, 1959) |

**Table 24 (contd)**

| Compound | Route | Species (No. at start) | Tumour incidence (no. of animals with tumours/effective number) | Reference |
|---|---|---|---|---|
| Nickel carbonyl | Inhalation | Rat | 1/71 lung tumour vs 0/32 control | Sunderman & Donnelly (1965) |
| Nickel carbonyl | Intravenous | Rat (121) | 19/120 lung tumours | Lau et al. (1972) |
| Nickel-enriched fly ash | Inhalation | Hamster (102) | No significant difference | Wehner et al. (1981, 1984) |
| Nickelocene | Intramuscular | Rat (50) | 144 mg, 18/50 local tumours 300 mg, 21/50 local tumours | Furst & Schlauder (1971) |
| Nickelocene | Intramuscular | Hamster (50) | 8×5 mg, 0/50 local tumour 25 mg, 4/29 local tumours | Furst & Schlauder (1971) |
| Nickel monoxide dust | Intratracheal | Rat (26) | 1/26 lung tumour vs 0/47 control | Saknyn & Blokhin (1978) |
| Nickel selenide | Intramuscular | Rat | 8/16 local tumours | Sunderman (1984) |
| Nickel selenide | Intramuscular | Rat | 1/12 local tumour vs 0/79 control | Sunderman et al. (1984b) |
| Nickel subselenide | Intramuscular | Rat | 21/23 local tumours | Sunderman (1984) |
| Nickel subselenide | Intrarenal | Rat | 2/23 local tumours vs 0/79 control | Sunderman et al. (1984b) |
| Nickel sulfarsenide | Intramuscular | Rat | 14/16 vs 0/40 control (p < 0.05) | Sunderman & McCully (1983) |
| Nickel sulfarsenide | Intrarenal | Rat | 3/15 local tumours vs 0/79 control | Sunderman et al (1984b) |
| Nickel telluride | Intramuscular | Rat | 14/26 vs 0/40 control (p < 0.05) | Sunderman & McCully (1983) |
| Nickel telluride | Intrarenal | Rat | 0/19 local tumour | Sunderman et al. (1984b) |
| Nickel titanate | Intramuscular | Rat | No local tumour | Sunderman & McCully (1983) |

**Table 24 (contd)**

| Compound | Route | Species (No. at start) | Tumour incidence (no. of animals with tumours/effective number) | Reference |
|---|---|---|---|---|
| Nickel titanate | Intrarenal | Rat | 0/19 local tumour | Sunderman *et al.* (1984b) |
| Refinery dust | Inhalation | Rat (5) | 1/5 lung tumour *vs* 0/47 control | Saknyn & Blokhin (1978) |
| Refinery dust | Intramuscular | Mouse (40) | 20/36 local tumours *vs* 0/48 control (*p* < 0.01) | Gilman & Ruckerbauer (1962) |
| Refinery dust | Intramuscular | Rat (35) | Dust, 19/27 local tumours Washed dust, 20/28 local tumours Controls, 0/30 local tumour | Gilman & Ruckerbauer (1962) |
| Refinery dust | Intraperitoneal | Rat (16, 23) | Dust 1, 3/16 local tumours Dust 2, 3/23 local tumours Controls, 0/47 local tumour | Saknyn & Blokhin (1978) |

## 3.2 Other relevant data in experimental systems

### (a) Absorption, distribution, excretion and metabolism

The results of studies on absorption, distribution, excretion, and metabolism of nickel compounds have been reviewed and/or summarized in several publications (National Research Council, 1975; Sunderman, 1977; Kasprzak, 1978; Bencko, 1983; Mushak, 1984; Sarkar, 1984; Fairhurst & Illing, 1987; Kasprzak, 1987; Sunderman, 1988; Maibach & Menné, 1989).

#### (i)  Nickel oxides and hydroxides

Male Wistar rats were exposed to 0.4-70 mg/m³ (0.6-4-μm particles) nickel monoxide aerosols for 6-7 h per day on five days per week for a maximum of three months. The clearance rate of nickel monoxide from the lung after a one-month exposure to 0.6-8 mg/m³ (1.2-μm particles) was estimated to be about 100 μg per year. The exposure did not increase background nickel levels in organs other than the lung (Kodama et al., 1985).

Electron microscopic examination of the lungs of male Wistar rats exposed to nickel monoxide aerosols (0.6-8 mg/m³; 1.2- or 2.2-μm particles) for a total of 140-216 h showed that the particles were trapped mainly by alveolar macrophages. One year after termination of exposure, the particles were distributed in the alveoli, hilar lymphoid apparatus and terminal bronchioli. Some nickel monoxide particles were present within the lysosomes of macrophages (Horie et al., 1985).

Female Wistar rats were given a single intratracheal injection of black nickel monoxide, prepared by heating nickel hydroxide at 250°C for 45 min (final product containing a mixture of nickel monoxide and nickel hydroxide; >90% insoluble in water; particles, 3.7 μm or less in diameter) in a normal saline suspension (100 nmol [7.5 μg] nickel monoxide in 0.2 ml). The highest concentrations of nickel were seen in the lungs and mediastinal lymph nodes, followed by the heart, femur, duodenum, kidney, pancreas, ovaries, spleen, blood and other tissues. Following injection, the concentration of nickel in the lung decreased at a much slower rate than in other tissues. By the third day after injection of nickel monoxide, about 17% of the nickel was excreted with the faeces and about 16% in the urine. By 90 days, about 60% of the dose of nickel had been excreted, half of it in the urine. The overall pattern indicates a partial transfer of nickel from lung to the mediastinal lymph nodes and slow solubilization of this product in tissue fluids (English et al., 1981).

#### (ii)  Nickel subsulfide

After intratracheal instillation of 11.7 μg α-[63]Ni-nickel subsulfide powder (1-66-μm particles) in a normal saline suspension to male strain A/J mice, 38% was cleared from the lungs with a half-time of 1.2 days, while 42% was cleared with a half-time of 12.4 days; 10% of the dose was retained in the lung 35 days after instillation. The highest amounts of nickel were found in the kidney, followed by blood > liver > femur up to seven days; at 35 days, levels were greatest in kidney, followed by femur > liver > blood; maximal levels occurred 4 h after dosing and decreased rapidly thereafter with biological half-times similar to those in the lung. The urine was the primary excretion pathway; after 35 days, 100% of the nickel dose was recovered in the excreta, 60% of which was in urine (Valentine & Fisher, 1984).

The cumulative eight-week urinary excretion of nickel following intramuscular injection of $^{63}$Ni-nickel subsulfide to male Fischer rats (1.2 mg/rat, 1.4-$\mu$m particles) was 67%, while faecal excretion during that time was only 7% of the dose. The residual nickel contents at the injection site at 22 and 31 weeks after injection were 13-17% and 13-14% of the dose, respectively. The kinetics of nickel disappearance were described by a three-compartmental model, with pool sizes of 60, 27 and 11% of the dose and half-times of 14, 60 and indefinite number of days, respectively (Sunderman *et al.*, 1976).

$\alpha$-Nickel subsulfide particles labelled with $^{63}$Ni and $^{35}$S injected intramuscularly into Fischer rats (Kasprzak, 1974) or intramuscularly and subcutaneously into NMRI mice of each sex (Oskarsson *et al.*, 1979) persisted at the injection site for several months, with a gradual loss of both $^{63}$Ni and $^{35}$S. In mice, nickel subsulfide was transferred to regional lymph nodes and to the reticuloendothelial cells of the liver and spleen. The presence of $^{63}$Ni in the kidney and $^{35}$S in the cartilage indicated solubilization of the subsulfide from the site of injection during tumorigenesis. There was no excessive or specific localization of the solubilized $^{63}$Ni or $^{35}$S in the tumours or in metastases. Most of the radioactivity in the tumours appeared to be associated with dust particles.

Elevated concentrations of nickel were detected in fetuses after intramuscular administration of $\alpha$-nickel subsulfide to Fischer rats on day 6 of gestation (Sunderman *et al.*, 1978a).

### (iii)  *Nickel salts*

Intratracheal instillation of nickel chloride (100 nmol[13 $\mu$g]/rat) to female Wistar rats resulted in a fast distribution of nickel throughout the body, followed by rapid clearance. During the first six days after injection, over 60% of the dose was excreted in the urine and approximately 5% in faeces; after 90 days, these amounts had increased only slightly, to 64% and 6%, respectively (English *et al.*, 1981). Similar distribution and excretion patterns were observed after intratracheal injection of nickel chloride (1.27 $\mu$g/rat Ni) to male Sprague-Dawley rats (Carvalho & Ziemer, 1982).

Pulmonary clearance and excretion of nickel following intratracheal instillation of nickel sulfate at doses of 17, 190 or 1800 nmol [1, 11 or 106 $\mu$g] Ni per rat to

Fischer 344 rats appeared to depend on the dose. At periods up to four days after instillation, lungs, trachea, larynx, kidney and urinary bladder contained the highest concentrations of nickel. The half-time for urinary excretion (the predominant route of excretion) varied from 23 h for the lowest dose to 4.6 h for the highest. Faecal excretion accounted for 30% (17- and 190-nmol doses) and 13% (1800-nmol) of the dose. The long-term half-time of nickel clearance from the lung varied from 21 h at the highest dose to 36 h at the lowest dose (Medinsky *et al.*, 1987).

In male Sprague-Dawley rats exposed to nickel chloride aerosols (90 µg/m³ Ni; 0.7-0.9-µm particles) for 2 h per day for 14 days, the nickel burden in the lung reached a steady level after five days. The maximal clearance velocity was calculated to be 34.6 ng/g.h. These data support the hypothesis of a saturable clearance mechanism for 'soluble nickel' in the lung (Menzel *et al.*, 1987).

After intratracheal administration of 'nickel carbonate' (0.05 mg/mouse Ni) to female Swiss albino mice, most of the dose was eliminated in the urine in about 12 days (Furst & Al-Mahrouq, 1981). [The Working Group noted that the compound tested was most probably basic nickel carbonate.]

After a single intravenous injection of 10 µg nickel as [63]Ni-nickel chloride per mouse (albino or brown mice [strains not specified], including pregnant mice), whole-body autoradiography at 30 min showed that nickel persisted in the blood, kidney, urinary bladder, lung, eye and hair follicles; at three weeks, nickel persisted in the lung, central nervous system, kidneys, hair follicles and skin (Bergman *et al.*, 1980). In C57Bl mice, nickel was also localized in the epithelium of the forestomach; in the kidney, it was present in the cortex at sites that probably corresponded to the distal convoluted tubules. Nickel was retained much longer in the lung than in other tissues (Oskarsson & Tjälve, 1979a).

A single intravenous injection of 1 mg/kg bw [63]Ni-nickel chloride to male Sprague-Dawley rats resulted in rapid urinary excretion of 87% of the dose in the first day after injection and 90% after four days. Faecal excretion was much lower, up to a total of approximately 3% of the dose after four days (Sunderman & Selin, 1968). Lung and spleen were ranked after kidney as nickel-accumulating organs in Sprague-Dawley rats given an intraperitoneal injection of 82 µg/kg bw [63]Ni-nickel chloride (Sarkar, 1980).

The kinetics of nickel metabolism in rats and rabbits after a single intravenous injection of [63]Ni-nickel chloride followed a two-compartmental mathematical model, with first-order kinetics of nickel elimination from plasma with half-times of 6 and 50 h for rats and 8 and 83 h for rabbits, respectively, for the two compartments (Onkelinx *et al.*, 1973).

Following a single intraperitoneal injection of [63]Ni-nickel chloride to BALB/c mice (100 µCi/mouse), nickel was found to remain in the lung much longer than in any other tissue (Herlant-Peers *et al.*, 1982). Preferential accumulation of nickel in the lung was also observed in Fischer 344 rats following daily subcutaneous injections of 62.5 or 125 μmol [8.1 or 16.3 mg]/kg bw nickel chloride for up to six weeks (Knight *et al.*, 1988). In contrast, multiple intraperitoneal injections of nickel acetate to male Swiss albino mice (0.5, 0.75 or 1.0 mg/mouse; 10, 20 or 30 daily injections each) resulted in preferential accumulation of nickel in the thymus (Feroz *et al.*, 1976).

Daily oral administration of 2.5 mg nickel sulfate per rat [strain unspecified] for 30 days resulted in accumulation of nickel in trachea > nasopharynx > skull > oesophagus > intestine > skin > liver = spleen > stomach > kidney > lung = brain > heart (Jiachen *et al.*, 1986).

Nickel was taken up from the lumen of male Sprague-Dawley rat jejunum *in vitro* at a rate proportional to the concentration of $^{63}$Ni-nickel chloride in the perfusate up to 20 μM [1.2 mg] Ni. At higher concentrations (6 and 12 mg Ni), apparent saturation was approached. Nickel was not retained by the mucosa and showed a very low affinity for metallothionein (Foulkes & McMullen, 1986).

Dermal absorption of 2 or 40 μCi $^{63}$Ni-nickel chloride was observed in guinea-pigs. After 1 h, nickel had accumulated in highly keratinized areas, the stratum corneum and hair shafts. Following exposure for 4-48 h, nickel also accumulated in basal and suprabasal epidermal cells. After 4 h, nickel appeared in blood and urine (Lloyd, 1980).

It has been demonstrated in several studies that nickel chloride crosses the placenta in mice (Jacobsen *et al.*, 1978; Lu *et al.*, 1979; Olsen & Jonsen, 1979; Lu *et al.*, 1981; Jasim & Tjälve, 1986) and rats (Sunderman *et al.*, 1977; Mas *et al.*, 1986).

(iv)    *Other nickel compounds*

In NMRI mice, high levels of nickel were found in the respiratory tract, brain, spinal cord, heart, diaphragm, adrenal cortex, brown fat, kidney and urinary bladder 5 min to 24 h following inhalation of $^{63}$Ni- and $^{14}$C-nickel carbonyl at 3.05 g/m$^3$ Ni for 10 min (Oskarsson & Tjälve, 1979b).

After exposure of rats to nickel carbonyl by inhalation, increased levels of nickel were found predominantly in microsomal and supernatant fractions of the lung and in the microsomal fraction of the liver (Sunderman & Sunderman, 1963).

After an intravenous injection of nickel carbonyl as 22 mg/kg bw Ni to Sprague-Dawley rats, most of the subcellular nickel in liver and lung was bound to supernatant fractions, followed by nuclei and debris, mitochondria and microsomes (Sunderman & Selin, 1968).

Twenty-four hours after an intravenous injection of $^{63}$Ni-nickel carbonyl (0.9 mg/kg bw Ni) to NMRI mice, nickel was found to be associated with both particulate and soluble cellular constituents of the lung, liver and kidneys. Radioactivity was detected in the gel chromatograms of cytosols from lung, kidney and blood serum of treated mice in the void volume and salt volume (Oskarsson & Tjälve, 1979c).

Following intravenous injection of 50 µl/kg bw nickel carbonyl (22 µg/kg bw Ni) to Sprague-Dawley rats, over 38% of the dose was exhaled during 6 h after injection and none after that time. Average total urinary excretion of nickel over four days was 31% (23% within the first 12 h), whereas total faecal excretion was 2.4% and biliary excretion was 0.2%. Total average excretion of nickel in four days was 72%. Most of the remaining nickel carbonyl underwent intracellular decomposition and oxidation to nickel[II] and carbon monoxide. Twenty-four hours after the injection, nickel injected as nickel carbonyl was distributed among organs and tissues, with the highest concentration in lung (Sunderman & Selin, 1968; Kasprzak & Sunderman, 1969).

### (b)  Dissolution and cellular uptake

#### (i)  Metallic nickel and nickel alloys

Slow dissolution and elimination of finely powdered nickel metal from the muscle injection site was observed in rats. In the local rhabdomyosarcomas that developed, nickel was recovered in the nuclear fraction and mitochondria; little or no nickel was found in the microsomes (Heath & Webb, 1967). The nuclear fraction of nickel is preferentially bound to nucleoli (Webb et al., 1972).

Slow dissolution of metallic nickel occurred when nickel metal powder was incubated at 37°C with horse serum or sterile homogenates of rat muscle, liver, heart or kidney prepared in Tyrode solution. The solubilization may have involved oxygen uptake and was faster for a freshly reduced powder than for an older commercial powder; over 97% of the dissolved nickel became bound to diffusible components of the tissue homogenates (mostly histidine, followed by nucleotides, nucleosides and free bases) (Weinzierl & Webb, 1972).

#### (ii)  Nickel oxides and hydroxides

The dissolution half-times of six differently prepared samples of nickel oxide and four samples of nickel-copper oxides in water were longer than 11 years. However, in rat serum and renal cytosol, the half-time dropped to about one year for a low-temperature nickel oxide and to 2.7-7.2 years for three nickel-copper oxides, the rest retaining the > 11-year value. Two preparations of nickel oxide obtained at temperatures ≤735°C and all four nickel-copper oxides appeared to be phagocytized by C3H/10T½ cells more actively than the other nickel oxides (Sunderman et al., 1987).

Kasprzak et al. (1983) found the half-times for two preparations of nickel hydroxide (air-dried colloidal and crystalline) in an 0.1 M ammonium acetate buffer of pH 7.4 to be 56 h and 225 h, respectively. Corresponding values in an artificial lung fluid were 360 h and 1870 h, respectively.

### (iii)   *Nickel sulfides*

The dissolution rate of α-nickel subsulfide depends on the particle size, the presence of oxygen and the dissolving medium (Gilman & Herchen, 1963; Kasprzak & Sunderman, 1977; Dewally & Hildebrand, 1980; Lee *et al.*, 1982).

Both *in vivo* and in cell-free systems *in vitro*, α-nickel subsulfide reacts with oxygen to yield insoluble crystalline β-nickel sulfide and soluble nickel[II] derivatives; β-nickel sulfide also dissolves through oxidation of its sulfur moiety (Kasprzak & Sunderman, 1977; Oskarsson *et al.*, 1979; Dewally & Hildebrand, 1980). It has been suggested that the transformation of nickel subsulfide into β-nickel sulfide under anaerobic conditions in the muscle might be due to reaction with sulfur from sulfhydryl groups in the host organism (Dewally & Hildebrand, 1980).

Particles of crystalline nickel sulfides, α-nickel subsulfide and β-nickel sulfide (<5 μm in diameter, 1-20 μg/ml) were phagocytized by cultured Syrian hamster embryo cells and Chinese hamster CHO cells, while particles of amorphous nickel sulfide were taken up only sparingly by the cells. Pretreatment of Syrian hamster embryo cells with benzo[*a*]pyrene enhanced the uptake of nickel subsulfide. The half-life of the engulfed particles was about 40 h in Syrian hamster cells; they disappeared from the cells through solubilization, and solubilized nickel was detected in the nuclear fraction (Costa & Mollenhauer, 1980a,b; Costa *et al.*, 1981a).

α-Nickel subsulfide and β-nickel sulfide were also incorporated into human embryonic L132 pulmonary cells in culture. β-Nickel sulfide was present within large intracellular vesicles; nickel subsulfide was generally bound to the membranes of intracellular vesicles, to lysosomal structures and to the outer cell membrane (Hildebrand *et al.*, 1985, 1986).

The soluble nickel derived from nickel subsulfide and β-nickel sulfide intracellularly undergoes subcellular distribution that differs from that following entry of nickel from outside the cells (Harnett *et al.*, 1982; Sen & Costa, 1986a). Treatment of cultured Chinese hamster CHO cells with β-nickel sulfide (10 μg/ml, three-day incubation) resulted in binding of nickel to DNA and RNA at a level 300-2000 times higher and to protein at a level 15 times higher than after similar treatment with nickel chloride (Harnett *et al.*, 1982). Cellular uptake of β-nickel sulfide facilitates a specific interaction of nickel with the heterochromatic long arm of the X chromosome of Chinese hamster CHO cells (Sen & Costa, 1986a). Lee *et al.* (1982) found that soluble nickel derived from nickel subsulfide forms an exceptionally stable ternary protein-nickel-DNA complex *in vitro* in the presence of DNA and rat liver microsomes.

(iv)  *Nickel salts*

Soluble nickel retained in the tissues of mice becomes bound to particulate and soluble cellular constituents, the distribution depending on the tissue. In lung and liver of NMRI mice, nickel was bound predominantly to a high-molecular-weight protein; in the kidney, it was bound mainly to low-molecular-weight ultrafiltrable ligands. No nickel was bound to metallothionein or superoxide dismutase (Oskarsson & Tjälve, 1979c).

Several nickel-binding proteins were found in lung and liver cytosol of BALB/c mice that were different after incorporation *in vivo* and *in vitro*. The composition and structures of these proteins were not identified (Herlant-Peers *et al.*, 1982).

Intracellular nickel concentrations in the lungs of strain A mice given intraperitoneal injections of nickel acetate were highest in the microsomes, followed by mitochondria, cytosol and nuclei (Kasprzak, 1987).

In blood serum, nickel was sequestered mainly by albumin, which had a high binding capacity for this metal in most species tested, except for dogs and pigs (Callan & Sunderman, 1973). Nickel in human serum is chelated by histidine, serum albumin or both in a ternary complex, although a small fraction is bound to a glycoprotein (Sarkar, 1980; Glennon & Sarkar, 1982).

Less nickel chloride was taken up by Chinese hamster CHO cells than insoluble nickel sulfides; moreover, nickel incorporated from nickel chloride had a much higher affinity for cellular proteins than for DNA or RNA (Harnett *et al.*, 1982). A greater effect on the heterochromatic long arm of the X chromosome was observed when Chinese hamster CHO cells were exposed to nickel-albumin complexes encapsulated in liposomes than to nickel chloride alone (Sen & Costa, 1986a).

Cellular binding and uptake of nickel depend on the hydro- and lipophilic properties of the nickel complexes to which the cells are exposed. Nickel-complexing ligands, L-histidine, human serum albumin, D-penicillamine and ethylenediaminetetraacetic acid, which form hydrophilic nickel complexes, inhibited the uptake of nickel by rabbit alveolar macrophages, human B-lymphoblasts and human erythrocytes. The same ligands also sequestered nickel from nickel-preloaded cells. Diethyldithiocarbamate, however, which forms a lipophilic nickel complex, enhanced the cellular uptake of nickel and prevented its removal from nickel-preloaded cells. It also induced transfer of nickel in a cell lysate from the cytosol to the residual pellet (Nieboer *et al.*, 1984b). Sodium pyridinethione, which forms a lipophilic nickel complex, behaved similarly (Jasim & Tjälve, 1986).

Nickel applied to rat liver and kidney nuclei as nickel chloride bound in a dose-related manner to the chromatin and as to polynucleosomes and to the DNA molecule. In the nuclear chromatin, nickel was associated with both the DNA and histone and non-histone proteins; a ternary nickel-DNA-protein complex more stable than binary nickel-DNA complexes was identified (Ciccarelli & Wetterhahn, 1985).

Calf thymus DNA appeared to have more than two types of binding site for nickel; DNA phosphate moieties were identified as having the highest affinity for nickel (Kasprzak *et al.*, 1986).

### (v) *Other nickel compounds*

'Nickel carbonate' particles were actively phagocytized by human embryonal lung epithelial cells L132 in culture and showed an increased affinity for cytoplasmic and cell membranes (Hildebrand *et al.*, 1986). [The Working Group noted that the compound tested was most probably basic nickel carbonate.]

Following an intraperitoneal injection of 'nickel carbonate' to male Sprague-Dawley rats, nickel was found to be associated with liver and kidney nuclear DNA as early as 3 h after injection, with a further increase by 20 h. The nickel concentration in kidney DNA was five to six times higher than that in liver. Significant differences were found in the distribution of nickel between nucleic acids and associated proteins in DNA samples extracted from kidney and liver (Ciccarelli & Wetterhahn, 1984a,b). [The Working Group noted that the compound tested was most probably basic nickel carbonate.]

Sunderman *et al.* (1984b) determined dissolution half-times in rat serum and renal cytosol and phagocytic indices in peritoneal macrophages *in vitro* of various water-insoluble nickel derivatives, including nickel selenide, nickel subselenide, nickel telluride, nickel sulfarsenide, nickel arsenide, nickel arsenide tetragonal, nickel arsenide hexagonal, nickel antimonide, nickel ferrosulfide matte, a ferronickel alloy ($NiFe_{1.6}$) and nickel titanate. No correlation was found between those two parameters and the carcinogenic activity of the tested compounds in the muscle of Fischer 344 rats.

### (c) *Interactions*

Parenteral administration of soluble nickel salts induced changes in the tissue distribution of other metal ions (Whanger, 1973; Nielsen, 1980; Chmielnicka *et al.*, 1982; Nieboer *et al.*, 1984b; Nielsen *et al.*, 1984).

Several physiological divalent cations appeared to affect nickel metabolism. Thus, manganese decreased the proportion of ultrafiltrable nickel constituents of muscle homogenates; the gross muscle uptake and excretion of nickel were not affected. Metallic manganese dust also inhibited the dissolution rate of nickel subsulfide in rat serum, serum ultrafiltrate and water (Sunderman *et al.*, 1976). Manganese dust reduced the phagocytosis of nickel subsulfide particles by Syrian hamster embryo cells *in vitro* (Costa *et al.*, 1981a). Magnesium decreased the uptake of nickel by pulmonary nuclei and cytosol of strain A mice and decreased nickel uptake by lung, kidney and liver of Fischer 344 rats (Kasprzak *et al.*, 1987). Both manganese and magnesium strongly antagonized the binding of nickel to the phosphate groups of calf thymus DNA *in vitro*, while copper, which did not inhibit nickel carcinogenesis, was a much weaker antagonist (Kasprzak *et al.*, 1986).

Nickel that accumulated in mouse tissues following administration of nickel carbonyl *in vivo* could be displaced from those tissues by treatment *in vitro* with other cations, including $H^+$, in proportion to their valence; $Mg^{2+}$ and $La^{3+}$ were the most effective (Oskarsson & Tjälve, 1979b).

Certain nickel[II]-peptide complexes in aqueous solution were found to react with ambient oxygen by a facile autocatalytic process in which nickel[III] intermediates played a major role. Such reactions may lead to degradation, e.g., decarboxylation, of the organic ligand (Bossu *et al.*, 1978). Nickel[III] was also identified in a nickel[II]-glycyl-glycyl-*n*-histidine complex, indicating possible redox effects of the nickel[III]/nickel[II] redox couple on that protein (Nieboer *et al.*, 1986).

### (d)  Toxic effects

The toxicity of nickel and its inorganic compounds has been reviewed (US Environmental Protection Agency, 1986; Fairhurst & Illing, 1987; World Health Organization, 1990), and the chemical basis of the biological reactivity of nickel has been discussed (Ciccarelli & Wetterhahn, 1984a; Nieboer *et al.*, 1984b,c).

### (i)  Metallic nickel and nickel alloys

The lungs of male rabbits exposed by inhalation to 1 mg/m³ nickel metal dust ( < 40 μm particles) for 6 h per day on five days per week for three and six months showed two- to three-fold increases in the volume density of alveolar type II cells. The six-month exposure caused focal pneumonia (Johansson *et al.*, 1981; Camner *et al.*, 1984).

Similar changes, resembling alveolar proteinosis, were observed in rabbits after exposure to nickel metal dust by inhalation for four weeks (Camner *et al.*, 1978). After three or six months of exposure at 1 mg/m³, phagocytic activity *in vitro* was increased upon challenge by *Escherichia coli* (Johansson *et al.*, 1980).

A single intramuscular injection of 20 mg nickel metal dust to male WAG rats resulted in long-lasting suppression of natural killer cell activity in peripheral blood mononuclear cells. Between eight and 18 weeks after the nickel injection, the activity decreased to 50-60% of that in the control rats (Judde *et al.*, 1987).

### (ii)  Nickel oxides

Exposure of female Wistar rats by inhalation to nickel monoxide aerosols (generated at 550°C from nickel acetate) at concentrations of 200, 400 and 800 μg/m³ for 24 h per day for 120 days resulted in a significant, dose-related reduction in growth rate, decreased kidney and liver weights and erythrocyte count, decreased activity of serum alkaline phosphatase, increased wet lung weight and leukocyte count and increased mean erythrocyte cell volume (Weischer et al., 1980a,b).

Male Wistar rats exposed continuously to nickel monoxide (generated at 550°C from nickel acetate) aerosols at 50 µg/m³ (median particle diameter, 0.35 µm) for 15 weeks showed no significant difference in the overall ability of the lungs to clear ferrous oxide up to day 7. After that time, lung clearance in nickel oxide-exposed rats decreased significantly. The half life of ferrous oxide clearance after day 6 was 58 days for control rats and 520 days for nickel oxide-exposed rats; in excised lungs, the values were 56 and 74 days, respectively (Oberdoerster & Hochrainer, 1980).

An increase in lung weight (six-fold) and alveolar proteinosis were observed in male Wistar rats that died during life-time exposure to an aerosol of nickel monoxide (produced by pyrolysis of nickel acetate [probably at 550°C] [particle size unspecified]) at 60 or 200 µg/m³, 23 h per day, seven days per week. With longer exposures, marked accumulation of macrophages and focal septal fibrosis were also observed (Takenaka et al., 1985).

No significant histopathological change was found in male Wistar rats exposed to green nickel oxide (0.6 µm particles) for up to 12 months at 0.3 or 1.2 mg/m³, 7 h per day on five days per week (Tanaka et al., 1988).

No mortality was observed following exposure by inhalation of Fischer 344/N rats and B6C3F₁ mice to nickel monoxide (formed at 1350°C; 3 µm particles) at 0.9-24 mg/m³ Ni for 6 h/day on five days per week for 12 days. Lung inflammation and hyperplasia of alveolar macrophages occurred primarily at the highest exposure concentration in both species; generally, the lung lesions in mice were less severe than those in rats. Atrophy of the olfactory epithelium was seen only in two rats at the highest dose, while atrophy of the thymus and hyperplasia of the lymph nodes were seen in both rats and mice exposed to the highest concentrations (Dunnick et al., 1988).

In Syrian golden hamsters, life-time inhalation of 53 mg/m³ nickel monoxide ([unspecified] 0.3 µm particles) for 7 h per day resulted in emphysema in animals that died early in the experiment. Other lung effects included interstitial pneumonitis and diffuse granulomatous pneumonia, fibrosis of alveolar septa, bronchiolar (basal-cell) hyperplasia, bronchiolization of alveolar epithelium, squamous metaplasia and emphysema and/or atelectasia of various degrees (Wehner et al., 1975).

The median lethal concentration for rat macrophages exposed in vitro to green nickel monoxide exceeded 12 µmol (708 µg)/ml Ni. The $LC_{50}$ for canine macrophages was 3.9 µmol (230 µg)/ml Ni as nickel monoxide for 20 h. Nickel monoxide was far less toxic to macrophages than nickel sulfate, nickel chloride or nickel subsulfide (Benson *et al.*, 1986a). The toxicity of six different preparations of nickel monoxide calcined at temperatures of < 650-1045 °C and four mixed nickel-copper oxides was tested *in vitro* on alveolar macrophages of beagle dogs, Fischer 344 rats and B6C3F$_1$ mice. Nickel oxides were less toxic to the macrophages than were the nickel-copper oxides; the toxicity of the nickel-copper oxides increased with increasing copper content. Generally, dog macrophages were more sensitive to the oxides than mouse and rat macrophages (Benson *et al.*, 1988a).

The ability of the same oxides to stimulate erythropoiesis in Fischer 344 rats correlated well with their cell transforming ability in Syrian hamster embryo cells (see also genetic and related effects; Sunderman *et al.*, 1987).

### (iii)   *Nickel sulfides*

The LD$_{50}$ after a single instillation in B6C3F$_1$ mice of nickel subsulfide (particle size, < 2 μm) in a normal saline suspension was 4 mg/kg bw (Fisher *et al.*, 1986).

Acute toxic effects of nickel subsulfide (1.8 μm particles) administered intratracheally to male BALB/c mice (12 μg/mouse) included pulmonary haemorrhaging, most evident three days after exposure. The number of polymorphonuclear cells in the pulmonary lavage fluid was increased, whereas the number of macrophages tended to decrease below the control values later (20 h to seven days) after the exposure (Finch *et al.*, 1987).

Alveolitis was observed in Fischer 344 rats following intratracheal instillation of nickel subsulfide as a saline/gelatin suspension (3.2-320 μg/kg bw). The effects closely resembled those of nickel chloride and nickel sulfate at comparable doses of nickel. Pulmonary lesions also included type II cell hyperplasia with epithelialization of alveoli and, in some animals, fibroplasia of the pulmonary interstitium (Benson *et al.*, 1986b).

Chronic active inflammation, fibrosis and alveolar macrophage hyperplasia were observed in Fischer 344 rats and B6C3F$_1$ mice exposed by inhalation to nickel subsulfide (low-temperature form) for 13 weeks (6 h per day, five days per week; 0.11-1.8 mg/m³ Ni). The toxicity of nickel subsulfide to the lung resembled that of nickel sulfate hexahydrate, and both were more toxic than nickel oxide. Rats were more sensitive than mice (Dunnick *et al.*, 1989).

Administration of nickel subsulfide to female rats as a single intrarenal injection caused pronounced erythrocytosis (Jasmin & Riopelle, 1976; Oskarsson *et al.*, 1981). A single intrarenal injection of nickel subsulfide to male rats also caused an increase in renal haem oxygenase activity; no correlation between the induction of haem oxygenase and erythrocytosis was observed (Sunderman *et al.*, 1983a). Administration of nickel sulfide [probably amorphous] in glycerine or saline into each pole of the kidney of female rats did not induce renal erythropoietic activity (Jasmin & Riopelle, 1976).

Under comparable exposure *in vitro*, beagle dog alveolar macrophages were more sensitive to the toxicity of nickel subsulfide than were those of Fischer 344 rats. Nickel subsulfide appeared to be much more toxic to the macrophages of both species than nickel chloride, nickel sulfate or nickel monoxide (Benson *et al.*, 1986a).

Nickel subsulfide incubated with calf thymus histones in the presence of molecular oxygen caused random polymerization of those proteins; this effect was not produced by soluble nickel acetate (Kasprzak & Bare, 1989).

### (iv) *Nickel salts*

The oral $LD_{50}$ of nickel acetate was 350 mg/kg bw in rats and 420 mg/kg bw in mice; the intraperitoneal $LD_{50}$ was 23 mg/kg bw in rats (National Research Council, 1975). The $LD_{50}$ of nickel acetate in ICR mice after an intraperitoneal injection was 97 mg/kg bw in females and 89 mg/kg bw in males at days 3 and 5 for three-week-old animals and 39-54 mg/kg bw in nine- or 14-week-old animals of either sex (Hogan, 1985). With nickel chloride, intraperitoneal $LD_{50}$ values of 6-9.3 mg/kg bw Ni were reported for female Wistar rats (Mas *et al.*, 1985), 11 mg/kg bw rats and 48 mg/kg bw for mice (National Research Council, 1975).

Exposure of $B6C3F_1$ mice and Fischer 344/N rats to nickel sulfate hexahydrate by inhalation for 6 h per day for 12 days (five days per week plus two consecutive days; 0.8-13 mg/m³ Ni; 2 μm particles) caused death of all mice at concentrations of ≥1.6 mg/m³ and of some rats at concentrations of 13 mg/m³. Lesions of the lung and nasal cavity were observed in both mice and rats after exposure to 0.8 mg/m³ nickel or more; these included necrotizing pneumonia, chronic inflammation and degeneration of the bronchiolar epithelium, atrophy of the olfactory epithelium, and hyperplasia of the bronchial and mediastinal lymph nodes (Benson *et al.*, 1988b; Dunnick *et al.*, 1988).

A single intratracheal instillation of nickel chloride hexahydrate or nickel sulfate hexahydrate to Fischer 344/Cr1 rats (0.01, 0.1 or 1.0 μmol [0.59, 5.9 or 59 μg Ni/rat) caused alveolitis and affected the activities of several enzymes measured in the pulmonary lavage fluid (Benson *et al.*, 1985, 1986b).

Rabbits were exposed to nickel chloride (0.2-0.3 mg/m³ Ni) for 6 h per day on five days per week for one to eight months. Nodular accumulation of macrophages was seen in lung tissue, and the volume density of alveolar type II cells was elevated. The phagocytic activity of macrophages was normal after one month of exposure but was decreased after three months (Camner *et al.*, 1984; Lundborg & Camner, 1984; Camner *et al.*, 1985).

Exposure of Syrian golden hamsters to a nickel chloride aerosol (100-275 μg/m³ Ni; < 2-μm particles) for 2 h per day for one or two days resulted in a dose-related decrease in the ciliary activity of the tracheal epithelium and in mucosal degeneration (Adalis *et al.*, 1978).

A single intramuscular injection of nickel chloride (18.3 mg/kg bw) to male CBA/J mice caused significant involution of the thymus within two days. Significant reduction in the mitogen-stimulated responses of B and T lymphocytes *in vitro* as well as significant suppression of the primary antibody response (T-cell-dependent) to sheep red blood cells were observed after the treatment. Natural killer cell activity was also suppressed. The immunosuppressive effects of nickel chloride lasted for a few days. The activity of peritoneal macrophages was not affected (Smialowicz *et al.*, 1984, 1985).

Following a single intramuscular injection of 10-20 mg/kg bw nickel chloride into Fischer 344 rats, the activity of natural killer cells was transiently suppressed for three days. In contrast to mice, rats showed no significant difference in the lymphoproliferative responses of splenocytes to B and T mitogens from those of controls (Smialowicz *et al.*, 1987).

Intramuscular injection of nickel chloride (20 mg/kg bw Ni) to Fischer 344 rats 4 h before death inhibited thymidine uptake into kidney DNA (Hui & Sunderman, 1980). An immediate, significant decrease, followed by a transient sharp increase of thymidine incorporation into pulmonary DNA was observed in strain A mice following intraperitoneal administration of nickel acetate (Kasprzak & Poirier, 1985).

After 90 daily intraperitoneal injections of nickel sulfate (3 mg/kg bw Ni) to male albino rats, focal necrosis of the proximal convoluted tubules in the kidneys and marked cellularity around periportal areas and necrotic areas in the liver were observed. Bile-duct proliferation and Kupffer-cell hyperplasia were also evident, and degenerative changes were observed in a few seminiferous tubules and in the inner wall of the myocardium (Mathur *et al.*, 1977a).

Subcutaneous injection of up to 0.75 mmol [98 mg]/kg bw nickel chloride to male Fischer 344 rats increased lipid peroxidation in the liver, kidney and lung in a dose-related manner (Sunderman *et al.*, 1985b).

Renal, hepatic, pulmonary and brain haem oxygenase activity was induced after subcutaneous injection of 15 mg/kg bw nickel chloride to male Fischer 344 rats. Induction of haem oxygenase was also observed in the kidneys of male BL6 mice, male Syrian golden hamsters and male guinea-pigs killed 17 h after subcutaneous injection of 0.25 mmol [32 mg]/kg bw nickel chloride (Sunderman *et al.*, 1983a).

The skin of male albino rats was painted once daily for up to 30 days with 0.25 ml nickel sulfate hexahydrate solution in normal saline (40, 60 and 100 mg/kg bw Ni). The 30-day painting caused atrophy in some areas and acanthosis in other areas of the epidermis, disorder in the arrangement of epidermal cells and hyperkeratinization. Liver damage, including focal necrosis, was seen in histological studies (Mathur *et al.*, 1977b).

The toxicity of nickel sulfate and nickel chloride to alveolar macrophages from beagle dogs and Fischer 344 rats *in vitro* was intermediate to that of nickel subsulfide and nickel monoxide (median lethal concentrations, 0.30-0.36 μmol [17.7-21.2 μg] and 3.1-3.6 μmol [183-212 μg]/ml Ni for dog and rat macrophages, respectively) (Benson *et al.*, 1986a). Macrophages lavaged from rabbit lungs and incubated for two days with 3-24 μg/ml Ni as nickel chloride showed a decrease of up to 50% in lysozyme activity with increasing concentrations of nickel (Lundborg *et al.*, 1987).

Although nickel salts inhibit the proliferation of normal mammalian cells in culture, nickel sulfate hexahydrate increased proliferation of some lymphoblastoid cell lines carrying the Epstein-Barr virus (Wu *et al.*, 1986).

Exposure of Syrian hamster embryo cells to nickel chloride or nickel sulfate at a concentration of 10 μmol [600 μg]/l Ni or more enhanced nucleoside excretion (Uziel *et al.*, 1986).

Nickel chloride inhibited the transcription of calf thymus DNA and phage T4 DNA with *Escherichia coli* RNA polymerase in a concentration-dependent manner (0.01-10 mM [0.6-600 mg] Ni). It also stimulated RNA chain initiation at very low concentrations (maximal at 0.6 mg), followed by a progressive decrease in initiation at concentrations that significantly inhibited overall transcription (Niyogi *et al.*, 1981).

### (v)   *Other nickel compounds*

Animals exposed to nickel carbonyl by inhalation developed pulmonary oedema within 1 h. $LC_{50}$ values (30-min exposure) reported include 67 mg/m³ for mice, 240 mg/m³ for rats and 190 mg/m³ for cats (National Research Council, 1975). Even after administration by other routes, the lung is the main target organ (Hackett & Sunderman, 1969); the $LD_{50}$ for rats was 65 mg/kg, 61 mg/kg and 38 mg/kg after intravenous, subcutaneous and intraperitoneal administration, respectively (National Research Council, 1975).

Male Wistar rats exposed by inhalation to 0.03-0.06 mg/l nickel carbonyl for 90 min three times a week for 52 weeks developed extensive inflammatory lesions in the lung, contiguous pericarditis and suppurative lesions of the thoracic walls. Squamous-cell metaplasia was present in bronchiectatic walls of several rats (Sunderman *et al.*, 1957).

Exposure of female Fischer 344 rats by inhalation to 1.2-6.4 μmol [0.2-1.1 mg]/l nickel carbonyl for 15 min caused acute hyperglycaemia (Horak *et al.*, 1978). Urinary excretion of proteins and amino acids indicated nephrotoxicity (Horak & Sunderman, 1980).

After exposure of rats to 0.6 mg/l nickel carbonyl by inhalation, RNA derived from the lung showed alterations in the phase transition curve, indicating disruption of hydrogen bonds (Sunderman, 1963). Nickel carbonyl administered intravenously at an $LD_{50}$ dose of 20 mg/kg bw nickel to Sprague-Dawley rats inhibited cortisone-induced hepatic tryptophan pyrrolase (Sunderman, 1967), orotic acid incorporation into liver RNA *in vivo* and *in vitro* (Beach & Sunderman, 1969, 1970) and incorporation of leucine into liver and lung protein (Witschi, 1972). Intravenous administration of nickel carbonyl to Fischer 344 rats (20 mg/kg bw nickel) caused a significant decrease in thymidine incorporation into liver and kidney DNA 4 h later (Hui & Sunderman, 1980).

The toxicity of 'nickel carbonate' to human embryo pulmonary epithelium L132 cells in culture did not differ significantly from that of nickel chloride at the same 25-150 μM concentration range applied (Hildebrand *et al.*, 1986). [The Working Group noted that the compound tested was most probably basic nickel carbonate.]

A highly significant correlation was found between carcinogenic potential and the incidence of erythrocytosis for various water-insoluble nickel compounds, including nickel selenide, nickel subselenide, nickel telluride, nickel sulfarsenide, nickel arsenide, nickel arsenide tetragonal, nickel arsenide hexagonal, nickel antimonide, nickel ferrosulfide matte, a ferronickel alloy ($NiFe_{1.6}$) and nickel titanate (Sunderman *et al.*, 1984b).

Dusts of nickel-converter mattes (58% nickel sulfide, 11% metallic nickel, 2% nickel monoxide, 1% copper, 0.5% cobalt, 0.2% soluble nickel salts), a nickel concentrate (67% total nickel, 57% nickel sulfide) and two nickel-copper mattes (27-33% nickel sulfides, ~3% metallic nickel, 23-36% copper) were administered to white rats and mice by inhalation or by intragastric, intratracheal or intraperitoneal routes and onto the skin. The intratracheal $LD_{50}$ was 200-210 mg/kg bw for the mattes and 220 mg/kg for the nickel concentrate. The intraperitoneal $LD_{50}$ varied from 940 mg/kg bw for the nickel concentrate to 1000 mg/kg bw for the nickel-copper mattes and 1100 mg/kg bw for the nickel matte. Mice and rats were almost equally sensitive. Chronic exposure of rats and mice by inhalation to the same dusts caused bronchitis, perivasculitis, bronchopneumonia and fibrosis. Haemorrhagic foci and atrophy were observed in the kidneys (Saknyn *et al.*, 1976).

### (e) *Effects on reproduction and prenatal toxicity*

The embryotoxicity and genotoxicity of nickel, both directly to the mammalian embryo and indirectly through maternal injury, have been reviewed (Léonard & Jacquet, 1984).

#### (i) *Metallic nickel and nickel alloys*

Treatment of chick embryo myoblasts with 20-40 μg nickel powder per litre of culture fluid prevented normal differentiation of cells, with only a few mitoses seen after five days' incubation. Reduction of cell division was coupled with cell degeneration, resulting in small colony size. At concentrations of 80 μg/l nickel, extensive degeneration of the cultures and complete suppression of mitosis occurred within five days (Daniel *et al.*, 1974).

### (ii)  *Nickel sulfides*

Nickel subsulfide (80 mg/kg bw Ni) administered intramuscularly to Fischer rats on day 6 of gestation reduced the mean number of live pups per dam. No anomaly was found, and no evidence of maternal toxicity was reported (Sunderman *et al.*, 1978a). In another study, intrarenal injection of nickel subsulfide (30 mg/kg bw Ni) to female rats prior to breeding produced intense erythrocytosis in pregnant dams but not in the pups, which had reduced blood haematocrits at two weeks (Sunderman *et al.*, 1983b).

Both rats and mice administered 5 or 10 mg/m$^3$ nickel subsulfide aerosols by inhalation for 12 days developed degeneration of testicular germinal epithelium (Benson *et al.*, 1987).

### (iii)  *Nickel salts*

Studies on the teratogenic effects of nickel chloride in chick embryos have produced conflicting results, perhaps due to differences in dose and route of administration. Cardiac anomalies (Gilani, 1982), exencephaly and distorted skeletal development (Gilani & Marano, 1980) have been reported, whereas some authors found no nickel-induced anomaly (Ridgway & Karnofsky, 1952; Anwer & Mehrotra, 1986).

Embryo cultures from BALB/c mice were used to determine the mechanism of preimplantation loss of embryos derived from matings three and four weeks after treatment of males with 40 or 56 mg/kg bw nickel nitrate. Treated and control animals were allowed to mate with superovulated females and the number of cleaved eggs and the development of embryos to blastocysts and implantations were counted. Neither the fertilizing capacity of spermatozoa nor the development of cultured embryos was influenced by a dose of 40 mg/kg bw. A dose of 56 mg/kg bw significantly reduced the fertilization rate but did not affect the development of two-cell embryos. The results suggest that preimplantation loss after exposure to nickel is due to toxic effects on spermatids and spermatogonia rather than to zygotic death (Jacquet & Mayence, 1982).

Following daily intragastric administration of 25 mg/kg bw nickel sulfate to male white rats over a period of 120 days, severe lesions in germ-cell development in the testis were observed (Waltscheva *et al.*, 1972). Rats administered nickel sulfate by inhalation for 12 days developed testicular degeneration (Benson *et al.*, 1988b).

Groups of three to five male albino rats received subcutaneous injections of 0.04 mmol [6.2 mg]/kg bw nickel sulfate either as a single dose or as daily doses for up to 30 days. Treatment interfered to some degree with spermatogenesis, but this was temporary, and the testes ultimately recovered (Hoey, 1966).

Preimplantation embryos from NMRI mice (two- and four- to eight-cell stages) were cultured with nickel chloride hexahydrate; 10 μM (2.5 mg) adversely affected the development of day 2 embryos (two-cell stage), whereas 300 μM (71.3 mg) were required to affect day 3 embryos (eight-cell stage) (Storeng & Jonsen, 1980). In order to compare the effects of nickel chloride hexahydrate on mouse embryos treated *in vivo* by intraperitoneal injection during the preimplantation period, a single injection of 20 mg/kg bw nickel chloride was given to groups of female mice on day 1, 2, 3, 4, 5 or 6 of gestation. On day 19 of gestation, the implantation frequency in females treated on day 1 was much lower than that of controls. The litters of the control group were larger, and significantly so, among mice treated on days 1, 3 and 5 of gestation; the body weight of fetuses was also decreased on day 19. Nickel chloride may thus adversely affect mouse embryos during the passage through the oviduct, with subsequent effects after implantation. Data on maternal effects were not presented (Storeng & Jonsen, 1981).

Long-Evans rats born in a laboratory especially designed to avoid environmental contamination from trace metals were administered nickel [salt unspecified] at 5 mg/l in the drinking-water in five pairs. About one-third of the offspring in the first generation were runts, and one maternal death occurred. In the second generation, there were 10% young deaths with only 5% runts and, in the third generation, 21% young deaths with 6% runts. Thus, the size of the litters decreased somewhat with each generation and, with some failures in breeding, the number of rats was reduced (Schroeder & Mitchener, 1971). A subsequent study, reported in an abstract, found similar effects on reproduction through two generations of rats following administration of 500 mg/l nickel chloride in drinking-water. There was no decrease in maternal weight gain or other maternal effect (Kimmel et al., 1986).

Nickel chloride was administered in the drinking-water to female rats at a concentration of 0.1 or 0.01 mg/l Ni for seven months and then during pregnancy. Embryonic mortality was 57% among nine rats exposed to the higher concentration, compared to 34% among eight controls. At the lower concentration no such difference was observed (Nadeenko et al., 1979).

Nickel chloride (1.2-6.9 mg/kg bw Ni) was administered intraperitoneally to pregnant ICR mice on single days between days 7-11 of gestation. Increased resorption, decreased fetal weight, delayed skeletal ossification and a high incidence of malformations were observed in a dose-related fashion on gestation day 18. The malformations consisted of acephaly, exencephaly, cerebral hernia, open eyelids, cleft palate, micromelia, ankylosis of the extremities, club foot and other skeletal abnormalities. Five of 27, 6/25 and 7/24 dams receiving 4.6 mg/kg bw or more died within 72 h after injection on days 9, 10 and 11 (Lu *et al.*, 1979).

Fischer rats were administered nickel chloride (16 mg/kg bw Ni) intramuscularly on day 8 of gestation. The body weight of fetuses on day 20 of gestation and of weanlings four to eight weeks after birth were reduced. No congenital anomaly was found in fetuses from nickel-treated dams, or in rats that received ten intramuscular injections of 2 mg/kg bw Ni as nickel chloride twice daily from day 6 to day 10 of gestation (Sunderman *et al.*, 1978a).

Groups of pregnant Wistar rats were given nickel chloride (1, 2 or 4 mg/kg bw Ni) by intraperitoneal injection on days 8, 12 and 16 of pregnancy and were sacrificed on day 20. More malformations occurred when nickel was administered during organogenesis than after, and their occurrence was maximal at dose levels that were toxic to dams. The abnormalities included hydrocephalus, haemorrhage, hydronephrosis, skeletal retardation and one heart defect (Mas *et al.*, 1985).

### (iv) *Other nickel compounds*

Nickel carbonyl (11 mg/kg bw Ni) was injected intravenously into pregnant Fischer rats on day 7 of gestation. On day 20, fetal mortality was increased, the body weight of live pups was decreased and there was a 16% incidence of fetal malformations, including anophthalmia, microphthalmia, cystic lungs and hydronephrosis. No information was given regarding maternal toxicity (Sunderman *et al.*, 1983b).

Fischer rats were exposed on day 7 or 8 of gestation by inhalation to nickel carbonyl at concentrations of 80, 160 or 360 mg/m³ for 15 min. Ophthalmic anomalies (anophthalmia and microphthalmia) were observed in 86/511 fetuses from 62 pregnancies; they were most prevalent at the highest dose level and were not observed when the compound was given on day 9 of gestation (Sunderman *et al.*, 1979b). In another experiment, pregnant rats exposed to 60 or 120 mg/m³ nickel carbonyl by inhalation for 15 min on day 8 of gestation also had a high incidence of ocular anomalies. Maternal toxicity was not reported (Sunderman *et al.*, 1978b).

Groups of pregnant hamsters were administered 60 mg/m³ nickel carbonyl by inhalation for 15 min on days 4, 5, 6, 7 or 8 of gestation. Dams were sacrificed on day 15 and the fetuses examined for malformation. Exposure on days 4 and 5 of gestation resulted in malformations in about 5.5% of the progeny, which included cystic lung, exencephaly, fused rib, anophthalmia, cleft palate and haemorrhage into the serous cavities. Nine of 14 dams lived until day 16 of gestation. Haemorrhages were not observed in controls. Among the fetuses of dams exposed to nickel carbonyl on day 6 or 7 of gestation, one fetus had fused ribs and two had hydronephrosis. For pregnancies allowed to reach full-term, there was no significant difference on the day of delivery between pups from nickel carbonyl-exposed litters and controls. Neonatal mortality was increased (Sunderman *et al.*, 1980).

### (f)  Genetic and related effects

Many reviews of the genetic effects of nickel compounds have been published (Heck & Costa, 1982; Christie & Costa, 1984; Costa & Heck, 1984; Hansen & Stern, 1984; Reith & Brøgger, 1984; Costa & Heck, 1986; Fairhurst & Illing, 1987; Sunderman, 1989).

The genotoxic effects of different nickel compounds are divided into five categories: (i) those for metallic nickel; (ii) those for nickel oxides and hydroxides; (iii) those for crystalline nickel sulfide, crystalline nickel subsulfide and amorphous nickel sulfide; (iv) those for nickel chloride, nickel sulfate, nickel acetate and nickel nitrate; and (v) those for nickel carbonate, nickelocene, nickel potassium cyanide and nickel subselenide. The studies on these compounds are summarized in Appendix 1 to this volume.

### (i)  Metallic nickel

Nickel powder was reported not to induce chromosomal aberrations in cultured human peripheral lymphocytes [details not given] (Paton & Allison, 1972).

Nickel powder ground to a mean particle size of 4-5 μm at concentrations of 5, 10 and 20 μg/ml caused a dose-dependent increase in morphological transformation of Syrian hamster embryo cells (Costa et al., 1981b). At 20 μg/ml, nickel powder produced a 3% incidence of transformation, while crystalline nickel subsulfide and crystalline nickel sulfide (at 10-20 μg/ml) produced a 10-13% incidence of transformation and 5 and 10 μg/ml of amorphous nickel sulfide induced none. Nickel powder inhibited progression through S phase in Chinese hamster CHO cells, as measured by flow cytometry (Costa et al., 1982).

Hansen and Stern (1984) reported that nickel powder transformed BHK 21 cells [see General Remarks for concern about this assay]. Proliferation in soft agar was used as the endpoint. At equally toxic doses, they found that nickel powder and crystalline nickel subsulfide had similar transforming activities; the toxicity of 200 μg/ml nickel powder was equal to that of 10 μg/ml nickel subsulfide.

### (ii)  Nickel oxides

Nickel monoxide and nickel trioxide in distilled water gave negative results in the Bacillus subtilis rec[+]/rec[-] assay for differential toxicity at concentrations ranging from 5 to 50 mM (Kanematsu et al., 1980). [The Working Group noted that since particulate nickel compounds such as these are relatively insoluble and their entry into mammalian cells requires phagocytosis (Costa & Mollenhauer, 1980a,b,c), it is unlikely that they were able to enter the bacteria.]

Chromosomal aberrations were not induced in human peripheral lymphocytes by treatment *in vitro* with nickel monoxide [details not given] (Paton & Allison, 1972).

Nickel monoxide and nickel trioxide transformed Syrian hamster embryo cells at concentrations of 5-20 µg/ml. The activity of the trioxide was about twice that of the monoxide, similar to that of metallic nickel and about 20% that of crystalline nickel sulfide (Costa *et al.*, 1981a,b).

Nickel monoxide that was calcined at a low temperature had greater transforming activity in this system than nickel monoxide calcined at a high temperature at concentrations of 5 and 10 µg/ml and was equivalent to that of crystalline nickel sulfide. The cell-transforming activity of these nickel compounds was reported to correlate well with their ability to induce preneoplastic changes in rats (Sunderman *et al.*, 1987).

Syrian hamster BHK 21 cells were transformed by nickel monoxide and by a nickel oxide catalyst identified as $NiO_{1.4}(3H_2O)$. At equally toxic doses, nickel monoxide had the same transforming activity as did nickel subsulfide. [See General Remarks for concern about this assay.] The nickel oxide catalyst, $NiO_{1.4}$, had similar toxicity and transforming capacity as nickel subsulfide (Hansen & Stern, 1983, 1984).

The ability of 50 µM nickel monoxide to induce anchorage-independent growth in primary human diploid foreskin fibroblasts was similar to that of 10 µM nickel subsulfide or nickel acetate. The absolute numbers of anchorage-independent colonies induced at these doses were 26 with nickel monoxide, 67 with nickel subsulfide, 79 with nickel sulfide (10 µM) and about 42 with nickel acetate, compared with none in cultures of untreated cells. The frequency of anchorage-independent growth induced by nickel monoxide was about three-fold less than with nickel subsulfide, but was equivalent to that obtained with nickel acetate. The tranformed cells had 33- to 429-fold higher plating efficiency in agar than the parental cells; anchorage-independence was stable for eight passages only (Biedermann & Landolph (1987).

Nickel oxide inhibited progression through S phase in Chinese hamster CHO cells, as measured by flow cytometry (Costa *et al.*, 1982).

(iii)  *Nickel sulfides (crystalline nickel sulfide, crystalline nickel subsulfide and amorphous nickel sulfide)*

Crystalline nickel sulfide and nickel subsulfide were actively phagocytized by cells at an early stage following their addition to tissue cultures. Phagocytosis was dependent upon the calcium concentration in the medium (Abbracchio *et al.*, 1982a) and particle size (particles > 5-6 µm were much less actively taken up and much less toxic than smaller particles) (Costa & Mollenhauer, 1980a,b,c). Particles are taken up in areas of active cell ruffling, internalized and moved about the cell in a saltatory motion; lysosomes repeatedly interact with the particles, which are contained in the perinuclear region and sometimes inside cytoplasmic vacuoles, where they slowly dissolve, releasing nickel ions (Evans *et al.*, 1982). Interaction between lysosomes and nickel sulfide particles may result in exposure of the particles to the acidic content of the lysosomes, and this interaction may accelerate intracellular dissolution of crystalline nickel sulfide to ionic nickel (Abbracchio *et al.*, 1982a). In contrast, amorphous nickel sulfide and nickel particles were not significantly taken up by cells *in vitro* (Costa *et al.*, 1981a). Crystalline nickel sulfide particles differ from amorphous particles in that they have a negative surface charge, as shown using Z-potential measurements and binding of the particles to filter-paper discs offering different charges (Abbracchio *et al.*, 1982b). Alteration of the positive charge of amorphous nickel sulfide particles by treatment with lithium aluminium hydride results in activation of phagocytosis (Abbracchio *et al.*, 1982b; Costa, 1983).

Crystalline nickel sulfide was actively phagocytized by the protozoan *Paramoecium tetraurelia* and induced lethal genetic damage in parent cells. The activity of nickel subsulfide was more consistent than that of nickel sulfide, but both compounds produced higher mutagenic activities than glass beads, used as a control. The concentrations used ranged from 0.5 to 54 µg/ml; both compounds showed greatest mutagenicity at 0.5 µg/ml, as higher levels were toxic (Smith-Sonneborn *et al.*, 1983).

Crystalline nickel subsulfide at 5, 10 and 50 µg/ml inhibited DNA synthesis in the rat liver epithelial cell line T51B (Swierenga & McLean, 1985). Nickel subsulfide inhibited progression through S phase in Chinese hamster CHO cells, as measured by flow cytometry (Costa *et al.*, 1982).

Crystalline nickel sulfide and nickel subsulfide were active in inducing DNA damage in cultured mammalian cells. Crystalline nickel sulfide induced DNA strand breaks in rat primary hepatocytes (Sina *et al.*, 1983) and, at 1-20 µg/ml, single-strand breaks in tritium-labelled DNA in cultured Chinese hamster ovary cells, as determined using alkaline sucrose gradients (Robison & Costa, 1982). Using the same technique, Robison *et al.* (1982) showed that crystalline nickel subsulfide also induced strand breaks, whereas amorphous nickel sulfide, which is not phagocytized by cells, did not. As observed with alkaline elution analysis, crystalline nickel sulfide induced two major types of lesion — single-strand breaks and DNA protein cross-links (Costa *et al.*, 1982; Patierno & Costa, 1985). Treatment of primary Syrian hamster embryo cells with crystalline nickel subsulfide at 10 µg/ml and Chinese hamster CHO cells with crystalline nickel sulfide at 1-5 µg/ml induced DNA repair, as determined by analysis with caesium chloride gradients. Amorphous nickel sulfide had no effect in either cell type (Robison *et al.*, 1983).

Crystalline nickel subsulfide and amorphous nickel sulfide induced a weak mutation response at the *hprt* (6-thioguanine and 8-azaguanine resistance) locus in Chinese hamster ovary cells (Costa *et al.*, 1980).

Mutation to 8-azaguanine resistance was induced in a cultured rat liver epithelial cell line T51B treated with particulate crystalline nickel subsulfide at concentrations ranging from 5 to 50 $\mu$g/ml. At noncytotoxic doses, the mutagenic activity was four-fold above background, and at cytotoxic doses it was 20-fold above background. The mutagenic activity of dissolved products of these particles (at 12.5-20 $\mu$g/ml) was about two-fold above background at noncytotoxic doses and 20-fold above background at cytotoxic doses. Neither dissolved nor particulate nickel subsulfide at 2-27 $\mu$g/ml induced unscheduled DNA synthesis in rat primary hepatocytes (Swierenga & McLean, 1985). Nickel subsulfide, however, was reported to inhibit unscheduled DNA synthesis induced in primary rat hepatocytes by methyl methane sulfonate [details not given] (Swierenga & McLean, 1985). Concentrations of 0.5-10 $\mu$M nickel subsulfide did not induce 8-azaguanine or 6-thioguanine resistance in primary human fibroblasts (Biedermann & Landolph, 1987).

Crystalline nickel sulfide (0.1-0.8 $\mu$g/cm$^2$) was mutagenic in monolayer cultures in Chinese hamster V79 cells in which the endogenous *hprt* gene had been inactivated by a mutation and a single copy of a bacterial *gpt* gene had been inserted (Christie *et al.*, 1990).

The frequency of sister chromatid exchange was increased in cultured human lymphocytes treated with nickel subsulfide at 1-10 $\mu$g/ml (Saxholm *et al.*, 1981).

Chromosomal aberrations were induced in cultured mouse mammary carcinoma Fm3A cells following treatment with $4-8\times 10^{-4}$M crystalline nickel sulfide dissolved in medium and filtered. The early chromosomal aberrations consisted of gaps; following reincubation in control medium after treatment, gaps, breaks, exchanges and other types of aberration were observed (Nishimura & Umeda, 1979; Umeda & Nishimura, 1979). [The Working Group noted that the chemical form of nickel used in this study is not known.]

Treatment of Chinese hamster ovary cells with crystalline nickel sulfide at 5-20 $\mu$g/ml for 6-48 h produced a dose- and time-dependent increase in the frequency of chromosomal aberrations, which were selective for heterochromatin and included mostly gaps and breaks, with some exchanges and dicentrics (Sen & Costa, 1985). Crystalline nickel sulfide at 1-10 $\mu$g/ml also increased the frequency of sister chromatid exchange in a dose-dependent fashion, selectively in heterochromatic regions, in both Chinese hamster ovary cells (Sen & Costa, 1986b) and mouse C3H/10T½ cells (Sen *et al.*, 1987).

A dose-dependent increase in the frequency of morphological transformation was induced in primary Syrian hamster embryo cells by treatment with crystalline nickel subsulfide at 1-5 μg/ml for nine days (DiPaolo & Casto, 1979) and by either crystalline nickel sulfide or nickel subsulfide at 0.1-10 μg/ml for 48 h (Costa *et al.*, 1979; Costa, 1980; Costa & Mollenhauer, 1980a,b,c; Costa *et al.*, 1981a,b, 1982). At the same dose range, amorphous nickel sulfide had no effect. Clones derived from the transformed cells had greater plating efficiency, saturation densities and proliferation rates than normal cells; they also had more inducibility of ornithine decarboxylase, were able to proliferate in soft agar and were tumorigenic in nude mice.

C3H/10T½ cells were transformed at equal frequencies by crystalline nickel subsulfide at concentrations of 0.001, 0.01 and 0.1 μg/ml; at concentrations higher than 1 μg/ml, there was no transformation due to cell lysis or death. Transformed cells also showed long microvilli. They were not characterized for their ability to form tumours in nude mice or for anchorage-independent growth (Saxholm *et al.*, 1981). [The Working Group questioned the induction of transformation by concentrations of crystalline nickel subsulfide as low as 0.001 μg/ml.]

Crystalline nickel subsulfide induced transformed properties in rat liver epithelial T51B cells that were related to cytokeratin lesions. Solutions prepared as leachates of nickel subsulfide (containing about 300 μg/ml Ni) induced large juxtanuclear cytokeratin aggregates within 24 h of exposure, which persisted after removal of the compounds and were passed on to daughter cells. After long-term exposure to 2.5 μg/ml crystalline nickel subsulfide (dissolution products), these lesions were related to concomitant induction of differentiation and transformation markers, loss of density dependence, ability to grow in calcium-deficient medium and increased growth rates. Altered cells formed differentiated benign tumours in nude mice (Swierenga *et al.*, 1989).

Crystalline nickel subsulfide at 5-20 μg/ml induced transformation to anchorage-independence of Syrian hamster BHK 21 cells (Hansen & Stern, 1983). [See General Remarks for concern about this assay.]

Human skin fibroblasts transformed by crystalline nickel subsulfide to anchorage-independent growth had a much higher plating efficiency than normal cells. The phenotype was stable for eight passages (Biedermann & Landolph, 1987).

Crystalline nickel sulfide, but not amorphous nickel sulfide, at doses of 1–20 μg/ml, inhibited the polyriboinosinic-polyribocytidylic acid-stimulated production of α/β interferon in mouse embryo fibroblasts (Sonnenfeld *et al.*, 1983).

Heterochromatic abnormalities were seen in early-passage cultures of cells from crystalline nickel sulfide-induced, mouse rhabdomyosarcomas (Christie *et al.*, 1988).

(iv) *Nickel salts (nickel chloride, nickel sulfate, nickel nitrate and nickel acetate)*

Nickel acetate induced λ prophage in *Escherichia coli* WP2$_s$, with a maximal effect at 0.04 mM (Rossmann *et al.*, 1984). Nickel sulfate at 300 μg/ml did not induce forward mutations in T4 phage (Corbett *et al.*, 1970).

Nickel chloride at 1-10 mM decreased the fidelity of DNA polymerase using a poly (c) template (Sirover & Loeb, 1976, 1977). Nickel acetate inhibited DNA synthesis in mouse mammary carcinoma Fm3A cells (Nishimura & Umeda, 1979).

Nickel chloride at 200-1000 μM induced a genotoxic response in a differential killing assay using *E. coli* WP2 (wild-type) and the repair-deficient derivative WP67 (*uvr*A⁻, *pol*A⁻) and CM871 (*uvr*A⁻, *rec*A⁻, *lex*A⁻) (Tweats *et al.*, 1981). De Flora *et al.* (1984) reported negative results with nickel chloride, nickel nitrate and nickel acetate using the same strains in a liquid micromethod test procedure, with and without an exogenous metabolic system.

Nickel chloride did not induce differential toxicity in *B. subtilis* H17 *rec*⁺ (*arg*⁻, *trp*⁻) or M45 *rec*⁻ (*arg*⁻, *trp*⁻) at 5-500 mM (Nishioka, 1975; Kanematsu *et al.*, 1980). No mutagenicity was induced by nickel chloride at 0.1-100 mM in *S. typhimurium* LT₂ or TA100 (Tso & Fung, 1981), by nickel chloride, nickel acetate or nickel nitrate in *S. typhimurium* TA1535, TA1537, TA1538, TA97, TA98 or TA100 (De Flora *et al.*, 1984) or by nickel chloride or nickel sulfate in *S. typhimurium* TA1535, TA1537, TA1538, TA98 or TA100, when trimethylphosphate was substituted for *ortho*-phosphate to allow nickel to be soluble in the media (Arlauskas *et al.*, 1985). Even when substantial quantities of nickel were demonstrated to enter the bacteria, there was still no mutagenic response in *S. typhimurium* strains TA1535, TA1538, TA1975 or TA1978 (0.5-2 mM) (Biggart & Costa, 1986).

Pikálek and Nečásek (1983), however, demonstrated mutagenic activity of nickel chloride at 0.5-10 μg/ml in homoserine-dependent *Corynebacterium* sp887, utilizing a fluctuation test. Dubins and LaVelle (1986) demonstrated co-mutagenesis of nickel chloride with alkylating agents in *S. typhimurium* strain TA100 and in *E. coli* strains WP2⁺ and WP2*uvr*A⁻; Ogawa *et al.* (1987) demonstrated co-mutagenesis with 9-aminoacridine. Nickel acetate at up to 100 μM was not co-mutagenic with ultraviolet light in *E. coli* WP2 (Rossman & Molina, 1986). Soluble nickel salts have been shown to be negative in host-mediated assays, using *S. typhimurium* G46 in NMRI mice and *Serratia marcescens* A21 in mice, at concentrations of 50 mg/kg (Buselmaier *et al.*, 1972).

Nickel chloride at 3 and 10 mM for 24 h induced gene conversion in *Saccharomyces cerevisiae* D7 (Fukunaga *et al.*, 1982). It also induced petite mutations in 13 *S. cerevisiae* haploid strains (Egilsson *et al.*, 1979).

Negative results were obtained in the *Drosophila melanogaster* somatic eye colour (zeste mutation) test with nickel chloride at 0.21 mM (Rasmuson, 1985) and at
4.2 mM (Vogel, 1976) and with nickel nitrate at 0.14 mM (Rasmuson, 1985).

Nickel sulfate induced sex-linked recessive lethal mutations in *D. melanogaster*
at concentrations of 200, 300 and 400 ppm and sex chromosomal loss at the highest
concentration tested. The injection volume was not stated, but the $LD_{50}$ was 400
ppm (Rodriguez-Arnaiz & Ramos, 1986). Nickel nitrate at 3.4-6.9 mM did not induce sex-linked recessive lethal mutations in *D. melanogaster* (Rasmuson, 1985).

Nickel chloride increased the frequency of strand breaks in Chinese hamster
ovary cells at 1 and 10 μg/ml with 2-h exposure (Robison & Costa, 1982) and at
10-100 μM for 16 and 48 h, with a decrease in the average molecular weight of DNA
from 7.2-5.7 × $10^{-7}$ Da (Robison *et al.*, 1982). Nickel chloride at 0.5-5 mM induced
both single-strand breaks and DNA-protein cross-links in the same cell line. The
extent of cross-linking was maximal during the late S phase of the cell cycle when
heterochromatic DNA is replicated (Patierno & Costa, 1985; Patierno *et al.*, 1985).

Nickel chloride at 0.05 mM for 30 min did not induce DNA strand breaks in
human lymphocytes as evaluated by alkaline unwinding (McLean *et al.*, 1982). [The
Working Group noted that the exposure period was very short and the dose very
low.] Nickel sulfate at 250 μg/ml did not induce DNA single-strand breaks in human fibroblasts (Ag 1522) (Fornace, 1982).

Nickel chloride at 0.1-1 mM induced DNA repair synthesis in Chinese hamster
ovary and primary Syrian hamster embryo cells, which have a very high degree of
density inhibition of growth and very little background replication synthesis (Robison *et al.*, 1983, 1984). It inhibited DNA synthesis in primary rat embryo cells at 1.0
μg/ml (Basrur & Gilman, 1967) and in T51B rat liver epithelial cells (Swierenga &
McLean, 1985).

Exposure of two human cell lines, HeLa and diploid embryonic fibroblasts,
and of Chinese hamster V79 cells and L-A mouse fibroblasts to nickel chloride *in
vitro* resulted in a dose-dependent depression of proliferation and mitotic rate. The
effects on viability were accompanied by a reduction in DNA, protein and, to a lesser degree, RNA synthesis. Cells in G1 and early S phases were most sensitive (Škreb
& Fischer, 1984). Nickel chloride also selectively blocked cell cycle progression in
the S phase in Chinese hamster ovary cells (Harnett *et al.*, 1982). Nickel chloride at
40-120 μM for one to several days of exposure prolonged S-phase in Chinese hamster ovary cells (Costa *et al.*, 1982).

Nickel chloride at 0.4 and 0.8 mM for 20 h induced 8-azaguanine-resistant mutations in Chinese hamster V79 cells, although 0.8 mM induced a very weak mutagenic response (Miyaki *et al.*, 1979). Nickel chloride at 0.5-2.0 mM induced a
dose-related increase in the frequency of mutation to 6-thioguanine resistance in

Chinese hamster V79 cells. At 2 mM, cell survival was 50% and the mutant fraction was 8.6-fold above background (Hartwig & Beyersmann, 1989). Trifluorothymidine-resistant mutants were induced in L5178Y tk$^{+/-}$ mouse lymphoma cells following exposure to nickel chloride at 0.17-0.71 mM for 3 h; dose-dependent two- to five-fold increases in mutation frequency were seen, survival ranging from 5 to 33.5% (Amacher & Paillet, 1980).

Nickel sulfate at 0.1 mM induced a two-fold increase in the frequency of mutation to 6-thioguanine resistance over the background level in Chinese hamster V79 cells (G12) containing a transfected bacterial *gpt* gene (Christie *et al.*, 1990). No gene mutation to ouabain resistance was seen, however, in primary Syrian hamster embryo cells exposed to 5 μg/ml nickel sulfate (Rivedal & Sanner, 1980).

As assessed in a mutation assay for the synthesis of P-85$^{gag-mos}$ viral proteins, nickel chloride at concentrations of 20-160 μM induced expression of the v-*mos* gene in MuSVts 110-infected rat kidney cells (6m2 cell line) (Biggart & Murphy, 1988).

Nickel chloride at 0.01-0.05 mM increased the incidence of sister chromatid exchange in Chinese hamster ovary cells (Sen *et al.*, 1987). An increased frequency was also seen with nickel sulfate at 0.1 mM in the P33 8D$_1$ macrophage cell line (Andersen, 1983), at 0.13 mM in Chinese hamster Don cells (Ohno *et al.*, 1982), at 0.004-0.019 mM in Syrian hamster embryo cells (Larramendy *et al.*, 1981), at 0.75 μg/ml (0.003 mM) in Chinese hamster ovary cells (Deng & Ou, 1981) and at 0.01 mM in human lymphocytes (Andersen, 1983). Dose-dependent increases in the frequency of sister chromatid exchange were seen in human peripheral blood lymphocytes with nickel sulfate at 0.01 mM and 0.019 mM (Larramendy *et al.*, 1981), 0.0023-2.33 mM (Wulf, 1980) and 0.95-2.85 μM (Deng & Ou, 1981).

Nickel chloride induced chromosomal aberrations in Fm3A mouse mammary carcinoma cells (Nishimura & Umeda, 1979; Umeda & Nishimura, 1979). It also induced aberrations (primarily gaps, breaks and exchanges) in Chinese hamster ovary cells at 0.001-1 mM, preferentially in heterochromatic regions (Sen & Costa, 1985, 1986b; Sen *et al.*, 1987); and aberrations in Syrian hamster embryo cells at 0.019 mM (Larramendy *et al.*, 1981). Increased frequencies were also reported in Syrian hamster embryo cells (0.019 mM) and human peripheral blood lymphocytes (0.019 mM) exposed to nickel sulfate hexahydrate (Larramendy *et al.*, 1981) and in Fm3A mouse mammary carcinoma cells exposed to nickel acetate at 0.6 mM for 48 h (Umeda & Nishimura, 1979) or at 1 mM for 24 h (Nishimura & Umeda, 1979).

Nickel sulfate at 1.0 mM reduced average chromosomal length in human lymphocytes, indicating its ability to act as a powerful spindle inhibitor at concentrations just below lethal levels (Andersen, 1985).

Nickel sulfate hexahydrate and nickel chloride induced a concentration-dependent increase in morphological transformation of Syrian hamster embryo cells (Pienta *et al.*, 1977; DiPaolo & Casto, 1979 [2.5-10 μg/ml]; Zhang & Barrett, 1988). Nickel sulfate transformed these cells at 5 μg/ml (Rivedal & Sanner, 1980; Rivedal *et al.*, 1980; Rivedal & Sanner, 1981, 1983), and concentrations of 10–40 μg/ml (38-154 μM) nickel sulfate enhanced transformation of normal rat kidney cells infected with Molony murine sarcoma virus (Wilson & Khoobyarian, 1982).

Nickel acetate at 100-400 μg/ml transformed Syrian hamster BHK21 cells (Hansen & Stern, 1983) [See General Remarks for concern about this assay.]

Nickel acetate and nickel sulfate at 10 μM induced transformation to anchorage-dependent growth of primary human foreskin fibroblasts (Biedermann & Landolph, 1987).

Continuous exposure of cultures of normal human bronchial epithelial cells to nickel sulfate at 5-20 μg/ml reduced colony-forming efficiency by 30-80%. After 40 days of incubation, 12 cell lines were derived which exhibited accelerated growth, aberrant squamous differentiation and loss of the requirement for epidermal growth factor for clonal growth. Aneuploidy was induced and marker chromosomes were found. However, none of these transformed cultures was anchorage-independent or produced tumours upon injection into athymic nude mice (Lechner *et al.*, 1984). Human fetal kidney cortex explants were exposed continuously to 5 μg/ml nickel sulfate. After 70-100 days, immortalized cell lines were obtained, with decreased serum dependence, increased plating efficiency, higher saturation density and ability to grow in soft agar. However, they were not tumorigenic (Tveito *et al.*, 1989).

Nickel sulfate disrupted cell-to-cell communication in a dose-related manner in NIH3T3 cells from a base level of 98% at 0.5 mM to 2% at 5mM; cell viability was not affected by these concentrations (Miki *et al.*, 1987). [The Working Group noted that the method for determining cell viability was not described.]

Intraperitoneal injections of nickel sulfate at 15-30% of the $LD_{50}$ to CBA mice *in vivo* suppressed DNA synthesis in hepatic epithelial cells and in the kidney (Amlacher & Rudolph, 1981). Nickel chloride given by intramuscular injection to rats at 20 mg/kg bw Ni inhibited DNA synthesis in the kidney (Hui & Sunderman, 1980).

Polychromatic erythrocytes were not induced in BALB/c mice after an intraperitoneal injection of 25 mg/kg bw nickel chloride or 56 mg/kg bw nickel nitrate (Deknudt & Léonard, 1982).

The frequency of chromosomal aberrations in bone-marrow cells and spermatogonia of male albino rats was not increased following intraperitoneal injections of 3 and 6 mg/kg bw nickel sulfate. Animals were sacrificed seven to 14 days after treatment (Mathur *et al.*, 1978).

Nickel chloride increased the frequency of chromosomal aberrations in bone-marrow cells of Chinese hamsters given intraperitoneal injections of concentrations that were 4-20% of the $LD_{50}$ (Chorvatovičová, 1983) and of Swiss mice given intraperitoneal injections of 6, 12 or 24 mg/kg bw (Mohanty, 1987).

Dominant lethal mutations were not induced in BALB/c mice after an intraperitoneal injection of 12.5-100 mg/kg bw nickel chloride or 28-224 mg/kg bw nickel nitrate (Deknudt & Léonard, 1982).

### (v)  Other nickel compounds

DNA-protein cross-linking in the presence of the nickel[II]- and nickel[III]-tetraglycine complexes and molecular oxygen was observed in vitro in calf thymus nucleohistone. The same complexes were also able to cause random polymerization of histones in vitro (Kasprzak & Bare, 1989).

Haworth et al. (1983) reported no mutation in S. typhimurium TA100, TA1535, TA1537 or TA98 following exposure to nickelocene at doses up to 666 μg/plate.

Nickel potassium cyanide at concentrations of 0.2-1.6 mM for 48 h increased the frequency of chromosomal aberrations in Fm3A mouse mammary carcinoma cells (Nishimura & Umeda, 1979; Umeda & Nishimura, 1979).

Crystalline nickel subselenide at 1-5 μg/ml inhibited cell progression through S phase, as seen with flow cytometry (Costa et al., 1982). Concentrations of 5-20 μg/ml crystalline nickel subselenide transformed primary Syrian hamster embryo cells (Costa et al., 1981a,b; Costa & Mallenhauer, 1980c).

Intravenous administration of nickel carbonyl to rats at 20 mg/kg bw Ni inhibited DNA synthesis in liver and kidney (Hui & Sunderman, 1980).

DNA-protein cross-links and single-strand breaks, as detected by alkaline elution, were found in rat kidney nuclei 20 h after intraperitoneal injection of 'nickel carbonate' at 10-40 mg/kg bw (Ciccarelli et al., 1981). After 3 and 20 h, single-strand breaks were detected in lung and kidney nuclei, and both DNA-protein and DNA interstrand cross-links were found in kidney nuclei. No DNA damage was observed in liver or thymus gland nuclei (Ciccarelli & Wetterhahn, 1982). [The Working Group noted that the compound tested was probably basic nickel carbonate.]

### 3.3  Other relevant data in humans

#### (a)  Absorption, distribution, excretion and metabolism

Recent reviews include those of Raithel and Schaller (1981), Sunderman et al. (1986a), the US Environmental Protection Agency (1986), Grandjean et al. (1988), Sunderman (1988) and the World Health Organization (1990).

A positive relation exists between air levels of nickel and serum/plasma concentrations of nickel after occupational exposure to various forms of nickel (see also

Tables 11, 12, 13). A considerable scattering of results was apparent, and the correlation was poor; a better correlation may be achieved in individual studies of well-defined exposure groups (Grandjean et al., 1988). Sparingly soluble compounds may be retained in the lungs for long periods of time. Thus, even three to four years after cessation of exposure, nickel concentrations in plasma and urine were elevated in retired nickel workers exposed to sparingly soluble compounds in the roasting/smelting department of a nickel refinery (Boysen et al., 1984). Respiratory uptake of nickel in welders is described in the monograph on welding.

Provided that pulmonary exposure to nickel can be excluded, the approximate fraction of nickel absorbed by the intestinal tract can be estimated from oral intake and faecal and urinary nickel elimination (Horak & Sunderman, 1973). Cumulative urinary excretion in non-fasting volunteers given a single oral dose of 5.6 mg Ni as nickel sulfate hexahydrate indicated an intestinal absorption of 1-5% (Christensen & Lagesson, 1981; Sunderman, 1988). After ingestion of nickel sulfate during fasting, 4-20% of the dose was excreted in the urine within 24 h (Cronin et al., 1980). Compartmental analysis of nickel levels in serum, urine and faeces in a study of intestinal absorption of nickel sulfate by human volunteers showed that an average of about 27% was absorbed when ingested as an aqueous solution after 12 h of fasting, while 0.7% was absorbed when the nickel was ingested with scrambled eggs (Sunderman et al., 1989b). Ingestion of food items with a high natural nickel content resulted in a urinary excretion corresponding to about 1% of the amount ingested (Nielsen et al., 1987). The bioavailability of nickel can be reduced by various dietary constituents and beverages. Drugs may influence intestinal nickel absorption. Ethylenediaminetetraacetic acid very efficiently prevented intestinal absorption of nickel (Solomons et al., 1982); and, as reported in an abstract, disulfiram increased the intestinal absorption of nickel, probably by forming a lipophilic complex between its metabolite diethyldithiocarbamate and nickel (Hopfer et al., 1984).

After intestinal absorption of nickel ingested as nickel sulfate hexahydrate in lactose by eight volunteers, most of the nickel present in blood was in serum; nickel concentrations in serum and blood showed a very high positive correlation ($r = 0.99$) (Christensen & Lagesson, 1981). In patients with chronic renal failure, a high nickel concentration was found in serum but no significant increase was observed in lymphocytes (Wills et al., 1985). However, in nickel refinery workers, plasma nickel concentrations were lower than those in whole blood, and about 63% appeared to be contained in the buffy coat (Barton et al., 1980).

As reported in an abstract, nickel levels in intercellular fluid were significantly lower in a group of nickel-allergic patients than in controls, possibly due to cell binding or uptake (Bonde et al., 1987). This finding may be related to the observation that incubation with nickel subsulfide in vitro caused considerable binding of nickel to the cell membrane of T-lymphocytes from nickel-sensitized patients but to very few cells from nonsensitized persons (Hildebrand *et al.*, 1987).

The lungs contain the highest concentration of nickel in humans with no known occupational nickel exposure; lower levels occur in the kidneys, liver and other tissues (Sumino *et al.*, 1975; Rezuke *et al.*, 1987). One study documented high levels in the thyroid and adrenals (Rezuke *et al.*, 1987) and another in bone (Sumino *et al.*, 1975). The pulmonary burden of nickel appears to increase with age (Kollmeier *et al.*, 1987), although this correlation was not confirmed in another study (Raithel *et al.*, 1988). The upper areas of the lungs and the right middle lobe contained higher nickel concentrations than the rest of the lung (Raithel *et al.*, 1988), and high concentrations were found in hilar lymph nodes (Rezuke *et al.*, 1987).

Lung tissue from three of four random cases of bronchial carcinoma from an area with particularly high local emissions of chromium and nickel contained increased concentrations of nickel and chromium (Kollmeier *et al.*, 1987), while no such tendency was seen in ten other cases with no known occupational exposure to nickel (Turhan *et al.*, 1985).

High nickel concentrations were found in biopsies of nasal mucosa from both active and retired workers from the Kristiansand, Norway, nickel refinery, particularly in workers from the roasting/smelting department. After retirement, increased nickel levels persisted for at least ten years, with slow release at a half-time of 3.5 years (Torjussen & Andersen, 1979). Biopsies from two nasal carcinomas in nickel refinery workers contained nickel concentrations similar to those seen in biopsies from workers without cancer (Torjussen *et al.*, 1978). Lung tissue obtained at autopsy of workers from the roasting and smelting department of the Norwegian nickel refinery contained higher nickel concentrations (geometric mean, 148 µg/g dry weight; n = 15) than tissue from workers from the electrolysis department (geometric mean, 16 µg/g; n = 24); nickel concentrations in lung tissue were not higher in workers who had died from lung cancer than in workers who had died of other causes (Andersen & Svenes, 1989).

In cases of nickel carbonyl poisoning, the highest nickel concentrations have been recorded in the lungs, with lower levels in kidneys, liver and brain (National Research Council, 1975).

The half-time of nickel in serum was 11 h (one-compartment model during the first 32 h) in eight volunteers after ingestion of 5.6 mg nickel sulfate hexahydrate in lactose; serum nickel concentration and urinary nickel excretion showed a highly positive correlation ($r = 0.98$) (Christensen & Lagesson, 1981). Possibly due to delayed absorption of inhaled nickel, somewhat longer half-times were reported for nickel concentrations in plasma and urine (20-34 h and 17-39 h, respectively) in nickel platers (Tossavainen *et al.*, 1980), glass workers (30-50 h in urine) (Raithel *et al.*, 1982; Sunderman *et al.*, 1986a) and welders (53 h in urine) (Zober *et al.*, 1984). Ten subjects who had accidentally ingested soluble nickel compounds and were treated the following day with intravenous fluids to induce diuresis, showed an average elimination half-time of 27 h, while the half-time was twice as high in untreated subjects with lower serum nickel concentrations (Sunderman *et al.*, 1988b).

Urinary excretion of nickel is frequently used to survey workers exposed to inorganic nickel compounds (Aitio, 1984; Sunderman *et al.*, 1986a; Grandjean *et al.*, 1988). The best indicator of current exposure to soluble nickel compounds is a 24-h urine sample (Sunderman *et al.*, 1986a). In cases of nickel carbonyl intoxication, urinary nickel level is an important diagnostic and therapeutic guide (Sunderman & Sunderman, 1958; Adams, 1980), but its use in biological monitoring of exposure to nickel carbonyl has not been evaluated in detail.

Systemically absorbed nickel may be excreted through sweat (Christensen *et al.*, 1979). Faecal excretion includes non-absorbed nickel and nickel secreted into the gastrointestinal tract (World Health Organization, 1990). Saliva contains nickel concentrations similar to those seen in plasma (Catalanatto & Sunderman, 1977). Secretin-stimulated pancreatic juice was reported to contain an average of 1.09 nmol [64 μg]/ml nickel, corresponding to a total nickel secretion of about 1.64-2.18 μmol [96-128 μg] per day at a pancreatic secretion rate of 1.5-2 l/day (Ishihara *et al.*, 1987). Bile obtained at autopsy contained an average nickel concentration of 2.3 μg/l, suggesting daily biliary excretion of about 2-5 μg (Rezuke *et al.*, 1987). A biliary nickel concentration of 62 μg/g was recorded at autopsy of a small girl who had swallowed about 15 g nickel sulfate crystals (Daldrup *et al.*, 1983); since biliary excretion in this case would correspond to about 0.1% of the dose, it was considered that this route of excretion would be of minimal importance in acute intoxication (Rezuke *et al.*, 1987). Nickel-exposed battery production workers showed high faecal nickel excretion, probably owing to direct oral intake of nickel (e.g., *via* contamination of food from exposed surfaces); faecal nickel content (24 μg/g dry weight) was correlated with the amount present in air (18 μg/m³) (Hassler *et al.*, 1983).

Nickel was found in cord blood from full-term infants at 3 μg/l (McNeely *et al.*, 1971). Tissue levels at 22-43 weeks of gestation were similar to those seen in adults (Casey & Robinson, 1978).

### (b)  *Toxic effects*

Nickel is an essential nutrient in several species, but no essential biochemical function has been established in humans. Recent reviews of nickel toxicity in humans include those of Raithel and Schaller (1981), the US Environmental Protection Agency (1986), Sunderman (1988) and the World Health Organization (1990).

Acute symptoms reported in 23 patients exposed to severe nickel contamination during haemodialysis included nausea, vomiting, weakness, headache and palpitations; the symptoms disappeared rapidly upon cessation of dialysis (Webster *et al.*, 1980). Twenty workers who accidentally ingested water contaminated with nickel sulfate and chloride hexahydrates at doses estimated at 0.5-2.5 g Ni developed nausea, abdominal pain or discomfort, giddiness, lassitude, headache, diarrhoea, vomiting, coughing and shortness of breath; no related sequela was observed on physical examination, and all individuals were asymptomatic within three days (Sunderman *et al.*, 1988b). In a study of fasting human volunteers, one subject who ingested nickel sulfate (as 50 μg/kg bw Ni) in water developed a transient hemianopsia at the time of peak nickel concentration in serum (Sunderman *et al.*, 1989b). One fatal case of oral intoxication with nickel sulfate has been reported (Daldrup *et al.*, 1983).

Biochemical indications of nephrotoxicity, mainly with tubular dysfunction, have been observed in nickel electrolysis workers (Sunderman & Horak, 1981). Increased haemoglobin and reticulocyte counts were reported in ten subjects three to eight days after they had accidentally ingested 0.5-2.5 g Ni as nickel sulfate and chloride hexahydrates in contaminated drinking-water (Sunderman *et al.*, 1988b).

Nickel is a common skin allergen—in recent studies, the most frequent cause of allergic contact dermatitis in women and one of the most common causes in men; about 10-15% of the female population and 1-2% of males show allergic responses to nickel challenge (Peltonen, 1979; Menné *et al.*, 1982). Nickel ions are considered to be exclusively responsible for the immunological effects of nickel (Wahlberg, 1976). Sensitization appears to occur mainly in young persons, usually due to non-occupational skin exposures to nickel alloys (Menné *et al.*, 1982). Subsequent provocation of hand eczema may be caused by occupational exposures, especially to nickel-containing fluids and solutions (Rystedt & Fischer, 1983). Oral intake of low doses of nickel may provoke contact dermatitis in sensitized individuals (Veien *et al.*, 1985). Inflammatory reactions to nickel-containing prostheses and implants may occur in nickel-sensitive individuals (Lyell *et al.*, 1978).

Several cases of nickel-associated asthma have been described (Cirla *et al.*, 1985). Case reports suggest that inhalation of nickel dusts may result in chronic respiratory diseases (asthma, bronchitis and pneumoconiosis) (Sunderman, 1988). [The Working Group was unable to determine the causal significance of nickel in this regard.]

Nickel carbonyl is the most acutely toxic nickel compound. Symptoms following nickel carbonyl intoxication occur in two stages, separated by an almost symptom-free interval which usually lasts for several hours. Initially, the major symptoms are nausea, headache, vertigo, upper airway irritation and substernal pain, followed by interstitial pneumonitis with dyspnoea and cyanosis. Prostration, pulmonary oedema, kidney toxicity, adrenal insufficiency and death may occur in severe cases (Sunderman & Kincaid, 1954; Vuopala *et al.*, 1970; Sunderman, 1977).

Frequent clinical findings included fever with leukocytosis, electrocardiographic abnormalities suggestive of myocarditis and chest X-ray changes (Zhicheng, 1986). Hyperglycaemia has also been reported (Sunderman, 1977). Neurasthenic signs and weakness may persist in survivors for up to six months (Zhicheng, 1986).

### (c)  Effects on reproduction and prenatal toxicity

No data were available to the Working Group.

### (d)  Genetic and related effects

Cytogenetic studies have been performed using peripheral blood lymphocytes from electroplating and nickel refining plant workers; they are summarized in Appendix 1 to this volume.

Waksvik and Boysen (1982) found elevated levels of chromosomal aberrations (mainly gaps; $p < 0.003$), but not of sister chromatid exchanges, in two groups of nickel refinery workers. One group of nine workers engaged in crushing/roasting/smelting processes and exposed mainly to nickel monoxide and nickel subsulfide for an average of 21.2 years (range, 3-33 years) at an air nickel content of 0.5 mg/m³ (range, 0.1-1.0 mg/m³) and with a mean plasma nickel level of 4.2 µg/l had 11.9% of metaphases with gaps. Another group of workers, engaged in electrolysis, who were exposed mainly to nickel chloride and nickel sulfate for an average of 25.5 years (range, 8-31 years) at an air nickel content of 0.2 mg/m³ (range, 0.1-0.5 mg/m³) and with a mean plasma level of 5.2 µg/l, had 18.3% of metaphases with gaps[1]. Mean control values of 3.7% of metaphases with gaps were seen in seven office workers in the same plant with plasma nickel levels of 1 µg/l, who were matched for age and sex. All subjects were nonsmokers and nonalcohol consumers, were free from overt viral disease, were not known to have cancer and had not received therapeutic radiation; none was a regular drug user and the groups were uniform as to previous exposure to diagnostic X-rays.

Waksvik et al. (1984) investigated nine ex-workers from the same plant who had been retired for an average of eight years who had had similar types of exposure to more than 1 mg/m³ atmospheric nickel for 25 years or more; they were selected from among a group of workers known to have nasal dysplasia and who still had plasma nickel levels of 2 µg/l plasma. These retired workers showed some retention of gaps ($p < 0.05$) and an increased frequency of chromatid breaks to 4.1% of metaphases versus 0.5% ($p < 0.001$) in 11 unexposed retired workers controlled for age, life style and medication status. All subjects were of similar socioeconomic status and had

---

[1]The exposures of these workers were clarified in an erratum to the original article, published subsequently (Mutat. Res., 104, 395 (1982)).

not had X-rays or overt viral disease recently; none smoked or drank alcohol. Four exposed and nine unexposed subjects were on medication but not with drugs known to influence chromosomal parameters.

Deng *et al.* (1983, 1988) studied the frequencies of sister chromatid exchange and chromosomal aberrations in lymphocytes from seven electroplating workers exposed to nickel. Air nickel concentrations were 0.0053-0.094 mg/m³ (mean, 0.024 mg/m³). Control subjects were ten administrative workers from the same plant matched for age and sex; the groups were uniform as to socioeconomic status, and none of the subjects smoked or used alcohol, had overt viral disease, had recently been exposed to X-rays or was taking medication known to have chromosomal effects. The exposed workers had an increased frequency of sister chromatid exchange (7.50 ± 2.19 (SEM) *versus* 6.06 ± 2.30 (SEM); $p < 0.05$). [The Working Group noted that this is a small difference between groups.] The frequency of chromosomal aberrations (gaps, breaks and fragments) was increased from 0.8% of metaphases in controls to 4.3% in nickel platers.

The frequencies of sister chromatid exchange and chromosomal aberrations were studied in workers in a nickel carbonyl production plant. The subjects were divided into four groups: exposed, exposed smokers, controls and control smokers. Controls were ex-employees. None of the subjects had a history of serious illness; none was receiving irradiation or was infected by viruses at the time of blood sampling. No significant difference in the frequency of chromosomal breaks or gaps was observed between the different groups, and there was no statistically significant difference in the frequency of sister chromatid exchange between unexposed and nickel-exposed workers (Decheng *et al.*, 1987). [The Working Group noted that several discrepancies in the description of this study make it difficult to evaluate.]

Studies of mutagenicity and chromosomal effects in humans are summarized in Table 25.

### 3.4 Epidemiological studies of carcinogenicity to humans

#### (a) Introduction

The report of the International Committee on Nickel Carcinogenesis in Man (ICNCM) (1990) presents updated results on nine cohort studies and one case-control study of nickel workers, one of which was previously unpublished. The industries include mining, smelting, refining and high-nickel alloy manufacture and one industry in which pure nickel powder was used. The report adds to or supersedes previous publications on most of these cohorts, as various new analyses are included, some cohorts have been enlarged, and follow-up has been extended. Nickel species were divided into four categories: metallic nickel, oxidic nickel, soluble nickel and sulfidic nickel (including nickel subsulfide). Soluble nickel was defined as

Table 25. Cytogenetic studies of people exposed occupationally to nickel and nickel compounds

| Occupational exposure | Reported principal components | Mean reported dose (range) | Sister chromatid exchange | Chromosomal aberrations | Reference |
|---|---|---|---|---|---|
| Crushing, roasting, smelting | Nickel monoxide, nickel subsulfide | Air: 0.5 (0.1–1.0) mg/m³ Exposure: 21.2 (3–33) years | None | Only gaps | Waksvik & Boysen (1982) |
| Electrolysis | Nickel chloride, nickel sulfate | Air: 0.2 (0.1–0.5) mg/m³ Exposure: 25.2 (8–31) years | None | Mainly gaps | Waksvik & Boysen (2982) |
| Crushing, roasting, smelting and/or electrolysis | Nickel monoxide, nickel subsulfide, nickel chloride, nickel sulfate | Air: 1 mg/m³ Exposure: > 25 years | None | Gaps and breaks in retired workers | Waksvik et al. (1984) |
| Nickel carbonyl production | Nickel carbonyl | Exposure: 7971 h | None | None | Decheng et al. (1987) |
| Electroplating | Nickel and chromium compounds | Air: 0.0053–0.094 mg/m³ Exposure: 2–27 years | Small increase | Mainly gaps, but also breaks and fragments | Deng et al. (1983, 1988) |

consisting 'primarily of nickel sulfate and nickel chloride but may in some estimates include the less soluble nickel carbonate and nickel hydroxide'.

The historical estimates of exposure cited in the reviews of the following studies were not based on contemporary measurements. Furthermore, total airborne nickel was estimated first, and this estimate was then divided into estimates for four nickel species (metallic, oxidic, sulfidic and soluble), as defined in the report of the committee (ICNCM, 1990). The procedures for dividing the exposure estimates are described in section 2 of this monograph (pp. 297-298). Because of the inherent error and uncertainties in the procedures for estimating exposures, the estimated concentrations of nickel species in workplaces in the ICNCM analysis must be interpreted as broad ranges indicating only estimates of the order of magnitude of the actual exposures.

In order to facilitate the interpretation of the epidemiological findings on mortality from lung cancer and nasal cancer, selected estimates of exposure are presented in Tables 26, 27 and 28 (pp. 402-404) for some of the plants and subcohorts. The exposure estimates presented in the tables should be used only to make qualitative comparisons of exposure among departments within a plant and should not be used to make comparisons of exposure estimates among plants, for the reasons given above.

### (b)   Nickel mining, smelting and refining

#### (i)   INCO Ontario, Canada (mining, smelting and refining)[1]

Follow-up of all sinter plant workers and of all men employed at the Ontario division of INCO for at least six months and who had worked (or been a pensioner) between 1 January 1950 and 31 December 1976 (total number of men, 54 509) was extended to the end of 1984 by record linkage to the Canadian Mortality Data Base (ICNCM, 1990). Sinter plant workers included men who had worked in two different sinter plants in the Sudbury area (the Coniston and Copper Cliff sinter plants) and in the leaching, calcining and sintering department at the Port Colborne nickel refinery. In the Coniston sinter plant, sulfidic nickel ore concentrates were partially oxidized at 600°C (Roberts et al., 1984) on sinter machines to remove about one-third of the sulfur and to agglomerate the fine material for smelting in a blast furnace. In the Copper Cliff sinter plant, nickel subsulfide was oxidized to nickel oxide at very high temperatures (1650°C). The leaching, calcining and sintering

---

[1]There are some discrepancies between the figures cited here and those reported by Roberts et al. (1990a,b), but the differences are not substantial.

department produced black and green nickel oxides from nickel subsulfide by a series of leaching and calcining operations. The department also included a sinter plant like that at Copper Cliff. Employment records for men employed in the department did not allow them to be assigned to individual leaching, calcining or sintering operations. Mortality up to the end of 1976 in this cohort of about 55 000 men was described by Roberts *et al.* (1984); an earlier study of 495 men employed at the Copper Cliff sinter plant was reported by Chovil *et al.* (1981). The nickel species to which men were exposed in dusty sintering operations were primarily oxidic and sulfidic nickel, and possibly soluble nickel at lower levels (see Table 26). High concentrations of nickel compounds were estimated in the Copper Cliff sinter plant, which ranged from 25-60 mg/m³ Ni as nickel oxide and 15-35 mg/m³ Ni as nickel subsulfide, with up to 4 mg/m³ Ni soluble nickel as anhydrous nickel sulfate between 1948 and 1954. Among the 3769 sinter plant workers, there were 148 lung cancer deaths (standardized mortality ratio (SMR), 261; 95% confidence interval (CI), 220-306) and 25 nasal cancer deaths (SMR, 5073; 95% CI, 3282-7489). Among the 50 977 nonsinter workers in the cohort, there were 547 lung cancer deaths (SMR, 110; 95% CI, 101-120) and six nasal cancer deaths (SMR, 142; 95% CI, 52-309). The only other site for which cancer mortality was significantly elevated was the buccal cavity and pharynx (12 deaths in sinter plant workers: SMR, 211; 95% CI, 109-369; 35 deaths in other workers: SMR, 71; 95% CI, 49-99). The sinter plant workers had little or no excess risk during the first 15 years after starting work (no nasal cancer death; five lung cancer deaths; SMR, 158 [95% CI, 51-370]), and their subsequent relative risk increased with increasing duration of employment. There were also statistically significant excesses of mortality from lung cancer in men employed for 25 or more years in the Sudbury area, both in mining (129 deaths; SMR, 134 [95% CI, 112-159]) and in copper refining (24 deaths; SMR, 207 [95% CI, 133-308]). In the electrolysis department of the Port Colborne plant, workers were estimated to be exposed to low concentrations of metallic, oxidic, sulfidic and soluble nickel. Seven nasal cancer deaths occurred (SMR, 5385; 95% CI, 2165-11 094) in men who had spent over 15 years in the electrolysis department at Port Colborne; all seven had spent some time in the leaching, sintering and calcining area at the Sudbury site, although two had spent only three and seven months, respectively. Lung cancer mortality among workers in the electrolysis department with no exposure in leaching, calcining and sintering, but with 15 or more years since first exposure, gave an SMR of 88 (19 deaths; 95% CI, 53-137). There was a marked difference in the ratio of lung to nasal cancer excess between the Copper Cliff sinter plant and the Port Colborne leaching, calcining and sintering plant: 7:1 at Copper Cliff (63 observed lung cancers, minus 20.5 expected, *versus* six nasal cancers) and only about 2:1 at Port Colborne (72 observed lung cancers, minus 30.0 expected, *versus* 19 nasal cancers).

## (ii) *Falconbridge, Ontario, Canada (mining and smelting)*

A cohort of 11 594 men employed at Falconbridge, Ontario, between 1950 and 1976, with at least six months' service, was previously followed up to the end of 1976 (Shannon *et al.*, 1984a,b). Follow-up has now been extended to the end of 1985 by record linkage to the Canadian Mortality Data Base (ICNCM, 1990). Expected numbers were calculated from Ontario provincial death rates. One death was due to nasal cancer, compared with 0.77 expected. The only cause of death showing a statistically significant excess in the overall analysis was lung cancer (114 deaths; SMR, 135; 95% CI, 111-162). Subdivision of the total cohort by duration of exposure in different areas and latency revealed no SMR for lung cancer that differed significantly from this moderate overall excess, but the highest SMRs occurred in men who had spent more than five years in the mines (46 deaths; SMR, 158; 95% CI, 116-211) or in the smelter (15 deaths; SMR, 163; 95% CI, 91-269). Men who had worked in the smelter are reported to have had low levels of exposure to pentlandite and pyrrhotite, sulfidic nickel, oxidic nickel and some exposure to nickel sulfate. Estimated total exposures to nickel in all areas of the facility were below 1 mg/m³ Ni (ICNCM, 1990).

## (iii) *INCO, Clydach, South Wales, UK (refining)*

The excess of lung and nasal sinus cancer among workers in the INCO refinery in Clydach, South Wales, which opened in 1902, was recognized over 50 years ago (Bridge, 1933). The first formal analyses of cancer mortality were carried out by Hill in 1939 and published by Morgan (1958), who identified calcining, furnaces and copper sulfate extraction as the most hazardous processes. Subsequent reports indicated that the risk had been greatly reduced by 1925 or 1930 (Doll, 1958; Doll *et al.*, 1970, 1977; Cuckle *et al.*, 1980); trends in risk with age at first exposure, period of first exposure and latency were analysed (Doll *et al.*, 1970; Peto *et al.*, 1984; Kaldor *et al.*, 1986). The cohort of 845 men employed prior to 1945 studied by Doll *et al.* (1970) has now been extended to include 2521 men employed for at least five years between 1902 and 1969, and followed up to the end of 1984 (ICNCM, 1990). Among 1348 men first employed before 1930 there were 172 lung cancer deaths (SMR, 393; 95% CI, 336-456) and 74 nasal cancer deaths (SMR, 21 120; 95% CI, 16 584-26 514); the highest risks were associated with calcining, furnaces and copper sulfate production. The calcining and furnace areas had high estimated levels of oxidic, sulfidic and metallic nickel (see Table 27). Until the late 1930s, the oxidic nickel consisted of nickel-copper oxide. Men in the copper plant were exposed to very high concentrations of nickel-copper oxide; they were also exposed to soluble nickel: the extraction of copper from the calcine involved the handling of large volumes of solutions containing 60 g/l nickel as nickel sulfate. Until 1923, arsenic present in sulfuric acid is believed to have accumulated at significant levels in several process departments, mainly as nickel arsenides. The only other significantly elevated risks were an excess of five lung cancer deaths (SMR, 333; 95% CI, 108-776) and four nasal cancer deaths (SMR, 36 363; 95% CI, 9891-93 089) in men employed before 1930 with less than one year in calcining, furnace or copper sulfate but over five years in hydrometallurgy, an area in which exposure to soluble nickel was similar to that in other high-risk areas and exposures to oxidic nickel were an order of magnitude lower than in other high-risk areas, with negligible exposure to sulfidic nickel (see Table 27); and in the small subgroup of nickel plant cleaners (12 lung cancer deaths; SMR, 784 [95% CI, 402-1361]), who were highly exposed to metallic nickel (5 mg/m³ Ni), oxidic nickel (6 mg /m³ Ni) and sulfidic nickel ( > 10 mg/m³ Ni), with negligible exposure to soluble nickel (ICNCM, 1990). A notable anomaly in the data for the whole refinery was the marked reduction in nasal cancer but not lung cancer mortality, when comparing men first exposed before 1920 and those first exposed between 1920 and 1925 (Peto et al., 1984). The risk, although greatly reduced, may not have been entirely eliminated by 1930, as there were 44 lung cancers (SMR, 125 [95% CI, 91-168]) and one nasal cancer (SMR, 526 [95% CI, 13-3028]) among the 1173 later employees.

(iv)  *Falconbridge, Kristiansand, Norway (refining)*

The cohort of 3250 men reported by ICNCM (1990) is restricted to men first employed in 1946-69 with at least one year's service and followed until the end of 1984. For each work area, average concentrations for the four categories of nickel (sulfidic nickel, metallic nickel, oxidic nickel and soluble nickel) were estimated as four ranges for three periods (1946-67, 1968-77 and 1978-84). The four ranges and the arithmetic average computed for each range were: low (0.3 mg/m³), medium (1.3 mg/m³), high (5 mg/m³) and very high (10 mg/m³). There were 77 lung cancer deaths (SMR, 262; 95% CI, 207-327), three nasal cancer deaths (SMR, 453; 95% CI, 93-1324) and a further four incident cases of nasal cancer. Five of the nasal cancer cases had spent their entire employment in the roasting, smelting and calcining department, where oxidic nickel was estimated to have been the predominant exposure, with lesser amounts of sulfidic and metallic nickel. Before 1953, arsenic was present in the feed materials, and significant contamination with nickel arsenides is believed to have occurred at various steps of the process. The remaining two cases were in electrolysis workers who were exposed mainly to soluble nickel (nickel sulfate until 1953 and nickel sulfate and nickel chloride solutions thereafter) and nickel-copper oxides. No other type of cancer occurred significantly in excess. Among men first employed after 1955, there have been 13 lung cancer deaths (SMR, 173 [95% CI, 92-296]) and no nasal cancer (0.2 expected). Several comparisons were made assuming 15 years' latency. The highest risk for lung cancer was seen among a group of workers who had worked in the electrolysis deparment but never in roasting and smelting (30 deaths; SMR, 385; 95% CI, 259-549). In the group of workers who had worked in roasting and smelting but never in the electrolysis department, 14 lung cancer deaths were seen (SMR, 225; 95% CI, 122-377) (see also Table 28). In those who had spent no time in either of these departments, the SMR was 187 (six cases [95% CI, 68-406]). Although exposure to soluble nickel in the roasting, calcining and smelting department was initially estimated to be negligible, it was noted that soluble nickel was certainly present in the Kristiansand roasting department in larger amounts than had been allowed for, and to some extent in all smelter and calcining plants (ICNCM, 1990).

The overlapping cohort reported by Pedersen *et al.* (1973) and Magnus *et al.* (1982) included 2247 men employed for at least three years from when the plant began operation in 1910. Results for cancers diagnosed up to 1979 were presented by Magnus *et al.* (1982). There were 82 lung cancers [standardized incidence ratio (SIR), 373; 95% CI, 296-463] and 21 nasal cancers (SIR, 2630 [95% CI, 1625-4013]). Of the nasal cancers, eight occurred in men involved in roasting-smelting, eight in electrolysis workers, two in workers in other specified processes and three in administration, service and unspecified workers. The incidence of no other type of cancer was significantly elevated overall, although there were four laryngeal cancers (SIR, 670) among roasting and smelting workers. An analysis of lung cancer incidence in relation to smoking suggested an additive rather than a synergistic effect. Adjustment for national trends in lung cancer rates, assuming an additive effect of nickel exposure, suggested little or no reduction in lung cancer risk between men first employed in 1930-39 and those first employed in 1950-59. This contrasts with the marked reduction in nasal cancer risk.

### (v)  *Hanna Mining and Nickel Smelting, Oregon, USA*

A total of 1510 men who had worked for at least six months between 1953, when the plant opened, and 1977 were followed up to the end of 1983 (ICNCM, 1990). Expected numbers of deaths were those for the state of Oregon. A statistically significant excess of lung cancer was observed among men with less than one year of exposure (seven deaths; SMR, 265 [95% CI, 107-546]) but not in men with longer exposure (20 deaths; SMR, 127 [95% CI, 77-196]) or in the subgroup who had worked in areas with potentially high exposures (smelting, 'skull plant', refining and ferrosilicon plant; seven deaths; SMR, 113; 95% CI, 45-233). There was no nasal cancer, and no excess of other cancers (21 deaths; SMR, 65 [95% CI, 41-100]). Average airborne concentrations were estimated to have been 1 mg/m$^3$ Ni or less, even in areas with potentially high exposure, and in most areas were below 0.1 mg/m$^3$ Ni. The principal nickel compounds to which workers were exposed were nickel-containing silicate ore and iron-nickel oxide, with very little soluble nickel and no sulfidic nickel.

### (vi)  *Societé Le Nickel, New Caledonia (mining and smelting)*

Approximately 25% of the adult male population of New Caledonia has worked in nickel mines (silicate-oxide nickel ores) or smelters. Since the local rates for cancer of the lung and upper respiratory tract are higher than those in neighbouring islands, a small hospital-based case-control study was conducted (Lessard *et al.*, 1978). Of the 68 cases identified in 1970-74, 29 cases and 22/109 controls had been exposed to nickel, giving an age- and smoking-adjusted relative risk (RR) of 3.0. [The Working Group noted that control subjects were selected from among patients seen in the laboratory of one hospital, while cases were identified through a variety of sources. Selection bias could have contributed to the apparent excess risk.]

Another study showed no difference in the incidence of lung cancer (RR, 0.9, not significant) or of upper respiratory tract cancer (RR, 1.4; not significant) between nickel workers and the general population. In a case-control study conducted among the nickel workers, no association was found between cancers at these sites and exposure to total dust, nickeliferous dust, raw ore or calcined ore (Goldberg *et al.*, 1987). Subsequent analyses (Goldberg *et al.*, 1990) provided little evidence that people with lung and upper respiratory tract cancer had had greater exposure to nickel than controls. Exposure was principally to silicate oxides, complex oxides, sulfides, metallic iron-nickel alloy and soluble nickel. The estimated total airborne nickel concentration in the facility was estimated to be low ( < 2 mg/m$^3$ Ni) (ICNCM, 1990).

### (vii)  *Other studies of mining, smelting and refining*

Several studies have been published in which the results were not described in sufficient detail for evaluation. Saknyn and Shabynina (1970, 1973) reported elevated lung cancer mortality among process workers in four nickel smelters in the USSR (SMRs, 200, 280, 380, 400 [no observed numbers given]). Electrolysis workers, exposed mainly to nickel sulfate and nickel chloride, were reported to be at particularly high risk for lung cancer (SMR, 820); excesses of stomach cancer and soft-tissue sarcoma were also observed. Tatarskaya (1965, 1967) reported an excess of nasal cancer among electrolysis workers in the USSR.

Olejár *et al.* (1982) reported a marginal excess of lung cancer (based on eight cases) among workers in a Czechoslovak refinery.

One nasal sinus cancer and one lung cancer occurred among 129 men at the Outokumpu Oy refinery in Finland, but expected numbers were not calculated. Workers were exposed primarily to soluble nickel; the highest measurement recorded was 1.1 mg/m$^3$ Ni (ICNCM, 1990).

Egedahl and Rice (1984) found no excess risk among workers in a refinery in Alberta, Canada, but there were only two cases of lung cancer in the cohort (SIR, 83 [95% CI, 10-301]).

### (c) Nickel alloy and stainless-steel production

#### (i) Huntington Alloys (INCO), W. Virginia (refining and manufacture of high-nickel alloys)

A cohort of 3208 men with at least one year's service before 1947 was followed up to the end of 1977 (Enterline & Marsh, 1982) and then to the end of 1984 (ICNCM, 1990). Workers were exposed to metallic, oxidic, sulfidic and soluble nickel at low levels, except in the calcining department where high levels of sulfidic nickel (4000 mg/m³ Ni) were present. Average airborne exposures were estimated to have been below 1 mg/m³ Ni in all areas except calcining. On the basis of the ICNCM report (1990), there was no significant overall excess of lung cancer (91 deaths; SMR, 97 [95% CI, 80-121]). There was a nonsignificant excess among men first employed before 1947 (when calcining ceased) with 30 or more years' service (40 deaths; SMR, 124; 95% CI, 88-169). The group who had worked in calcining for five or more years was too small for useful analysis (two lung cancers; SMR, 100; 95% CI, 12-361). Four deaths from nasal cancer occurred in the whole cohort, all in persons employed before 1948; two were coded on death certificates as nasal cancer (expected, 0.9) and two were classified on the death certificates as bone cancer. Two had not worked in calcining and three had never been exposed to nickel sulfides; one had also worked as a heel finisher in a shoe factory. There was no excess mortality from nonrespiratory cancers.

#### (ii) Henry Wiggin, UK (high-nickel alloy plant)

Mortality up to 1978 in a cohort of 1925 men employed for at least five years in a plant that opened in 1953 was reported by Cox *et al.* (1981). Follow-up has now been extended to April 1985 for 1907 men (ICNCM, 1990). Average exposures from 1975 on rarely exceeded 1 mg/m³ Ni in any area, with an overall average of the order of 0.5 mg/m³ Ni. Measurements taken since 1975 were stated probably to be underestimates of the level of exposure to oxidic and metallic nickel of workers in earlier periods. Soluble nickel was reported to constitute 14-49% of total nickel in various departments (Cox *et al.*, 1981). Thirty deaths were due to lung cancer (SMR, 98; 95% CI, 57-121), including 13 deaths among men employed for ten years or more in areas where they were exposed to nickel (SMR, 91; 95% CI, 57-149). Subdivision by duration of exposure or latency produced no evidence of increased lung cancer risk, and there was no nasal cancer. An excess of soft-tissue sarcoma was found, based on two cases (SMR, 769; 95% CI, 92-2769) (ICNCM, 1990).

(iii)    *Twelve high-nickel alloy plants in the USA*

Mortality up to the end of 1977 among 28 261 workers (90% male) employed for at least one year in 12 high-nickel alloy plants in the USA, and still working at some time between 1956 and 1960, was reported by Redmond (1984). There were 332 lung cancer deaths (SMR, 109 [95% CI, 98-122]) and two nasal sinus cancer deaths (SMR, 93 [95% CI, 12-358]). The excess of lung cancer was confined to men employed for five or more years in 'allocated services', most of whom were maintenance workers (197 deaths; SMR, 127 [95% CI, 110-146]). Excess mortality was observed from liver cancer (31 deaths; SMR, 182 [95% CI, 124-259]) in all men, and from cancer of the large intestine (SMR, 223 [95% CI, 122-375]) among non-white men. No data on exposure were available, but the authors noted that there may have been exposure to asbestos in these plants.

(iv)    *Twenty-six nickel-chromium alloy foundries in the USA*

A proportionate mortality analysis of 851 deaths among men ever employed in 26 nickel-chromium alloy foundries in the USA in 1968-79 (Cornell & Landis, 1984) showed no statistically significant excess of lung cancer (60 deaths; proportionate mortality ratio (PMR, 105 [95% CI, 80-135]) or other cancers (103 deaths; PMR, 87 [95% CI, 71-106]) in comparison with US males. No death was due to nasal cancer.

Lung cancer mortality in a cohort of foundry workers was investigated by Fletcher and Ades (1984). The cohort consisted of men hired between 1946 and 1965 in nine steel foundries in the UK and employed for at least one year. The 10 250 members of the cohort were followed up until the end of 1978 and assigned to 25 occupational categories according to information from personnel officers. Lung cancer mortality for the subcohort of fettlers and grinders in the fettling shop was higher than expected on the basis of mortality rates for England and Wales (32 cases; SMR, 195; 95% CI, 134-276). [The Working Group noted that these workers may have been exposed to chromium- and nickel-containing dusts.]

(v)    *Seven stainless-steel and low-nickel alloy production plants in the USA*

A proportionate mortality analysis of 3323 deaths among white males ever employed in areas with potential exposure to nickel in seven stainless-steel and low-nickel alloy production plants (Cornell, 1984) showed no excess of lung cancer (218 deaths; PMR, 97 [95% CI, 85-111]) or of other cancers (419 deaths; PMR 91 [95% CI, 83-100]). There was no death from nasal cancer.

(d)    *Other industrial exposures to nickel*

(i)    *Two nickel-cadmium battery factories in the UK*

Kipling and Waterhouse (1967) reported an excess of prostatic cancer based on four cases among 248 men exposed for one year or longer in a nickel-cadmium battery factory. The cohort was enlarged to include 3025 workers (85% men) employed for at least one month (Sorahan & Waterhouse, 1983, 1985), and the most recent report included deaths up to the end of 1984 (Sorahan, 1987). Exposure categories were defined on the basis of exposure to cadmium. The authors commented that almost all jobs with high exposure to cadmium also entailed high exposure to nickel hydroxide, and there was also possible exposure to welding fumes (Sorahan & Waterhouse, 1983). The excess of prostatic cancer cases was confined to highly exposed workers, among whom there were eight cases (SIR, 402 [95% CI, 174-792]); in the remainder of the cohort there were seven (SIR, 78 [95% CI, 31-160]) (Sorahan & Waterhouse, 1985). An excess of cancer of the lung was seen (110 deaths; SMR, 130 [95% CI, 107-157]), and this showed a significant association with duration in 'high exposure' jobs, particularly among men first employed before 1947 (Sorahan, 1987).

### (ii)   *A nickel-cadmium battery factory in Sweden*

A total of 525 male workers in a Swedish nickel-cadmium battery factory employed for at least one year were followed up to 1980 (Andersson *et al.*, 1984). Six deaths were due to lung cancer (SMR, 120 [95% CI, 44-261]), four to prostatic cancer (SMR, 129 [95% CI, 35-330]) and one to nasopharyngeal cancer (SMR, > 1000). Cadmium levels prior to 1950 were said to have been about 1 mg/m³ in some areas; nickel levels were reported as 'about five times higher', although no actual measurement was reported.

### (iii)   *A nickel and chromium plating factory in the UK*

A total of 2689 workers (48% male) employed in a nickel-chromium plating factory in the UK were followed to the end of 1983 by Sorahan *et al.* (1987). There was excess mortality from lung cancer (72 deaths; SMR, 150 [95% CI, 117-189]) and nasal cancer (three deaths; SMR, 1000 [95% CI, 206-2922]), but this was confined to workers whose initial employment had been as chrome bath platers, and the lung cancer excess was significantly related to duration of chrome bath work. An earlier study of 508 men employed only as nickel platers in the factory (Burges, 1980) showed no excess for any cancer except that of the stomach (eight deaths; SMR, 267); among men with more than one year's employment, the SMR for stomach cancer was 476 (adjusted for social class and region; four deaths [95% CI, 130-1219]). The SMR for lung cancer was 122 [95% CI, 59-224].

### (iv)   *A die-casting and electroplating plant in the USA*

A proportionate mortality analysis of 238 deaths (79% male) in workers employed for at least ten years in a die-casting and electroplating plant in the USA was reported by Silverstein *et al.* (1981). There was excess mortality from lung cancer (28 deaths; PMR 191 [95% CI, 127-276]) among white men, but not for cancer at any other site. The PMRs for lung cancer by duration of employment were 165 ( < 15 years) and 209 (≥15 years), and those by latency were 178 (<22.5 years) and 211 (≥ 22.5 years). The authors noted that the workers had been exposed to chromium[VI], polycyclic aromatic hydrocarbons and various compounds of nickel.

### (v) *Oak Ridge gaseous diffusion plant, Tennessee, USA*

Fine pure nickel powder is used as barrier material in uranium enrichment by gaseous diffusion. A cohort of 814 white men employed at any time before 1954 in the production of this material was followed up from 1948 to 1972 by Godbold and Tompkins (1979). Exposure was thus entirely to metallic nickel. Follow-up was extended to the end of 1977 by Cragle *et al.* (1984), and mortality up to the end of 1982 was reported by ICNCM (1990). The median concentration of nickel was about 0.13 mg/m³, but high concentrations occurred in some areas. About 300 of the 814 men had been employed for a total of less than two years. There was no excess of lung cancer, either overall (nine deaths; SMR, 54; 95% CI, 25-103) or among men employed for 15 years or longer (five deaths; SMR, 109 [95% CI, 35-254]), and mortality from other cancers was close to that expected (29 deaths; SMR, 96 [95% CI, 64-137]) for the whole cohort. No death from nasal cancer occurred, but only 0.22 were expected. [The Working Group noted that measurements made in 1948-63 (Godbold & Tompkins, 1979) suggest that the average exposure may have been to 0.5 mg/m³ Ni.]

### (vi) *Aircraft engine factory, Connecticut, USA*

Bernacki *et al.* (1978b) compared the employment histories of 42 men at an aircraft engine factory in the USA who had died of lung cancer with those of 84 age-matched men who had died of causes other than cancer. The proportion classified as nickel-exposed was identical (26%) among cases and controls. Atmospheric nickel concentrations in the past were believed to have been <1 mg/m³.

### (e) *Other studies*

Several studies have been reported in which occupational histories of nasal cancer patients were sought by interview with patients or relatives, from medical or other records, or from death certificates. Acheson *et al.* (1981), in a study of 1602 cases diagnosed in England and Wales over a five-year period, found an excess (29 cases; SMR, 250 [95% CI, 167-359]) in furnace and foundry workers, which was partly (but not entirely) due to the inclusion of seven process workers from the INCO (Clydach) nickel refinery (see above). Hernberg *et al.* (1983) studied 287 cases diagnosed in Denmark, Finland or Sweden over a 3.5-year period. The association with exposure to nickel (12 cases, five matched controls among 167 matched case-control pairs who were interviewed; odds ratio, 2.4; 95% CI, 0.9-6.6) was not statistically significant. All except one of the nickel-exposed cases (a nickel refinery worker) had also been classified as having exposure to chromium (odds ratio, 2.7;

95% CI, 1.1-6.6), which was significantly associated with nasal cancer risk. Brinton *et al.* (1984) recorded exposure to nickel in only one (RR, 1.8; 95% CI, 0.1-27.6) of 160 cases and one of 290 controls in a hospital-based study between 1970 and 1980 in North Carolina and Virginia. Roush *et al.* (1980) examined exposure to nickel, cutting oils and wood dust in a case-control study based on all sinonasal cancer deaths in Connecticut in 1935-75. Job titles were obtained from deaths certificates and city directories and were classified according to estimated airborne exposures. Ten of 216 cases and 49 of 662 controls were classified as having been exposed to nickel (RR, 0.71; 95% CI, 0.4-1.5).

Gérin *et al.* (1984) reported significantly more frequent exposure to nickel among 246 Canadian lung cancer patients (29 exposed; odds ratio, 3.1; 95% CI, 1.9-5.0) than among patients with other cancers. All 29 cases had also been exposed to chromium, and 20 (69%) had been exposed to stainless-steel welding fumes. In a case-control study of 326 Danish laryngeal cancer patients, Olsen and Sabroe (1984) found a statistically significant association with exposure to nickel from alloys, battery chemicals and chemicals used in plastics production (RR, 1.7; 95% CI, 1.2-2.5; adjusted for age, tobacco and alcohol consumption and sex).

# 4. Summary of Data Reported and Evaluation

## 4.1 Exposure data

Nickel, in the form of various alloys and compounds, has been in widespread commercial use for over 100 years. Several million workers worldwide are exposed to airborne fumes, dusts and mists containing nickel and its compounds. Exposures by inhalation, ingestion or skin contact occur in nickel and nickel alloy production plants as well as in welding, electroplating, grinding and cutting operations. Airborne nickel levels in excess of 1 mg/m³ have been found in nickel refining, in the production of nickel alloys and nickel salts, and in grinding and cutting of stainless-steel. In these industries, modern control technologies have markedly reduced exposures in recent years. Few data are available to estimate the levels of past exposures to total airborne nickel, and the concentrations of individual nickel compounds were not measured.

Occupational exposure has been shown to give rise to elevated levels of nickel in blood, urine and body tissues, with inhalation as the main route of uptake. Non-occupational sources of nickel exposure include food, air and water, but the levels found are usually several orders of magnitude lower than those typically found in occupational situations.

Table 26. INCO Ontario (Canada) nickel refinery facilities – average nickel exposure levels and cancer risks in workers with 15 or more years since first exposure[a]

| Plant | Department | Estimated airborne concentration (mg/m³ Ni) | | | | | Duration in department | | | | | | | |
| | | Metallic nickel | Oxidic nickel | Sulfidic nickel | Soluble nickel | Total nickel | Ever | | | | ≥5 years | | | |
| | | | | | | | Lung cancer | | Nasal cancer | | Lung cancer | | Nasal cancer | |
| | | | | | | | Obs | SMR (95% CI) | Obs | SMR (95% CI) | Obs | SMR (95% CI) | Obs | SMR (95% CI) |
|---|---|---|---|---|---|---|---|---|---|---|---|---|---|---|
| Coniston | Sinter | Negl.[b] | 0.1-0.5 | 1-5 | Negl. | 1-5 | 8 | 292 (126-576) | 0 | - | 6 | 492 (181-1073) | 0 | - |
| Copper Cliff | Sinter | | | | | | | | | | | | | |
| 1948-54 | | Negl. | 25-60 | 15-35 | <4 | 40-100 | 63 | 307 (238-396) | 6 | 3617 (1327-7885) | 33 | 789 (543-1109) | 4 | 13 146 (3576-33 654) |
| 1955-63 | | Negl. | 5-25 | 3-15 | <2 | 8-40 | | | | | | | | |
| Port Colborne | Leaching, calcining, sintering | | | | | | | | | | | | | |
| 1926-35 | | Negl. | 20-40 | 10-20 | <3 | 30-80 | 72 | 239 (187-302) | 19 | 7776 (4681-12 144) | 38 | 366 (259-502) | 15 | 18 750 (10 500-30 537) |
| 1936-45 | | Negl. | 3-15 | 2-10 | <3 | 5-25 | | | | | | | | |
| 1946-58 | | Negl. | 5-25 | 3-15 | <3 | 8-40 | | | | | | | | |
| | Electrolysis | <0.5 | <0.2 | <0.5 | <0.3 | <1 | 19 | 88[d] (53-137) | 0[c,d] | - | 104[e] | 89 | 0[c,d] | - |

[a]From ICNCM (1990), estimated average airborne concentrations of nickel species and mortality from lung cancer and nasal cancer by department; standardized mortality ratio (SMR) and 95% confidence interval (CI)

[b]Negl, negligible exposure

[c]Two nasal cancer deaths occurred in men with >20 years in electrolysis and only short exposure (three months and seven months) in leaching, calcining and sintering

[d]Never worked in leaching, calcining and sintering

[e]Workers with ≥10 years in electrolysis

**Table 27. MOND/INCO (Clydach, South Wales, UK) nickel refinery – average nickel exposure levels and cancer risks in 'high-risk' departments in workers with 15 or more years since first exposure[a]**

| Department | Estimated airborne concentration (mg/m³ Ni)[b] | | | | Duration in department | | | | | | | |
| --- | --- | --- | --- | --- | --- | --- | --- | --- | --- | --- | --- | --- |
| | | | | | Ever | | | | ≥5 years | | | |
| | | | | | Lung cancer | | Nasal cancer | | Lung cancer | | Nasal cancer | |
| | Metallic nickel | Oxidic nickel | Sulfidic nickel | Soluble nickel | Obs | SMR (95% CI) | Obs | SMR (95% CI) | Obs | SMR (95% CI) | Obs | SMR (95% CI) |
| Furnaces, 1905–63 | 5.6 | 6.4 | 2.6 | 0.4 | 9 | 409 | 3 | 24 781 | 1 | 370 | 3 | 1000 |
| Linear calciners, 1902–30; milling and grinding, 1902–36 | 5.3 | 18.8 | 6.8 | 0.8 | 16 | 725 | 7 | 44 509 | 12 | 1244 | 6 | 78 280 |
| Copper plant, before 1937 | – | 13.1 | 0.4 | 1.1 | 17 | 317 (185–507) | 5 | 13 912 (4507–32 415) | 8 | 541 (233–1066) | 2 | 14 541 (1759–52 493) |
| 1938–60 | – | 0.4 | 0.01 | 0.01 | – | | – | | – | | – | |
| Hydrometallurgy 1902–79 | 0.5 | 0.9 | 0.05 | 1.3 | 7 | 196 (79–404) | 4 | 18 779 (5108–48 074) | 5 | 333 (108–776) | 4 | 36 363 (9891–93 089) |

[a]From ICNCM (1990); estimated average airborne concentrations of nickel species and mortality from lung cancer and nasal cancer by department. In each row, observations are restricted to men with < 1 year employment in other high–risk departments. Standardized mortality ratio (SMR) and 95% confidence interval (CI)

[b]The Working Group expressed reservations about the accuracy of these estimates, as discussed on p. 391.

Table 28. Falconbridge (Kristiansand, Norway) nickel refinery – average nickel exposure levels and cancer risks in workers with 15 or more years since first exposure[a]

| Department | Estimated airborne concentration (mg/m³ Ni) | | | | Duration in department | | | | | | | |
|---|---|---|---|---|---|---|---|---|---|---|---|---|
| | | | | | Ever | | | | ≥5 years | | | |
| | | | | | Lung cancer | | Nasal cancer[b] | | Lung cancer | | Nasal cancer[b] | |
| | Metallic nickel | Oxidic nickel | Sulfidic nickel | Soluble nickel | Obs | SMR (95% CI) | Obs | SMR (95% CI) | Obs | SMR (95% CI) | Obs | SMR (95% CI) |
| Calcining, roasting, smelting; never in electrolysis | 0.3–1.3 | 5.0–10.0 | 0.3 | Negl.[c] | 14 | 225 (122–377) | 5 | – | 8 | 254 (109–500) | 5 | – |
| Electrolysis; never in calcining, roasting smelting | 0.3–1.3 | 0.3–1.3 | Negl.–1.3 | 1.3–5.0 | 30 | 385 (259–549) | 2 | – | 19 | 476 (287–744) | 2 | – |

[a]From ICNCM (1990); estimated average airborne concentrations of nickel species and mortality from or incidence of lung cancer and nasal cancer by department; standardized mortality ratio (SMR) and 95% confidence interval (CI)
[b]Three deaths and four incident cases
[c]Negl., negligible exposure

## 4.2 Experimental carcinogenicity data

### Metallic nickel and nickel alloys

*Metallic nickel* was tested by inhalation exposure in mice, rats and guinea-pigs, by intratracheal instillation in rats, by intramuscular injection in rats and hamsters, and by intrapleural, subcutaneous, intraperitoneal and intrarenal injection in rats. The studies by inhalation exposure were inadequate for an assessment of carcinogenicity. After intratracheal instillation, it produced significant numbers of squamous-cell carcinomas and adenocarcinomas of the lung. Intrapleural injections induced sarcomas. Subcutaneous administration of metallic nickel pellets induced sarcomas in rats, intramuscular injection of nickel powder induced sarcomas in rats and hamsters, and intraperitoneal injections induced carcinomas and sarcomas. No significant increase in the incidence of local kidney tumours was seen following intrarenal injection.

*Nickel alloys* were tested by intramuscular, intraperitoneal and intrarenal injection and by subcutaneous implantation of pellets in rats. A ferronickel alloy did not induce local tumours after intramuscular or intrarenal injection. Two powdered nickel alloys induced malignant tumours following intraperitoneal injection, and one nickel alloy induced sarcomas following subcutaneous implantation in pellets.

### Nickel oxides and hydroxides

*Nickel monoxide* was tested by inhalation exposure in rats and hamsters, by intratracheal instillation in rats, by intramuscular administration in two strains of mice and two strains of rats, and by intrapleural, intraperitoneal and intrarenal injection in rats. The two studies by inhalation exposure in rats were inadequate for an assessment of carcinogenicity; lung tumours were not induced in the study in hamsters. Intratracheal instillation resulted in a significant incidence of lung carcinomas. Local sarcomas were induced at high incidence after intrapleural, intramuscular and intraperitoneal injection. No renal tumour was seen following intrarenal injection.

Two studies in rats in which *nickel trioxide* was injected intramuscularly or intracerebrally were inadequate for evaluation.

In a study in which *nickel hydroxide* was tested in three physical states by intramuscular injection in rats, local sarcomas were induced by dry gel and crystalline forms. Local sarcomas were induced in one study in which nickel hydroxide was tested by intramuscular injection in rats.

### Nickel sulfides

*Nickel subsulfide* was tested by inhalation exposure and by intratracheal instillation in rats, by subcutaneous injection to mice and rats, by intramuscular administration to mice, rats, hamsters and rabbits, by intrapleural, intraperitoneal, intrarenal, intratesticular, intraocular and intra-articular administration in rats, by injection into retroperitoneal fat in rats, by implantation into rat heterotopic tracheal transplants and by administration to pregnant rats.

After exposure by inhalation, rats showed a significant increase in the incidence of benign and malignant lung tumours. Multiple intratracheal instillations resulted in malignant lung tumours (adenocarcinomas, squamous-cell carcinomas and mixed tumours).

A high incidence of local sarcomas was observed in rats after intrapleural administration. Subcutaneous injection induced sarcomas in mice and rhabdomyosarcomas and fibrous histiocytomas in rats. Nickel subsulfide has been shown consistently to induce local sarcomas following intramuscular administration, and dose-response relationships were demonstrated in rats and hamsters. The majority of the sarcomas induced were of myogenic origin, and the incidences of metastases were generally high. In rats, strain differences in tumour incidence and local tissue responses were seen. After intramuscular implantation of millipore diffusion chambers containing nickel subsulfide, a high incidence of local sarcomas was induced.

Mesotheliomas were included among the malignancies induced by intraperitoneal administration. Intrarenal injections resulted in a dose-related increase in the incidence of renal-cell neoplasms. A high incidence of sarcomas (including some rhabdomyosarcomas) was seen after intratesticular injection, and a high incidence of eye neoplasms (including retinoblastomas, melanomas and gliomas) after intraocular injection. Intra-articular injection induced sarcomas (including rhabdomyosarcomas and fibrous histiocytomas), and injection into retroperitoneal fat induced mainly fibrous histiocytomas. Implantation of pellets containing nickel subsulfide into rat heterotopic tracheal transplants induced both carcinomas and sarcomas; in the group given the highest dose, sarcomas predominated. The study in which pregnant rats were injected with nickel subsulfide early in gestation was inadequate for evaluation.

*Nickel disulfide* was tested by intramuscular and intrarenal injection in rats. High incidences of local tumours were induced.

*Nickel monosulfide* was tested by intramuscular and intrarenal injection in rats. The crystalline form induced local tumours, but the amorphous form did not.

*Nickel ferrosulfide matte* induced local sarcomas after administration by intramuscular injection in rats.

**Nickel salts**

*Nickel sulfate* was tested for carcinogenicity by intramuscular and intraperitoneal injection in rats. Repeated intramuscular injections did not induce local tumours; however, intraperitoneal injections induced malignant tumours in the peritoneal cavity.

*Nickel chloride* was tested by repeated intraperitoneal injections in rats, inducing malignant tumours in the peritoneal cavity.

*Nickel acetate* was tested by intraperitoneal injection in mice and rats. After repeated intraperitoneal injections in rats, malignant tumours were induced in the peritoneal cavity. In strain A mice, lung adenocarcinomas were induced in one study and an increased incidence of pulmonary adenomas in two studies.

Studies in rats in which *nickel carbonate* was tested for carcinogenicity by intraperitoneal administration and *nickel fluoride* and *nickel chromate* by intramuscular injection could not be evaluated.

### Other forms of nickel

*Nickel carbonyl* was tested for carcinogenicity by inhalation exposure and intravenous injection in rats. After inhalation exposure, a few lung carcinomas were observed two years after the initial treatment. Intravenous injection induced an increase in the overall incidence of neoplasms, which were located in several organs.

*Nickelocene* induced some local tumours in rats and hamsters following intramuscular injection.

One sample of *dust collected in nickel refineries*, containing nickel subsulfide and various proportions of nickel monoxide and nickel sulfate, induced sarcomas in mice and rats following intramuscular injection. Intraperitoneal administration of two samples of dust, containing unspecified nickel sulfides and various proportions of nickel oxide, soluble nickel and metallic nickel, induced sarcomas in rats. In a study in which hamsters were given prolonged exposure to a *nickel-enriched fly ash* by inhalation, the incidence of tumours was not increased.

Intramuscular administration to rats of *nickel sulfarsenide*, two *nickel arsenides*, *nickel antimonide*, *nickel telluride* and two *nickel selenides* induced significant increases in the incidence of local sarcomas, whereas administration of *nickel monoarsenide* and *nickel titanate* did not. None of these compounds increased the incidence of renal-cell tumours in rats after intrarenal injection.

### 4.3  Human carcinogenicity data

Increased risks for lung and nasal cancers were found to be associated with exposures during high-temperature oxidation of nickel matte and nickel-copper matte (roasting, sintering, calcining) in cohort studies in Canada, Norway (Kristiansand) and the UK (Clydach), with exposures in electrolytic refining in a study in Norway, and with exposures during leaching of nickel-copper oxides in acidic solution (copper plant) and extraction of nickel salts from concentrated solution (hydrometallurgy) in the UK (see Table 26).

The substantial excess risk for lung and nasal cancer among Clydach hydro-metallurgy workers seems likely to be due, at least partly, to their exposure to 'soluble nickel'. Their estimated exposures to other types of nickel (metallic, sulfidic and oxidic) were up to an order of magnitude lower than those in several other areas of the refinery, including some where cancer risks were similar to those observed in hydrometallurgy. Similarly, high risks for lung and nasal cancers were observed among electrolysis workers at Kristiansand. These men were exposed to high estimated levels of soluble nickel and to lower levels of other forms of nickel. Nickel sulfate was the only or predominant soluble nickel species present in these areas.

The highest risks for lung and nasal cancers were observed among calcining workers, who were heavily exposed to both sulfidic and oxidic nickel. A high lung cancer rate was also seen among nickel plant cleaners at Clydach, who were heavily exposed to these insoluble compounds, with little or no exposure to soluble nickel. The separate effects of oxides and sulfides cannot be estimated, however, as high exposure was always either to both, or to oxides together with soluble nickel. Workers in calcining furnaces and nickel plant cleaners were also exposed to high levels of metallic nickel.

Among hard-rock sulfide nickel ore miners in Canada, there was some increase in lung cancer risk, but exposure to other substances could not be excluded. In studies of open-cast miners of silicate-oxide nickel ores in the USA and in New Caledonia, no significant increase in risk was seen, but the numbers of persons studied were small and the levels of exposure were reported to be low.

No significant excess of respiratory tract cancer was observed in three studies of workers in high-nickel alloy manufacture or in a small study of users of metallic nickel powder. No increase in risk for lung cancer was observed in one small group of nickel electroplaters in the UK with no exposure to chromium.

In a case-control study, an elevated risk for lung cancer was found among persons exposed to nickel together with chromium-containing materials.

The results of epidemiological studies of stainless-steel welders are consistent with the finding of excess mortality from lung cancer among other workers exposed to nickel compounds, but they do not contribute independently to the evaluation of nickel since welders are also exposed to other compounds. (See also the monograph on welding.)

## 4.4  Other relevant data

Nickel and nickel compounds are absorbed from the respiratory tract, and to a smaller extent from the gastrointestinal tract, depending on dissolution and cellular uptake. Absorbed nickel is excreted predominantly in the urine. Nickel tends to persist in the lungs of humans and of experimental animals, and increased concentrations are seen notably in workers after inhalation of nickel. The nasal mucosa may retain nickel for many years.

Nickel carbonyl is the most acutely toxic nickel compound and causes severe damage to the respiratory system in experimental animals and in humans. Nickel causes contact dermatitis in humans. In experimental animals, adverse effects have also been documented in the respiratory system and in the kidney.

In four studies, the frequency of sister chromatid exchange did not appear to be increased in peripheral blood lymphocytes of nickel workers exposed during various processes. Enhanced frequencies of chromosomal gaps and/or anomalies were observed in single studies in peripheral blood lymphocytes of employees engaged in: (i) crushing, roasting and smelting (exposure mainly to nickel oxide and nickel subsulfide); (ii) electrolysis (exposure mainly to nickel chloride and nickel sulfate); and (iii) electroplating (exposure to nickel and chromium compounds). Enhanced frequencies were also seen in lymphocytes from retired workers who had previously been exposed in crushing, roasting and smelting and/or electrolysis.

Some nickel compounds have adverse effects on reproduction and prenatal development in rodents. Decreased fertility, reduction in the number of pups per litter and birth weight per pup, and a pattern of anomalies, including eye malformations, cystic lungs, hydronephrosis, cleft palate and skeletal deformities, have been demonstrated.

In one study, metallic nickel did not induce chromosomal aberrations in cultured human cells, but it transformed animal cells *in vitro*. Nickel oxides induced anchorage-independent growth in human cells *in vitro* and transformed cultured rodent cells; they did not induce chromosomal aberrations in cultured human cells in one study.

Crystalline nickel subsulfide induced anchorage-independent growth and increased the frequency of sister chromatid exchange but did not cause gene mutation in human cells *in vitro*. Crystalline nickel sulfide and subsulfide induced cell transformation, gene mutation and DNA damage in cultured mammalian cells; the sulfide also induced chromosomal aberrations and sister chromatid exchange. Amorphous nickel sulfide did not transform or produce DNA damage in cultured mammalian cells. In one study, crystalline nickel sulfide and crystalline nickel subsulfide produced DNA damage in *Paramoecium*.

Nickel chloride and nickel nitrate were inactive in assays *in vivo* for induction of dominant lethal mutation and micronuclei, and nickel sulfate did not induce chromosomal aberrations in bone-marrow cells; however, nickel chloride induced chromosomal aberrations in Chinese hamster and mouse bone-marrow cells.

Soluble nickel compounds were generally active in the assays of human and animal cells *in vitro* in which they were tested.

Nickel sulfate and nickel acetate induced anchorage-independent growth in human cells *in vitro*. Nickel sulfate increased the frequency of chromosomal aberrations in human cells, and nickel sulfate and nickel chloride increased the frequency of sister chromatid exchange. Nickel sulfate did not induce single-strand DNA breaks in human cells. Nickel sulfate and nickel chloride transformed cultured mammalian cells. Chromosomal aberrations were induced in mammalian cells by nickel chloride, nickel sulfate and nickel acetate, and sister chromatid exchange was induced by nickel chloride and nickel sulfate. Nickel chloride and nickel sulfate also induced gene mutation, and nickel chloride caused DNA damage in mammalian cells. In one study, nickel sulfate inhibited intercellular communication in cultured mammalian cells.

Nickel sulfate induced aneuploidy and gene mutation in a single study in *Drosophila*; nickel chloride and nickel nitrate did not cause gene mutation. Nickel chloride induced gene mutation and recombination in yeast.

In single studies, nickel acetate produced DNA damage in bacteria, while nickel nitrate did not; the results obtained with nickel chloride were inconclusive. In bacteria, neither nickel acetate, sulfate, chloride nor nitrate induced gene mutation.

Nickel carbonate induced DNA damage in rat kidney *in vivo*. Crystalline nickel subselenide transformed cultured mammalian cells, and nickel potassium cyanide increased the frequency of chromosomal aberrations. Nickelocene did not induce bacterial gene mutation. DNA damage was induced in calf thymus nucleohistone by nickel[III]-tetraglycine complexes.

## 4.5 Evaluation[1]

There is *sufficient evidence* in humans for the carcinogenicity of nickel sulfate, and of the combinations of nickel sulfides and oxides encountered in the nickel refining industry.

There is *inadequate evidence* in humans for the carcinogenicity of metallic nickel and nickel alloys.

There is *sufficient evidence* in experimental animals for the carcinogenicity of metallic nickel, nickel monoxides, nickel hydroxides and crystalline nickel sulfides.

There is *limited evidence* in experimental animals for the carcinogenicity of nickel alloys, nickelocene, nickel carbonyl, nickel salts, nickel arsenides, nickel antimonide, nickel selenides and nickel telluride.

---

[1]For descriptions of the italicized terms, see Preamble, pp. 33–37.

There is *inadequate evidence* in experimental animals for the carcinogenicity of nickel trioxide, amorphous nickel sulfide and nickel titanate.

The Working Group made the overall evaluation on nickel compounds as a group on the basis of the combined results of epidemiological studies, carcinogenicity studies in experimental animals, and several types of other relevant data, supported by the underlying concept that nickel compounds can generate nickel ions at critical sites in their target cells.

**Overall evaluation**

Nickel compounds *are carcinogenic to humans* (Group 1).
Metallic nickel *is possibly carcinogenic to humans* (Group 2B).

# 5. References

Abbracchio, M.P., Heck, J.D., Caprioli, R.M. & Costa, M. (1981) Differences in surface properties of amorphous and crystalline metal sulfides may explain their toxicological potency. *Chemosphere, 10*, 897-908

Abbracchio, M.P., Simmons-Hansen, J. & Costa, M. (1982a) Cytoplasmic dissolution of phagocytized crystalline nickel sulfide particles: a prerequisite for nuclear uptake of nickel. *J. Toxicol. environ. Health, 9*, 663-676

Abbracchio, M.P., Heck, J.D. & Costa, M. (1982b) The phagocytosis and transforming activity of crystalline metal sulfide particles are related to their negative surface charge. *Carcinogenesis, 3*, 175-180

Acheson, E.D., Cowdell, R.H. & Rang, E.H. (1981) Nasal cancer in England and Wales: an occupational survey. *Br. J. ind. Med., 38*, 218-224

Adalis, D., Gardner, D.E. & Miller, F.J. (1978) Cytotoxic effects of nickel on ciliated epithelium. *Am. Rev. respir. Dis., 118*, 347-354

Adams, D.B. (1980) The routine determination of nickel creatinine in urine. In: Brown, S.S. & Sunderman, F.W., Jr, eds, *Nickel Toxicology*, London, Academic Press, pp. 99-102

Adamsson, E., Lind, B., Nielsen, B. & Piscator, M. (1980) Urinary and fecal elimination of nickel in relation to airborne nickel in a battery factory. In: Brown, S.S. & Sunderman, F.W., Jr, eds, *Nickel Toxicology*, London, Academic Press, pp. 103-106

Aitio, A. (1984) Biological monitoring of occupational exposure to nickel. In: Sunderman, F.W., Jr, ed., *Nickel in the Human Environment* (IARC Scientific Publications No. 53), Lyon, IARC, pp. 497-505

Aitio, A., Tossavainen, A., Gustafsson, T., Kiilunen, M., Haapa, K. & Järvisalo, J. (1985) Urinary excretion of nickel and chromium in workers of a steel foundry. In: Brown, S.S. & Sunderman, F.W., Jr, eds, *Progress in Nickel Toxicology*, Oxford, Blackwell Scientific Publishers, pp. 149-152

Albert, D.M., Gonder, J.R., Papale, J., Craft, J.L., Dohlman, H.G., Reid, M.C. & Sunderman, F.W., Jr (1980) Induction of ocular neoplasms in Fischer rats by intraocular injection of nickel subsulfide. In: Brown, S.S. & Sunderman, F.W., Jr, eds, *Nickel Toxicology*, London, Academic Press, pp. 55-58

Aldrich Chemical Co., Inc. (1988) *Aldrich Catalog/Handbook of Fine Chemicals*, Milwaukee, WI, pp. 1097-1099

Alexander, A.J., Goggin, P.L. & Cooke, M. (1983) A Fourier-transform infrared spectrometric study of the pyrosynthesis of nickel tetracarbonyl and iron pentacarbonyl by combustion of tobacco. *Anal. chim. Acta, 151,* 1-12

Amacher, D.E. & Paillet, S.C. (1980) Induction of trifluorothymidine-resistant mutants by metal ions in L5178Y/TK$^{+/-}$ cells. *Mutat. Res., 78,* 279-288

Amavis, R., Hunter, W.J. & Smeets, J.G.P.M., eds (1976) *Hardness of Drinking Water and Public Health. Proceedings of the European Scientific Colloquium, Luxembourg, May 1975* (EUR 5447), Oxford, Pergamon Press, p. 194

American Conference of Governmental Industrial Hygienists (1988) *Threshold Limit Values and Biological Exposure Indices for 1988-1989*, Cincinnati, OH, p. 28

American Tokyo Kasei (1988) *Organic Chemicals 88/89 Catalog*, Portland, OR, p. 913

Amlacher, E. & Rudolph, C. (1981) The thymidine incorporation inhibiting screening system (TSS) to test carcinogenic substances: a nuclear DNA synthesis suppressive short term test. *Arch. Geschwulstforsch., 51,* 605-610

Andersen, O. (1983) Effects of coal combustion products and metal compounds on sister chromatid exchange (SCE) in a macrophage-like cell line. *Environ. Health Perspect., 47,* 239-253

Andersen, O. (1985) Evaluation of the spindle-inhibiting effect of Ni$^{++}$ by quantitation of chromosomal super-contraction. *Res. Commun. chem. Pathol. Pharmacol., 50,* 379-386

Andersen, I. & Svenes, K.B. (1989) Determination of nickel in lung specimens of thirty-nine autopsied nickel workers. *Int. Arch. occup. environ. Health, 61,* 289-295

Andersen, J.R., Gammelgaard, B. & Reimert, S. (1986) Direct determination of nickel in human plasma by Zeeman-corrected atomic absorption spectrometry. *Analyst, 3,* 721-722

Andersson, K., Elinder, C.G., Høgstedt, C., Kjellström, T. & Spång, G. (1984) Mortality among cadmium and nickel-exposed workers in a Swedish battery factory. *Toxicol. environ. Chem., 9,* 53-62

Angerer, J. & Heinrich-Ramm, R. (1988) Nickel in blood (Ger.). In: *Analytische Methoden zur Prüfung gesundheitsschädlicher Arbeitsstoffe — Analysen in biologischem Material* (Analytical Methods for Investigation of Noxious Occupational Substances. Analysis in Biological Material), Vol. 2/3, Part 9, Weinheim, VCH-Verlagsgesellschaft, pp. 1-11

Angerer, J. & Schaller, K.H. (1985) *Analyses of Hazardous Substances in Biological Materials*, Vol. 1, Weinheim, VCH-Verlagsgesellschaft, pp. 177-188

Angerer, J., Heinrich-Ramm, R. & Lehnert, G. (1989) Occupational exposure to cobalt and nickel. Biological monitoring. *Int. J. environ. anal. Chem.*, *35*, 81-88

Antonsen, D.H. (1981) Nickel compounds. In: Mark, H.F., Othmer, D.F., Overberger, C.G., Seaborg, G.T. & Grayson, M., eds, *Kirk-Othmer Encyclopedia of Chemical Technology*, 3rd ed., Vol. 15, New York, John Wiley & Sons, pp. 801-819

Anwer, J. & Mehrotra, N.K. (1986) Effect of simultaneous exposure to nickel chloride and benzo(*a*)pyrene on developing chick embryos. *Drug chem. Toxicol.*, *9*, 171-183

Arbeidsinspectie (Labour Inspection) (1986) *De Nationale MAC-Lijst 1986* (National MAC-List 1986), Voorburg, p. 18

Arbejdstilsynet (Labour Inspection) (1988) *Graensevaerdier for Stoffer og Materialer* (Limit Values for Compounds and Materials) (No. 3.1.0.2), Copenhagen, p. 25

Arbetarskyddsstyrelsens (National Board of Occupational Safety and Health) (1987) *Hygieniska Gränsvärden* (Hygienic Limit Values), Stockholm, p. 35

Archer, F.C. (1980) Trace elements in soils in England and Wales. In: *Inorganic Pollution and Agriculture*, London, Her Majesty's Stationery Office, pp. 184-190

Arlauskas, A., Baker, R.S.U., Bonin, A.M., Tandon, R.K., Crisp, P.T. & Ellis, J. (1985) Mutagenicity of metal ions in bacteria. *Environ. Res.*, *36*, 379-388

Barton, R.T., Andersen, I. & Høgetveit, A.C. (1980) Distribution of nickel in blood fractions. In: Brown, S.S. & Sunderman, F.W., Jr, eds, *Nickel Toxicology*, London, Academic Press, pp. 85-88

Basrur, P.K. & Gilman, J.P.W. (1967) Morphologic and synthetic response of normal and tumor muscle cultures to nickel sulfide. *Cancer Res.*, *27*, 1168-1177

Beach, D.J. & Sunderman, F.W., Jr (1969) Nickel carbonyl inhibition of $^{14}$C-orotic acid incorporation into rat liver RNA. *Proc. Soc. exp. Biol. Med.*, *131*, 321-322

Beach, D.J. & Sunderman, F.W., Jr (1970) Nickel carbonyl inhibition of RNA synthesis by a chromatin-RNA polymerase complex from hepatic nuclei. *Cancer Res.*, *30*, 48-50

Bencko, V. (1983) Nickel: a review of its occupational and environmental toxicology. *J. Hyg. Epidemiol. Microbiol. Immunol.*, *27*, 237-247

Bennett, B.G. (1984) Environmental nickel pathways to man. In: Sunderman, F.W., Jr, ed., *Nickel in the Human Environment* (IARC Scientific Publications No. 53), Lyon, IARC, pp. 487-495

Benson, J.M., Henderson, R.F., McClellan, R.O. & Rebar, A.H. (1985) Comparative toxicity of nickel salts to the lung. In: Brown, S.S. & Sunderman, F.W., Jr, eds, *Progress in Nickel Toxicology*, Oxford, Blackwell Scientific Publications, pp. 85-88

Benson, J.M., Henderson, R.F. & McClellan, R.O. (1986a) Comparative cytotoxicity of four nickel compounds to canine and rodent alveolar macrophages *in vitro*. *J. Toxicol. environ. Health*, *19*, 105-110

Benson, J.M., Henderson, R.F., McClellan, R.O., Hanson, R.L. & Rebar, A.H. (1986b) Comparative acute toxicity of four nickel compounds to F344 rat lung. *Fundam. appl. Toxicol.*, *7*, 340-347

Benson, J.M., Carpenter, R.L., Hahn, F.F., Haley, P.J., Hanson, R.L., Hobbs, C.H., Pickrell, J.A. & Dunnick, J.K. (1987) Comparative inhalation toxicity of nickel subsulfide to F344/N rats and B6C3F$_1$ mice exposed for 12 days. *Fundam. appl. Toxicol.*, *9*, 251-265

Benson, J.M., Henderson, R.F. & Pickrell, J.A. (1988a) Comparative in vitro cytotoxicity of nickel oxides and nickel-copper oxides to rat, mouse, and dog pulmonary alveolar macrophages. *J. Toxicol. environ. Health, 24*, 373-383

Benson, J.M., Burt, D.G., Carpenter, R.L., Eidson, A.F., Hahn, F.F., Haley, P.J., Hanson, R.L., Hobbs, C.H., Pickrell, J.A. & Dunnick, J.K. (1988b) Comparative inhalation toxicity of nickel sulfate to F344/N rats and B6C3F$_1$ mice exposed for 12 days. *Fundam. appl. Toxicol., 10*, 164-178

Bergman, B., Bergman, M., Magnusson, B., Söremark, R. & Toda, Y. (1980) The distribution of nickel in mice. An autoradiographic study. *J. oral Rehabil., 7*, 319-324

Bernacki, E.J., Parsons, G.E., Roy, B.R., Mikac-Devic, M., Kennedy, C.D. & Sunderman, F.W., Jr (1978a) Urine nickel concentrations in nickel-exposed workers. *Ann. clin. Lab. Sci., 8*, 184-189

Bernacki, E.J., Parsons, G.E. & Sunderman, F.W., Jr (1978b) Investigation of exposure to nickel and lung cancer mortality. Case control study at a aircraft engine factory. *Ann. clin. Lab. Sci., 8*, 190-194

Bernacki, E.J., Zygowicz, E. & Sunderman, F.W., Jr (1980) Fluctuations of nickel concentrations in urine of electroplating workers. *Ann. clin. Lab. Sci., 10*, 33-39

Berry, J.P., Galle, P., Poupon, M.F., Pot-Deprun, J., Chouroulinkov, I., Judde, J.G. & Dewally, D. (1984) Electron microprobe in vitro study of interaction of carcinogenic nickel compounds with tumour cells. In: Sunderman, F.W., Jr, ed., *Nickel in the Human Environment* (IARC Scientific Publications No. 53), Lyon, IARC, pp. 153-164

Biedermann, K.A. & Landolph, J.R. (1987) Induction of anchorage independence in human diploid foreskin fibroblasts by carcinogenic metal salts. *Cancer Res., 47*, 3815-3823

Biggart, N.W. & Costa, M. (1986) Assessment of the uptake and mutagenicity of nickel chloride in *Salmonella* tester strains. *Mutat. Res., 175*, 209-215

Biggart, N.W. & Murphy, E.C., Jr (1988) Analysis of metal-induced mutations altering the expression or structure of a retroviral gene in a mammalian cell line. *Mutat. Res., 198*, 115-129

Blakeley, St J.H. & Zatka, V.J. (1985) *Report to the NiPERA Scientific Advisory Committee on Interlaboratory Test Program on Nickel Phase Speciation in Dust Samples. First Test on Bulk Dust Samples — Summer 1985*, Toronto, Nickel Producers Environmental Research Association

Boldt, J. & Queneau, P. (1967) *The Winning of Nickel*, New York, Van Nostrand

Bonde, I., Beck, H.-I., Jørgensen, P.J. & Grandjean, P. (1987) Nickel levels in intercellular fluid from nickel-allergic patients and controls. In: *Trace Elements in Human Health and Disease, Abstracts, Second Nordic Symposium, August 1987, Odense, University of Copenhagen*, Copenhagen, World Health Organization, p. D12

Bossu, F.P., Paniago, E.B., Margerum, D.W., Kirksey, S.T., Jr & Kurtz, J.L. (1978) Trivalent nickel catalysis of the autooxidation of nickel(II) tetraglycine. *Inorg. Chem., 17*, 1034-1042

Boysen, M., Solberg, L.A., Torjussen, W., Poppe, S. & Høgetveit, A.C. (1984) Histological changes, rhinoscopical findings and nickel concentration in plasma and urine in retired nickel workers. *Acta otolaryngol., 97*, 105-115

Bridge, J.C. (1933) *Annual Report of the Chief Inspector of Factories and Workshops for the Year 1932*, London, His Majesty's Stationery Office, pp. 103-109

Brinton, L.A., Blot, W.J., Becker, J.A., Winn, D.M., Browder, J.P., Farmer, J.C., Jr & Fraumeni, J.F., Jr (1984) A case-control study of cancers of the nasal cavity and paranasal sinuses. *Am. J. Epidemiol.*, *119*, 896-906

Brown, S.S., Nomoto, S., Stoeppler, M. & Sunderman, F.W., Jr (1981) IUPAC reference method for analysis of nickel in serum and urine by electrothermal atomic absorption spectrometry. *Clin. Biochem.*, *14*, 295-299

Burges, D.C.L. (1980) Mortality study of nickel platers In: Brown, S.S. & Sunderman, F.W., Jr, eds, *Nickel Toxicology*, London, Academic Press, pp. 15-18

Burgess, W.A. (1981) *Recognition of Health Hazards in Industry. A Review of Materials and Processes*, New York, John Wiley & Sons

Buselmaier, M., Röhrborn, G. & Propping, P. (1972) Mutagenicity testing with pesticides in the host-mediated assay and in the dominant lethal test in mouse (Ger.). *Biol. Zbl.*, *91*, 311-325

Callan, W.M. & Sunderman, F.W., Jr (1973) Species variations in binding of $^{63}$Ni(II) by serum albumin. *Res. Commun. chem. Pathol. Pharmacol.*, *5*, 459-472

Camner, P., Johansson, A. & Lundborg, M. (1978) Alveolar macrophages in rabbits exposed to nickel dust. Ultrastructural changes and effect on phagocytosis. *Environ. Res.*, *16*, 226-235

Camner, P., Casarett-Bruce, M., Curstedt, T., Jarstrand, C., Wiernik, A., Johansson, A., Lundborg, M. & Robertson, B. (1984) Toxicology of nickel. In: Sunderman, F.W., Jr, ed., *Nickel in the Human Environment* (IARC Scientific Publications No. 53), Lyon, IARC, pp. 267-276

Camner, P., Curstedt, T., Jarstrand, C., Johansson, A., Robertson, B. & Wiernik, A. (1985) Rabbit lung after inhalation of manganese chloride: a comparison with the effects of chlorides of nickel, cadmium, cobalt, and copper. *Environ. Res.*, *38*, 301-309

Carvalho, S.M.M. & Ziemer, P.L. (1982) Distribution and clearance of $^{63}$Ni administered as $^{63}$NiCl$_2$ in the rat: intratracheal study. *Arch. environ. Contam. Toxicol.*, *11*, 245-248

Casey, C.E. & Robinson, M.F. (1978) Copper, manganese, zinc, nickel, cadmium and lead in human foetal tissues. *Br. J. Nutr.*, *39*, 639-646

Catalanatto, F.A. & Sunderman, F.W., Jr (1977) Nickel concentrations in human parotid saliva. *Ann. clin. Lab. Sci.*, *7*, 146-151

Cawse, P.A. (1978) *A Survey of Atmospheric Trace Elements in the UK: Results for 1977* (Harwell Report AERE-R 9164), Harwell, Environmental and Medical Sciences Division, Atomic Energy Authority

Chamberlain, P.G. (1988) Nickel. In: *Minerals Yearbook 1986* (Preprint from Bulletin 675), Vol. I, *Metals and Minerals*, Washington DC, Bureau of Mines, US Government Printing Office, pp. 1-17

Chemical Information Services Ltd (1988) *Directory of World Chemical Producers 1989/90 Edition*, Oceanside, NY, pp. 49, 287, 426-427, 489-490

Chmielnicka, J., Szymanska, J.A. & Tyfa, J. (1982) Disturbances in the metabolism of endogenous metals (Zn and Cu) in nickel-exposed rats. *Environ. Res.*, *27*, 216-221

Chorvatovičová, D. (1983) The effect of NiCl$_2$ on the level of chromosome aberrations in Chinese hamster *Cricetulus griseus* (Czech.). *Biológia (Bratislava)*, *38*, 1107-1112

Chovil, A., Sutherland, R.B. & Halliday, M. (1981) Respiratory cancer in a cohort of nickel sinter plant workers. *Br. J. ind. Med.*, *38*, 327-333

Christensen, O.B. & Lagesson, V. (1981) Nickel concentration of blood and urine after oral administration. *Ann. clin. Lab. Sci.*, *11*, 119-125

Christensen, O.B. & Möller, H. (1978) Release of nickel from cooking utensils. *Contact Dermatitis*, *4*, 343-346

Christensen, O.B., Möller, H., Andrasko, L. & Lagesson, V. (1979) Nickel concentration of blood, urine and sweat after oral administration. *Contact Dermatitis*, *5*, 312-316

Christie, N.T. & Costa, M. (1984) In vitro assessment of the toxicity of metal compounds. IV. Disposition of metals in cells: interactions with membranes, glutathione, metallothionein, and DNA. *Biol. Trace Elem. Res.*, *6*, 139-158

Christie, N.T., Tummolo, D.M., Biggart, N.W. & Murphy, E.C., Jr (1988) Chromosomal changes in cell lines from mouse tumors induced by nickel sulfide and methylcholanthrene. *Cell Biol. Toxicol.*, *4*, 427-445

Christie, N.T., Tummolo, D.M., Klein, C.B. & Rossman, T.G. (1990) The role of Ni(II) in mutation. In: Nieboer, E. & Aitio, A., eds, *Advances in Environmental Science and Technology, Nickel and Human Health: Current Perspectives*, New York, John Wiley & Sons (in press)

Ciccarelli, R.B. & Wetterhahn, K.E. (1982) Nickel distribution and DNA lesions induced in rat tissues by the carcinogen nickel carbonate. *Cancer Res.*, *42*, 3544-3549

Ciccarelli, R.B. & Wetterhahn, K.E. (1984a) Molecular basis for the activity of nickel. In: Sunderman, F.W., Jr, ed., *Nickel in the Human Environment* (IARC Scientific Publications No. 53), Lyon, IARC, pp. 201-213

Ciccarelli, R.B. & Wetterhahn, K.E. (1984b) Nickel-bound chromatin, nucleic acids, and nuclear proteins from kidney and liver of rats treated with nickel carbonate *in vivo*. *Cancer Res.*, *44*, 3892-3897

Ciccarelli, R.B. & Wetterhahn, K.E. (1985) In vitro interaction of 63-nickel(II) with chromatin and DNA from rat kidney and liver nuclei. *Chem.-biol. Interact.*, *52*, 347-360

Ciccarelli, R.B., Hampton, T.H. & Jennette, K.W. (1981) Nickel carbonate induces DNA-protein crosslinks and DNA strand breaks in rat kidney. *Cancer Lett.*, *12*, 349-354

Cirla, A.M., Bernabeo, F., Ottoboni, F. & Ratti, R. (1985) Nickel induced occupational asthma: immunological and clinical aspects. In: Brown, S.S. & Sunderman, F.W., Jr, eds, *Progress in Nickel Toxicology*, Oxford, Blackwell Scientific Publications, pp. 165-168

Considine, D.M., ed. (1974) *Chemical and Process Technology Encyclopedia*, New York, McGraw Hill Book, pp. 394, 613, 765-769

Cook, W.A. (1987) *Occupational Exposure Limits — Worldwide*, Washington DC, American Industrial Hygiene Association, pp. 124, 147, 203

Corbett, T.H., Heidelberger, C. & Dove, W.F. (1970) Determination of the mutagenic activity to bacteriophage T4 of carcinogenic and noncarcinogenic compounds. *Mol. Pharmacol.*, *6*, 667-679

Cornell, R.G. (1984) Mortality patterns among stainless-steel workers. In: Sunderman, F.W., Jr, ed., *Nickel in the Human Environment* (IARC Scientific Publications No. 53), Lyon, IARC, pp. 65-71

Cornell, R.G. & Landis, J.R. (1984) Mortality patterns among nickel/chromium alloy foundry workers. In: Sunderman, F.W., Jr, ed., *Nickel in the Human Environment* (IARC Scientific Publications No. 53), Lyon, IARC, pp. 87-93

Costa, M. (1980) Biochemical and morphological transformation of hamster embryo cells in tissue culture by specific metal compounds. In: Bhatnagar, R.E., ed., *Molecular Basis of Environmental Toxicity*, Ann Arbor, MI, Ann Arbor Science Publishers, pp. 373-389

Costa, M. (1983) Sequential events in the induction of transformation in cell culture by specific nickel compounds. *Biol. Trace Elem. Res.*, 5, 285-295

Costa, M. & Heck, J.D. (1984) Perspectives on the mechanism of nickel carcinogenesis. In: Eichhorn, G.L. & Marzilli, L., eds, *Advances in Organic Biochemistry*, Vol. 6, Berlin (West), Springer-Verlag, pp. 285-309

Costa, M. & Heck, J.D. (1986) Metal ion carcinogenesis: mechanistic aspects. In: Sigel, H., ed., *Metal Ions in Biological Systems*, Vol. 20, *Concepts on Metal Ion Toxicity*, New York, Marcel Dekker, pp. 259-278

Costa, M. & Mollenhauer, H.H. (1980a) Carcinogenic activity of particulate nickel compounds is proportional to their cellular uptake. *Science*, 209, 515-517

Costa, M. & Mollenhauer, H.H. (1980b) Phagocytosis of nickel subsulfide particles during the early stages of neoplastic transformation in tissue culture. *Cancer Res.*, 40, 2688-2694

Costa, M. & Mollenhauer, H.H. (1980c) Phagocytosis of particulate nickel compounds is related to their carcinogenic activity. In: Brown, S.S. & Sunderman, F.W., Jr, eds, *Nickel Toxicology*, New York, Academic Press, pp. 43-46

Costa, M., Nye, J.S., Sunderman, F.W., Jr, Allpass, P.R. & Gondos, B. (1979) Induction of sarcomas in nude mice by implantation of Syrian hamster fetal cells exposed *in vitro* to nickel subsulfide. *Cancer Res.*, 39, 3591-3597

Costa, M., Jones, M.K. & Lindberg, O. (1980) Metal carcinogenesis in tissue culture systems. In: Martell, A.E., ed., *Inorganic Chemistry in Biology and Medicine* (ACS Symposium Series No. 140), Washington DC, American Chemical Society, pp. 45-73

Costa, M., Simmons-Hansen, J., Bedrossian, C.W.M., Bonura, J. & Caprioli, R.M. (1981a) Phagocytosis, cellular distribution, and carcinogenic activity of particulate nickel compounds in tissue culture. *Cancer Res.*, 41, 2868-2876

Costa, M., Abbracchio, M.P. & Simmons-Hansen, J. (1981b) Factors influencing the phagocytosis, neoplastic transformation, and cytotoxicity of particulate nickel compounds in tissue culture systems. *Toxicol. appl. Pharmacol.*, 60, 313-323

Costa, M., Heck, J.D. & Robison, S.H. (1982) Selective phagocytosis of crystalline metal sulfide particles and DNA strand breaks as a mechanism for the induction of cellular transformation. *Cancer Res.*, 42, 2757-2763

Cotton, F.A. & Wilkinson, G. (1988) *Advanced Inorganic Chemistry*, 5th ed., New York, John Wiley & Sons, pp. 741-755

Cox, J.E., Doll, R., Scott, W.A. & Smith, S. (1981) Mortality of nickel workers: experience of men working with metallic nickel. *Br. J. ind. Med.*, *38*, 235-239

Cragle, D.L., Hollis, D.R., Newport, T.H. & Shy, C.M. (1984) A retrospective cohort mortality study among workers occupationally exposed to metallic nickel powder at the Oak Ridge gaseous diffusion plant. In: Sunderman, F.W., Jr, ed., *Nickel in the Human Environment* (IARC Scientific Publications No. 53), Lyon, IARC, pp. 57-63

Cronin, E., Di Michiel, A.D. & Brown, S.S. (1980) Oral challenge in nickel-sensitive women with hand eczema. In: Brown, S.S. & Sunderman, F.W., Jr, eds, *Nickel Toxicology*, London, Academic Press, pp. 149-152

Cuckle, H., Doll, R. & Morgan, L.G. (1980) Mortality study of men working with soluble nickel compounds. In: Brown, S.S. & Sunderman, F.W., Jr, eds, *Nickel Toxicology*, London, Academic Press, pp. 11-14

Daldrup, T., Haarhoff, K. & Szathmary, S.C. (1983) Fetal nickel sulfate intoxication (Ger.). *Beitr. gerichtl. Med.*, *41*, 141-144

Damjanov, I., Sunderman, F.W., Jr, Mitchell, J.M. & Allpass, P.R. (1978) Induction of testicular sarcomas in Fischer rats by intratesticular injection of nickel subsulfide. *Cancer Res.*, *38*, 268-276

Daniel, M.R. (1966) Strain differences in the response of rats to the injection of nickel sulphide. *Br. J. Cancer.*, *20*, 886-895

Daniel, M., Edwards, M. & Webb, M. (1974) The effect of metal-serum complexes on differentiating muscle *in vitro*. *Br. J. exp. Pathol.*, *55*, 237-244

Decheng, C., Ming, J., Ling, H., Shan, W., Ziqing, Z. & Xinshui, Z. (1987) Cytogenetic analysis in workers occupationally exposed to nickel carbonyl. *Mutat. Res.*, *188*, 149-152

De Flora, S., Zanacchi, P., Camoirano, A., Bennicelli, C. & Badolati, G.S. (1984) Genotoxic activity and potency of 135 compounds in the Ames reversion test and in a bacterial DNA-repair test. *Mutat. Res.*, *133*, 161-198

Deknudt, G. & Léonard, A. (1982) Mutagenicity tests with nickel salts in the male mouse. *Toxicology*, *25*, 289-292

Deng, C. & Ou, B. (1981) The cytogenetic effects of nickel sulphate (Chin.). *Acta genet. sin.*, *8*, 212-215

Deng, C.Z., Ou, B., Huang, J., Zhuo, Z., Xian, H., Yao, M.C., Chen, M.Y., Li, Z.X., Sheng, S.Y. & Yei, Z.F. (1983) Cytogenetic effects of electroplating workers (Chin.). *Acta sci. circumst.*, *3*, 267-271

Deng, C.Z., Lee, H.C.H., Xian, H.L., Yao, M.C., Huang, J.C. & Ou, B.X. (1988) Chromosomal aberrations and sister chromatid exchanges of peripheral blood lymphocytes in Chinese electroplating workers: effect of nickel and chromium. *J. trace Elements exp. Med.*, *1*, 57-62

Dewally, D. & Hildebrand, H.F. (1980) The fate of nickel subsulphide implants during carcinogenesis. In: Brown, S.S. & Sunderman, F.W., Jr, eds, *Nickel Toxicology*, London, Academic Press, pp. 51-54

DiPaolo, J.A. & Casto, B.C. (1979) Quantitative studies of in vivo morphological transformation of Syrian hamster cells by inorganic metal salts. *Cancer Res.*, *39*, 1008-1013

Doll, R. (1958) Cancer of the lung and nose in nickel workers. *Br. J. ind. Med.*, *15*, 217-223

Doll, R., Morgan, L.G. & Speizer, F.E. (1970) Cancers of the lung and nasal sinuses in nickel workers. *Br. J. Cancer*, *24*, 623-632

Doll, R., Mathews, J.D. & Morgan, L.G. (1977) Cancers of the lung and nasal sinuses in nickel workers: a reassessment of the period of risk. *Br. J. ind. Med.*, *34*, 102-105

Drazniowsky, M., Channon, S.M., Parkinson, I.S., Ward, M.K., Poon, T.F.-H. & Kerr, D.N.S. (1985) The measurement of nickel in chronic renal failure. In: Brown, S.S. & Sunderman, F.W., Jr, eds, *Progress in Nickel Toxicology*, Oxford, Blackwell Scientific Publications, pp. 141-144

Dubins, J.S. & LaVelle, J.M. (1986) Nickel(II) genotoxicity: potentiation of mutagenesis of simple alkylating agents. *Mutat. Res.*, *162*, 187-199

Dunnick, J.K., Benson, J.M., Hobbs, C.H., Hahn, F.F., Cheng, Y.S. & Eidson, A.F. (1988) Comparative toxicity of nickel oxide, nickel sulfate hexahydrate, and nickel subsulfide after 12 days of inhalation exposure to F344/N rats and B6C3F$_1$ mice. *Toxicology*, *50*, 145-156

Dunnick, J.K., Elwell, M.R., Benson, J.M., Hobbs, C.H., Hahn, F.F., Haly, P.J., Cheng, Y.S. & Eidson, A.F. (1989) Lung toxicity after 13-week inhalation exposure to nickel oxide, nickel subsulfide, or nickel sulfate hexahydrate in F344/N rats and B6C3F$_1$ mice. *Fundam. appl. Toxicol.*, *12*, 584-594

Egedahl, R. & Rice, E. (1984) Cancer incidence at a hydrometallurgical nickel refinery. In: Sunderman, F.W., Jr, ed., *Nickel in the Human Environment* (IARC Scientific Publications No. 53), Lyon, IARC, pp. 47-55

Egilsson, V., Evans, I.H. & Wilkie, D. (1979) Toxic and mutagenic effects of carcinogens on the mitochondria of *Saccharomyces cerevisiae*. *Mol. gen. Genet.*, *174*, 39-46

English, J.C., Parker, R.D.R., Sharma, R.P. & Oberg, S.G. (1981) Toxicokinetics of nickel in rats after intratracheal administration of a soluble and insoluble form. *Am. ind. Hyg. Assoc. J.*, *42*, 486-492

Enterline, P.E. & Marsh, G.M. (1982) Mortality among workers in a nickel refinery and alloy manufacturing plant in West Virginia. *J. natl Cancer Inst.*, *68*, 925-933

ERAMET-SLN (Entreprise de Recherches et d'Activités — Métaux — Société le Nickel) (1985) *Electroplating. Nickel Chloride Hexahydrate. Liquid Nickel Chloride*, Paris

ERAMET-SLN (Entreprise de Recherches et d'Activités — Métaux — Société le Nickel) (1986) *Ferronickel*, Paris

ERAMET-SLN (Entreprise de Recherche et d'Activités — Métaux — Société le Nickel) (1989a) *Stainless-steel Production*, Paris

ERAMET-SLN (Entreprise de Recherches et d'Activités — Métaux — Société le Nickel) (1989b) *Nickel Sulfate. Nickel Chloride. Estimated Quantity of Product per Year*, Paris

Eurométaux (1986) *Data Relating to Nickel Production, Consumption and Application in Europe*, Brussels

European Chemical Industry Ecology and Toxicology Centre (1989) *Nickel and Nickel Compounds. Review of Toxicology and Epidemiology with Special Reference to Carcinogenesis* (ECETOC Technical Report No. 33), Brussels

Evans, W.H., Read, J.I. & Lucas, B.E. (1978) Evaluation of a method for the determination of total cadmium, lead and nickel in foodstuffs using measurement by flame atomic absorption spectrophotometry. *Analyst*, *103*, 580-594

Evans, D.J.I., Shoemaker, R.S. & Veltman, H., eds, (1979) *International Laterite Symposium, New Orleans, LA, February 19-21 1979*, New York, Society of Mining Engineers of the American Institute of Mining, Metallurgical and Petroleum Engineers

Evans, R.M., Davies, P.J.A. & Costa, M. (1982) Video time-lapse microscopy of phagocytosis and intracellular fate of crystalline nickel sulfide particles in cultured mammalian cells. *Cancer Res.*, *42*, 2729-2735

Fairhurst, S. & Illing, H.P.A. (1987) *The Toxicity of Nickel and Its Inorganic Compounds* (Health and Safety Executive Toxicity Review 19), London, Her Majesty's Stationery Office

Farrell, R.L. & Davis, G.W. (1974) The effects of particulates on respiratory carcinogenesis by diethylnitrosamine. In: Karbe, E. & Park, J.F., eds, *Experimental Lung Cancer, Carcinogenesis and Bioassays*, New York, Springer, pp. 219-233

Fassett, J.D., Moore, L.J., Travis, J.C. & DeVoe, J.R. (1985) Laser resonance ionization mass spectrometry. *Science*, *230*, 262-267

Feroz, M., Mughal, M.S. & Malik, M.A. (1976) Studies on accumulation of nickel ions in various tissues of the mouse (*Mus musculus*) injected with nickel acetate. *Biologia*, *22*, 181-192

Finch, G.L., Fisher, G.L. & Hayes, T.L. (1987) The pulmonary effects and clearance of intratracheally instilled $Ni_3S_2$ and $TiO_2$ in mice. *Environ. Res.*; *42*, 83-93

Fisher, G.L., Crisp, C.E. & McNeill, D.A. (1986) Lifetime effects of intratracheally instilled nickel subsulfide on B6C3F1 mice. *Environ. Res.*, *40*, 313-320

Fletcher, A.C. & Ades, A. (1984) Lung cancer mortality in a cohort of English foundry workers. *Scand. J. Work Environ. Health*, *10*, 7-16

Flora, C.J. & Nieboer, E. (1980) Determination of nickel by differential pulse polarography at a dropping mercury electrode. *Anal. Chem.*, *52*, 1013-1020

Fornace, A.J., Jr (1982) Detection of DNA single-strand breaks produced during the repair of damage by DNA-protein cross-linking agents. *Cancer Res.*, *42*, 145-149

Foulkes, E.C. & McMullen, D.M. (1986) On the mechanism of nickel absorption in the rat jejunum. *Toxicology*, *38*, 35-42

Fukunaga, M., Kurachi, Y. & Mizuguchi, Y. (1982) Action of some metal ions on yeast chromosomes. *Chem. pharm. Bull.*, *30*, 3017-3019

Furst, A. & Al-Mahrouq, H. (1981) Excretion of nickel following intratracheal administration of the carbonate. *Proc. west. Pharmacol. Soc.*, *24*, 119-121

Furst, A. & Cassetta, D. (1973) Carcinogenicity of nickel by different routes (Abstract No. 121). *Proc. Am. Assoc. Cancer Res*, *14*, 31

Furst, A. & Schlauder, M.C. (1971) The hamster as a model for metal carcinogenesis. *Proc. west. Pharmacol. Soc.*, *14*, 68-71

Furst, A., Cassetta, D.M. & Sasmore, D.P. (1973) Rapid induction of pleural mesotheliomas in the rat. *Proc. west. Pharmacol. Soc.*, *16*, 150-153

Gentry, S.J., Howarth, S.R. & Jones, A. (1983) Catalysts. In: Parmeggiani, L., ed., *Encyclopaedia of Occupational Health and Safety*, Geneva, International Labour Office, Vol. 1, pp. 421-426

Gérin, M., Siemiatycki, J., Richardson, L., Pellerin, J., Lakhani, R. & Dewar, R. (1984) Nickel and cancer associations from a multicancer occupation exposure case-referent study: preliminary findings. In: Sunderman, F.W., Jr, ed., *Nickel in the Human Environment* (IARC Scientific Publications No. 53), Lyon, IARC, pp. 105-115

Gilani, S.H. (1982) The effect of nickel upon chick embryo cardiogenesis (Abstract). *Teratology*, *25*, 44A

Gilani, S.H. & Marano, M. (1980) Congenital abnormalities in nickel poisoning in chick embryos. *Arch. environ. Contam. Toxicol.*, *9*, 17-22

Gilman, J.P.W. (1962) Metal carcinogenesis. II. A study of the carcinogenic activity of cobalt, copper, iron, and nickel compounds. *Cancer Res.*, *22*, 158-162

Gilman, J.P.W. (1966) Muscle tumorigenesis. *Can. Cancer Conf.*, *6*, 209-223

Gilman, J.P.W. & Herchen, H. (1963) The effect of physical form of implant on nickel sulphide tumourigenesis in the rat. *Acta unio. int. cancrum*, *19*, 615-619

Gilman, J.P.W. & Ruckerbauer, G.M. (1962) Metal carcinogenesis. I. Observations on the carcinogenicity of a refinery dust, cobalt oxide and colloidal thorium dioxide. *Cancer Res.*, *22*, 152-157

Glaser, U., Hochrainer, D., Oldiges, H. & Takenaka, S. (1986) Long-term inhalation studies with NiO and $As_2O_3$ aerosols in Wistar rats. *Excerpta med. int. Congr. Sci.*, *676*, 325-328

Glennon, J.D. & Sarkar, B. (1982) Nickel(II) transport in human blood serum. Studies of nickel(II) binding to human albumin and to native-sequence peptide, and ternary-complex formation with L-histidine. *Biochem. J.*, *203*, 15-23

Godbold, J.H., Jr & Tompkins, E.A. (1979) A long-term mortality study of workers occupationally exposed to metallic nickel at the Oak Ridge gaseous diffusion plant. *J. occup. Med.*, *21*, 799-806

Goldberg, M., Goldberg, P., Leclerc, A., Chastang, J.F., Fuhrer, R., Brodeur, J.M., Segnan, N., Floch, J.J. & Michel, G. (1987) Epidemiology of respiratory cancers related to nickel mining and refining in New Caledonia (1978-1984). *Int. J. Cancer*, *40*, 300-304

Goldberg, M., Goldberg, P., Leclerc, A., Chastang, J.F., Marne, M.J., Gueziec, J., Lavigne, F., Dubourdrieu, D. & Huerre, M. (1990) A seven-year survey of respiratory cancers among nickel workers in New Caledonia (1978-1984). In: Nieboer, E. & Aitio, A., eds, *Advances in Environmental Science and Technology, Nickel and Human Health: Current Perspectives*, New York, John Wiley & Sons (in press)

Grandjean, P. (1984) Human exposure to nickel. In: Sunderman, F.W., Jr, ed., *Nickel in the Human Environment* (IARC Scientific Publications No. 53), Lyon, IARC, pp. 469-485

Grandjean, P. (1986) *Health Effects Document on Nickel*, Odense, Department of Environmental Medicine, Odense University

Grandjean, P., Selikoff, I.J., Shen, S.K. & Sunderman, F.W., Jr (1980) Nickel concentrations in plasma and urine of shipyard workers. *Am. J. ind. Med.*, *1*, 181-189

Grandjean, P., Andersen, O. & Nielsen, G.D. (1988) Nickel. In: Alessio, L., Berlin, A., Boni, M. & Roi, R., eds, *Biological Indicators for Assessment of Human Exposure to Industrial Chemicals,* Luxembourg, Commission of the European Communities, pp. 57-81

Grandjean, P., Nielsen, G.D. & Andersen, O. (1989) Human nickel exposure and chemobiokinetics. In: Maibach, H.I. & Menné, T., eds, *Nickel and the Skin: Immunology and Toxicology,* Boca Raton, FL, CRC Press, pp. 9-28

Grice, J.D. & Ferguson, R.B. (1974) Crystal structure refinement of millerite (beta-NiS). *Can. Mineral., 12,* 248-252

Gross, H. (1987) Carcinogenic effect of nickel in industry? Conclusions from industrial-medical and epidemiological research, workplace analysis in the steel industry, and legal instructions (Ger.). *Zbl. Arbeitsmed., 37,* 170-183

Hackett, R.L. & Sunderman, F.W., Jr (1969) Nickel carbonyl. Effects upon the ultrastructure of hepatic parenchymal cells. *Arch. environ. Health, 19,* 337-343

Hansen, K. & Stern, R.M. (1983) In vitro toxicity and transformation potency of nickel compounds. *Environ. Health Perspect., 51,* 223-226

Hansen, K. & Stern, R.M. (1984) Toxicity and transformation potency of nickel compounds in BHK cells *in vitro.* In: Sunderman, F.W., Jr, ed., *Nickel in the Human Environment* (IARC Scientific Publications No. 53), Lyon, IARC, pp. 193-200

Harnett, P.B., Robison, S.H., Swartzendruber, D.E. & Costa, M. (1982) Comparison of protein, RNA, and DNA binding and cell-cycle-specific growth inhibitory effects of nickel compounds in cultured cells. *Toxicol. appl. Pharmacol., 64,* 20-30

Hartwig, A. & Beyersmann, D. (1989) Enhancement of UV mutagenesis and sister-chromatid exchanges by nickel ions in V79 cells: evidence for inhibition of DNA repair. *Mutat. Res., 217,* 65-73

Hassler, E., Lind, B., Nilsson, B. & Piscator, M. (1983) Urinary and fecal elimination of nickel in relation to air-borne nickel in a battery factory. *Ann. clin. Lab. Sci., 13,* 217-224

Hauptverband der gewerblichen Berufsgenossenschaften (Principal Union of Industrial Occupational Associations) (1981) *Von den Berufsgenossenschaften anerkannte Analysenverfahren zur Feststellung der Konzentrationen Krebserzeugender Arbeitsstoffe in der Luft in Arbeitsbereichen* (Occupational associations for recognized analytical methods to identify concentrates of carcinogenic occupational substances in the air of work environments) (ZH 1/120.10), Cologne, Carl Heymanns, pp. 151-158

Haworth, S., Lawlor, T., Mortelmans, K., Speck, W. & Zeiger, E. (1983) *Salmonella* mutagenicity test results for 250 chemicals. *Environ. Mutagenesis, 5 (Suppl. 1),* 3-142

Hayashi, Y., Takahashi, M., Maekawa, A., Kurokawa, Y. & Kokubo, T. (1984) Screening of environmental pollutants for promotion effects on carcinogenesis (Jpn.). In: *Annual Report of the Ministry of Health and Welfare, Japan, for Fiscal Years 1982-1984,* Vol. 20, Tokyo, Ministry of Health and Welfare, pp. 20-1–20-10

Health and Safety Executive (1987) *Occupational Exposure Limits 1987* (Guidance Note EH 40/87), London, Her Majesty's Stationery Office, pp. 18, 21

Heath, J.C. & Daniel, M.R. (1964) The production of malignant tumours by nickel in the rat. *Br. J. Cancer, 18,* 261-264

Heath, J.C. & Webb, M. (1967) Content and intracellular distribution of the inducing metal in the primary rhabdomyosarcomata induced in the rat by cobalt, nickel and cadmium. *Br. J. Cancer*, *21*, 768-779

Heck, J.D. & Costa, M. (1982) In vitro assessment of the toxicity of metal compounds. II. Mutagenesis. *Biol. Trace Elem. Res.*, *4*, 319-330

Heidermanns, G., Wolf, D. & Hoffmann, E. (1983) Nickel exposure on grinding and polishing nickel alloys with nickel proportions below 80% (Ger.). *Staub-Reinhalt. Luft*, *43*, 374-376

Herchen, H. & Gilman, J.P.W. (1964) Effect of duration of exposure on nickel sulphide tumorigenesis. *Nature*, *202*, 306-307

Herlant-Peers, M.C., Hildebrand, H.F. & Biserte, G. (1982) $^{63}$Ni(II) incorporation into lung and liver cytosol of Balb/C mouse. An in vitro and in vivo study. *Zbl. Bakt. Hyg., I. Abt. Orig. B*, *176*, 368-382

Hernberg, S., Westerholm, P., Schultz-Larsen, K., Degerth, R., Kuosma, E., Englund, A., Engzell, U., Hansen, H.S. & Mutanen, P. (1983) Nasal and sinonasal cancer. Connection with occupational exposures in Denmark, Finland and Sweden. *Scand. J. Work Environ. Health*, *9*, 315-326

Hildebrand, H.F. & Biserte, G. (1979a) Nickel subsulphide-induced leiomyosarcoma in rabbit white skeletal muscle — a light microscopical and ultrastructural study. *Cancer*, *43*, 1358-1374

Hildebrand, H.F. & Biserte, G. (1979b) Cylindrical laminated bodies in nickel subsulphide-induced rhabdomyosarcoma in rabbits. *Eur. J. Cell Biol.*, *19*, 276-280

Hildebrand, H.F., Collyn-D'Hooghe, M. & Herlant-Peers, M.-C. (1985) Incorporation of $\alpha$-Ni$_3$S$_2$ and $\beta$-NiS into human embryonic pulmonary cells in culture. In: Brown, S.S. & Sunderman, F.W., Jr, eds, *Progress in Nickel Toxicology*, Oxford, Blackwell Scientific Publications, pp. 61-64

Hildebrand, H.F., Collyn-D'Hooghe, M. & Herlant-Peers, M.-C. (1986) Cytotoxicity of nickel derivatives and their incorporation into human embryonic pulmonary epithelial cells (Fr.). *Larc med.*, *6*, 249-251

Hildebrand, H.F., Decaestecker, A.M. & Hetuin, D. (1987) Binding of nickel sulfides to lymphocyte subcellar structures. In: *Trace Elements in Human Health and Disease (Extended Abstracts) from the Second Nordic Symposium, August 1987, Odense* (WHO Environmental Health Series No. 20), Copenhagen, World Health Organization, pp. 82-85

Hoey, M.J. (1966) The effects of metallic salts on the histology of functioning of the rat testis. *J. Reprod. Fertil.*, *12*, 461-471

Hogan, G.R. (1985) Nickel acetate-induced mortality in mice of different ages. *Bull. environ. Contam. Toxicol.*, *34*, 446-450

Høgetveit, A.C., Barton, R.T. & Kostøl, C.O. (1978) Plasma nickel as a primary index of exposure in nickel refining. *Ann. occup. Hyg.*, *21*, 113-120

Hopfer, S.M., Linden, J.V., Crisostomo, C., O'Brien, J.E. & Sunderman, F.W., Jr (1984) Hypernickelemia in patients receiving disulfiram (Abstract No. 18). *Ann. clin. Lab. Sci.*, *14*, 319-320

Hopfer, S.M., Linden, J.V., Crisostomo, C., Catalanatto, F.A., Galen, M. & Sunderman, F.W., Jr (1985) Hypernickelemia in hemodialysis patients. In: Brown, S.S. & Sunderman, F.W., Jr, eds, *Progress in Nickel Toxicology*, Oxford, Blackwell Scientific Publishers, pp. 133-136

Horak, E. & Sunderman, F.W., Jr (1973) Fecal nickel excretion by healthy adults. *Clin. Chem.*, *19*, 429-430

Horak, E. & Sunderman, F.W., Jr (1980) Nephrotoxicity of nickel carbonyl in rats. *Ann. clin. Lab. Sci.*, *10*, 425-431

Horak, E., Zygowicz, E.R., Tarabishy, R., Mitchell, J.M. & Sunderman, F.W., Jr (1978) Effect of nickel chloride and nickel carbonyl upon glucose metabolism in rats. *Ann. clin. Lab. Sci.*, *8*, 476-482

Horie, A., Haratake, J., Tanaka, I., Kodama, Y. & Tsuchiya, K. (1985) Electron microscopical findings with special reference to cancer in rats caused by inhalation of nickel oxide. *Biol. Trace Elem. Res.*, *7*, 223-239

Hueper, W.C. (1952) Experimental studies in metal carcinogenesis. I. Nickel cancers in rats. *Texas Rep. Biol. Med.*, *16*, 167-186

Hueper, W.C. (1955) Experimental studies in metal carcinogenesis. IV. Cancer produced by parenterally introduced metallic nickel. *J. natl Cancer Inst.*, *16*, 55-67

Hueper, W.C. (1958) Experimental studies in metal carcinogenesis. IX. Pulmonary lesions in guinea pigs and rats exposed to prolonged inhalation of powdered metallic nickel. *Arch. Pathol.*, *65*, 600-607

Hueper, W.C. & Payne, W.W. (1962) Experimental studies in metal carcinogenesis. Chromium, nickel, iron, arsenic. *Arch. environ. Health*, *5*, 445-462

Hui, G. & Sunderman, F.W., Jr (1980) Effects of nickel compounds on incorporation of [$^3$H]-thymidine into DNA in rat liver and kidney. *Carcinogenesis*, *1*, 297-304

IARC (1973) *IARC Monographs on the Evaluation of Carcinogenic Risk of Chemicals to Man*, Vol. 2, *Some Inorganic and Organometallic Compounds*, Lyon, pp. 126-149

IARC (1976) *IARC Monographs on the Evaluation of Carcinogenic Risk of Chemicals to Man*, Vol. 11, *Cadmium, Nickel, Some Epoxides, Miscellaneous Industrial Chemicals and General Considerations on Volatile Anaesthetics*, Lyon, pp. 87-112

IARC (1977) *IARC Monographs on the Evaluation of Carcinogenic Risk of Chemicals to Man*, Vol. 14, *Asbestos*, Lyon

IARC (1979) *IARC Monographs on the Evaluation of the Carcinogenic Risk of Chemicals to Humans*, Suppl. 1, *Chemicals and Industrial Processes Associated with Cancer in Humans, IARC Monographs Volumes 1 to 20*, Lyon, p. 38

IARC (1982) *IARC Monographs on the Evaluation of the Carcinogenic Risk of Chemicals to Humans*, Suppl. 4, *Chemicals, Industrial Processes and Industries Associated with Cancer in Humans. IARC Monographs Volumes 1 to 29*, Lyon, pp. 167-170

IARC (1984) *IARC Monographs on the Evaluation of the Carcinogenic Risk of Chemicals to Humans*, Vol. 34, *Polynuclear Aromatic Compounds, Part 3, Industrial Exposures in Aluminium Production, Coal Gasification, Coke Production, and Iron and Steel Founding*, Lyon, pp. 133-190

IARC (1987) *IARC Monographs on the Evaluation of Carcinogenic Risks to Humans*, Suppl. 7, *Overall Evaluations of Carcinogenicity: An Updating of* IARC Monographs *Volumes 1 to 42*, Lyon, pp. 264-269

IARC (1988a) *IARC Monographs on the Evaluation of Carcinogenic Risks to Humans*, Vol. 43, *Man-made Mineral Fibres and Radon*, Lyon, pp. 173-259

IARC (1988b) *Information Bulletin on the Survey of Chemicals Being Tested for Carcinogenicity*, No. 13, Lyon, pp. 19, 42-43, 250-251

IARC (1989) *IARC Monographs on the Evaluation of Carcinogenic Risks to Humans*, Vol. 46, *Diesel and Gasoline Engine Exhausts and Some Nitroarenes*, Lyon, pp. 41-185

INCO (1981-82) *INCOMOND, Nickel Plating Chemicals*, New York, The International Nickel Company

INCO (1988) *INCO Specialty Powder Products*, New York, The International Nickel Company

Institut National de Recherche et de Sécurité (National Institute of Research and Safety) (1986) *Valeurs Limites pour les Concentrations de Substances Dangereuses dans l'Air des Lieux de Travail* (Limit Values for Concentrations of Dangerous Substances in Occupational Air) (DN 1609-125-86), Paris, p. 572

International Committee on Nickel Carcinogenesis in Man (1990) Report of the International Committee on Nickel Carcinogenesis in Man. *Scand. J. Work Environ. Health, 16,* 1-84

Ishihara, N., Koizumi, M. & Yoshida, A. (1987) Metal concentrations in human pancreatic juice. *Arch. environ. Health, 42,* 356-360

Ivankovic, S., Seller, W.J., Lehmann, E., Komitowski, D. & Frölich, N. (1987) Different carcinogenicity of two nickel alloys following intratracheal administration in the hamster (Abstract No. 103). *Naunyn-Schniederberg's Arch. Pharmacol., 335,* R26

Jacobsen, N., Alfheim, I. & Jonsen, J. (1978) Nickel and strontium distribution in some mouse tissues. Passage through placenta and mammary glands. *Res. Commun. chem. Pathol. Pharmacol., 20,* 571-584

Jacquet, P. & Mayence, A. (1982) Application of the in vitro embryo culture to the study of the mutagenic effects of nickel in male germ cells. *Toxicol. Lett., 11,* 193-197

Jasim, S. & Tjälve, H. (1986) Effects of sodium pyridinethione on the uptake and distribution of nickel, cadmium and zinc in pregnant and non-pregnant mice. *Toxicology, 38,* 327-350

Jasmin, G. & Riopelle, J.L. (1976) Renal carcinomas and erythrocytosis in rats following intrarenal injection of nickel subsulfide. *Lab. Invest., 35,* 71-78

Jiachen, H., Yifen, L., Guazhen, L., Guosan, Z., Chengen, M., Zengxi, L., Shaoyu, S. & Zifeng, Y. (1986) The distribution of trace elements in rats (Chin.). *Acta zool. sin., 32,* 35-39

Johansson, A., Camner, P., Jarstrand, C. & Wiernik, A. (1980) Morphology and function of alveolar macrophages after long-term nickel exposure. *Environ. Res., 23,* 170-180

Johansson, A., Camner, P. & Robertson, B. (1981) Effects of long-term nickel dust exposure on rabbit alveolar epithelium. *Environ. Res., 25,* 391-403

J.T. Baker (1988) *Reagents and Laboratory Products (Catalog 880C)*, Phillipsbury, NJ, pp. 142-143

Judde, J.G., Breillout, F., Clemenceau, C., Poupon, M.F. & Jasmin, C. (1987) Inhibition of rat natural killer cell function by carcinogenic nickel compounds: preventive action of manganese. *J. natl Cancer Inst., 78,* 1185-1190

Kaldor, J., Peto, J., Easton, D., Doll, R., Hermon, C. & Morgan, L. (1986) Models for respiratory cancer in nickel refinery workers. *J. natl Cancer Inst.*, 77, 841-848

Kanematsu, N., Hara, M. & Kada, T. (1980) Rec assay and mutagenicity studies on metal compounds. *Mutat. Res.*, 77, 109-116

Kasprzak, K.S. (1974) An autoradiographic study of nickel carcinogenesis in rats following injection of $^{63}Ni_3S_2$ and $Ni_3{}^{35}S_2$. *Res. Commun. chem. Pathol. Pharmacol.*, 8, 141-150

Kasprzak, K.S. (1978) *Problems of Metabolism of the Carcinogenic Nickel Compounds* (Pol.), Poznań, Technical University of Poznań Press

Kasprzak, K.S. (1987) Nickel. In: Fishbein, L., Furst, A. & Mehlman, M.A., eds, *Advances in Modern Environmental Toxicology*, Vol. XI, *Genotoxic and Carcinogenic Metals: Environmental and Occupational Occurrence and Exposure*, Princeton, NJ, Princeton Scientific Publishing, pp. 145-183

Kasprzak, K.S. & Bare, R.M. (1989) In vitro polymerization of histones by carcinogenic nickel compounds. *Carcinogenesis*, 10, 621-624

Kasprzak, K.S. & Poirier, L.A. (1985) Effects of calcium(II) and magnesium(II) on nickel(II) uptake and stimulation of thymidine incorporation into DNA in the lungs of strain A mice. *Carcinogenesis*, 6, 1819-1821

Kasprzak, K.S. & Sunderman, F.W., Jr (1969) The metabolism of nickel carbonyl-$^{14}$C. *Toxicol. appl. Pharmacol.*, 15, 295-303

Kasprzak, K.S. & Sunderman, F.W., Jr (1977) Mechanisms of dissolution of nickel subsulfide in rat serum. *Res. Commun. chem. Pathol. Pharmacol.*, 16, 95-108

Kasprzak, K.S., Marchow, L. & Breborowicz, J. (1973) Pathological reactions in rat lungs following intratracheal injection of nickel subsulfide and 3,4-benzpyrene. *Res. Commun. chem. Pathol. Pharmacol.*, 6, 237-245

Kasprzak, K.S., Gabryel, P. & Jarczewska, K. (1983) Carcinogenicity of nickel(II) hydroxides and nickel(II) sulfate in Wistar rats and its relation to the in vitro dissolution rates. *Carcinogenesis*, 4, 275-279

Kasprzak, K.S., Waalkes, M.P. & Poirier, L.A. (1986) Antagonism by essential divalent metals and amino acids of nickel(II)-DNA binding *in vitro*. *Toxicol. appl. Pharmacol.*, 82, 336-343

Kasprzak, K.S., Waalkes, M.P. & Poirier, L.A. (1987) Effects of essential divalent metals on carcinogenicity and metabolism of nickel and cadmium. *Biol. Trace Elem. Res.*, 13, 253-273

Kettrup, A., Mühlen, T. & Angerer, J. (1985) *Luftanalysen. Analytische Methoden zur Prüfung gesundheitsschädlicher Arbeitsstoffe* (Air Analysis. Analytical Method for Estimating Noxious Workplace Substances), Vol. 1, Weinheim, VCH-Verlagsgesellschaft

Kiilunen, M., Järvisalo, J., Mäkitie, O. & Aitio, A. (1987) Analysis, storage stability and reference values for urinary chromium and nickel. *Int. Arch. occup. environ. Health*, 59, 43-50

Kimmel, G.L., Price, C.J., Sonawane, B.R., Rubenstein, R. & Bellin, J.S. (1986) The effect of nickel chloride in drinking water on reproductive and developmental parameters (Abstract No. T12). *Teratology*, 33, 90C

Kipling, M.D. & Waterhouse, J.A.H. (1967) Cadmium and prostatic carcinoma. *Lancet, i*, 730-731

Klus, H, & Kuhn, H. (1982) Distribution of different tobacco smoke constituents in mainstream and sidestream smoke (A review) (Ger.). *Beitr. Tabakforsch.*, *11*, 229-265

Knight, J.A., Rezuke, W.N., Gillies, C.G., Hopfer, S.M. & Sunderman, F.W., Jr (1988) Pulmonary histopathology of rats following parenteral injections of nickel chloride. *Toxicol. Pathol.*, *16*, 350-359

Knutti, R. & Zimmerli, B. (1985) Analysis of daily rations from Swiss canteens and restaurants. III. Lead, cadmium, mercury, nickel and aluminium (Ger.). *Mittel Geb. lebensmittelhyg.*, *76*, 206-232

Kodama, Y., Tanaka, I., Matsuno, K., Ishimatsu, S., Horie, A. & Tsuchiya, K. (1985) Pulmonary deposition and clearance of inhaled nickel oxide aerosol. In: Brown, S.S. & Sunderman, F.W., Jr, eds, *Progress in Nickel Toxicology*, Oxford, Blackwell Scientific Publications, pp. 81-84

Kollmeier, H., Seemann, J.W., Müller, K.-M., Rothe, G., Wittig, P. & Schejbal, V.B. (1987) Increased chromium and nickel content in lung tissue and bronchial carcinoma. *Am. J. ind. Med.*, *11*, 659-669

Kollmeier, H., Seemann, J., Müller, K.-M., Schejbal, V., Rothe, G., Wittig, P. & Hummelsheim, G. (1988) Associations between high chromium and nickel concentrations in lung tissue and lung cancer (Ger.). *Prax. klin. Pneumol.*, *42*, 142-148

König, W., Meis, F.U., Neder, L., Sartori, P., Holtus, G. & Johannsen, H. (1985) *Schadstoffe beim Schleifvorgang* (Hazardous Agents in Grinding Process) (Research No. 427), Dortmund, Bundesanstalt für Arbeitsschutz

Kretzschmar, J.G., Delespaul, I. & De Rijck, T. (1980) Heavy metal levels in Belgium: a five-year survey. *Sci. total Environ.*, *14*, 85-97

Kurokawa, Y., Matsushima, M., Imazawa, T., Takamura, N., Takahashi, M. & Hayashi, Y. (1985) Promoting effect of metal compounds on rat renal tumorigenesis. *J. Am. Coll. Toxicol.*, *4*, 321-330

Larramendy, M.L., Popescu, N.C. & DiPaolo, J.A. (1981) Induction by inorganic metal salts of sister chromatid exchanges and chromosome aberrations in human and Syrian hamster cell strains. *Environ. Mutagenesis*, *3*, 597-606

Lau, T.J., Hackett, R.L. & Sunderman, F.W., Jr (1972) The carcinogenicity of intravenous nickel carbonyl in rats. *Cancer Res.*, *32*, 2253-2258

Leach, C.N., Jr & Sunderman, F.W., Jr (1985) Nickel contamination of human serum albumin solutions (Letter to the Editor). *New Engl. J. Med.*, *313*, 1232

Leach, C.A., Jr & Sunderman, F.W., Jr (1987) Hypernickelemia following coronary arteriography caused by nickel in the radiographic contrast medium. *Ann. clin. Lab. Sci.*, *17*, 137-144

Lechner, J.F., Tokiwa, T., McClendon, I.A. & Haugen, A. (1984) Effects of nickel sulfate on growth and differentiation of normal human bronchial epithelial cells. *Carcinogenesis*, *5*, 1697-1703

Lee, J.E., Ciccarelli, R.B. & Wetterhahn-Jennette, K. (1982) Solubilization of the carcinogen nickel subsulfide and its interaction with deoxyribonucleic acid and protein. *Biochemistry, 21*, 771-778

Léonard, A. & Jacquet, P. (1984) Embryotoxicity and genotoxicity of nickel. In: Sunderman, F.W., Jr, ed., *Nickel in the Human Environment* (IARC Scientific Publications No. 53), Lyon, IARC, pp. 277-291

Lessard, R., Reed, D., Maheux, B. & Lambert, J. (1978) Lung cancer in New Caledonia, a nickel smelting island. *J. occup. Med., 20*, 815-817

Linden, J.V., Hopfer, S.M., Crisostomo, C., Catalanatto, F., Galen, M. & Sunderman, F.W., Jr (1984) Hypernickelemia in hemodialysis patients (Abstract No. 19). *Ann. clin. Lab. Sci., 14*, 320

Liu, T. *et al.* (1983) The role of nickel sulfate in inducing nasopharyngeal carcinoma (NPC) in rats (Abstract). In: *Cancer Research Reports — WHO Collaborating Centre for Research on Cancer*, Vol. 4, Guangzhou, China, Cancer Institute of Zhongshan Medical College, pp. 48-49

Lloyd, G.K. (1980) Dermal absorption and conjugation of nickel in relation to the induction of allergic contact dermatitis — preliminary results. In: Brown, S.S. & Sunderman, F.W., Jr, eds, *Nickel Toxicology*, Oxford, London Academic Press, pp. 145-148

Lu, C.-C., Matsumoto, N. & Iijima, S. (1979) Teratogenic effects of nickel chloride on embryonic mice and its transfer to embryonic mice. *Teratology, 19*, 137-142

Lu, C.-C., Matsumoto, N. & Iijima, S. (1981) Placental transfer and body distribution of nickel chloride in pregnant mice. *Toxicol. appl. Pharmacol., 59*, 409-413

Lundborg, M. & Camner, P. (1984) Lysozyme levels in rabbit lung after inhalation of nickel, cadmium, cobalt, and copper chlorides. *Environ. Res., 34*, 335-342

Lundborg, M., Johansson, A. & Camner, P. (1987) Morphology and release of lysozyme following exposure of rabbit lung macrophages to nickel or cadmium *in vitro. Toxicology, 46*, 191-203

Lyell, A., Bain, W.H. & Thomson, R.M. (1978) Repeated failure of nickel-containing prosthetic heart valves in a patient allergic to nickel. *Lancet, ii*, 657-659

Maenza, R.M., Pradhan, A.M. & Sunderman, F.W., Jr (1971) Rapid induction of sarcomas in rats by combination of nickel sulfide and 3,4-benzpyrene. *Cancer Res., 31*, 2067-2071

Magnus, K., Andersen, A. & Høgetveit, A.C. (1982) Cancer of respiratory organs among workers at a nickel refinery in Norway. *Int. J. Cancer, 30*, 681-685

Maibach, H.I. & Menné, T. (1989) *Nickel and the Skin: Immunology and Toxicology*, Boca Raton, FL, CRC Press

Malcolm, D. (1983) Batteries, secondary or rechargeable, or accumulators. In: Parmeggiani, L., ed., *Encyclopaedia of Occupational Health and Safety*, 3rd ed., Geneva, International Labour Office, pp. 249-253

Mallinckrodt, Inc. (1987) *Reagent and Laboratory Chemicals Catalog 1987-88*, St Louis, MO, pp. 167-168

Mart, L. (1983) Seasonal variations of cadmium, lead, copper and nickel levels in snow from the eastern Arctic Ocean. *Tellus Ser. B, 35B*, 131-141 [*Chem. Abstr., 99*, 163271x]

Mas, A., Holt, D. & Webb, M. (1985) The acute toxicity and teratogenicity of nickel in pregnant rats. *Toxicology*, *35*, 47-57

Mas, A., Peligero, M.J., Arola, L. & Alemany, M. (1986) Distribution and kinetics of injected nickel in the pregnant rat. *Clin. exp. Pharmacol. Physiol.*, *13*, 91-96

Mason, M.M. (1972) Nickel sulfide carcinogenesis. *Environ. Physiol. Biochem.*, *2*, 137-141

Mastromatteo, E. (1986) Nickel. *Am. ind. Hyg. Assoc. J.*, *47*, 589-601

Mathur, A.K. & Tandon, S.K. (1981) Urinary excretion of nickel and chromium in occupational workers. *J. environ. Biol.*, *2*, 1-6

Mathur, A.K., Chandra, S.V., Behari, J. & Tandon, S.K. (1977a) Biochemical and morphological changes in some organs of rats in nickel intoxication. *Arch. Toxicol.*, *37*, 159-164

Mathur, A.K., Datta, K.K., Tandon, S.K. & Dikshith, T.S.S. (1977b) Effect of nickel sulphate on male rats. *Bull. environ. Contam. Toxicol.*, *17*, 241-248

Mathur, A.K., Dikshith, T.S.S., Lal, M.M. & Tandon, S.K. (1978) Distribution of nickel and cytogenetic changes in poisoned rats. *Toxicology*, *10*, 105-113

McLean, J.R., McWilliams, R.S., Kaplan, J.G. & Birnboim, H.C. (1982) Rapid detection of DNA strand breaks in human peripheral blood cells and animal organs following treatment with physical and chemical agents. *Prog. Mutat. Res.*, *3*, 137-141

McNeely, M.D., Sunderman, F.W., Jr, Nechay, M.W. & Levine, H. (1971) Abnormal concentrations of nickel in serum in cases of myocardial infarction, stroke, burns, hepatic cirrhosis, and uremia. *Clin. Chem.*, *17*, 1123-1128

McNeely, M.D., Nechay, M.W. & Sunderman, F.W., Jr (1972) Measurements of nickel in serum and urine as indices of environmental exposure to nickel. *Clin. Chem.*, *18*, 992-995

Medinsky, M.A., Benson, J.M. & Hobbs, C.H. (1987) Lung clearance and disposition of [63]Ni in F344/N rats after intratracheal instillation of nickel sulfate solutions. *Environ. Res.*, *43*, 168-178

Menné, T., Borgan, Ø. & Green, A. (1982) Nickel allergy and hand dermatitis in a stratified sample of the Danish female population: an epidemiological study including a statistic appendix. *Acta dermatovenerol.*, *62*, 35-41

Menzel, D.B., Deal, D.L., Tayyeb, M.I., Wolpert, R.L., Boger, J.R., III, Shoaf, C.R., Sandy, J., Wilkinson, K. & Francovitch, R.J. (1987) Pharmacokinetic modeling of the lung burden from repeated inhalation of nickel aerosols. *Toxicol. Lett.*, *38*, 33-43

Méranger, J.C., Subramanian, K.S. & Chalifoux, C. (1981) Survey for cadmium, cobalt, chromium, copper, nickel, lead, zinc, calcium and magnesium in Canadian drinking water supplies. *J. Assoc. off. anal. Chem.*, *64*, 44-53

Meyer, A. & Neeb, R. (1985) Determination of cobalt and nickel in some biological matrices — comparison between chelate-gas-chromatography and adsorption-voltammetry (Ger.). *Fresenius Z. anal. Chem.*, *321*, 235-241

Miki, H., Kasprzak, K.S., Kenney, S. & Heine, U.I. (1987) Inhibition of intercellular communication by nickel(II): antagonistic effect of magnesium. *Carcinogenesis*, *8*, 1757-1760

Mitchell, D.F., Shankwalker, G.B. & Shazer, S. (1960) Determining the tumorigenicity of dental materials. *J. dent. Res.*, *31*, 1023-1028

Miyaki, M., Akamatsu, N., Ono, T. & Koyama, H. (1979) Mutagenicity of metal cations in cultured cells from Chinese hamster. *Mutat. Res.*, *68*, 259-263

Mohanty, P.K. (1987) Cytotoxic effect of nickel chloride on the somatic chromosomes of Swiss albino mice *Mus musculus. Curr. Sci.*, *56*, 1154-1157

Morgan, J.G. (1958) Some observations on the incidence of respiratory cancer in nickel workers. *Br. J. ind. Med.*, *15*, 224-234

Morgan, L.G. & Rouge, P.J.C. (1979) A study into the correlation between atmospheric and biological monitoring of nickel in nickel refinery workers. *Ann. occup. Hyg.*, *22*, 311-317

Morgan, L.G. & Rouge, P.J.C. (1984) Biological monitoring in nickel refinery workers. In: Sunderman, F.W., Jr, ed., *Nickel in the Human Environment* (IARC Scientific Publications No. 53), Lyon, IARC, pp. 507-520

Muhle, H., Bellmann, B., Takenaka, S., Fuhst, R., Mohr, U. & Pott, F. (1990) Chronic effects of intratracheally instilled nickel containing particles in hamsters. In: Nieboer, E. & Aitio, A., eds, *Advances in Environmental Science and Technology, Nickel and Human Health: Current Perspectives*, New York, John Wiley & Sons (in press)

Mukubo, K. (1978) Studies on experimental lung tumor by the chemical carcinogens and inorganic substances. III. Histopathological studies on lung tumor in rats induced by pertracheal vinyl tube infusion of 20-methylcholanthrene combined with chromium and nickel powder, (Jpn.). *J. Nara med. Assoc.*, *29*, 321-340

Mushak, P. (1984) Nickel metabolism in health and disease. *Clin. Lab. Ann. Sci.*, *3*, 249-269

Myron, D.R., Zimmerman, T.J., Shuler, T.R., Klevay, L.M., Lee, D.E. & Nielsen, F.H. (1978) Intake of nickel and vanadium by humans. A survey of selected diets. *Am. J. clin. Nutr.*, *31*, 527-531

Nadeenko, V.G., Lenchenko, B.T., Arkhipenko, G.A. & Saichenko, S.P. (1979) Embryotoxic effect of nickel entering the organism by drinking water (Russ.). *Gig. Sanit.*, *6*, 86-88

National Institute for Occupational Safety and Health (1977a) *National Occupational Hazard Survey 1972-74*, Cincinnati, OH

National Institute for Occupational Safety and Health (1977b) *Criteria for a Recommended Standard: Occupational Exposure to Inorganic Nickel* (DHEW-NIOSH Document, No. 77-164), Washington DC, US Government Printing Office

National Institute for Occupational Safety and Health (1981) Inorganic nickel, metal and compounds. Method No. 298. In: Taylor, D.G., ed., *NIOSH Manual of Analytical Methods*, Vol. 7, Cincinnati, OH, US Department of Health, Education, and Welfare, pp. 82-100

National Institute for Occupational Safety and Health (1984) *Manual of Analytical Methods*, 3rd ed., Cincinnati, OH, US Department of Health, Education and Welfare, pp. 7300-1 — 7300-5

National Institute for Occupational Safety and Health (1988) NIOSH recommendations for occupational safety and health standards. *Morbid. Mortal. Wkly Rep.*, *Suppl. 37*, S-20

National Research Council (1975) *Medical and Biological Effects of Environmental Pollutants. Nickel*, Washington DC, Committee on Medical and Biological Effects of Environmental Pollutants, National Academy of Sciences

Nickel Development Institute (1987a) *High-temperature High-strength Nickel Base Alloys*, Toronto

Nickel Development Institute (1987b) *Design Guidelines for the Selection and Use of Stainless Steel*, Toronto

Nieboer, E., Yassi, A., Jusys, A.A. & Muir, D.C.F. (1984a) *The Technical Feasibility and Usefulness of Biological Monitoring in the Nickel Producing Industry (Final Report)*, Toronto, Nickel Producers Environmental Research Association

Nieboer, E., Maxwell, R.I. & Stafford, A.R. (1984b) Chemical and biological reactivity of insoluble nickel compounds and the bioinorganic chemistry of nickel. In: Sunderman, F.W., Jr, ed., *Nickel in the Human Environment* (IARC Scientific Publications No. 53), Lyon, IARC, pp. 439-458

Nieboer, E., Stafford, A.R., Evans, S.L. & Dolovich, J. (1984c) Cellular binding and/or uptake of nickel(II) ions. In: Sunderman, F.W., Jr, ed., *Nickel in the Human Environment* (IARC Scientific Publications No. 53), Lyon, IARC, pp. 321-331

Nieboer, E., Maxwell, R.I., Rossetto, F.E., Stafford, A.R. & Stetsko, P.I. (1986) Concepts in nickel carcinogenesis. In: Xavier, A.V., ed., *Frontiers in Bioinorganic Chemistry*, Weinheim, VCH Verlag, pp. 142-151

Nielsen, F.H. (1980) Interactions of nickel with essential minerals. In: Nriagu, J.O., ed., *Nickel in the Environment*, New York, John Wiley & Sons, pp. 611-634

Nielsen, G.D. & Flyvholm, M. (1984) Risks of high nickel intake with diet. In: Sunderman, F.W., Jr, ed., *Nickel in the Human Environment* (IARC Scientific Publications No. 53), Lyon, IARC, pp. 333-338

Nielsen, F.H., Shuler, T.R., McLeod, T.G. & Zimmerman, T.J. (1984) Nickel influences iron metabolism through physiologic, pharmacologic and toxicologic mechanisms in the rat. *J. Nutr., 114*, 1280-1288

Nielsen, G.D., Jørgensen, P.J., Keiding, K. & Grandjean, P. (1987) Urinary nickel excretion before and after loading with naturally occurring nickel. In: *Trace Elements in Human Health and Disease, Abstracts, Second Nordic Symposium, August 1987, Odense University*, Copenhagen, World Health Organization, p. C3

Nishimura, M. & Umeda, M. (1979) Induction of chromosomal aberrations in cultured mammalian cells by nickel compounds. *Mutat. Res., 68*, 337-349

Nishioka, H. (1975) Mutagenic activities of metal compounds in bacteria. *Mutat. Res., 31*, 185-189

Niyogi, S.K., Feldman, R.P. & Hoffman, D.J. (1981) Selective effects of metal ions on RNA synthesis rates. *Toxicology, 22*, 9-21

Norseth, T. (1984) Chromium and nickel. In: Aitio, A., Riihimäti, V. & Vainio, H., eds, *Biological Monitoring and Surveillance of Workers Exposed to Chemicals*, Washington DC, Hemisphere Publishing Corp., pp. 49-59

Oberdoerster, G. & Hochrainer, D. (1980) Effect of continuous nickel oxide exposure on lung clearance. In: Brown, S.S. & Sunderman, F.W., Jr, eds, *Nickel Toxicology*, London, Academic Press, pp. 125-128

Odense University (1986) *Health Effects Document on Nickel*, Odense, Department of Environmental Medicine

Ogawa, H.I., Tsuruta, S., Niyitani, Y., Mino, H., Sakata, K. & Kato, Y. (1987) Mutagenicity of metal salts in combination with 9-aminoacridine in *Salmonella typhimurium*. *Jpn. J. Genet.*, *62*, 159-162

Ohno, H., Hanaoka, F. & Yamada, M.-A. (1982) Inducibility of sister-chromatid exchanges by heavy-metal ions. *Mutat. Res.*, *104*, 141-145

Okamoto, M. (1987) Induction of ocular tumor by nickel subsulfide in the Japanese common newt, *Cynops pyrrhogaster*. *Cancer Res.*, *47*, 5213-5217

Olejár, S., Olejárová, E. & Vrábel, K. (1982) Neoplasia of the lungs in the workers of a nickel smelting plant (Czech.). *Pracov. Lék.*, *34*, 280-282

Olsen, I. & Jonsen, J. (1979) Whole body autoradiography of $^{63}$Ni in mice throughout gestation. *Toxicology*, *12*, 165-172

Olsen, J. & Sabroe, S. (1984) Occupational causes of laryngeal cancer. *J. Epidemiol. Commun. Health*, *38*, 117-121

Onkelinx, C., Becker, J. & Sunderman, F.W., Jr (1973) Compartmental analysis of the metabolism of $^{63}$Ni(II) in rats and rabbits. *Res. Commun. chem. Pathol. Pharmacol.*, *6*, 663-676

Oskarsson, A. & Tjälve, H. (1979a) An autoradiographic study on the distribution of $^{63}$NiCl$_2$ in mice. *Ann. clin. Lab. Sci.*, *9*, 47-59

Oskarsson, A. & Tjälve, H. (1979b) The distribution and metabolism of nickel carbonyl in mice. *Br. J. ind. Med.*, *36*, 326-335

Oskarsson, A. & Tjälve, H. (1979c) Binding of $^{63}$Ni by cellular constituents in some tissues of mice after the administration of $^{63}$NiCl$_2$ and $^{63}$Ni(CO)$_4$. *Acta pharmacol. toxicol.*, *45*, 306-314

Oskarsson, A., Andersson, Y. & Tjälve, H. (1979) Fate of nickel subsulfide during carcinogenesis studied by autoradiography and X-ray powder diffraction. *Cancer Res.*, *39*, 4175-4182

Oskarsson, A., Reid, M.C. & Sunderman, F.W., Jr (1981) Effect of cobalt chloride, nickel chloride, and nickel subsulfide upon erythropoiesis in rats. *Ann. clin Lab. Sci.*, *11*, 165-172

Ostapczuk, P., Valenta, P., Stoeppler, M. & Nürnberg, H.W. (1983) Voltammetric determination of nickel and cobalt in body fluids and other biological materials. In: Brown, S.S. & Savory, J., eds, *Chemical Toxicology and Clinical Chemistry of Metals*, London, Academic Press, pp. 61-64

Ottolenghi, A.D., Haseman, J.K., Payne, W.W., Falk, H.L. & MacFarland, H.N. (1974) Inhalation studies of nickel sulfide in pulmonary carcinogenesis of rats. *J. natl Cancer Inst.*, *54*, 1165-1172

Ou, B., Lu, Y., Huang, X. & Feng, G. (1980) The promoting action of nickel in the induction of nasopharyngeal carcinoma in rats (Chin.). In: *Cancer Research Reports — WHO Collaborating Centre for Research on Cancer*, Vol. 2, Guangzhou, Cancer Institute of Zhongshan Medical College, pp. 3-8

Ou, B., Liu, Y. & Zheng, G. (1983) Tumor induction in next generation of dinitropiperazine-treated pregnant rats (Abstract). In: *Cancer Research Reports — WHO Collaborat-*

*ing Centre for Research on Cancer*, Vol. 4, Guangzhou, Cancer Institute of Zhongshan Medical College, pp. 44-45

Patierno, S.R. & Costa, M. (1985) DNA-protein cross-links induced by nickel compounds in intact cultured mammalian cells. *Chem.-biol. Interactions*, *55*, 75-91

Patierno, S.R., Sugiyama, M., Basilion, J.P. & Costa, M. (1985) Preferential DNA-protein cross-linking by $NiCl_2$ in magnesium-insoluble regions of fractionated Chinese hamster ovary cell chromatin. *Cancer Res.*, *45*, 5787-5794

Paton, G.R. & Allison, A.C. (1972) Chromosome damage in human cell cultures induced by metal salts. *Mutat. Res.*, *16*, 332-336

Payne, W.W. (1964) Carcinogenicity of nickel compounds in experimental animals (Abstract No. 197). *Proc. Am. Assoc. Cancer Res.*, *5*, 50

Pedersen, E., Høgetveit, A.C. & Andersen, A. (1973) Cancer of respiratory organs among workers at a nickel refinery in Norway. *Int. J. Cancer*, *12*, 32-41

Peltonen, L. (1979) Nickel sensitivity in the general population. *Contact Dermatitis*, 5, 27-32

Peto, J., Cuckle, H., Doll, R., Hermon, C. & Morgan, L.G. (1984) Respiratory cancer mortality of Welsh nickel refinery workers. In: Sunderman, F.W., Jr, ed., *Nickel in the Human Environment* (IARC Scientific Publications No. 53), Lyon, IARC, pp. 37-46

Pfeiffer, W. & Willert, G. (1986) *Thermisches Spritzen* (Thermal Spraying) (BIA-Report 6), St Augustin, Berufsgenossenschaftliches Institut für Arbeitssicherheit

Pharmacie Centrale (1988) *Nickel Carbonate*, Paris

Pienta, R.J., Poiley, J.A. & Lebherz, W.B., III (1977) Morphological transformation of early passage golden Syrian hamster embryo cells derived from cryopreserved primary cultures as a reliable in vitro bioassay for identifying diverse carcinogens. *Int. J. Cancer*, *19*, 642-655

Pihlar, B., Valenta, P. & Nürnberg, H.W. (1981) New high-performance analytical procedure for the voltammetric determination of nickel in routine analysis of waters, biological materials and food. *Fresenius Z. anal. Chem.*, *307*, 337-346

Pikálek, P. & Nečásek, J. (1983) The mutagenic activity of nickel in *Corynebacterium* sp. *Folia Microbiol.*, *28*, 17-21

Poirier, L.A., Theiss, J.C., Arnold, L.J. & Shimkin, M.B. (1984) Inhibition by magnesium and calcium acetates of lead subacetate- and nickel acetate-induced lung tumors in strain A mice. *Cancer Res.*, *44*, 1520-1522

Pott, F., Ziem, U., Reiffer, F.-J., Huth, F., Ernst, H. & Mohr, U. (1987) Carcinogenicity studies on fibres, metal compounds and some other dusts in rats. *Exp. Pathol.*, *32*, 129-152

Pott, F., Rippe, R.M., Roller, M., Csicsaky, M., Rosenbruch, M. & Huth, F. (1989) Tumours in the abdominal cavity of rats after intraperitoneal injection of nickel compounds. In: Vernet, J.-P., ed., *Proceedings of the International Conference on Heavy Metals in the Environment, Geneva, 12-15 September 1989*, Vol. 2, Geneva, World Health Organization, pp. 127-129

Pott, F., Rippe, R.M., Roller, M., Csicsaky, M., Rosenbruch, M. & Huth, F. (1990) Carcinogenicity studies on nickel compounds and nickel alloys after intraperitoneal injection in rats. In: Nieboer, E. & Aitio, A., *Advances in Environmental Sciences and Toxicology, Nickel and Human Health: Current Perspectives*, New York, John Wiley & Sons (in press)

Punsar, S., Erämetsä, O., Karvonen, M.J., Ryhänen, A., Hilska, P. & Vornamo, H. (1975) Coronary heart disease and drinking water. A search in two Finnish male cohorts for epidemiologic evidence of a water factor. *J. chron. Dis.*, *28*, 259-287

Queensland Nickel Sales Pty Ltd (1989) *On Nickel Oxide Sinter (90% Ni)*, London

Raithel, H.J. (1987) *Untersuchungen zur Belastung und Beanspruchung von 837 beruflich Nickel-exponierten Personen* (Studies of Exposure and Effects in 837 Persons Occupationally Exposed to Nickel), St Augustin, Hauptverband der gewerblichen Berufsgenossenschaften

Raithel, H.-J. & Schaller, K.H. (1981) Toxicity and carcinogenicity of nickel and its compounds. A review of the current status (Ger.). *Zbl. Bakteriol. Hyg. I. Abt. Orig.*, *B 173*, 63-91

Raithel, H.-J., Schaller, K.H., Mohrmann, W., Mayer, P. & Henkels, U. (1982) Study of elimination kinetics of nickel during injury in the glass and electroplating industry (Ger.). In: Fliedner, T.M., ed., *Bericht über die 22. Jahrestagung der Deutschen Gesellschaft für Arbeitsmedizin* (Report on the 22nd Anniversary of the German Society of Occupational Medicine), Stuttgart, Gentner, pp. 223-228

Raithel, H.J., Ebner, G., Schaller, K.H., Schellmann, P. & Valentin, H. (1987) Problems in establishing norm values for nickel and chromium concentrations in human pulmonary tissue. *Am. J. ind. Med.*, *12*, 55-70

Raithel, H.J., Schaller, K.H., Reith, A., Svenes, K.B. & Valentin, H. (1988) Investigations on the quantitative determination of nickel and chromium in human lung tissue. Industrial medical, toxicological, and occupational medical expertise aspects. *Int. Arch. occup. environ. Health*, *60*, 55-66

Rasmuson, Å. (1985) Mutagenic effects of some water-soluble metal compounds in a somatic eye-color test system in *Drosophila melanogaster. Mutat. Res.*, *157*, 157-162

Redmond, C.K. (1984) Site-specific cancer mortality among workers involved in the production of high nickel alloys. In: Sunderman, F.W., Jr, ed., *Nickel in the Human Environment* (IARC Scientific Publications No. 53), Lyon, IARC, pp. 73-86

Reith, A. & Brøgger, A. (1984) Carcinogenicity and mutagenicity of nickel and nickel compounds. In: Sunderman, F.W., Jr, ed., *Nickel in the Human Environment* (IARC Scientific Publications No. 53), Lyon, IARC, pp. 175-192

Rezuke, W.N., Knight, J.A. & Sunderman, F.W., Jr (1987) References values for nickel concentrations in human tissues and bile. *Am. J. ind. Med.*, *11*, 419-426

Ridgway, L.P. & Karnofsky, D.A. (1952) The effects of metals on chick embryos: toxicity and production of abnormalities in development. *Ann. N.Y. Acad. Sci.*, *55*, 203-215

Riedel-de Haën (1986) *Laboratory Chemicals*, Hanover, pp. 72, 756-760

Rigaut, J.P. (1983) *Rapport Préparatoire sur les Critères de Santé pour le Nickel* (Preparatory Report on Health Criteria for Nickel) (Doc. CCE/Lux/V/E/24/83), Luxembourg, Commission of the European Communities

Rivedal, E. & Sanner, T. (1980) Synergistic effect on morphological transformation of hamster embryo cells by nickel sulphate and benz[a]pyrene. *Cancer Lett.*, *8*, 203-208

Rivedal, E. & Sanner, T. (1981) Metal salts as promoters of *in vitro* morphological transformation of hamster embryo cells initiated by benzo(a)pyrene. *Cancer Res.*, *41*, 2950-2953

Rivedal, E. & Sanner, T. (1983) Evaluation of tumour promotors by the hamster embryo cell transformation assay. In: Bartsch, H. & Armstrong, B., eds, *Host Factors in Human Carcinogenesis* (IARC Scientific Publications No. 39), Lyon, IARC, pp. 251-258

Rivedal, E., Hemstad, J. & Sanner, T. (1980) Synergistic effects of cigarette smoke extracts, benz(a)pyrene and nickel sulphate on morphological transformation of hamster embryo cells. In: Holmstedt, B., Lauwerys, R., Mercier, M. & Roberfroid, M., eds, *Mechanisms of Toxicity and Hazard Evaluation*, Amsterdam, Elsevier, pp. 259-263

Roberts, R.S., Julian, J.A., Muir, D.C.F. & Shannon, H.S. (1984) Cancer mortality associated with the high-temperature oxidation of nickel subsulphide. In: Sunderman, F.W., Jr, ed., *Nickel in the Human Environment* (IARC Scientific Publications No. 53), Lyon, IARC, pp. 23-34

Roberts, R.S., Julian, J.A., Sweezey, D., Muir, D.C.F., Shannon, H.S. & Mastromatteo, E. (1990a) A study of mortality in workers engaged in the mining, smelting, and refining of nickel. I. Methodology and mortality by major case groups. *Toxicol. ind. Health* (in press)

Roberts, R.S., Julian, J.A., Muir, D.C.F. & Shannon, H.S. (1990b) A study of mortality in workers engaged in the mining, smelting and refining of nickel. II. Mortality from cancer of the respiratory tract and kidney. *Toxicol. ind. Health* (in press)

Robison, S.H. & Costa, M. (1982) The induction of DNA strand breakage by nickel compounds in cultured Chinese hamster ovary cells. *Cancer Lett., 15*, 35-40

Robison, S.H., Cantoni, O. & Costa, M. (1982) Strand breakage and decreased molecular weight of DNA induced by specific metal compounds. *Carcinogenesis, 5*, 657-662

Robison, S.H., Cantoni, O., Heck, J.D. & Costa, M. (1983) Soluble and insoluble nickel compounds induce DNA repair synthesis in cultured mammalian cells. *Cancer Lett., 17*, 273-279

Robison, S.H., Cantoni, O. & Costa, M. (1984) Analysis of metal-induced DNA lesions and DNA-repair replication in mammalian cells. *Mutat. Res., 131*, 173-181

Rodriguez-Arnaiz, R. & Ramos, P.M. (1986) Mutagenicity of nickel sulphate in *Drosophila melanogaster*. *Mutat. Res., 170*, 115-117

Rossman, T.G. & Molina, M. (1986) The genetic toxicology of metal compounds: II. Enhancement of ultraviolet light-induced mutagenesis in *Escherichia coli* WP2. *Environ. Mutagenesis, 8*, 263-271

Rossman, T.G., Molina, M. & Meyer, L.W. (1984) The genetic toxicology of metal compounds: I. Induction of $\lambda$ prophage in *E. coli* WP2$_s$ ($\lambda$). *Environ. Mutagenesis, 6*, 59-69

Roush, G.C., Meigs, J.W., Kelly, J.A., Flannery, J.T. & Burdo, H. (1980) Sinonasal cancer and occupation: a case-control study. *Am. J. Epidemiol., 111*, 183-193

Rystedt, I. & Fischer, T. (1983) Relationship between nickel and cobalt sensitization in hard metal workers. *Contact Dermatitis, 9*, 195-200

Saknyn, A.V. & Blokhin, V.A. (1978) Development of malignant tumours in rats exposed to nickel containing aerosols (Russ.). *Vopr. Onkol., 24*, 44-48

Saknyn, A.V. & Shabynina, N.K. (1970) Some statistical data on the carcinogenous hazards for workers engaged in the production of nickel from oxidized ores (Russ.). *Gig. Tr. prof. Zabol., 14*, 10-13

Saknyn, A.V. & Shabynina, N.K. (1973) Epidemiology of malignant neoplasms in nickel smelters (Russ.). *Gig. Tr. prof. Zabol.*, *17*, 25-29

Saknyn, A.V., Elnichnykh, L.N., Vorontsova, A.S. & Frash, V.N. (1976) General toxic action of dusts generated in the manufacture of crude nickel (Russ.). *Gig. Tr. prof. Zabol.*, *12*, 29-32

Salmon, L., Atkins, D.H.F., Fisher, E.M.R., Healy, C. & Law, D.V. (1978) Retrospective trend analysis on the content of UK air particulate material 1957-1974. *Sci. total Environ.*, *9*, 161-200

Sarkar, B. (1980) Nickel in blood and kidney. In: Brown, S.S. & Sunderman, F.W., Jr, eds, *Nickel Toxicology*, London, Academic Press, pp. 81-84

Sarkar, B. (1984) Nickel metabolism. In: Sunderman, F.W., Jr, ed., *Nickel in the Human Environment* (IARC Scientific Publications No. 53), Lyon, IARC, pp. 367-384

Savory, J., Brown, S., Bertholf, R.L., Ross, R. & Wills, M.R. (1985) Serum and lymphocyte nickel and aluminium concentrations in patients with extracorporeal hemodialysis. In: Brown, S.S. & Sunderman, F.W., Jr, eds, *Progress in Nickel Toxicology*, Oxford, Blackwell Scientific Publications, pp. 137-140

Sax, N.I. & Lewis, R.J., Sr (1987) *Hawley's Condensed Chemical Dictionary*, 11th ed., New York, Van Nostrand Reinhold, pp. 818-821

Saxholm, J.J.K., Reith, A. & Brøgger, A. (1981) Oncogenic transformation and cell lysis in C3H/10T1/2 cells and increased sister chromatid exchange in human lymphocytes by nickel subsulfide. *Cancer Res.*, *41*, 4136-4139

Schaller, K.H. & Zober, A. (1982) Renal elimination of toxicologically relevant metals in occupationally non-exposed individuals (Ger.). *Ärztl. Lab.*, *28*, 209-214

Schaller, K.H., Stoeppler, M. & Raithel, H.J. (1982) Analytical determination of nickel in biological matrices. A summary of present knowledge and experience (Ger.). *Staub-Reinhalt. Luft*, *42*, 137-140

Scheller, R., Strahlmann, B. & Schwedt, G. (1988) Chemical and technological aspects of food for a diet poor in nickel for endogenous nickel contact eczema (Ger.). *Hautarzt*, *39*, 491-497

Scholz, R.C. & Holcomb, M.L. (1980) *Feasibility Study for Reduction of Workers Exposures to Nickel and Chromium in Alloy Foundries* (Report submitted to OSHA Docket H-110 by the Foundry Nickel Committee), Washington DC, US Occupational Safety and Health Administration

Schramel, P., Lill, G. & Hasse, S. (1985) Mineral and trace elements in human urine (Ger.). *J. clin. Chem. clin. Biochem.*, *23*, 293-301

Schroeder, H.A. & Mitchener, M. (1971) Toxic effects of trace elements on the reproduction of mice and rats. *Arch. environ. Health*, *23*, 102-106

Seemann, J., Wittig, P., Kollmeier, H. & Rothe, G. (1985) Analytical measurements of Cd, Pb, Zn, Cr and Ni in human tissues (Ger.). *Lab. Med.*, *9*, 294-299

Sen, P. & Costa, M. (1985) Induction of chromosomal damage in Chinese hamster ovary cells by soluble and particulate nickel compounds: preferential fragmentation of the heterochromatic long arm of the X-chromosome by carcinogenic crystalline NiS particles. *Cancer Res.*, *45*, 2320-2325

Sen, P. & Costa, M. (1986a) Pathway of nickel uptake influences its interaction with heterochromatic DNA. *Toxicol. appl. Pharmacol.*, *84*, 278-285

Sen, P. & Costa, M. (1986b) Incidence and localization of sister chromatid exchanges induced by nickel and chromium compounds. *Carcinogenesis*, *7*, 1527-1533

Sen, P., Conway, K. & Costa, M. (1987) Comparison of the localization of chromosome damage induced by calcium chromate and nickel compounds. *Cancer Res.*, *47*, 2142-2147

Shannon, H.S., Julian, J.A. & Roberts, R.S. (1984a) A mortality study of 11,500 nickel workers. *J. natl Cancer Inst.*, *73*, 1251-1258

Shannon, H.S., Julian, J.A., Muir, D.C.F. & Roberts, R.S. (1984b) A mortality study of Falconbridge workers. In: Sunderman, F.W., Jr, ed., *Nickel in the Human Environment* (IARC Scientific Publications No. 53), Lyon, IARC, pp. 117-124

Shibata, M., Izumi, K., Sano, N., Akagi, A. & Otsuka, H. (1989) Induction of soft tissue tumours in F344 rats by subcutaneous, intramuscular, intra-articular, and retroperitoneal injection of nickel sulphide ($Ni_3S_2$). *J. Pathol.*, *157*, 263-274

Sibley, S.F. (1985) Nickel. In: *Mineral Facts and Problems, 1985 ed.* (*Preprint from Bulletin 675*), Washington DC, Bureau of Mines, pp. 1-17

Silverstein, M., Mirer, F., Kotelchuck, D., Silverstein, B. & Bennett, M. (1981) Mortality among workers in a die-casting and electroplating plant. *Scand. J. Work Environ. Health*, *7* (*Suppl. 4*), 156-165

Sina, J.F., Bean, C.L., Dysart, G.R., Taylor, V.I. & Bradley, M.O. (1983) Evaluation of the alkaline elution/rat hepatocyte assay as a predictor of carcinogenic/mutagenic potential. *Mutat. Res.*, *113*, 357-391

Sirover, M.A. & Loeb, L.A. (1976) Infidelity of DNA synthesis *in vitro*: screening for potential metal mutagens or carcinogens. *Science*, *194*, 1434-1436

Sirover, M.A. & Loeb, L.A. (1977) On the fidelity of DNA replication: effects of metal activators during synthesis with avian myeloblastosis virus DNA polymerase. *J. biol. Chem.*, *252*, 3605-3610

Skaug, V., Gylseth, B., Reiss, A.-L.P. & Norseth, T. (1985) Tumor induction in rats after intrapleural injection of nickel subsulfide and nickel oxide. In: Brown, S.S. & Sunderman, F.W., Jr, *Progress in Nickel Toxicology*, Oxford, Blackwell Scientific Publications, pp. 37-41

Škreb, Y. & Fischer, A.B. (1984) Toxicity of nickel for mammalian cells in culture. *Zbl. Bakt. Hyg. I. Abt. Orig. B*, *178*, 432-445

Smart, G.A. & Sherlock, J.C. (1987) Nickel in foods and the diet. *Food Addit. Contam.*, *4*, 61-71

Smialowicz, R.J., Rogers, R.R., Riddle, M.M. & Stott, G.A. (1984) Immunologic effects of nickel: I. Suppression of cellular and humoral immunity. *Environ. Res.*, *33*, 413-427

Smialowicz, R.J., Rogers, R.R., Riddle, M.M., Garner, R.J., Rowe, D.G. & Luebke, R.W. (1985) Immunologic effects of nickel: II. Suppression of natural killer cell activity. *Environ. Res.*, *36*, 56-66

Smialowicz, R.J., Rogers, R.R., Rowe, D.G., Riddle, M.M. & Luebke, R.W. (1987) The effects of nickel on immune function in the rat. *Toxicology*, *44*, 271-281

Smith-Sonneborn, J., Palizzi, R.A., McCann, E.A. & Fisher, G.L. (1983) Bioassay of geno-toxic effects of environmental particles in a feeding ciliate. *Environ. Health Perspect.*, *51*, 205-210

Solomons, N.W., Viteri, F., Shuler, T.R. & Nielsen, F.H. (1982) Bioavailability of nickel in man: effects of foods and chemically-defined dietary constituents on the absorption of inorganic nickel. *J. Nutr.*, *112*, 39-50

Sonnenfeld, G., Streips, U.N. & Costa, M. (1983) Differential effects of amorphous and crys-talline nickel sulfide on murine α/β interferon production. *Environ. Res.*, *32*, 474-479

Sorahan, T. (1987) Mortality from lung cancer among a cohort of nickel cadmium battery workers: 1946-84. *Br. J. ind. Med.*, *44*, 803-809

Sorahan, T. & Waterhouse, J.A.H. (1983) Mortality study of nickel-cadmium battery workers by the method of regression models in life tables. *Br. J. ind. Med.*, *40*, 293-300

Sorahan, T. & Waterhouse, J.A.H. (1985) Cancer of prostate among nickel-cadmium battery workers (Letter). *Lancet*, *i*, 459

Sorahan, T., Burges, D.C.L. & Waterhouse, J.A.H. (1987) A mortality study of nickel/chro-mium platers. *Br. J. ind. Med.*, *44*, 250-258

Sosinksi, E. (1975) Morphological changes in rat brain and skeletal muscle in the region of nickel oxide implantation. *Neuropathol. Pol.*, *13*, 479-483

Stedman, D.H., Tammaro, D.A., Branch, D.K. & Pearson, R., Jr (1979) Chemiluminescence detector for the measurement of nickel carbonyl in air. *Anal. Chem.*, *51*, 2340-2342

Stettler, L.E., Donaldson, H.M. & Grant, G.C. (1982) Chemical composition of coal and other mineral slags. *Am. ind. Hyg. Assoc. J.*, *43*, 235-238

Stoeppler, M. (1980) Analysis of nickel in biological materials and natural waters. In: Nriagu, J.O., ed., *Nickel in the Environment*, New York, John Wiley & Sons, pp. 661-822

Stoeppler, M. (1984a) Analytical chemistry of nickel. In: Sunderman, F.W., Jr, ed., *Nickel in the Human Environment* (IARC Scientific Publications No. 53), Lyon, IARC, pp. 459-468

Stoeppler, M. (1984b) Recent improvements for nickel analysis in biological materials. In: *Trace Element Analytical Chemistry*, Vol. 3, Berlin (West), Walter de Gruyter & Co., pp. 539-557

Stoner, G.D., Shimkin, M.B., Troxell, M.C., Thompson, T.L. & Terry, L.S. (1976) Test for carcinogenicity of metallic compounds by the pulmonary tumor response in strain A mice. *Cancer Res.*, *36*, 1744-1747

Storeng, R. & Jonsen, J. (1980) Effect of nickel chloride and cadmium acetate on the devel-opment of preimplantation mouse embryos *in vitro*. *Toxicology*, *17*, 183-187

Storeng, R. & Jonsen, J. (1981) Nickel toxicity in early embryogenesis in mice. *Toxicology*, *20*, 45-51

Sumino, K., Hayakawa, K., Shibata, T. & Kitamura, S. (1975) Heavy metals in normal Japa-nese tissues. Amount of 15 heavy metals in 30 subjects. *Arch. environ. Health*, *30*, 487-494

Sunderman, F.W., Jr (1963) Studies of nickel carcinogenesis: alterations of ribonucleic acid following inhalation of nickel carbonyl. *Am. J. clin. Pathol.*, *39*, 549-561

Sunderman, F.W., Jr (1967) Nickel carbonyl inhibition of cortisone induction of hepatic tryptophan pyrrolase. *Cancer Res.*, 27, 1595-1599

Sunderman, F.W., Jr (1977) A review of the metabolism and toxicology of nickel. *Ann. clin. Lab. Sci.*, 7, 377-398

Sunderman, F.W., Jr (1981) Recent research on nickel carcinogenesis. *Environ. Health Perspect.*, 40, 131-141

Sunderman, F.W., Jr (1983a) Potential toxicity from nickel contamination of intravenous fluids. *Ann. clin. Lab. Sci.*, 3, 1-4

Sunderman, F.W., Jr (1983b) Organ and species specificity in nickel subsulfide carcinogenesis. *Basic Life Sci.*, 24, 107-127

Sunderman, F.W., Jr (1984) Carcinogenicity of nickel compounds in animals. In: Sunderman, F.W., Jr, ed., *Nickel in the Human Environment* (IARC Scientific Publications No. 53), Lyon, IARC, pp. 127-142

Sunderman, F.W., Jr (1986a) Nickel. In: Seiler, H.G., Sigel, H. & Sigel, A., eds, *Handbook on Toxicity of Inorganic Compounds*, New York, Marcel Dekker, pp. 453-468

Sunderman, F.W., Jr (1986b) Nickel determination in body fluids, tissues, excreta and water. In: O'Neill, I.K., Schuller, P. & Fishbein, L., eds, *Environmental Carcinogens: Selected Methods of Analysis*, Vol. 8, *Some Metals: As, Be, Cd, Cr, Ni, Pb, Se, Zn* (IARC Scientific Publications No. 72), Lyon, IARC, pp. 319-334

Sunderman, F.W., Jr (1988) Nickel. In: Clarkson, T.W., Friberg, L., Nordberg, G.F. & Sager, P.R., eds, *Biological Monitoring of Toxic Metals*, New York, Plenum Press, pp. 265-282

Sunderman, F.W., Jr (1989) Mechanisms of nickel carcinogenesis. *Scand. J. Work Environ. Health*, 15, 1-12

Sunderman, F.W. & Donnelly, A.J. (1965) Studies on nickel carcinogenesis: metastasizing pulmonary tumors induced by the inhalation of nickel carbonyl. *Am. J. clin. Pathol.*, 46, 1027-1041

Sunderman, F.W., Jr & Horak, E. (1981) Biochemical indices of nephrotoxicity exemplified by studies of nickel nephropathy. In: Brown, S.S. & Davies, D.S., eds, *Organ-directed Toxicity: Chemical Indices and Mechanisms*, Oxford, Pergamon Press, pp. 55-67

Sunderman, F.W. & Kincaid, J.F. (1954) Nickel poisoning. II. Studies on patients suffering from acute exposure to vapors of nickel carbonyl. *J. Am. med. Assoc.*, 155, 889-895

Sunderman, F.W., Jr & Maenza, R.M. (1976) Comparisons of carcinogenicities of nickel compounds in rats. *Res. Commun. chem. Pathol. Pharmacol.*, 14, 319-330

Sunderman, F.W., Jr & McCully, K.S. (1983) Carcinogenesis tests of nickel arsenides, nickel antimonide, and nickel telluride in rats. *Cancer Invest.*, 1, 469-474

Sunderman, F.W., Jr & Selin, C.E. (1968) The metabolism of nickel-63 carbonyl. *Toxicol. appl. Pharmacol.*, 12, 207-218

Sunderman, F.W. & Sunderman, F.W., Jr (1958) Nickel poisoning. VIII. Dithiocarb: a new therapeutic agent for persons exposed to nickel carbonyl. *Am. J. med. Sci.*, 236, 26-31

Sunderman, F.W. & Sunderman, F.W., Jr (1961) Nickel poisoning. XI. Implication of nickel as a pulmonary carcinogen in tobacco smoke. *Am. J. clin. Pathol.*, 35, 203-209

Sunderman, F.W., Jr & Sunderman, F.W. (1963) Studies on pulmonary carcinogenesis: the subcellular partition of nickel and the binding of nickel by ribonucleic acids (Abstract No. 1592). *Fed. Proc., 22*, 427

Sunderman, F.W., Kincaid, J.F., Donnelly, A.J. & West, B. (1957) Nickel poisoning. IV. Chronic exposure of rats to nickel carbonyl: a report after one year observation. *Arch. environ. Health, 16*, 480-485

Sunderman, F.W., Donnelly, A.J., West, B. & Kincaid, J.F. (1959) Nickel poisoning. IX. Carcinogenesis in rats exposed to nickel carbonyl. *Arch. environ. Health, 20*, 36-41

Sunderman, F.W., Jr, Roszel, N.O. & Clark, R.J. (1968) Gas chromatography of nickel. *Arch. environ. Health, 16*, 836-843

Sunderman, F.W., Jr, Kasprzak, K.S., Lau, T.J., Minghetti, P.P., Maenza, R.M., Becker, N., Onkelinx, C. & Goldblatt, P.J. (1976) Effects of manganese on carcinogenicity and metabolism of nickel subsulfide. *Cancer Res., 36*, 1790-1800

Sunderman, F.W., Jr, Shen, S., Mitchell, J., Allpass, P. & Damjanov, I. (1977) Fetal toxicity and transplacental transport of Ni(II) in rats (Abstract No. 176). *Toxicol. appl. Pharmacol., 41*, 205

Sunderman, F.W., Jr, Shen, S.K., Mitchell, J.M., Allpass, P.R. & Damjanov, I. (1978a) Embryotoxicity and fetal toxicity of nickel in rats. *Toxicol. appl. Pharmacol., 43*, 381-390

Sunderman, F.W., Jr, Mitchell, J., Allpass, P. & Baselt, R. (1978b) Embryotoxicity and teratogenicity of nickel carbonyl in rats (Abstract No. 295). *Toxicol. appl. Pharmacol., 45*, 345

Sunderman, F.W., Jr, Maenza, R.M., Hopfer, S.M., Mitchell, J.M., Allpass, P.R. & Damjanov, I. (1979a) Induction of renal cancers in rats by intrarenal injection of nickel subsulfide. *J. environ. Pathol. Toxicol., 2*, 1511-1527

Sunderman, F.W., Jr, Allpass, P.R., Mitchell, J.M., Baselt, R.C. & Albert, D.M. (1979b) Eye malformations in rats: induction by prenatal exposure to nickel carbonyl. *Science, 203*, 550-553

Sunderman, F.W., Jr, Shen, S.K., Reid, M.C. & Allpass, P.R. (1980) Teratogenicity and embryotoxicity of nickel carbonyl in Syrian hamsters. *Teratog. Carcinog. Mutagenesis, 1*, 223-233

Sunderman, F.W., Jr, McCully, K.S. & Rinehimer, L.A. (1981) Negative test for transplacental carcinogenicity of nickel subsulfide in Fischer rats. *Res. Commun. chem. Pathol. Pharmacol., 31*, 545-554

Sunderman, F.W., Jr, Reid, M.C., Bibeau, L.M. & Linden, J.V. (1983a) Nickel induction of microsomal heme oxygenase activity in rodents. *Toxicol. appl. Pharmacol., 68*, 87-95

Sunderman, F.W., Jr, Reid, M.C., Shen, S.K. & Kevorkian, C.B. (1983b) Embryotoxicity and teratogenicity of nickel compounds. In: Clarkson, T.W., Nordberg, G.F. & Sager, P.R., eds, *Reproductive and Developmental Toxicity of Metals*, New York, Plenum Press, pp. 399-416

Sunderman, F.W., Jr, Crisostomo, M.C., Reid, M.C., Hopfer, S.M. & Nomoto, S. (1984a) Rapid analysis of nickel in serum and whole blood by electrothermal atomic absorption spectrophotometry. *Ann. clin. Lab. Sci., 14*, 232-241

Sunderman, F.W., Jr, McCully, K.S. & Hopfer, S.M. (1984b) Association between erythrocytosis and renal cancers in rats following intrarenal injection of nickel compounds. *Carcinogenesis*, 5, 1511-1517

Sunderman, F.W., Jr, Marzouk, A., Crisostomo, M.C. & Weatherby, D.R. (1985a) Electrothermal atomic absorption spectrometry of nickel in tissue homogenates. *Ann. clin. Lab. Sci.*, 15, 299-307

Sunderman, F.W., Jr, Marzouk, A., Hopfer, S.M., Zaharia, O. & Reid, M.C. (1985b) Increased lipid peroxidation in tissues of nickel chloride-treated rats. *Ann. clin. Lab. Sci.*, 15, 229-236

Sunderman, F.W., Jr, Aitio, A., Morgan, L.G. & Norseth, T. (1986a) Biological monitoring of nickel. *Toxicol. ind. Health*, 2, 17-78

Sunderman, F.W., Jr, Hopfer, S.M., Crisostomo, M.C. & Stoeppler, M. (1986b) Rapid analysis of nickel in urine by electrothermal atomic absorption spectrophotometry. *Ann. clin. Lab. Sci.*, 16, 219-230

Sunderman, F.W., Jr, Hopfer, S.M., Knight, J.A., McCully, K.S., Cecutti, A.G., Thornhill, P.G., Conway, K., Miller, C., Patierno, S.R. & Costa, M. (1987) Physicochemical characteristics and biological effects of nickel oxides. *Carcinogenesis*, 8, 305-313

Sunderman, F.W., Jr, Hopfer, S.M. & Crisostomo, M.C. (1988a) Nickel analysis by atomic absorption spectrometry. *Methods Enzymol.*, 158, 382-391

Sunderman, F.W., Jr, Dingle, B., Hopfer, S.M. & Swift, T. (1988b) Acute nickel toxicity in electroplating workers who accidently ingested a solution of nickel sulfate and nickel chloride. *Am. J. ind. Med.*, 14, 257-266

Sunderman, F.W., Jr, Hopfer, S.M., Swift, T., Rezuke, W.N., Ziebka, L., Highman, P., Edwards, B., Folcik, M. & Gossling, H.R. (1989a) Cobalt, chromium, and nickel concentrations in body fluids of patients with porous-coated knee or hip prostheses. *J. orthopaed. Res.*, 7, 307-315

Sunderman, F.W., Jr, Hopfer, S.M., Sweeney, K.R., Marcus, A.H., Most, B.M. & Creason, J. (1989b) Nickel absorption and kinetics in human volunteers. *Proc. Soc. exp. Biol. Med.*, 191, 5-11

Swierenga, S.H.H. & McLean, J.R. (1985) Further insights into mechanisms of nickel-induced DNA damage: studies with cultured rat liver cells. In: Brown, S.S. & Sunderman, F.W., Jr, eds, *Progess in Nickel Toxicology*, Oxford, Blackwell Scientific Publications, pp. 101-104

Swierenga, S.H.H., Marceau, N., Katsuma, Y., French, S.W., Mueller, R. & Lee, F. (1989) Altered cytokeratin expression and differentiation induction during neoplastic transformation of cultured rat liver cells by nickel subsulfide. *Cell Biol. Toxicol.*, 5, 271-286

Szadkowski, D., Schultze, H., Schaller, K.-H. & Lehnert, G. (1969) On the ecological significance of heavy metal contents of cigarettes (Ger.) *Arch. Hyg.*, 153, 1-8

Takenaka, S., Hochrainer, D. & Oldiges, H. (1985) Alveolar proteinosis induced in rats by long-term inhalation of nickel oxide. In: Brown, S.S. & Sunderman, F.W., Jr, eds, *Progress in Nickel Toxicology*, Oxford, Blackwell Scientific Publications, pp. 89-92

Tanaka, I., Horie, A., Haratake, J., Kodama, Y. & Tsuchiya, K. (1988) Lung burden of green nickel oxide aerosol and histopathological findings in rats after continuous inhalation. *Biol. Trace Elem. Res.*, *16*, 19-26

Tandon, S.K., Mathur, A.K. & Gaur, J.S. (1977) Urinary excretion of chromium and nickel among electroplaters and pigment industry workers. *Int. Arch. occup. environ. Health*, *40*, 71-76

Tatarskaya, A.A. (1965) Occupational cancer of the upper respiratory tract in the nickel-refining industry (Russ.). *Gig. Tr. prof. Zabol.*, *9*, 22-25

Tatarskaya, A.A. (1967) Cancer of the respiratory tract in people engaged in nickel industry (Russ.). *Vopr. Onkol.*, *13*, 58-60

Tien, J.K. & Howson, T.E. (1981) Nickel and nickel alloys. In: Mark, H.F., Othmer, D.F., Overberger, C.G., Seaborg, G.T. & Grayson, M., eds, *Kirk-Othmer Encyclopedia of Chemical Technology*, 3rd ed., Vol. 15, New York, John Wiley & Sons, pp. 787-801

Tissot, B.P. & Weltle, D. (1984) *Petroleum Formation and Occurrence*, 2nd ed., Berlin (West), Springer

Tola, S., Kilpiö, J. & Virtamo, M. (1979) Urinary and plasma concentrations of nickel as indicators of exposure to nickel in an electroplating shop. *J. occup. Med.*, *21*, 184-188

Torjussen, W. & Andersen, I. (1979) Nickel concentrations in nasal mucosa, plasma and urine in active and retired nickel workers. *Ann. clin. Lab. Sci.*, *9*, 289-298

Torjussen, W., Haug, F.-M.S. & Andersen, I. (1978) Concentration and distribution of heavy metals in nasal mucosa of nickel-exposed workers and of controls, studied with atomic absorption spectrophotometric analysis and with Timm's sulphide silver method. *Acta otolaryngol.*, *86*, 449-463

Tossavainen, A., Nurminen, M., Mutanen, P. & Tola, S. (1980) Application of mathematical modelling for assessing the biological half-times of chromium and nickel in field studies. *Br. J. ind. Med.*, *37*, 285-291

Tso, W.-W. & Fung, W.-P. (1981) Mutagenicity of metallic cations. *Toxicol. Lett.*, *8*, 195-200

Turhan, U., Wollburg, C., Angerer, J. & Szadkowski, D. (1985) Nickel content of human lungs and its significance for occupational bronchial carcinoma (Ger.). *Arbeitsmed. Sozialmed. Präventivmed.*, *20*, 277-281

Tveito, G., Hansteen, I.-L., Dalen, H. & Haugen, A. (1989) Immortalization of normal human kidney epithelial cells by nickel (II). *Cancer Res.*, *49*, 1829-1835

Tweats, D.J., Green, M.H.L. & Muriel, W.J. (1981) A differential killing assay for mutagens and carcinogens based on an improved repair-deficient strain of *Escherichia coli*. *Carcinogenesis*, *2*, 189-194

Työsuojeluhallitus (National Finnish Board of Occupational Safety and Health) (1987) *HTP-Azvot 1987* (TLV-Values 1987) (Safety Bull. 25), Helsinki, p. 21

Tyroler, G.P. & Landolt, C.A., eds (1988) *Extractive Metallurgy of Nickel and Cobalt*, Phoenix, AZ, Metallurgical Society

Umeda, M. & Nishimura, M. (1979) Inducibility of chromosomal aberrations by metal compounds in cultured mammalian cells. *Mutat. Res.*, *67*, 221-229

US Environmental Protection Agency (1986) *Health Assessment Document for Nickel and Nickel Compounds*, Washington DC, Office of Environmental Health Assessment, pp. 1-83

US Occupational Safety and Health Administration (1987) Air contaminants. *US Code Fed. Regul., Title 29*, Part 1910.1000, p. 680

Uziel, M., Owen, B. & Butler, A. (1986) Toxic response of hamster embryo cells on exposure to mixtures of $Ni^{2+}$ and benzo(a)pyrene. *J. appl. Toxicol.*, 6, 167-170

Valentine, R. & Fisher, G.L. (1984) Pulmonary clearance of intratracheally administered $^{63}Ni_3S_2$ in strain A/J mice. *Environ. Res.*, 34, 328-334

Veien, N.K. & Andersen, M.R. (1986) Nickel in Danish food. *Acta dermato-venerol.*, 66, 502-509

Veien, N.K., Hattel, T., Justesen, O. & Nørholm, A. (1985) Dietary treatment of nickel dermatitis. *Acta dermatovenerol.*, 65, 138-142

Vogel, E. (1976) The relation between mutational pattern and concentration by chemical mutagens in *Drosophila*. In: Montesano, R., Bartsch, H. & Tomatis, L., eds, *Screening Tests in Chemical Carcinogenesis* (IARC Scientific Publications No. 12), Lyon, IARC, pp. 117-137

Vuopala, U., Huhti, E., Takkunen, J. & Huikko, M. (1970) Nickel carbonyl poisoning. Report of 25 cases. *Ann. clin. Res.*, 2, 214-222

Waalkes, M.P., Rehm, S., Kasprzak, K.S. & Issaq, H.J. (1987) Inflammatory, proliferative and neoplastic lesions at the site of metallic identification ear tags in Wistar [Crl:(WI)BR] rats. *Cancer Res.*, 47, 2445-2450

Wahlberg, J.E. (1976) Immunoglobulin E, atopy, and nickel allergy. *Cutis*, 18, 715-716, 720

Waksvik, H. & Boysen, M. (1982) Cytogenetic analyses of lymphocytes from workers in a nickel refinery. *Mutat. Res.*, 103, 185-190

Waksvik, H., Boysen, M. & Hogetveit, A.C. (1984) Increased incidence of chromosomal aberrations in peripheral lymphocytes of retired nickel workers. *Carcinogenesis*, 5, 1525-1527

Waltscheva, W., Slatewa, M. & Michailow, I. (1972) Testicular changes due to long-term administration of nickel sulfate in rats (Ger.). *Exp. Pathol.*, 6, 116-120

Warner, J.S. (1984) Occupational exposure to airborne nickel in producing and using primary nickel products. In: Sunderman, F.W., Jr, ed., *Nickel in the Human Environment* (IARC Scientific Publications No. 53), Lyon, IARC, pp. 419-437

Weast, R.C. (1986) *CRC Handbook of Chemistry and Physics*, 67th ed., Boca Raton, FL, CRC Press, pp. B-118–B-119

Webb, M., Heath, J.C. & Hopkins, T. (1972) Intranuclear distribution of the inducing metal in the primary rhabdomyosarcomata induced in the rat by nickel, cobalt and cadmium. *Br. J. Cancer*, 26, 274-278

Webster, J.D., Parker, T.F., Alfrey, A.C., Smythe, W.R., Kubo, H., Neal, G. & Hull, A.R. (1980) Acute nickel intoxication by dialysis. *Ann. intern. Med.*, 92, 631-633

Wehner, A.P., Busch, R.H., Olson, R.J. & Craig, D.K. (1975) Chronic inhalation of nickel oxide and cigarette smoke by hamsters. *Am. ind. Hyg. Assoc. J.*, 36, 801-810

Wehner, A.P., Stuart, B.O. & Sanders, C.L. (1979) Inhalation studies with Syrian golden hamsters. *Prog. exp. Tumor Res.*, *24*, 177-198

Wehner, A.P., Dagle, G.E. & Milliman, E.M. (1981) Chronic inhalation exposure of hamsters to nickel-enriched fly ash. *Environ. Res.*, *26*, 195-216

Wehner, A.P., Dagle, G.E. & Busch, R.H. (1984) Pathogenicity of inhaled nickel compounds in hamsters. In: Sunderman, F.W., Jr, ed., *Nickel in the Human Environment* (IARC Scientific Publications No. 53), Lyon, IARC, pp. 143-151

Weinzierl, S.M. & Webb, M. (1972) Interaction of carcinogenic metals with tissue and body fluids. *Br. J. Cancer*, *26*, 279-291

Weischer, C.H., Kördel, W. & Hochrainer, D. (1980a) Effects of $NiCl_2$ and NiO in Wistar rats after oral uptake and inhalation exposure respectively. *Zbl. Bakt. Hyg. I Abt. Orig. B*, *171*, 336-351

Weischer, C.H., Oldiges, H., Hochrainer, D. & Kördel, W. (1980b) Subchronic effects induced by NiO-inhalation in Wistar rats. In: Holmstedt, B., Lauwerys, R., Mercier, M. & Roberfroid, M., eds, *Mechanisms of Toxicity and Hazard Evaluation*, Amsterdam, Elsevier, pp. 555-558

Whanger, P.D. (1973) Effects of dietary nickel on enzyme activities and mineral contents in rats. *Toxicol. appl. Pharmacol.*, *25*, 323-331

Wills, M.R., Brown, C.S., Bertholf, R.L., Ross, R. & Savory, J. (1985) Serum and lymphocyte, aluminium and nickel in chronic renal failure. *Clin. chim. Acta*, *145*, 193-196

Wilson, W.W. & Khoobyarian, N. (1982) Potential identification of chemical carcinogens in a viral transformation system. *Chem.-biol. Interactions*, *38*, 253-259

Windholz, M., ed. (1983) *The Merck Index*, 10th ed., Rahway, NJ, Merck & Co., pp. 932-933

Witschi, H. (1972) A comparative study of in vivo RNA and protein synthesis in rat liver and lung. *Cancer Res.*, *32*, 1686-1694

World Health Organization (1990) *Nickel* (Environmental Health Criteria Document), Geneva (in press)

Wu, Y., Luo, H. & Johnson, D.R. (1986) Effect of nickel sulfate on cellular proliferation and Epstein-Barr virus antigen expression in lymphoblastoid cell lines. *Cancer Lett.*, *32*, 171-179

Wulf, H.C. (1980) Sister chromatid exchanges in human lymphocytes exposed to nickel and lead. *Dan. med. Bull.*, *27*, 40-42

Yamashiro, S., Gilman, J.P.W., Hulland, T.J. & Abandowitz, H.M. (1980) Nickel sulphide-induced rhabdomyosarcomata in rats. *Acta pathol. jpn.*, *30*, 9-22

Yarita, T. & Nettesheim, P. (1978) Carcinogenicity of nickel subsulfide for respiratory tract mucosa. *Cancer Res.*, *38*, 3140-3145

Zatka, V.J. (1987) *Chemical Speciation of Nickel Phases in Industrial Dusts*, Mississauga, Ontario, INCO Ltd

Zatka, V.J. (1988) *Report to the NiPERA Scientific Advisory Committee on Interlaboratory Test Programme on Nickel Phase Speciation in Bulk Dust Samples by Sequential Leaching (Phase 3 — Fall 1987)*, Toronto, Nickel Producers Environmental Research Association

Zatka, V.J., Maskery, D. & Warner, J.S. (undated) *Chemical Speciation of Nickel in Airborne Dusts*, Toronto, Nickel Producers Environmental Research Association

Zhang, Q. & Barrett, J.C. (1988) Dose-response studies of nickel-induced morphological transformation of Syrian hamster embryo fibroblasts. *Toxicol. In Vitro*, 2, 303-307

Zhicheng, S. (1986) Acute nickel carbonyl poisoning: a report of 179 cases. *Br. J. ind. Med.*, 43, 422-424

Zober, A., Weltle, D., Schaller, K.-H. & Valentin, H. (1984) Study on the kinetics of chromium and nickel in biological samples during weekly arc welding with raw materials containing nickel and chromium (Ger.). *Schweissen Schneiden*, 36, 461-464

Zwennis, W.C.M. & Franssen, A.G. (1983) Exposure to insoluble nickel compounds in a plant for nickel catalysts. Relation between concentrations of nickel in urine and plasma (Abstract). In: *Proceedings of the Second International Conference on Clinical Chemistry and Clinical Toxicology of Metals, Montreal*, p. 128

# WELDING

## 1. Historical Perspectives and Process Description

### 1.1 Introduction

'Welding' is a term used to describe a wide range of processes for joining any materials by fusion or coalescence of the interface. It involves bringing two surfaces together under conditions of pressure or temperature which allow bonding to occur at the atomic level. Usually, this is accompanied by diffusion or mixing across the boundary, so that in the region of the weld an alloy is formed between the two pieces that have been joined. Welding and other methods of joining, such as soldering or brazing, can be distinguished clearly (Lancaster, 1980). In the latter, a low-melting alloy is heated until it flows and fills the gap between the two pieces of metal to be joined; the workpieces do not melt, and there is negligible diffusion or mixing of the metal across the boundaries. Metal can be welded by the application of energy in many forms: mechanical energy is utilized in forge, friction, ultrasonic and explosive welding; chemical energy in oxy-gas and thermit welding; electrical energy in arc welding, various forms of resistance welding and electron beam welding; and optical energy in laser welding. The term 'welding' is applicable equally to metals, thermoplastics and various other materials.

Many of the techniques used in welding can also be used for other purposes. Oxy-gas flames and electric arcs are used for cutting. Various processes, including flame spraying, plasma spraying and manual metal arc and metal inert gas hard surfacing, are used for depositing hard metal surface coatings and for building up worn machine components.

### 1.2 Development of welding in the twentieth century

Welding of metals has its origins in pre-history: at least 5000 years ago, metal was welded by heating and hammering overlapping pieces. The same principles are employed to this day in forge welding and other modern forms of 'solid state welding' (Lancaster, 1980; Lindberg & Braton, 1985). The development of modern welding technology began in the late nineteenth century with the application of oxy-fuel flames, electric arcs and electrical resistance welding. The industrial application of oxy-fuel combustion for cutting and welding was facilitated by the availability of calcium carbide, from which acetylene gas could be generated as required, and by the commercial availability from about 1895 of bottled oxygen produced by the liquefaction of air (Skriniar, 1986). Oxy-fuel welding underwent rapid development in the early years of the twentieth century, and by the middle of the First World War good quality welds could be made in steel plate, aluminium and other metals.

The phenomenon of the electric arc was first discovered in 1802 by Petrov; its first recorded use for welding was in 1882 by Bernardos (Skriniar, 1986), who used an electric arc struck between carbon electrodes to melt ferrous metals to effect repairs and make joints. The results were often brittle and unsatisfactory because of oxidation and nitrogen absorption from the surrounding air, and consequently arc welding developed only slowly at first. To fill larger gaps, metal wire had to be fed by hand into the molten metal of the weld pool. Early attempts to use the filler metal itself as a 'consumable' electrode, and to strike the arc onto the workpiece, produced poor results, largely because of nitrogen embrittlement (Lancaster, 1980). Electrodes consisting of wire wrapped in paper or asbestos string were found to produce better results (Brillié, 1990), and a range of materials was experimented with as 'flux' coatings. Flux compositions gradually evolved, and the resulting weld quality was improved as minerals were added to act as gas and slag formers, deoxidants and scavengers. A variety of binding agents was used to attach the flux coating to the electrode, but water-glass (sodium and potassium silicates) was quickly discovered to be most effective. By about 1930, the modern welding rod had been developed and weld quality was adequate for many structural and manufacturing purposes. The process came to be known as manual metal arc (MMA) (Morgan, 1989) or shielded metal arc welding (Lancaster, 1980). Throughout the 1930s, asbestos continued to be added to a small proportion of electrodes in the form of powder in the flux mixture, or as asbestos string wrapped around the electrodes. This practice declined after the Second World War and ceased in the 1950s.

Electrical resistance welding was also developed before the turn of the century. This process was found to be relatively immune to the embrittlement problems that usually accompanied early arc welding. Spot welding was developed for fastening thin sheet, and butt welding for joining bars and making chains. These and the related process of seam welding, used for making unbroken joints in sheet metal, were well developed by about 1920 (Lancaster, 1980).

Before 1914, welding was not a common industrial process and was often restricted to repair applications. It received a spur during the First World War in armament manufacture. Later, the car industry, particularly in the USA, adopted resistance welding techniques, and these were taken up for other production line manufacture; however, riveting remained the principal method of joining metal plates in buildings, bridges, ships, tanks and armaments until the late 1930s.

The Second World War provided a major impetus to the heavy manufacturing industry and heralded the widespread adoption of welding technology. Tanks and heavy armaments were built in large numbers using MMA welding, and this method of assembly was also applied to shipbuilding. Early welded ships were prone to catastrophic fractures due to hydrogen embrittlement, but this was overcome in the early 1940s when basic low-hydrogen MMA electrodes were developed (Lancaster, 1980). Other, newer welding processes also found applications in the war years. In 1936, submerged arc welding was patented in the USA (Skriniar, 1986). This differs from the MMA process in that the electrode is in the form of a continuous wire which is driven mechanically into the arc as it melts. A granulated flux is poured from a hopper so that it surrounds the arc region and melts to form a slag layer over the weld metal. This process was used extensively for the manufacture of tanks in the final years of the war. Tungsten inert gas (TIG) welding (gas tungsten arc welding; Lindberg & Braton, 1985), the first successful gas-shielded welding process, was introduced in 1943 (Lancaster, 1980). In this technique, a non-consumable tungsten electrode is used, and the arc is shielded with argon gas delivered by a nozzle which surrounds the electrode. The process was used initially instead of rivets for the assembly of aluminium and magnesium alloy aircraft frames (Skriniar, 1986). When filler metal was required, wire was fed by hand into the weld pool. A variant of TIG welding, developed in the late 1960s, is the plasma arc process, in which some of the shield gas is forced through the arc and ejected as a high velocity jet of ionized gas (plasma). Plasma arcs can be used either for cutting or welding, and higher welding speeds can be achieved than with TIG welding (Lindberg & Braton, 1985).

After the Second World War, welding became the principal means of joining metal throughout the manufacturing, shipbuilding and construction industries, and welding technology research and development accelerated. Metal inert gas (MIG) welding, the first gas-shielded welding process to involve a consumable metal electrode, was put into use in 1948 (Skriniar, 1986). As in submerged arc welding, the wire electrode is driven mechanically into the arc region at the same rate as it is consumed. The arc region is bathed in an inert gas mixture based on argon or helium to protect the molten weld metal from atmospheric gases. Attempts to use cheaper shield gases such a carbon dioxide were not very successful at first because of weld porosities; however, the development of special welding wires containing antioxidants in the early 1950s overcame this problem. As carbon dioxide cannot be described as an inert gas, the new process was referred to as metal active gas (MAG) welding. The terms MIG and MAG are loosely interchangeable, but, as argon- and helium-based shield gases usually contain some oxygen or carbon dioxide, MAG is the more accurate description. In the USA, both MIG and MAG welding are usually referred to as gas metal arc welding (Lindberg & Braton, 1985).

In the late 1950s, tubular electrodes were introduced for semi-automatic welding. Hand-held tubular electrodes had first appeared in the 1920s and were used to a limited extent after the Second World War for oxy-fuel welding. The new 'flux-cored' tubular electrodes were incorporated into MIG-type welding torches with a carbon dioxide shield gas. Their adoption was gradual, but by the mid 1960s the advantage of flux-cored wires over the solid-wire carbon dioxide process was generally appreciated. The flux contents of tubular wires can be used to control oxidation and alloying of the weld metal and gives it more effective protection during cooling. Tubular electrodes that contained gas-forming compounds and could be used without an external shield gas were introduced in the late 1950s. In the 1960s, such 'self-shielded' flux-cored welding wires rapidly gained popularity in the USA, the USSR and Japan but saw only limited use in Europe until the 1970s and 1980s (Widgery, 1988).

Recent developments in welding technology have involved refinements of the existing welding processes and the introduction of new, often more automated processes. Welding power supplies, once little more than heavy transformers and rectifiers, are increasingly sophisticated (Wilkinson, 1988): since the late 1970s, development of transistorized 'solid state' power sources has been dramatic; voltage and current profiles can be computer-programmed to give precise drop-by-drop delivery of weld metal to the weld pool. This can improve weld quality and productivity in MIG welding and related processes. The 1970s and 1980s have witnessed increasing use of electron beam and laser welding and in particular a marked increase in automated and robot welding. The automotive industry has for many years been highly automated, and few welds on motor vehicles are made by human welders. This type of automation is very inflexible and car production lines are usually built for a single product. Robot automation, in contrast, can be highly flexible and can be used for a variety of products. Computer-aided design and manufacture is now increasing, and this will gradually reduce the number of human welders employed in manufacturing industries in countries with advanced economies.

## 1.3 Description of major welding processes

### (a)  Introduction

Despite the many different types of welding process that have been developed, the large majority of welding still involves MMA, MAG, TIG, flux-cored and submerged arc processes (Stern, 1983; Lindberg & Braton, 1985). MMA has been the dominant welding process since the 1930s but is now declining in importance (Wilkinson, 1988). Since the late 1970s, the market for MMA electrodes in Europe has fallen markedly, partly due to the recession in heavy industry and the reduction in shipbuilding and off-shore construction, but also because of increasing use of other welding processes, particularly MIG. Cored wires have been important in the USA since the 1960s and are of rapidly increasing importance in Japan and the newly industrialized nations of the far east (Widgery, 1988).

Although welding is a recognized profession, many other workers, not employed specifically as welders, also carry out some welding. Most welders are familiar with the majority of the common industrial welding processes but usually have extensive work experience with only a few. Most welders have experience with MMA and many are also experienced with MIG. Fewer have much experience with TIG, submerged arc and the many other forms of welding. Some welders use a wide range of processes routinely, while others are employed to specialize in certain welding processes, such as TIG, and many specialize in welding certain types of metal such as stainless-steel and aluminium.

The fabrication of large structures, such as ships and heavy bridge girders, can involve long periods of continuous welding. Small, intricate assemblies require more manipulation of the workpieces and shorter, more intermittent periods of welding. Before a workpiece is welded, it usually requires some preparation including cutting, shaping and grinding of the edges to be joined. Such preparation is not usually carried out by welders; however, they might have to spend time positioning the parts to be joined and tacking them at intervals along the seam prior to welding, again reducing the overall arcing time. The proportion of the working day involved in arcing is sometimes referred to as the 'duty cycle'. Duty cycles rarely exceed 70% of the day and can be very much less. For MMA welding, the average duty cycle rarely exceeds 50% on average, and a figure of 20% is reported to be typical (Widgery, 1986).

The speed with which a weld can be made is determined by many factors, including the rate at which weld metal can be deposited. Metal deposition rates depend upon the type of welding process being used, the welding current, electrode diameter and characteristics, and upon the position of the weld being made. For all welding processes, the highest rates of deposition are achieved when horizontal welds are made from above (downhand welding). Vertical, overhead and other 'positional' welding require lower welding speeds to avoid sagging of the weld metal (Widgery, 1986). It is often necessary to finish the weld by chipping away residual flux or grinding away excess weld metal. Sometimes it is necessary to cut out areas of weld metal that contain flaws such as cracks and flux inclusions. This can be done by grinding, but often an electric arc gouging process is used. The most common of these is arc-air gouging which involves a carbon arc and a compressed air jet to blow away the molten metal.

Welding can be carried out in almost any setting, including under water and in hyperbaric conditions. It is often carried out on benches in engineering workshops, but much structural welding is done outdoors; some assemblies, such as ships, boilers, tanks and pipes, often require welding in confined spaces.

### (b) Manual metal arc welding

MMA (or shielded metal arc) welding equipment is relatively simple, consisting of a heavy source of electric current, such as a transformer, transformer-rectifier or generator, and a simple spring-loaded holder for the electrode (welding rod). A heavy cable carries the current to the electrode holder, and a similar cable provides a return or earth connection which is clamped to the workpiece or to a heavy metal bench on which the workpiece is placed. The welder strikes an electric arc between the tip of the electrode and the workpiece by brief contact and then withdraws the electrode tip several millimetres to maintain an arc gap, which must be adjusted continually as the electrode is consumed. Each electrode must be replaced after only a few minutes. The weld that is produced by the MMA process is covered by a layer of slag resulting from the flux coating on the electrode. This must be removed before the work is completed or before another layer of weld metal can be laid to build up a large joint, usually by use of a chipping hammer. Some types of slag systems are designed to peel off the weld easily, while other types adhere strongly and must be chipped vigorously. This cleaning task further slows the welding operation. The metal deposition rates achieved by MMA welding during continuous arcing are usually in the range 1-3 kg/h, although higher rates can be achieved with some electrodes. MMA electrodes in a wide range dimensions and compositions are available for welding different types of metal and for obtaining different mechanical and corrosion resistant properties. Most metals are welded with electrodes of similar composition; for example, stainless-steel electrodes are used to weld stainless-steel components. A notable exception to this general rule is the use of nickel consumables to weld cast iron. Three types of MMA flux system are commonly used: cellulosic — containing mostly cellulose, rutile (titanium dioxide) sand and magnesium silicate; rutile — containing mostly rutile sand and calcium carbonate plus a small amount of cellulose; and basic — containing mostly calcium carbonate. Many other ingredients are added to fluxes, including calcium fluoride (Brillié, 1990), sodium and potassium silicates and iron powder (Lancaster, 1980).

### (c) Metal inert gas welding

MIG/MAG (or gas metal arc) welding equipment is considerably more complicated than MMA equipment and consists of a special power source, an automatic wire feed unit and a gas-shielded welding torch. The welding wire is stored coiled on a drum and is fed automatically to the welding torch by a 'wire feed unit'. The power source is usually a 'constant potential' transformer-rectifier designed to provide a welding current proportional to the rate of consumption of the welding wire. A heavy cable carries the current to the torch, where it is delivered to the welding wire by a tubular copper 'contact tip' through which the wire passes. A heavy return cable is used, as in the MMA process. The power supply is activated by a trigger-like switch on the torch, and the arc is struck between the wire tip and the workpiece after a brief contact. At the same time, the shield gas flow and the wire feed unit are activated. Shield gases may be based on carbon dioxide, argon or helium; pure inert gases are rarely used as they do not result in a stable arc, and shield gases usually contain small amounts of carbon dioxide or oxygen. Because the welding wire must be replaced only occasionally and there is no slag to remove from the weld, duty cycles for MIG welding may be considerably longer than for MMA. Metal deposition rates may also be higher — from about 1 to 10 kg/h or more (Widgery, 1988). Some welding torches are water cooled to permit continuous operation at high power.

### (d)  Flux-cored wire welding

Flux-cored wire welding involves almost the same type of equipment as MIG welding, and the processes are technically similar. Self-shielded tubular electrodes do not need a shield gas, but a shield gas must be used for those flux-cored wires that do not contain gas-forming agents. In Japan, carbon dioxide is the gas most commonly used for this purpose, whereas in Europe argon-rich gas mixtures are preferred. The slag layer that is left on the weld is usually self-detaching or is relatively easy to detach mechanically. Flux-cored wires are easier to use in vertical welds because the slag can help to support the molten weld metal. Duty cycles are comparable with those of MIG welding, but weld metal deposition rates can be higher, particularly in positional welding. Deposition rates considerably in excess of 10 kg/h are possible in downhand welding (Widgery, 1988). A variety of fluxes is used in tubular electrodes including many (such as rutile sand) that are used in MMA electrodes. Self-shielded tubular electrodes frequently contain barium carbonate or barium fluoride (Dare *et al.*, 1984), but these are not usually found in gas-shielded flux-cored welding wires.

### (e)  Tungsten inert gas welding

TIG (or gas tungsten arc) welding involves use of a gas-shielded welding torch with a tungsten electrode. As the melting-point of tungsten is nearly 3500°C, the electrode does not melt during welding, provided that a high frequency alternating current is used or that a negative electrode is used in direct current welding. The arc region is shielded by argon, helium or a mixture of the two. The TIG process can be used for spot welding, or a filler wire can be used to produce larger welds. In simple TIG welding, a filler wire can be fed by hand into the molten weld pool. To obtain higher rates of metal deposition, mechanical wire feed units are used similar to those used in the MIG process. Higher heat inputs can be obtained by attaching a second power supply to deliver current to the filler wire. This process, sometimes referred to as 'hot wire TIG' is in fact a combination of the TIG and MIG processes (Lindberg & Braton, 1985). TIG welding gives high quality welds and is suitable for a wide range of metals including stainless-steel, aluminium, magnesium alloys and titanium.

### (f)   Submerged arc welding

In the submerged arc process, the welding arc and the still molten weld metal are entirely buried in granulated flux. The welding wire is delivered mechanically by a wire feed unit mounted directly above the welding torch, and the flux is fed continuously from a hopper ahead of the advancing arc. Loose flux granules are usually recovered by a vacuum attachment which follows the torch and recycled to the flux hopper. The welding torch, wire feed unit, flux hopper and vacuum unit are all mounted on a carriage which travels on wheels along the length of the weld. Metal deposition rates of several tens of kilograms per hour can be attained with a single torch and wire feed unit. Sometimes, several wires are used in line to give multiple weld layers at one pass. Submerged arc welding is almost automatic, and the welders' task is to set up the equipment to make each joint and to ensure weld quality with minimal intervention. Because the equipment must be repositioned to make each weld, the overall duty cycle is reduced; however, metal deposition rates can be very high, particularly if multiple wires are used.

### 1.4  Number and distribution of welders

A comparison of the industrial economies of the world suggests that there might be of the order of 3 million workers worldwide who perform some welding. In the USA, more than 185 000 workers are employed as welders, brazers or thermal cutters, and it is estimated that up to 700 000 US workers carry out some welding during their work (National Institute for Occupational Safety and Health, 1988).

The balance of different welding processes is difficult to estimate, partly because manufacturers do not publish figures of sales of welding equipment and materials. Such figures are available for Sweden in 1974 (Ulfvarson, 1981), and these are summarized in Table 1. Approximately 22% of Swedish welders were reported to be stainless-steel welders. This is a higher proportion than in countries of the European Economic Community, as the average for France, the Federal Republic of Germany, Spain and the UK was about 10% prior to 1979; and the proportion is even lower in less developed countries (Stern, 1980a).

In western Europe, MIG welding has a greater market share than in the USA because it usually allows greater productivity than MMA welding, since fewer welders are needed to lay the same amount of weld metal. This affects estimates not only

**Table 1. Distribution of Swedish welders by process and material in 1974[a]**

| Process[b] | Material | | | | |
|---|---|---|---|---|---|
| | Total | Mild–steel | Stainless–steel | Aluminium | Other |
| MMA | 25 585 | 16 854 | 5 896 | 1 496 | 1 339 |
| MIG + MAG | 9 143 | 6 232 | 1 594 | 1 141 | 176 |
| TIG | 4 216 | 1 547 | 1 529 | 913 | 233 |
| Gas | 3 823 | 2 762 | 479 | 325 | 257 |
| Submerged arc | 783 | 540 | 210 | 32 | 1 |
| Total | 43 550 | 27 935 | 9 708 | 3 907 | 2 006 |

[a]From Ulfvarson (1981)
[b]MMA, manual metal arc; MIG, metal inert gas; TIG, tungsten inert gas

of total numbers of welders but also of the relative importance of different welding processes. Sales of MMA electrodes in the major economies represent about 46% by weight of the total for all consumables. In terms of weld metal sales, i.e. excluding the weight of flux, MMA represents about 41% of the total. Assuming weld metal deposition rates of 3 kg/h for MMA and 7 kg/h for MIG welding, MMA must represent about two-thirds of welding in terms of arcing time. Furthermore, as the duty cycle for MMA might be only about half that for semi-automatic processes, MMA welding might represent about 80% of welders' payroll time (Jefferson, 1988).

Many types of metal are welded, including stainless-steel, high chromium armour plate, aluminium, copper and nickel; however, the large majority of welding is on mild and low alloy steels. Stainless-steel represents only about 4-5% of MMA electrode sales and about 3% of MAG and TIG wire sales in western Europe. Similarly, about 2-3% of MAG and TIG wire sales are aluminium.

## 2. Welding Fumes and Gases

### 2.1 Introduction

Welders are exposed to a variety of airborne contaminants arising from the welding process and other operations in the work place. In the literature, the term 'welding fume' is applied variously to some or all of the emissions from welding. In this monograph, the term is applied only to the particulate emissions intrinsic to the various welding processes, to distinguish these from gaseous emissions. Incidental particulate emissions, for example, from the pyrolysis of paint on metal being welded, are excluded from this definition.

The chemical composition and physical properties of welding fumes and gases and details of occupational exposures of welders in the work place have been reviewed (American Welding Society, 1973; Ulfvarson, 1981; Tinkler, 1983; Stern, R.M. *et al.*, 1986; National Institute for Occupational Safety and Health, 1988). The aerosol contains contributions from a number of sources: (*a*) vaporization of the wire, rod or metallic/alloying coatings; (*b*) decomposition and vaporization of the flux materials; (*c*) spatter from the arc region and weld pool and fumes therefrom; and (*d*) evaporation from the molten weld metal.

The consumable is the major source of fume, the workpiece making only a minor contribution unless it bears a surface coating.

The elemental composition of a welding aerosol reflects the composition of the consumable used, while the relative abundance of the elements in the aerosol is a function of the physics and chemistry of the arc and geometry of the weld: low-melting-point metals are relatively enriched in the fume (Mn by a factor of 2-6, Cu and Pb by a factor of 3-5), while the more refractory metals are depleted by factors of e.g., 0.07-0.5 for Fe, 0.2-0.7 for Cr and 0.03-0.4 for Ni (when present) (see e.g., Malmqvist *et al.* 1986).

Potential occupational exposure to fumes from a given consumable can be estimated by combining information on the relative elemental abundance of the aerosol, as determined from a chemical analysis of welding fumes produced in the laboratory under controlled conditions, with the total aerosol concentration expected on the basis of work-place measurements. Actual elemental exposures can be determined on the basis of fume samples collected at the work place by stationary samplers placed on the shop floor or by personal samplers placed in the breathing zone. Detailed descriptions of standard sampling methods have been proposed by a number of sources (e.g., American Welding Society, 1973; British Standards Institution, 1986), and the general characteristics of welding fumes have been studied under controlled conditions (e.g., American Welding Society, 1973; Evans *et al.*, 1979; Mayer & Salsi, 1980). Although a welder usually works for long periods with a single type of consumable, changing conditions may result in variations in the chemical composition of the fume with time over a working shift. In addition, the presence of other process applications in the vicinity contributes to the chemical composition of the background: under certain conditions, e.g., TIG (see below), the background may contribute significantly to the fume collected in the breathing zone, although typically the background fume concentration as measured with stationary samplers is about one-tenth that found in the breathing zone (Ulfvarson, 1981). Hence, the presence of specific elements determined by chemical analysis of samples obtained in the work place may not be corroborated by laboratory measurements of nominally the same welding process.

Each consumable produces a unique fume in terms of elemental composition (see, e.g., Mayer & Salsi, 1980), particle size distribution and identifiable stoichiometric compounds (see, e.g., Fasiska *et al.*, 1983). Since there are thousands of different consumables, the only way to review data on composition and exposure derived from laboratory and work-place measurements is by use of tables of ranges of elemental concentration for very general classes of processes, applications and consumables. This technique has the disadvantage that one cannot determine from the tables the actual composition of a specific welding fume; on the other hand, since welders use many consumables during a working week, their actual exposure is properly reflected in the logarithm of the median values so obtained.

Not only particulate matter but also a wide range of gaseous pollutants is produced by welding, either through decomposition of compounds in the flux coating or core of the consumable or through oxidation, dissociation or other chemical reactions in the air mixed into the arc or surrounding the arc region.

Estimates of exposure to potentially toxic gases (ozone, carbon monoxide, nitrogen oxides) based on production rates measured in the laboratory may be unreliable because of the influence of local ventilation and work-place design on the actual concentrations found in the welders' breathing zone. Determination of occupational exposures to gases must be based on work-place measurements.

## 2.2 Chemical composition and physical properties of welding fumes

### (a) Elemental composition

Fasiska *et al.* (1983) identified 38 individual types of covered electrodes (MMA/steel) and 20 classes of MIG/Al fume, the fumes from which contain one or more elements in high abundance. The detailed chemical composition of a number of classes of welding fume are summarized in Table 2. The range (when available) of elemental distributions is given, together with an indication of the analytical method used. Fumes for chemical analysis are typically produced in a 'fume box', standards for which have been reviewed recently (Moreton, 1986).

A description of work-place exposures and the chemistry of welding fumes can be considerably simplified by recognizing that each couplet of process technology-application represents a source of a broad class of welding fume that is similar in constituents if not in concentration. Three major process technologies (MMA, MIG/MAG, TIG) applied to two classes of metal (mild steel (MS) and stainless steel (SS)), plus a few additional couplets (e.g., MIG/Al), however, account for perhaps 80% of all exposures in welding (Stern, 1983). In addition, MIG/Ni and MMA/Ni processes, with wire or electrodes (i.e., consumables) containing high levels of nickel, are used on cast iron and low-alloy steel. MIG/MAG processes produce fume with components from the metal/alloy wire alone, while fume from flux-producing

**Table 2. Average or range (%) of elemental distribution of welding fumes by type**

| Element | Manual metal arc fume | | Metal inert gas fume | | Method[a] | Reference |
|---|---|---|---|---|---|---|
| | Mild steel | Stainless steel | Mild steel | Stainless steel | | |
| Si | 2.7–8.1 | 2.9–5.6 | 1.6–3.3 | 0.9 | XRF | Mayer & Salsi (1980) |
| | – | 10 | – | 1.7 | XRF | Moreton et al. (1986) |
| F | 7–14 | 16–24 | ND | ND | PIXE | Malmqvist et al. (1986) |
| | – | 14.9 | – | – | XRF | Moreton et al. (1986) |
| | 0.6–17 | 7–11.5 | 0.05–14 | – | XRF | Mayer & Salsi (1980) |
| Cl | ND–0.54 | ND–0.34 | ND | ND | PIXE | Malmqvist et al. (1986) |
| K | 9–19 | 18–22 | ND | ND | PIXE | Malmqvist et al. (1986) |
| | – | 19.9 | – | <0.1 | XRF | Moreton et al. (1986) |
| | 5.1–15 | 8.7–15.4 | 0.11–5.7 | – | XRF | Mayer & Salsi (1980) |
| Ca | 0.62–2.6 | 1.3–10 | ND | ND | PIXE | Malmqvist et al. (1986) |
| | – | 0.4 | – | <0.2 | XRF | Moreton et al.(1986) |
| | 0.09–10.8 | 3.8–6.8 | 0.01–13.6 | – | XRF | Mayer & Salsi (1980) |
| Ti | ND–0.54 | 0.62–2.3 | ND | ND | PIXE | Malmqvist et al. (1986) |
| | – | 2.1 | – | 0.1 | XRF | Moreton et al. (1986) |
| | 0.6–2.4 | 7.7–12.7 | 0.006–2.8 | – | XRF | Mayer & Salsi (1980) |
| Cr | ND–0.07 | 3.0–3.4 | 0.07 | 10–12 | PIXE | Malmqvist et al. (1986) |
| | – | 5.0 | – | 13.4 | XRF | Moreton et al. (1986) |
| | 0.11–0.7 | 6.5–9.2 | 0.2–0.6 | – | XRF | Mayer & Salsi (1980) |
| Mn | 2.8–5.9 | 2.4–14 | 7.3 | 4.8–5.3 | PIXE | Malmqvist et al. (1986) |
| | – | 5.0 | – | 12.6 | XRF | Moreton et al. (1986) |
| | 2.7–5.6 | 4.3–5.0 | 3.9–7.0 | – | XRF | Mayer & Salsi (1980) |
| Fe | 11–32 | 3.3–3.7 | 45 | 28–31 | PIXE | Malmqvist et al. (1986) |
| | – | 5.1 | – | 33.3 | XRF | Moreton et al. (1986) |
| | 14.4–31.8 | 6.0–15.9 | 33–55 | – | XRF | Mayer & Salsi (1980) |
| Ni | ND | 0.22–0.44 | ND | 4.5–4.8 | PIXE | Malmqvist et al. (1986) |
| | – | 0.4 | – | 4.9 | XRF | Moreton et al. (1986) |
| | 0.01–0.32 | 0.48–2.9 | 0.01–0.06 | – | XRF | Mayer & Salsi (1980) |
| Cu | ND–0.08 | ND–0.01 | 0.26 | 0.06–0.09 | PIXE | Malmqvist et al. (1986) |
| | – | <0.1 | – | 0.6 | XRF | Moreton et al. (1986) |
| | 0.04–0.24 | 0.09–0.14 | 0.01–0.18 | – | XRF | Mayer & Salsi (1980) |
| Zn | 0.04–0.29 | 0.11–0.25 | 0.04 | 0.17–0.18 | PIXE | Malmqvist et al. (1986) |
| | 0.04–0.07 | 0.007–0.10 | 0.08–0.40 | – | XRF | Mayer & Salsi (1980) |

**Table 2 (contd)**

| Element | Manual metal arc fume | | Metal inert gas fume | | Method[a] | Reference |
|---|---|---|---|---|---|---|
| | Mild steel | Stainless steel | Mild steel | Stainless steel | | |
| As | ND–0.06 | ND | ND | ND | PIXE | Malmqvist et al. (1986) |
| | 0.005–0.05 | 0.003–0.01 | 0.009–0.12 | – | XRF | Mayer & Salsi (1980) |
| Rb | ND | ND–0.02 | ND | ND | PIXE | Malmqvist et al. (1986) |
| Zr | ND–0.54 | ND | ND | ND | PIXE | Malmqvist et al. (1986) |
| Mo | ND | ND–0.09 | ND | 0.92–0.95 | PIXE | Malmqvist et al. (1986) |
| | – | <0.02 | – | 0.6 | XRF | Moreton et al. (1986) |
| | 0.005–0.3 | 0.2–1.4 | 0.1–0.2 | – | XRF | Mayer & Salsi (1980) |
| Pb | <0.07 | ND–0.04 | ND | ND | PIXE | Malmqvist et al. (1986) |
| | 0.03–0.28 | 0.08–0.55 | 0.05–0.22 | – | XRF | Mayer & Salsi (1980) |

[a]XRF, X-ray fluorescent spectrometry; PIXE, proton–induced X–ray spectrometry; –, no data; ND, not detected

processes (flux-cored electrode welding, MMA) contains significant contributions from the vaporization and decomposition of the flux-forming components of the filler or coating. For simplicity, the following list indicates the elements that occur in more than trace (i.e., 1%) quantities in the respective fumes of general–purpose electrodes:

| | |
|---|---|
| MIG/Al | Al |
| MIG/Ni | Ni, Fe |
| MIG-MAG/MS | Fe, Mn, Si |
| MIG-MAG/SS | Fe, Mn, Cr, Ni |
| MIG/MS | Fe, Mn, Si, K |
| MMA/Ni | Ni, Fe, Ba |
| MMA/MS | Fe, Mn, Ca, K, Si, F, Ti |
| MMA/SS | Fe, Mn, Ca, Si, F, K, Ti, Cr, Ni |

In addition to the elements listed above and in Table 2, many other trace elements (e.g., Ag, Ga, Nb, Se, Sn, Sr) have been identified in special-purpose welding fumes (Pedersen et al., 1987).

*(b)   Oxidation state of chromium*

Considerable attention has been given to the oxidation state of chromium in welding fumes. (See Pedersen et al., 1987, for a recent review.) The only soluble species of chromium in welding fumes is Cr[VI]. (For a discussion of the definition of solubility for Cr[VI] compounds, see p. 55 of the monograph on chromium, and the General Remarks, pp. 42-43). Table 3 gives information on the solubility and oxidation state of chromium in MMA/SS, MIG/SS and TIG/SS welding fumes. For all practical purposes, the (long-term) insoluble Cr[VI] content of SS welding fumes is less than 0.5% and is more typically of the order of 0.2-0.3%, and is thus negligible from the point of view of exposure. The high Cr[VI] content of MMA fumes is attributed to the presence of alkaline metals in the flux coating; hence, flux cord electrode fume resembles MMA fume with regard to chromium chemistry due to the presence of the flux forming materials in the core, although the technique resembles MIG. Numerous attempts have been made to alter the Cr[VI] content of MMA/SS fume; in a recent approach, potassium was replaced by sodium in a modified electrode (Kobayashi & Tsutsumi, 1986), resulting in a significant reduction in the relative Cr[VI] content (see below).

The concentration of Cr[VI] and the Cr[VI]/Cr (total) ratio in MIG(MAG)/SS welding fumes has been the subject of considerable discussion. Stern *et al.* (1984) showed that collection of MIG/SS fume in an impinger can result in fixation of 30% and more of the total Cr as Cr[VI] (compared to a maximum of 3% in membrane-collected fumes). The Cr[VI]:Cr(total) is heavily dependent on welding parameters (current, voltage, arc length) and time after welding (Thomsen & Stern, 1979; Stern, 1983). Maximal concentrations of Cr[VI] occur after about 10 s and then fall by about a factor of 3 within 3 min (Hewitt & Madden, 1986).

Occupational exposure to Cr[VI] also occurs in stainless-steel processes other than welding. Sawatari and Serita (1986) showed that the fumes from plasma spraying contain 27% Cr[VI]. Flame spraying, electric arc spraying and plasma spraying of additives containing mixtures of Fe, Cr and Ni produced fumes with approximately 6-8% Cr, of which 22-69% was Cr[VI] (Malmqvist *et al.*, 1981).

A problem with respect to chromium speciation has been lack of standardized collection and analytical methods. Reduction of fume during dry membrane collection and reduction or oxidation of fume during analysis could lead to under- or over-reporting of Cr[VI] concentrations (Pedersen *et al.*, 1987).

### (c)  Crystalline materials

Chemical analysis of welding fume is usually based on methods which allow determination only of the elemental content. Frequently, composition is given in terms of the putative oxide (e.g., $Fe_2O_3$, $Fe_3O_4$, $CrO_3$) although such assignment of compound is not justified without additional crystallographic evidence. Recently, a number of authors have begun to investigate the presence of crystallographic compounds in a range of welding fumes.

Fasiska *et al.* (1983) found $Fe_3O_4$, $(Fe, Mn)_3O_4$, $KF-CaF_2$, $CaF_2$, $MnFe_2O_4$, $(Fe,Cu)Fe_2O_4$, $K_2CrO_4$, $K_2FeO_8$, NaF, $K_2FeO_4$, $K_2(Cr,Fe)O_4$, $(Fe,Ni)Fe_2O_4$ and

Table 3. Distribution (%) of chromium by oxidation state and solubility and of nickel as a function of type of welding fume

| Type of fume[a] | Cr (total) | Cr[VI] | | | Cr[VI]: Cr (total) | Cr[VI] soluble: Cr (total) | Ni (total) | Reference |
|---|---|---|---|---|---|---|---|---|
| | | Total | Soluble | Insoluble | | | | |
| MMA/SS | 2.9–4.4 | – | 1.5–3.2 | <0.5–0.92 | – | 0.50–0.73 | 0.22–0.44 | Malmqvist et al. (1986) |
| MMA/SS | 5.0 | 4.1 | 3.8 | 0.3 | 0.82 | – | 0.4 | Moreton et al. (1986) |
| MMA/SS | 3.0–5.3 | 1.8–3.9 | – | – | 0.36–1.0 | – | 0.3–1.3 | Eichhorn & Oldenburg (1986) |
| MMA/SS (modified)[b] | 4.9–7.3[c] | – | 4.4–5.4 | 0.4–1.8 | – | 0.74–0.91 | 0.03–0.6[d] | Kobayashi & Tsutsumi (1986) |
| | 11.4 | – | 0.66 | 11.2 | – | 0.056 | 0.9 | |
| MMA/SS | 2.4–6.4 | – | 2.2–4.3 | 0.03–0.42 | – | 0.7–0.9 | 0.38–1.9 | Stern (1980b) |
| MMA/Ni[e] | 0.02 | – | – | – | – | – | 1.4 | Stern (1980b) |
| MIG/SS | 12 | – | 0.23 | <2 | – | 0.019 | 4.5 | Malmqvist et al. (1986) |
| MIG/SS | 13.4 | – | 0.2 | <0.1 | – | 0.015 | 4.9 | Moreton et al. (1986) |
| MIG/SS | 4.1–15.6 | 0.02–2.9 | – | 0.01–0.42 | 0.005–0.19[f] | – | 3.5–6.7 | Stern (1980b) |
| FCW/SS | 5.1 | 2.7 | 2.5 | 0.2 | 0.53 | – | 1.3 | Moreton et al. (1986) |
| MIG/Ni | 0.04 | – | <0.004 | 0.04 | – | – | 53–60 | Stern (1980b) |

[a]MMA, manual metal arc; SS, stainless steel; MIG, metal inert gas; FCW, flux-cored electrode
[b]Covering comprises modified lime–titania
[c]Total $Cr_2O_3$
[d]Total NiO
[e][Ba = 40%; 6% water-soluble]
[f][Impinger collection]

$PbCrO_4$ in a wide range of MMA fumes; and Kobayashi and Tsutsumi (1986) found the following compounds in different MMA welding fumes:

| | |
|---|---|
| Non-lime MMA/MS | $Fe_3O_4$, $MnFe_2O_4$, $Fe_2O_3$ |
| Lime-type MMA/MS | $K_2CO_3$, $Fe_3O_4$, $MnFe_2O_4$, NaF, $CaF_2$, $KCaF_3$, KCl (and MgO and $Na_2CO_3$ in a modified type) |
| MMA/SS | $K_2CrO_4$, $Fe_3O_4$. NaF, $CaF_2$, $Na_2CrO_4$ (and LiF in a modified type) |

Combined X-ray diffraction analysis and Mössbauer spectroscopy showed that Fe in welding fume occurs as $\alpha$-Fe (metallic) as well as in an iron oxide spinel ($Fe_3O_4$) with some degree of impurities and imperfection. MIG/MS and MIG/SS welding fumes contained approximately 7% $\alpha$-Fe and 12% $\gamma$-Fe, respectively (Stern *et al.*, 1987). Although welding fumes contain considerable amounts of silicium in oxidized form, the presence of crystalline silica has not been reported; only amorphous silica is observed (Mayer & Salsi, 1980), presumably because the physical/ chemical conditions for the formation of crystalline silica are not met during welding (Fasiska *et al.*, 1983; Kobayashi & Tsutsumi, 1986; Stern *et al.*, 1987). Previously asbestos and currently clays are used to provide elemental Al, Mg and Si; however, these originally crystalline materials are decomposed in the high temperature of the arc, and corresponding crystalline substances do not appear in the fumes.

*(d)   Physical properties*

The most important physical characteristic of welding fumes is their particulate size distribution, as this property determines the degree to which fumes are respirable and how they are deposited within the respiratory tract. Aerodynamic mass median diameters of welding fumes have been determined with cascade impactors; typical values are as follows: MMA fumes: 0.35-0.6 µm for total fume (Malmqvist *et al.* 1986); 0.23-0.52 µm aerodynamic diameter (Eichhorn & Oldenberg, 1986); 0.2 µm for metallic parts (Mn, Fe) and 2.0 µm for slag components (Ca) (Stern, 1982); MIG fumes: <0.2 µm (Stern, 1980b) and 0.11-0.23 µm aerodynamic diameter (Eichhorn & Oldenburg, 1986). Stern *et al.* (1984) and Malmqvist *et al.* (1986) showed by means of electron spectroscopy for chemical analysis and transmission electron microscopy that the outer layers of the amorphous matrix of MMA/SS fume particles are soluble in water and contain only Cr[VI]. With most digestion procedures, there is almost always an insoluble residue consisting of refractory cores from MIG/SS fume (Pedersen *et al.*, 1987). Transmission electrom microscopy showed that the particles of MIG fumes can be very crystalline and tend to form long chains, clusters and rafts, most of which, however, break up in solution (Stern, 1979; Grekula *et al.*, 1986; Farrants *et al.*, 1988). For MMA fumes, the situation is complex, since there are several sources of the aerosol. Slag particles make up a separate aerosol with a relatively large median diameter, and a certain fraction consists of particles similar to those found in MIG fumes. A third class of particles consist of an amorphous matrix containing droplets of metal-rich material, which in turn can contain a large number of crystalline precipitates, mostly of an impure, imperfect iron oxide (magnetic) spinel (Stern *et al.*, 1984).

Studies using energy dispersive analysis of X-rays in the electron microscope (Stern, 1979; Minni *et al.*, 1984; Grekula *et al.*, 1986; Gustafsson *et al.* 1986) show that individual particles, especially of MMA fume, can have widely varying chemistry; the particles of MIG fumes may be somewhat more homogeneous, the average particle chemistry resembling that of the fume.

Studies of the chemistry of fumes collected in liquid-filled impingers indicate that the elemental distribution varies as a function of particle size (Stern *et al.*, 1984).

### 2.3 Occupational exposures of welders

Exposures of welders that have been evaluated for carcinogenicity in previous IARC Monographs are listed in Table 4.

#### (a) *Exposures to welding fumes*

Occupational exposures in the welding industry have been measured for decades. Ambient concentrations of welding fumes are determined by the rates of formation of fume during the process and the extent of ventilation. Steady-state concentrations of fumes in work-room/work-space air are determined by the ratio of fume formation rate (in mg/s) to the ventilation rate ($m^3$/s). In small, confined spaces with poor ventilation, the concentration increases with time: a single welder working with a process producing 10 mg/s of fume in a ship double-bottom section or container with a volume of 10 $m^3$ will be exposed to an environment containing 60 mg/$m^3$ fume after 1 min of arcing time. Typical 4-mm diameter electrodes produce 0.5-4 g total fume and have a burning time of 30-45 s. In most contemporary shops in industrialized countries, ventilation rates are designed to maintain the background level well below 5-10 mg/$m^3$; present levels usually average 2-4 mg/$m^3$ and have been decreasing by a factor of two per decade since the 1940s, as can be seen from a comparison of recent data with measurements of working place concentrations in the 1960s (e.g., Caccuri & Fournier, 1969).

In order to compare fume production from different welding techniques, two entities can be defined — total fume emission rate, E (g/min), and the relative fume formation index, R, which is the total mass of emitted fume standardized to the mass of the deposited consumable (excluding slag) in mg/g (Malmqvist *et al.*, 1986).

**Table 4. Occupational exposures of welders, other than to nickel and chromium compounds (evaluated elsewhere in this volume) that were evaluated for carcinogenicity in *IARC Monographs* Volumes 1–48**

| Agent | Degree of evidence for carcinogenicity[a] | | Overall evaluation[a] | Occurrence |
|-------|-------|--------|-------|-------|
| | Human | Animal | | |
| Lead and lead compounds | | | | Welding fumes from special-purpose electrodes |
|   Inorganic | I | S | 2B | |
| Arsenic and arsenic compounds | S | L | 1* | Impurity in some mild stainless-steel welding fumes |
| Asbestos | S | S | 1 | Insulation material, e.g., in shipyards |
| Toluene | I | I | 3 | Welding fumes from painted steel |
| Xylene | I | I | 3 | Welding fumes from painted steel |
| Phenol | I | I | 3 | Welding fumes from painted steel |
| Benzene | S | S | 1 | Welding fumes from painted steel |
| 1,4–Dioxane | I | S | 2B | Welding fumes from painted steel |
| Formaldehyde | L | S | 2A | Welding fumes from painted steel |
| Acetaldehyde | I | S | 2B | Welding fumes from painted steel |
| Acrolein | I | I | 3 | Welding fumes from painted steel |
| Methyl methacrylate | ND | I | 3 | Welding fumes from painted steel |

[a]S, sufficient evidence; L, limited evidence; I, inadequate evidence, ND, no adequate data. For definitions of the overall evaluations, see Preamble, pp. 36-37.

*This evaluation applies to the group of chemicals as a whole and not necessarily to all individual chemicals within the group.

For a particular welding technique and typical welding parameters, the rate of fume formation does not vary by more than a factor of 3 from the average. In MMA, the amount of fume produced per electrode is independent of the current but roughly proportional to the length of the arc, and hence welding voltage. Poor welding technique can result in twice the fume production per rod. The burn time of an electrode is inversely proportional to the current, so welding at twice the current produces twice the fume formation rate (see Stern, 1977; Malmqvist *et al.*, 1986). Under most open and shipyard conditions, exposure is determined by the relationship between the position of the welder's face mask and the rising plume; typically, the mask effectively reduces exposure by a factor of 3-6 (American Welding Society, 1973).

One way of describing welders' exposures is to present data in terms of cumulative distribution curves for various welding processes. Stern (1980a) generalized the data for Swedish and Danish workplaces (Ulfvarson *et al.*, 1978a,b,c; Ulfvarson,

1979, 1981) and found that the median reported 8-h TWA total dust concentration in the breathing zone was 10 mg/m³ for MIG/Al; that for MMA and MIG processes was 1.5-10 mg/m³. Within the 10-90% range, the distribution curves are parallel: the 90% limit is typically four times greater than the 50% value. Ulfvarson (1986) reviewed many of the general principles that relate to fume concentrations and pointed out that actual fume formation rates are quite similar in different welding processes (with the exception of TIG) and that most of the variation comes from differences in arcing time, which can be as low as 20% for certain MMA operations requiring considerable work-piece preparation, and close to 85% for certain MIG operations. Rutile electrodes emit higher fume concentrations than do basic electrodes, and, with the exception of ozone formation during MIG welding, working postures do not affect fume emissions from mild steel. General ventilation affects exposure considerably: low ventilation rates in the winter lead to a strong seasonal variation (by a factor of 2-3) in Scandinavian work places. Local exhaust, on average, reduces fume concentrations by only 58% in MMA welding and 35% in MIG welding, and by much less if not used properly (close to the arc) or if poorly maintained (Ulfvarson, 1986).

An indication of the range of exposures to total particles was provided by Ulfvarson (1981): the 50% and 90% exposures (in mg/m³) were: TIG/Al, 1 and 4; MIG/Al, 9 and 43; MMA/SS, 4 and 10; TIG/SS, 2 and 6; MMA/Ni, 2 and 10; MMA/MS, 10 and 28; MIG(MAG)/MS, 7 and 18; and MIG/SS, 2 and 5. Most of the results of studies in factories and shipyards are in agreement with the upper limits, as can be seen in Tables 5 and 6. Table 5 also shows total chromium, hexavalent chromium and nickel concentrations in various stainless-steel welding processes. The concentration of hexavalent chromium (mostly water-soluble) ranged from 25 to 1550 µg/m³ in MMA/SS, from < 1 µg/m³ to < 20 µg/m³ in MIG/SS and was ≤1– < 6 µg/m³ in TIG/SS. The nickel levels were 10 to 970 µg/m³, 30 to < 570 µg/m³ and 10 to < 70 µg/m³, respectively. Higher levels of chromium and nickel occur during special process applications and during welding in confined spaces. The levels of other air contaminants are summarized in Tables 5-7 for mild-steel and stainless-steel welding.

(b)   *Biological monitoring of exposure* (see also pp. 484-485)

(i)   *Chromium*

Both blood and urine levels of chromium are found to be elevated in stainless-steel welders compared to control populations (Gylseth *et al.*, 1977; Tola *et al.*, 1977; Kalliomäki *et al.*, 1981; Rahkonen *et al.*, 1983; Sjögren *et al.*, 1983a; Welinder *et al.*, 1983; Littorin *et al.*, 1984; Cavalleri & Minoia, 1985; Gustavsson & Welinder, 1986; Schaller *et al.*, 1986). Typical levels of chromium in biological fluids of stainless-steel welders are presented in Table 8.

**Table 5. Occupational exposures within the stainless-steel welding industry by process and application (average and/or range)**

| Reference (country) | Process[a] | Total fume (mg/m³) | Total Cr (μg/m³) | Cr[VI] (μg/m³) or % of total Cr | Ni (μg/m³) | Cu (μg/m³) |
|---|---|---|---|---|---|---|
| Åkesson & Skerfving (1985) (Sweden) | MMA/SS | - | 101 (26-220) | - | 440 (70-970) | - |
| van der Wal (1985) (Netherlands) | MMA/SS | 2-40 | 30-1600 | 25-1550 | 10-210 | - |
| | MIG/SS | 1.5-3 | 60 | <1 | 30 | - |
| | TIG/SS[b] | 0.8-4.2 | 10-55 | <1 | 10-40 | - |
| | Background | 0.5-1.2 | - | - | - | - |
| | TIG/Monel | 1.3-5 | - | - | 330 | 215 |
| | MMA,TIG/Cu-Ni-Fe | 0.6-5.5 | - | - | 20-120 | 40-320 |
| Froats & Mason (1986)[b] (Canada) | MIG/SS (1st plant) | 0.3-2.25 | - | 0.1-0.6 | - | - |
| | MIG/SS (2nd plant) | 0.67-8.32 | 8-37 | 1-3.4 | - | - |
| | SS grinders | 1.6-21.6 | 17-108 | 1-3 | - | - |
| Coenen et al. (1985, 1986) (German Democratic Republic) | MMA/SS[b] | 90%, <13.4 | 90%, <350 | 90%, <400 | 90%, <240 | - |
| | Small MMA/SS | - | 90%, <210 | 90%, <30 | 90%, <70 | - |
| | Large MMA/SS | - | 90%, <1200 | 90%, <980 | 90%, <570 | - |
| | Background | 90%, <8 | 90%, <170 | 90%, <60 | 90%, <220 | - |
| | TIG/SS[b] | 90%, <5.4 | 90%, <40 | 90%, <6 | 90%, <70 | - |
| | Background | 90%, <1 | 90%, <40 | 90%, <2 | 90%, <26 | - |
| | MIG/SS[b] | 90%, <12.8 | 90%, <190 | 90%, <20 | 90%, <160 | - |
| | Background | 90%, <3.5 | 90%, <80 | 90%, <10 | 90%, <80 | - |
| | MAG/SS[b] | 90%, <41 | 90%, <340 | 90%, <30 | 90%, <190 | - |
| | Background | 90%, <14.4 | 90%, <30 | 90%, <3 | 90%, <20 | - |
| Ulfvarson et al. (1978b) (Sweden) | MMA/SS | 75%, <6.3 | 75%, 400 | 98% | 75%, <40 | - |
| | Background | 75%, <4 | 75%, <50 | 11.5% | 75%, <22 | - |
| | MIG/SS | 75%, <2.65 | 75%, <94 | - | - | - |
| | Background | 75%, <2 | 75%, <50 | - | - | - |
| van der Wal (1986)[b] (Netherlands) | PC/SS | 1.0-7.5 | 30-440 | <1-40 | <10-260 | - |
| | PW/SS | 0.2-1.1 | 20-30 | <1 | 1-20 | - |

[a]MMA, manual metal arc; SS, stainless-steel; MIG, metal inert gas; TIG, tungsten inert gas; AIB, aluminium bronze; PC, plasma cutting; PW, plasma welding
[b]Breathing zone

**Table 6. Occupational exposures of welders during various processes and applications in the mild–steel and non-ferrous industry**

| Reference (country) | Process[a] | Total fume (mg/m³) | CO (ppm) | $NO_2$ or $NO_x$ (mg/m³) | F (mg/m³) | Cu (mg/m³) | Mn (mg/m³) |
|---|---|---|---|---|---|---|---|
| Casciani et al.[c] (1986) (Italy) | MMA/MS: | | | | | | |
| | No exhaust | 8.8–90.6 | 1–47 | 0–6.5[d] | | | |
| | Average | 32.0 | 6.0 | 1.09 | 0.83 | | |
| | With exhaust | | | | | | |
| | Average | 4.34 | | | | | |
| Ulfvarson et al. (1978c) (Sweden) | MMA/MS | 1.3–53 | <5–10 | <0.5–2.5 | | 0.007–0.094 | 0.089–0.77 |
| | Average | 7.7 | | | | 0.016 | 0.26 |
| | MAG, MIG, TIG/MS | 1.3–52 | <5–150 | <0.5–0.5 | | 0.008–0.14 | 0.066–1.8 |
| | Average | 7.0 | 3 | | | 0.027 | 0.30 |
| van der Wal (1985) (Netherlands) | MMA/MS[c] | 1.3–13.2 | | 0.09[b] | | | |
| | Average | 5.3 | | | | | |
| | Background | 0.6–3.1 | | | | | |
| | MIG–MAG/MS[c] | 0.9–12.9 | | 0.09 | | | |
| | Average | 4.4 | | | | | |
| | Background | 0.4–6.7 | | | | | |

[a]MMA, manual metal arc; MS, mild steel; FCW, flux–cored electrode; MAG, metal active gas; MIG, metal inert gas
[b]$NO_2$
[c]Breathing zone
[d]$NO_x$

**Table 7. Concentrations of gaseous pollutants in welding fume**

| Reference (country) | Process[a] | CO | $O_3$ | $NO_2$ | $NO_x$ | NO | $Ni(CO)_4$ |
|---|---|---|---|---|---|---|---|
| Sipek & Smårs (1986) (Sweden) | TIG/SS | | 0.97 ppm | 0.21 ppm | | 0.005 ppm | |
| | TIG/SS | | 0.31 ppm | 2.0 ppm | | 0.44 ppm | |
| Hallne & Hallberg (1982) (Sweden) | MMA/Ni | 15–100 ppm | | 0.1–0.2 ppm | | 0.6–2.6 ppm | 0.02 ppm |
| Wiseman & Chapman (1986) (Canada) | TIG/Ni | | | | | | $\leq$0.00011 ppm |
| | MIG/Ni | | | | | | < 0.0001 ppm |
| | MIG/SS | | | | | | < 0.0001 ppm |
| | TIG/SS | | | | | | < 0.0001 ppm |
| van der Wal (1985) (Netherlands) | | | | (breathing zone) | | (background) | |
| | MMA/MS | | < 5 µg/m³ | ND–0.4 mg/m³ | | ND–0.7 mg/m³ | |
| | MIG–MAG/MS | | < 5 µg/m³ | ND–0.3 mg/m³ | | ND–0.7 mg/m³ | |
| | TIG/SS | | < 5 µg/m³ | ND–0.8 mg/m³ | | ND–1.1 mg/m³ | |
| | MIG/SS | | $\leq$100 µg/m³ | ND–17 mg/m³ | | ND–0.6 mg/m³ | |
| | MIG/Al bronze | | > 1000 µg/m³ | ND–0.1 mg/m³ | | ND–0.1 mg/m³ | |
| | MIG/Al | | | | | | |
| van der Wal (1986) (Netherlands) (breathing zone) | PC/SS | | | < 0.01–2 mg/m³ | | | |
| | PW/SS | | | 0.03–0.2 mg/m³ | | | |
| Ulfvarson (1981) (Sweden) | | | (50%,90%) | | (50%,90%) | | |
| | TIG/Al | | $\leq$0.02, 0.08 ppm | | $\leq$1, 7.6 ppm | | |
| | MIG/Al | | $\leq$0.08, 0.43 ppm | | $\leq$0.5, 3.2 ppm | | |
| | MMA/MS | | | | $\leq$0.2, 1.1 ppm | | |
| | MMA/SS | | < 0.01 ppm | | $\leq$0.5, 3.0 ppm | | |
| | MIG–MAG/SS | | $\leq$0.02, 0.2 ppm | | $\leq$0.5, 2.0 ppm | | |
| | MIG–MAG/MS | | $\leq$0.03, 0.08 ppm | | $\leq$0.5 ppm | | |

[a]TIG, tungsten inert gas; SS, stainless–steel; MMA, manual metal arc; MIG, metal inert gas; MAG, metal active gas; PC, plasma cutting; PW, plasma welding

**Table 8. Concentrations of chromium in biological fluids from stainless–steel welders**

| Reference (population)[a] | Concentration of chromium | | |
|---|---|---|---|
| | In urine | In serum (plasma) | In erythrocytes |
| Verschoor et al. (1988)[b] | | | |
| MMA/SS welders | 3 (1–62) µg/g creatinine | 0.2 (0.04–2.9) µg/l | – |
| SS Boilermakers | 1 (0.3–1.5) µg/g creatinine | 0.2 (0.07–0.7) µg/l | – |
| Controls | 0.4 (0.1–2.0) µg/g creatinine | 0.2 (0.01–0.9) µg/l | – |
| Angerer et al. (1987)[b] | | | |
| MMA–MIG/SS welders | 33 (5.4–229) µg/l | 9 (2.2–69) µg/l | 0.3 (<0.6–39) µg/l |
| Gustavsson & Welinder (1986)[c] | | | |
| MMA/SS welders | 15.6–61.1 µmol/mol creatinine | 52–190 nmol/l | 27–188 nmol/l |
| After summer vacation | 2–11.3 µmol/mol creatinine | <13–58 nmol/l | <20–65 nmol/l |
| Schaller et al. (1986)[d] | | | |
| MMA + TIG + MIG/SS welders | 8.3 (0.4–67.4) µg/g creatinine | 2.5 (0.4–7.8) µg/l | – |
| Zschiesche et al. (1987)[e] | | | |
| MMA/SS welders | 6.7 (2.2–34.8) µg/g creatinine | | |
| | 11.6 (2.4–42) µg/l | | |
| MAG–MIG/SS welders | 4.9 (3.2–10.9) µg/g creatinine | | |
| | 6.3 (3.4–21.9) µg/l | | |
| TIG/SS welders | 2.7 (2.3–4.5) µg/g creatinine | | |
| | 4.5 (4.1–8.6) µg/l | | |
| Controls | 1.4 (0.8–2.4) µg/g creatinine | | |
| | 1.6 (0.8–3.4) µg/l | | |
| Emmerling et al. (1987)[e] | | | |
| MMA/SS welders | 28 (8.1–54) µg/l | 10.7 (5.3–20.8) µg/l | 3.6 (1.3–12.5) µg/l |
| MIG–MAG/SS welders | 14.8 (4.9–30.7) µg/l | 5.7 (2.7–13.3) µg/l | 0.6 (0.4–1.4) µg/l |
| TIG welders | 8.7 (4.7–14.5) µg/l | 5.5 (3.0–8.1) µg/l | 1.5 (0.6–3.4) µg/l |

[a]MMA, manual metal arc; SS, stainless–steel; MIG, metal inert gas; TIG, tungsten inert gas; MAG, metal active gas
[b]Geometric mean, range
[c]Range
[d]Median, 90% range
[e]Median, 68% range

(ii) *Nickel*

Consistent results have been difficult to obtain with regard to the levels of nickel in blood and urine of persons exposed during welding, although levels are elevated when compared to unexposed individuals (Table 9).

**Table 9. Concentrations of nickel in work–room air and in the urine of stainless–steel welders**

| Reference (population)[a] | Concentration of nickel | | |
|---|---|---|---|
| | In air ($\mu$g/m³) | In plasma ($\mu$g/l) | In urine[a] (mean $\pm$ SD or range) |
| Åkkeson & Skerfving (1985)[b] | 440 | | |
| MMA/SS welders Monday morning before work | | | 12 (4.2–34) $\mu$g/l; 8.8 (3.1–14.1) $\mu$g/g creatinine |
| MMA/SS welders Thursday p.m. | | | 18 (8.1–38 $\mu$g/l); 12.4 (4.1–50.4) $\mu$g/g creatinine |
| Zschiesche *et al.* (1987)[c] | | | |
| MMA/SS welders post–shift | 19 | | 7.5 (2.5–15) $\mu$g/l; 4.5 (2.5–12) $\mu$g/g creatinine |
| MIG/SS welders | 66 | | 11.2 (4.1–28) $\mu$g/l; 8.1 (3.5–21.4) $\mu$g/g creatinine |
| Controls | – | | 2.3 (1.2–5.1) $\mu$g/g creatinine; 1.8 (1.1–5.0) $\mu$g/g creatinine |
| Angerer & Lehnert (1990)[d] | | | |
| MMA/SS welders | 72 $\pm$ 82 (< 50–260) | 4.3 $\pm$ 3.9 (< 1.8–18.1) | 13.2 $\pm$ 26.5 (0.6–164.7) $\mu$g/l |
| MIG/SS welders | 100 $\pm$ 82 (< 50–320) | 3.9 $\pm$ 4.2 (< 1.8–14.6) | 26.8 $\pm$ 53.6 (1.2–209.4) $\mu$g/l |
| MMA/SS and MIG/SS welders | – | 5.6 $\pm$ 4.1 (< 1.8–19.6) | 20.3 $\pm$ 18.3 (0.1–85.2) $\mu$g/l |
| Controls | – | < 1.8 | 0.9 $\pm$ 1.4 (< 0.1–13.3) $\mu$g/l |

[a]MMA, manual metal arc; SS, stainless–steel; MIG, metal inert gas; TIG, tungsten inert gas
[b]Median and range; welding of high–nickel alloy (75% Ni)
[c]Median and 68% range
[d]Mean $\pm$ SD (range)

(iii) *Manganese*

Most ferrous welding fumes contain manganese, and the range of manganese concentrations in blood and urine of exposed welders is considerably higher than the range in unexposed individuals, although there is considerable overlap (Järvisalo *et al.*, 1983; Zschiesche *et al.*, 1986). Cutters of manganese steel had elevated plasma levels of Mn (up to 28 nmol/l) compared to baseline levels (11 nmol/l) (Knight *et al.*, 1985).

### (iv)  *Fluoride*

Increased urinary fluoride excretion levels were detected in arc welders using basic electrodes; the fluoride levels correlated with the total dust exposures (Sjögren *et al.*, 1984; see Table 6).

### (v)  *Lead*

High blood lead concentrations may occur after thermal cutting or welding of lead oxide-coated steel (Rieke, 1969). Increased concentrations of lead in blood were seen in welders in a ship repair yard (Grandjean & Kon, 1981).

### (vi)  *Aluminium*

Welders utilizing the MIG/Al technique had elevated blood and urinary levels of aluminium (Sjögren *et al.*, 1983b). After exposure to air concentrations of 1.1 (0.2-5.3) mg/m$^3$ aluminium, the urinary aluminium level was 82 (6-564) μg/l (54 (6-322) μg/g creatine); after an exposure-free period, the concentration had decreased to 29 (3-434) μg/l among welders with more than ten years' exposure (Sjögren *et al.*, 1988).

### (vii)  *Barium*

Barium is found as a constituent in the coating of electrodes with a high nickel content for use on cast iron, and fumes from MMA/Ni welding can contain up to 40% barium (Stern, 1980b). Oldenburg (1988) found that up to 60% of barium in welding fumes was water-soluble. The concentration of barium in poorly ventilated spaces was about 20 mg/m$^3$ (Zschiesche *et al.*, 1989); increased exposure to barium resulted in higher urinary excretion of barium (Dare *et al.*, 1984).

### (c)  *Exposures to welding gases*

Welding processes produce not only particulate matter but also some gaseous pollutants. The high temperature of the arc and the presence of large surface areas of metal at temperatures above 600°C lead to the production of various oxides of nitrogen from the atmosphere. Decomposition of carbonates present in MMA electrode coatings and flux cores produces a protective shield of active carbon dioxide; this gas is also used in MIG/MAG welding as a shield component. Carbon monoxide is also produced, and in some cases has been used as an experimental shield gas component, together with either argon or helium (American Welding Society, 1973, 1979). It has been postulated that the presence of carbon monoxide in the vicinity of welding in which nickel is present, either in the work piece or in the consumable, could result in the formation of nickel carbonyl, which is extremely toxic (see pp. 387-388). Measurements with an instrument with a detection limit of 0.0001 ppm, however, indicated that nickel carbonyl is produced only occasionally in amounts that just exceed the detection threshold (Wiseman & Chapman, 1986).

Occupational exposures to gases have been described for the US industry by the American Welding Society (1973) and for the Swedish industry by Ulfvarson (1981). The results of the latter (see Table 7) reveal that most exposures to ozone arise during MIG and TIG welding of aluminium. Electric arc welding, and particularly MIG/SS, TIG/SS and MIG/Al welding, produce ozone by the ultra-violet decomposition of atmospheric oxygen; high concentrations are found mostly within 50 cm of the arc. The highest exposures to ozone are found in MIG welding of AlSi alloys: emission rates are 5-20 times those for MIG/SS. The presence of nitrogen monoxide, produced in large amounts by MMA welding, acts as a sink for ozone $(NO + O_3 = NO_2 + O_2)$ so that little or no residual ozone is produced in this process (Sipek & Smårs, 1986).

Tables 6 and 7 provided an indication of the ranges of gases found with various processes and working conditions. A major problem in interpreting occupational measurements is that sometimes continuous recording instruments are used to sample concentrations behind the face shield, and sometimes grab samples are taken using sampling tubes placed in front of the shield.

### (d)  Exposures to organic constituents of welding fumes

Welding is frequently performed on mild-steel base plates coated with shop primer, and although welders are usually instructed to remove the primer from the welding zone, this is frequently not done. Welding on primed plate can significantly increase the total fume concentration, especially if a zinc-based primer has been used. Primers frequently contain organic binders based on alkyl, epoxy, phenolic or polyvinyl butyral. A significant amount of organic material occurs in the fumes originating from pyrolytic decomposition of the plastic. Benzo[a]pyrene is frequently found, its distribution being approximately log-normal: 50% of observed values lie below 10 ng/m³, while 98% lie below 1000 ng/m³ (Ulfvarson, 1981). Table 10 gives a summary of the concentrations of some of the organic substances identified in welding fume.

### (e)  Other exposures

Because welding can be performed under a wide variety of industrial settings, welders (or those engaged in welding) are potentially exposed to a great number of substances derived from the welding process itself or from other industrial activities being performed in the immediate vicinity (bystander effect). The range of incidental exposures during welding was reviewed by Zielhuis and Wanders (1986).

**Table 10. Organic substances found during welding of painted mild steel**

| Paint type | Organic compound identified | Mean concentration (mg/m³) | Reference |
|---|---|---|---|
| Not reported | Aldehydes, ketones, methylbenzofurane, phenol, dioxane, 2,4–hexadienal, 2–hexanone, alcohols, naphthalene, cresol, pyridine, saturated and unsaturated aliphatic and aromatic hydrocarbons ($C_6$–$C_{14}$), etc. | | Bille *et al.* (1976) |
| Not reported | Toluene<br>Methylethylketone<br>Ethanol<br>Xylene<br>Benzene<br>Ethylbenzene<br>Isobutanol<br>*n*–Decane | 0.07<br>0.02<br>0.2<br>2.8<br>< 0.05<br>1.2<br>< 0.006<br>0.1 | Ulfvarson *et al.* (1978c) |
| Epoxy | Alkylated benzenes[a], aliphatic alcohols ($C_1$–$C_4$)[a], bisphenol A[a], phenol[a], aliphatic ketones ($C_3$–$C_5$), acetophenone, aliphatic aldehydes ($C_1$–$C_4$), aliphatic amines ($C_1$–$C_2$) | | Engström *et al.* (1988) |
| Ethyl silicate | Aliphatic alcohols ($C_1$–$C_4$)[a], butyraldehyde[a], butyric acid, aliphatic aldehydes ($C_6$–$C_9$), formaldehyde, acetaldehyde, acetic acid | | |
| Polyvinyl butyral | Aliphatic alcohols ($C_1$–$C_4$)[a], butyraldehyde[a], butyric acid[a], formaldehyde[a], acetaldehyde, acetic acid, phenol | | |
| Modified epoxy ester | Aliphatic aldehydes ($C_1$–$C_9$)[a], aliphatic acids ($C_6$–$C_9$)[a], methyl methacrylate[a], butyl methacrylate[a], phenol[a], bisphenol A[a], alkylated benzenes, aliphatic alcohols ($C_1$–$C_4$), phthalic anhydride, acrolein, aliphatic hydrocarbons ($C_6$–$C_7$) | | |
| Modified alkyd | Aliphatic aldehydes ($C_6$–$C_9$)[a], acrolein[a], phthalic anhydride[a], aliphatic acids ($C_5$–$C_9$)[a], alkylated benzenes, aliphatic alcohols ($C_1$–$C_4$), formaldehyde, benzaldehyde | | |

[a]Major compound

Ultra-violet radiation is produced during all electric arc welding. The ranking order for emission is MIG > MMA > TIG, with typical fluxes of the order of 22 W/m² for MIG (at 1 m from the arc) and 0.7-2.5 W/m² for MMA welding (American Welding Society, 1979; Moss & Murray, 1979). Infra-red radiation is also produced, and emissions in excess of 3500 W/m² were found in a number of allied processes

(Grozdenko & Kuzina, 1982). Extremely low frequency and radio frequency radiation are produced by the 50-60-Hz currents used in welding, the interruption of current by metal transfer in the arc, and by the radio frequency generators used for igniting MIG and TIG arcs. Typical magnetic flux densities near welding generators range from 2 to 200 μT (Stuchly & Lecuyer, 1989), and current pulses of up to 100 000 A have been found to produce magnetic flux densities of upward of 10 000 μT at distances of 0.2-1.0 m from cables of transformers (Stern, 1987).

Most welders prepare their own work piece by mechanical grinding. This produces an aerosol which, although it has a relatively large aerodynamic diameter, is frequently directed towards the face of the welder. Aerosols from stainless-steel grinding can contain appreciable amounts of metallic nickel and chromium (Koponen et al., 1981).

Asbestos may be encountered by welders in shipbuilding and construction, either from the spraying of asbestos coatings (as a fireproofing measure) or during repair and removal of insulation from pipes, ducts and bulkheads (Sheers & Coles, 1980; Stern, 1980a; Newhouse et al., 1985). Asbestos gloves and heat-protective cloth have been traditionally used by welders.

Sand blasting, as used extensively in the past for surface preparation, can contribute to exposure to free silica, although such exposures have not been studied systematically; glass beads are usually now used.

### (f)    Regulatory status and guidelines

Occupational exposure limits for airborne chromium and nickel in various forms are given in the respective monographs. The occupational exposure limit (time-weighted average) in the USA for welding fume (total particulate) is 5 mg/m³ (American Conference of Governmental Industrial Hygienists, 1988).

## 2.4  Chemical analysis of welding fumes and gases

Within recent years, standard practices have been developed for monitoring exposures in order to comply with occupational exposure limits for elements, compounds and nuisance dusts. Most measurements are made using personal monitoring systems with a small battery-driven pump at a flow of about 1 l/min connected to a cassette containing a membrane filter, which is mounted on the lapel or behind the face mask of welders for one or two periods of 3 h. Values are derived for time-weighted average concentrations of total fumes by weighing the filter before and after exposure; elemental concentrations are determined by chemical analysis of the filters (see American Welding Society, 1973; British Standards Institution, 1986). Attempts have also been made to make time-resolved analyses of exposures using special techniques (Barfoot et al., 1981).

A wide range of methods has been used to analyse welding fumes. Proton-induced X-ray emission fluorescence energy analysis has been used for total analysis of the elements (Malmqvist *et al.*, 1986; Pedersen *et al.*, 1987). This is an inexpensive method for providing information on all elements heavier than phosphorus, but one disadvantage is that special calibration methods are necessary which are not always accurate, and no detailed comparison has been reported between the results of this method and wet chemical methods. Special methods can be used to determine specific elements: Malmqvist *et al.* (1986) used a nuclear reaction to determine fluorine and electron spectroscopy to determine the relative distribution of Cr[VI] to total Cr on particle surfaces. The diphenyl carbazide technique, sometimes as adapted by Thomsen and Stern (1979), has been used widely to determine the Cr[VI] content of soluble fractions (Abell & Carlberg, 1984; National Institute for Occupational Safety and Health, 1985). Energy dispersive X-ray analysis has been used to identify the elemental content of individual particles under the electron microscope (Grekula *et al.*, 1986), and X-ray diffraction methods have been used to identify crystalline species. X-Ray photoelectron spectroscopy and Auger electron spectroscopy have been used to identify chemical species on the surface of particles and, together with argon sputtering, to analyse deeper within the particles (Minni, 1986).

In only a few cases have systematic comparisons been made of the results of various techniques on the same fume samples. Oláh and Tölgyessy (1985) showed that the results of X-ray fluorescence and neutron activation methods with regard to MMA fume composition agreed to within 5%.

It is becoming common practice to collect two filters for analysis of SS fumes — one for speciation of chromium and analysis of nickel and the other for total elemental analysis. Gas fibre filters without organic binders or polyvinylchloride filters are recommended (e.g., van der Wal, 1985; Pedersen *et al.*, 1987) to avoid reduction of Cr[VI], which can be as much as 95% if cellulose acetate filters are used. Typical procedures for the analysis of SS fumes are as follows. One part of the filter is leached with distilled water or 1% sodium carbonate at room temperature for 30 min to extract the soluble fraction. Soluble Cr[VI] in the leachate (filtered through a 0.45-$\mu$M Duropore membrane) is then determined by the diphenyl carbazide method (or by atomic absorption spectrometry). A second part of the filter is leached with 3% sodium carbonate and 2% sodium hydroxide in water (heated with a cover glass and avoiding formation of white fumes), and total Cr[VI] content is determined by the diphenyl carbazide method in the leachate. A third part of the filter is leached with nitric and hydrochloric acids for 1 h at 175°C and analysed by atomic absorption spectrometry to determine other elements and total chromium. A fourth part of the filter is fused with sodium carbonate for determination of total chromium in the melt solution (van der Wal, 1985).

Digestion of MIG/SS fumes in phosphoric acid:sulfuric acid (3:1) avoids the formation of insoluble residues, which can be as much as 20% of total fume mass for certain types, prior to analysis by atomic absorption spectroscopy for total metallic content (Pedersen *et al.*, 1987).

# 3. Biological Data Relevant to the Evaluation of Carcinogenic Risk to Humans

## 3.1 Carcinogenicity studies in animals

### (a) Intratracheal instillation

*Hamster*: Groups of 35 male Syrian golden hamsters, six weeks of age, received weekly intratracheal instillations of either (i) 2.0 mg of the particulate fraction of MIG/SS fume (containing 0.4% chromium and 2.4% nickel) in 0.2 ml saline; (ii) 0.5 mg or 2 mg of MMA/SS fume (containing 5% chromium and 0.4% nickel) in 0.2 ml saline; (iii) 0.2 ml saline alone; or (iv) 0.1 mg calcium chromate in 0.2 ml saline (see also the monograph on chromium, p. 123). The group receiving 2.0 mg MMA/SS fume had an acute toxic reaction to treatment, and, from week 26 onwards, the dose was given monthly. Following the 56 weeks of treatment, all animals were maintained for a further 44 weeks, at which time the study was terminated [survival figures were not given]. At 12 months, a single anaplastic tumour of the lung, probably a carcinoma, according to the authors, was found in the group that received 0.5 mg MMA/SS; and, at termination of the study, a single mixed epidermoid/adenocarcinoma of the lung was found in the group given 2 mg MMA/SS fume. No lung tumour was reported in the saline control, MIG/SS fume or calcium chromate-treated groups (Reuzel *et al.*, 1986).

### (b) Intrabronchial implantation

*Rat*: Groups of 51 male and 49 female Sprague-Dawley rats, weighing 140-330 g (males) and 115-195 g (females), received surgical implants of five 1-mm stainless-steel mesh pellets into the left bronchus. The pellets were loaded with either (i) 7.0 mg of the particulate fraction of shielded metal arc welding fume (comparable to MMA/SS fume) containing 3.6% total chromium, of which 0.7% was of low solubility, with a particle size of 0.3-0.6 μm as mass median aerodynamic diameter and suspended in cholesterol (50:50 by weight); (ii) 6.7 mg of a thermal spray fume (a mixture of chromic oxide[III] and [VI], containing a total of 56% chromium, of which 40% was of low solubility, produced by blowing an air-jet containing chromic oxide through a flame) suspended in cholesterol (50:50 by weight); or (iii) cholesterol alone (about 5.0 mg). A further three rats received intrabronchial pellets loaded with 40% benzo[a]pyrene (4.9-5.65 mg) in cholesterol as a positive control group. The experiment was terminated at 34 months; about 50% of animals were still alive at two years. No lung tumour was seen in the cholesterol control group, while all three benzo[a]pyrene-treated treated rats developed squamous-cell carcinomas or carcinomas *in situ* around the site of pellet implantation. A single, microscopic, subpleural squamous-cell carcinoma was found in the right lung of a rat given shielded metal arc welding fume, but the authors considered this to be unrelated to treatment (Berg *et al.*, 1987)

### 3.2 Other relevant data in experimental systems

(a) *Absorption, distribution, excretion and metabolism*

(i) *Mild-steel welding*

Male Wistar rats were exposed by inhalation to 43 mg/m³ (particle size, 0.12 μm mass median average diameter) MMA/MS welding fumes for 1 h per work day for up to four weeks; a saturation level of 550 μg/g dry lung of the welding fumes was observed. Clearance of the welding fume particles from the lung followed a two-phase exponential equation; most of the accumulated particles were excreted within a half-time of six days and the remainder with a half-time of 35 days. The two major components of the mild steel — iron and manganese — had similar pattern of saturable lung retention, but manganese was cleared much faster initially (the first half-time was 0.5 day). Some of the inhaled manganese was apparently soluble and was quickly absorbed from the lung, whereas the absorption of exogenous iron was slower and was obscured by a simultaneous occurrence of endogenous iron in lung tissue. Under the same exposure conditions, alveolar retention of the mild-steel welding fumes was much lower and its clearance much faster than the corresponding parameters for stainless-steel (Kalliomäki *et al.*, 1983a,b).

Male Sprague-Dawley rats were exposed for 46 min by inhalation to MMA/MS welding fumes (1178 mg/m³; particles, 0.13 μm mass median average diameter) containing < 0.1% chromium and cobalt. The immediate retention of the fume particles totalled 1.5 mg/lung, and the elemental composition of the fumes retained was slightly different from that of the original airborne fumes, indicating some selective retention/clearance. Iron was cleared from the lungs substantially more slowly than chromium or cobalt, and pulmonary retention of iron was represented as a three-phase exponential curve with half-times of 0.2 (50% of the deposit), 1.6 (32%) and 34 (18%) days (Lam *et al.*, 1979).

(ii) *Stainless-steel welding*

Dunkin-Hartley guinea-pigs were exposed by inhalation for 256 min to MIG/SS welding fumes (990 mg/m³; particle size, 0.064 μm median diameter as determined by electron microscopy). The initial fractional deposit of the fume was 17%; the proportions of iron, cobalt, nickel and chromium retained in the lung were different from those in airborne fumes. During 80 days after exposure, the metals were cleared from the lungs at different rates: chromium > nickel > cobalt > iron, according to individual three-phase kinetic curves, with half-times ranging from 0.4-0.6 days for the first phase to 72-151 days for the third phase, depending on the metal. Iron, chromium and cobalt were eliminated mostly with faeces (maximal at days 2-3 after exposure) (Lam *et al.*, 1979).

Wistar rats were exposed to MMA/SS welding fumes (43 mg/m³; 0.3 μm mass median diameter determined by electron microscopy) for 2 h per day for up to five days. The concentrations of chromium, nickel and exogenous iron in the lungs correlated well with the cumulative exposure time. No saturation trend was found for any of the metals. The average pulmonary concentration of chromium after the maximal exposure of 10 h was 39 ppm (mg/kg), that of nickel was 5.7 ppm (mg/kg) and that of exogenous iron, 132 ppm (mg/kg). The level of chromium was also elevated in the blood, kidneys, liver and spleen, while those of nickel and iron did not increase significantly in these tissues (Kalliomäki *et al.*, 1982a).

Male Wistar rats were exposed to 43 mg/m³ MMA/SS welding fumes for 1 h per work day for up to four weeks. Median particle size of the fume was 0.3-0.6 μm mass median average diameter as determined by electron microscopy. A linear relationship was observed between the duration of exposure and the concentration of exogenous iron, chromium and nickel in the lung. A simplified single exponential lung clearance model gave the following half-times: exogenous iron, 50 days; chromium, 40 days; and nickel, 20 days. The concentration of chromium in the blood was significantly elevated only during exposure, and it decreased rapidly after termination of exposure; concentrations of exogenous iron and nickel were near the detection limits (Kalliomäki *et al.*, 1983c). Use of the MIG/SS welding technique instead of the MMA/SS technique under comparable exposure conditions did not substantially change the pulmonary retention patterns of the welding fumes, but it markedly changed the clearance patterns, especially for chromium. After exposure to MMA welding fume, chromium, manganese and nickel were cleared at half-times of 40, 40 and 30 days, respectively; with the MIG fumes, the half-time for chromium was 240 days, while the clearance of manganese and nickel obeyed the double-exponential model with half-times of two and 125 days for manganese and three and 85 days for nickel (Kalliomäki *et al.*, 1983d, 1984).

Welding fumes collected from the MMA/SS and MIG/SS assemblies were suspended in normal saline (1% suspension) and instilled intratracheally into male Wistar rats at a dose of 0.2 ml/rat, and the fate of the metals contained in the fumes was followed for up to 106 days. After exposure to the MMA/SS fumes, iron, chromium and nickel were cleared with half-times of 73, 53 and 49 days, respectively; but with MIG/SS fume, practically none of the metal was cleared within two months. The disposition of chromium in the MMA/SS fume closely resembled that of intra-tracheally instilled soluble chromates, whereas the very slow lung clearance of chromium from the MIG/SS fumes was still slower than that of water-insoluble chromates or Cr[III] salts. Thus, the clearance of chromium strongly depends on the physicochemical form of chromium in the welding fume (Kalliomäki *et al.*, 1986).

The dissolution of MMA/SS and MIG/SS welding fumes was studied in the lungs of male Wistar rats following one to four weeks' exposure by inhalation to 50 mg/m³ for 1 h per day. Two particle populations with different behaviours were found in the lungs of rats exposed to the MMA/SS fumes. The particles of the principal population (0.1-0.25 µm mass median average diameter as determined by electron microscopy) dissolved in both alveolar macrophages and type-1 epithelial cells in about two months; quickly and slowly dissolving forms of chromium, manganese and iron were detected in these particles. The particles of the minor population (0.005-0.1 µm determined as above) showed no signs of dissolution during the three-month observation period; they were found to contain very stable mixed spinels. Inhalation of the MIG/SS fumes resulted in lung deposition of only one particle population, which was very similar to the minor population in the MMA/SS fumes; no dissolution of these particles was observed within three months (Anttila, 1986).

### (b)  Toxic effects

#### (i)  Mild-steel welding

Deposition of MMA/MS welding fumes in the lungs of male CFE rats following single exposures by inhalation or by intratracheal injection resulted in the development of reticulin fibres in the particle-laden macrophage aggregates, with only sparse collagen fibre formation, which did not increase markedly up to 450 days (Hicks *et al.*, 1983). The particles caused alveolar epithelial thickening with proliferation of granular pneumocytes and exudation of lamellar material. Foam cells appeared in alveoli. Formation of nodular aggregates of particle-laden macrophages and giant cells was observed as a delayed effect 80-300 days after exposure (Hicks *et al.*, 1984). Similar nonspecific pulmonary changes were seen in the lungs of Sprague-Dawley rats exposed to MMA/MS welding fumes (mass median diameter, 0.62 µm) as a single exposure to 1000 mg/m³ for 1 h or to 400 mg/m³ for 30 min per day on six days per week during two weeks (Uemitsu *et al.*, 1984).

In MRC hooded rats, single intratracheal instillations (0.5-5 mg/rat) of either 'basic' (18% $SiO_2$, 30% F, 23% Fe, 6% Mn) or 'rutile' (41% $SiO_2$, 2% Ti, 39% Fe, 3% Mn) MMA/MS welding particles, suspended in saline increased the ribonuclease and protease activity of lavaged cells by one week after administration (White *et al.*, 1981).

Cultured alveolar macrophages from the lavaged lungs of male Brown-Norway rats were exposed for one day to total dust or to the water-insoluble fraction of fume particles [size unspecified] from MMA/MS and MIG/MS welding (15, 25 or 50 μg/ml). Both dusts were toxic to the cells in a concentration-related manner; MMA/MS dust was more toxic than that of the MIG/MS. The toxicity of the MMA/MS and MIG/MS particles was not related to the water-soluble components (Pasanen et al., 1986).

In rat peritoneal macrophages in vitro, none of three welding fumes derived from MS showed fibrogenic potential; pure magnetite dust was also inactive (Stern & Pigott, 1983; Stern et al., 1983).

When alveolar macrophages from bovine lungs were exposed in vitro to MMA/MS welding particles (both 'basic' and 'rutile'; up to 40 μg/ml) for 17 h, dose-related detachment of cells, morphological changes and a decrease in viability were seen. Toxicity was reduced significantly by supplementation of the cell culture with 10% calf serum, but not by bovine serum albumin. Release of lactic dehydrogenase, but not of N-acetyl-β-glucosaminidase, was also observed. The 'basic' fumes were slightly more active than the 'rutile' fumes (White et al., 1983).

### (ii)   Stainless-steel welding

Two days after a single exposure of male Sprague-Dawley rats to MMA/SS welding fumes (1000 mg/m³ for 1 h or 400 mg/m³ for 30 min per day, six days per week during two weeks; mass median diameter, 0.8 μm), hyperplasia of mucous cells was seen in the bronchial epithelium which tended to increase with time (maximal at day 7). No other significant pathological effect was observed (Uemitsu et al., 1984).

In the study of White et al. (1981; see above), MMA/SS welding particles (containing 16% $SiO_2$, 13% F, 2% Fe, 3% Mn, 2% Cu and 2.5% Cr (nearly all in a water-soluble Cr[VI] form)) suspended in saline also increased the ribonuclease and protease activity of lavaged cells from MRC hooded rats.

Male Sprague-Dawley rats received a single intratracheal instillation of the soluble or insoluble fraction of MMA/SS welding fume particles containing 3.5% chromium (nearly all soluble Cr[VI]) or potassium dichromate at doses equivalent to those found in the fume particles. One week after instillation, most of the toxicity of the welding particles could be related to the content of soluble Cr[VI], although the insoluble particles also produced some changes at the alveolar surface (White et al., 1982).

MIG/SS welding fume deposited in the lungs of male CFE rats had similar effects to those of MMA/MS fume, reported above (Hicks et al., 1983, 1984). MIG/SS particles injected intradermally or given by topical application to Dunkin-Hartley guinea-pigs had moderate sensitizing properties, which were stronger than those of MMA/MS particles but weaker than those of chromates (Hicks *et al.*, 1979). After intramuscular injection to CFE rats and Dunkin-Hartley guinea-pigs, the MIG/SS and MMA/MS materials were much less toxic and irritant than the MMA/SS material. The differences in fibrogenic properties were less pronounced, but MMA/SS still had the greatest effect (Hicks *et al.*, 1987).

The toxic effects of MMA/SS fume in baby hamster kidney and Syrian hamster embryo cells were more pronounced than that of MIG/SS fume. The effect of MMA/SS fume corresponded to the content of soluble chromates (potassium dichromate), while that of MIG/SS fume was greater, implying phagocytosis of less soluble chromium particles. Freshly produced welding fume appeared to be more active than stored samples (Hansen & Stern, 1985).

Cultured alveolar macrophages from the lavaged lungs of male Brown-Norway rats were exposed for one day to the total dust or to the water-insoluble fraction of fume particles [size unspecified] from MMA/SS and MIG/SS (15, 25 or 50 µg/ml). Both dusts were toxic in a concentration-related manner, but the MMA/SS dust was more toxic than that of MIG/SS. MMA/SS particles, but not MIG/SS particles, were less toxic after prewashing. The effects of MMA/SS on cell viability were similar to those observed after exposure of cells to potassium chromate at equivalent concentrations (Pasanen *et al.*, 1986).

In rat peritoneal macrophages *in vitro*, MMA/SS had distinct fibrogenic potential (Stern & Pigott, 1983; Stern *et al.*, 1983).

When alveolar macrophages from bovine lungs were exposed *in vitro* to MMA/SS welding particles, chromium[III] chloride or potassium dichromate (at up to 30 nmol (1.6 µg) chromium/ml) for 17 h, dose-related detachment of cells, morphological changes and a decrease in viability were seen. Within the concentration range tested, the MMA/SS fume particles were more toxic than potassium dichromate, while Cr[III] had no effect on cell viability. Toxicity was reduced significantly by supplementation of the cell culture with 10% calf serum, but not by bovine serum albumin. Release of lactic dehydrogenase, but not of *N*-acetyl-β-glucosaminidase, was also observed (White *et al.*, 1983).

The cytotoxic effects of two MIG/SS and one MMA/SS welding fumes were tested at concentrations of 5-200 µg/ml in normal human embryonic pulmonary epithelium cells (L132) in culture. At equal concentrations, the two MIG/SS fumes had comparable cytotoxicity which was somewhat greater for the fume containing more nickel (60% *versus* 4% nickel). The MMA/SS fume was much more toxic, probably because it contained high proportions of soluble Cr[VI], fluorine and potassium; a comparable effect was obtained with an equivalent concentration of sodium chromate. The particles were phagocytized by the cells. Changes in cell morphology were also observed (Hildebrand *et al.*, 1986).

(c)  *Effects on reproduction and prenatal toxicity*

No data were available to the Working Group.

(d)  *Genetic and related effects*

The Working Group noted that the evaluation of genetic effects of welding fumes is complicated not only by many variations in welding techniques but also by variations in collection and storage methods prior to testing. In the studies reported, several different methods of sample collection and application were used. Particulate fractions were collected on filters and then suspended in water (Hedenstedt *et al.*, 1977; Knudsen, 1980; Hansen & Stern, 1985; Baker *et al.*, 1986), in dimethyl sulfoxide (Maxild *et al.*, 1978), in culture media (Koshi, 1979; Niebuhr *et al.*, 1980; de Raat & Bakker, 1988) or in phosphate buffer (Biggart *et al.*, 1987). In one study, particulate and volatile fractions were separated and the latter passed into a chamber containing bacteria on petri dishes (Biggart & Rinehart, 1987). Studies for genetic and related effects of welding fumes are summarized in Appendix 1 to this volume.

(i)  *Mild-steel welding*

MMA and MIG welding fumes did not inhibit growth of either *Escherichia coli* W3110 *pol*A$^+$ or the repair-deficient *E. coli* P3478 *pol*A$^-$ strain (Hedenstedt *et al.*, 1977).

MS welding fumes were not mutagenic to *Salmonella typhimurium* TA97, TA98, TA100 or TA102 (Hedenstedt *et al.*, 1977; Maxild *et al.*, 1978; Etienne *et al.*, 1986). The gaseous phase from MMA/MS welding induced mutation in *S. typhimurium* TA1535 but not in TA1538, while the particulate fraction (in phosphate buffer) induced mutation in TA1538 but not in TA1535 (Biggart & Rinehart, 1987; Biggart *et al.*, 1987).

MMA/MS and MIG/MS did not increase the incidence of chromosomal aberrations in Chinese hamster ovary cells at doses up to 32 μg/ml (MMA) or 1000 μg/ml (MIG) (Etienne *et al.*, 1986) and did not induce morphological transformation of Syrian baby hamster kidney cells at doses up to 600 μg/ml (MMA) or 600 μg/ml (MIG) (Hansen & Stern, 1985). [See General Remarks for concern about this assay.] Relatively high doses of MMA/MS (50-300 μg/ml), but not of MIG/MS (250-1000 μg/ml), fumes increased the frequency of sister chromatid exchange in Chinese hamster ovary cells (Etienne *et al.*, 1986; de Raat & Bakker, 1988).

Neither MMA/MS (at 64-217 mg/m³ for 6 h per day, five days per week for two weeks) nor MIG/MS (at 144 mg/m³ for 6 h per day, five days per week for two weeks) fumes increased the frequency of sister chromatid exchange in peripheral blood lymphocytes or of chromosomal aberrations in either peripheral blood lymphocytes or bone-marrow cells of rats after exposure by inhalation (Etienne *et al.*, 1986).

### (ii)   *Mild-steel and cast-iron welding with nickel-rich electrodes*

With MMA welding fumes from cast iron employing a nickel-rich (95% Ni) electrode, no mutagenicity was detected in four strains of *S. typhimurium* (TA97, TA98, TA100 and TA102) at up to 20 mg/plate; no *hprt* locus mutation and no induction of chromosomal aberrations, but an increased frequency of sister chromatid exchange, were observed in Chinese hamster ovary cells (Etienne *et al.*, 1986). In another study, an increased frequency of sister chromatid exchange was seen in an unspecified cell line [probably human peripheral lymphocytes] exposed to 100-500 µg/ml MIG/MS welding fume from a 95%-nickel electrode (Niebuhr *et al.*, 1980). The same type of fume caused anchorage-independent growth of baby hamster kidney fibroblasts at 100-400 µg/ml (Hansen & Stern, 1984). [See General Remarks for concerns about this assay.]

MMA welding fumes from cast iron employing a nickel-rich (95% Ni) electrode did not increase the frequency of sister chromatid exchange in peripheral blood lymphocytes or of chromosomal aberrations in either peripheral blood lymphocytes or bone–marrow cells of rats after exposure by inhalation to 57 mg/m$^3$ for 6 h per day, five days per week for two weeks (Etienne *et al.*, 1986).

### (iii)   *Stainless-steel welding*

Growth of the repair-deficient *E. coli* P347S *pol*A$^-$ mutant was selectively inhibited, as compared to *E. coli* W3110 *pol*A$^+$, by MMA/SS but not by MIG/SS fumes, demonstrating that MMA/SS has a greater DNA damaging potential (Hedenstedt *et al.*, 1977).

Both MMA/SS and MIG/SS fumes were mutagenic to *S. typhimurium* TA97, TA98, TA100 and TA102 (Hedenstedt *et al.*, 1977; Maxild *et al.*, 1978; Etienne *et al.*, 1986). The mutagenicity of some but not all fume samples was diminished by addition of an exogenous metabolic system from rat livers.

It was reported that MMA/SS fumes did not enhance unscheduled DNA synthesis in human cells (Reuzel *et al.*, 1986) [details not given]. MMA/SS fumes induced a significant response at the *hprt* locus (6-thioguanine resistance) at 10 µg/ml in one experiment of three in the Chinese hamster V79 cell line (Hedenstedt *et al.*, 1977). [The Working Group considered the overall effect to be negative.] Responses at the *hprt* locus varied according to the way in which fume was generated (Etienne *et al.*, 1986).

Sister chromatid exchange was induced by MMA/SS and MIG/SS fumes in Chinese hamster ovary cells (Etienne *et al.*, 1986; de Raat & Bakker, 1988) and Don hamster cells (Koshi, 1979; Baker *et al.*, 1986); these fumes also induced chromosomal aberrations in Don (Koshi, 1979) and Chinese hamster ovary (Etienne *et al.*, 1986) cell lines, and mitotic delay was found after treatment of hamster Don cells with the water-soluble and -insoluble fractions of MMA/SS fumes (Baker *et al.*, 1986).

MMA/SS (50 μg/ml) and MIG/SS (400-800 μg/ml) welding fumes induced anchorage-independent growth of Chinese baby hamster kidney cells, and 5 μg/ml MMA/SS and 18 μg/ml MIG/SS fumes caused morphological transformation of Syrian hamster embryo cells (Hansen & Stern, 1985).

MMA/SS fumes were mutagenic *in vivo* following intraperitoneal injection of 100 mg/kg bw over days 8, 9 and 10 of gestation, as observed in the mouse fur spot test (Knudsen, 1980); however, no increase in the frequency of either sister chromatid exchange in peripheral blood lymphocytes or of chromosomal aberrations in either peripheral blood lymphocytes or bone-marrow cells of rats was found after inhalation of MMA/SS fumes (60-100 mg/m³ for 6 h per day, five days per week for two weeks) or MIG/SS fumes (124-172 mg/m³ for 6 h per day, five days per week for two weeks) (Etienne *et al.*, 1986).

[The greater genotoxic activity *in vitro* of MMA/SS fumes as compared with MIG/SS welding fumes generally corresponds to their higher content of Cr[VI]. In the absence of chromium, the presence of nickel is sufficient to account for the observed activity *in vitro*.]

### 3.3  Other relevant data in humans

#### (a)  *Absorption, distribution, excretion and metabolism*

In human lungs on autopsy, welding-fume particles seemed to be preferentially retained in central regions, mainly behind but also in front of the hilus (Kalliomäki *et al.*, 1979). Characteristic stainless-steel particles could be identified by electron probe analysis in lung tissue from two deceased arc welders (Stettler *et al.*, 1977). Analysis by energy-dispersive X-ray technique of lung tissue from one welder revealed intracellular particles containing both iron and silicon (Guidotti *et al.*, 1978), while tissue samples from ten other welders revealed large amounts of iron in fibrotic septa, but no increase in the content of silicon (Funahashi *et al.*, 1988). Lung tissue from two SS welders contained up to 500 times more nickel and 60 times more chromium than in controls, but the high nickel levels may have been due in part to exposures at a nickel refinery (Raithel *et al.*, 1988).

Urinary chromium excretion after work in active welders using MMA/SS or MIG/SS correlated with concentrations of soluble chromium compounds in the air during the work day (Tola *et al.*, 1977; Sjögren *et al.*, 1983a; Welinder *et al.*, 1983; Mutti *et al.*, 1984; see Table 8). Concentrations of chromium in urine and plasma obtained from 103 MMA/SS and MIG/SS welders at the end of the shift were strongly correlated; chromium concentrations in erythrocytes, though much lower, correlated better with plasma levels than with urinary chromium concentrations

(Angerer et al., 1987). In ten MMA/SS welders, airborne chromium exposures correlated poorly with chromium concentrations in whole blood and plasma, but correlated significantly with increases occurring in blood and plasma concentrations during the shift (Rahkonen et al., 1983). In welders using exclusively gas-shielded welding techniques, chromium concentrations in urine and blood were barely increased above background levels (Angerer et al., 1987).

In welders with a long exposure history, urinary chromium excretion remained high during three exposure-free weeks, possibly due to slow excretion of previously retained chromium (Mutti et al., 1979). Accumulation of chromium is suggested by the observation that urine and plasma chromium concentrations may not return to background levels in MMA/SS welders over a weekend (Schaller et al., 1986). Increased excretion of chromium was also seen in nine retired welders (average, four years since cessation of exposure) who had done mainly MMA/SS but also some MIG and TIG welding (Welinder et al., 1983). Good correlations were found in ten MMA/SS welders between chromium levels in body fluids and the retention rate for magnetic dust, as estimated by magnetopneumography (Rahkonen et al., 1983).

Increased urinary nickel excretion was seen in MMA/SS welders but not in TIG welders, perhaps due to differences in the solubility of the airborne nickel compounds (Kalliomäki et al., 1981). Urinary nickel excretion of ten MMA/SS welders correlated significantly with airborne exposures (Rahkonen et al., 1983). Increased nickel concentrations were also seen in plasma and urine of shipyard (Grandjean et al., 1980) and other welders (Bernacki et al., 1978).

Increased concentrations of aluminium (Sjögren et al., 1985), barium (Dare et al., 1984), fluoride (Sjögren et al., 1984), lead (Grandjean & Kon, 1981) and manganese (Järvisalo et al., 1983) have been measured in samples of blood and urine from some groups of welders (see section 2.3).

(b)    Toxic effects

Adverse health effects of exposures during welding have been reviewed by Zober (1981a,b), Stern et al. (1983) and the National Institute for Occupational Safety and Health (1988).

Sensitivity to chromate resulted in contact dermatitis in five welders exposed to chromate-containing welding fumes (Fregert & Övrum, 1963). Cutaneous exposure to sparks and radiation may cause burns and other damage to the skin (Roquet-Doffiny et al., 1977), and localized cutaneous erythema and small cutaneous scars are frequent in welders. The ultra-violet radiation from welding operations can cause acute keratoconjunctivitis in the absence of eye protection, but such episodes normally cause no apparent lasting clinical abnormality or decrease in visual acuity (Emmett et al., 1981).

Metal fume fever is a nonspecific, acute illness characterized by fever, muscle pain and leukocytosis; it is fairly common among welders. For example, 23/59 ship repair welders had experienced metal fume fever during the previous year, and 4/59 had suffered more than six incidents of the illness during that time (Grandjean & Kon, 1981). In another study, 31% of 530 welders aged 20-59 had experienced metal fume fever at least once (Ross, 1974). This condition may rarely be associated with angioedema and urticaria (Farrell, 1987). Several cases of asthmatic reactions due to components of welding fume have been recorded (Keskinen *et al.*, 1980; Bjørnerem *et al.*, 1983). Acute inhalation of metal fumes containing cadmium or ozone may result in chemical pneumonitis and pulmonary oedema (Beton *et al.*, 1966; Anthony *et al.*, 1978).

Welders who had used electrodes with a high chromium content for many years showed signs of erosion of the nasal septum (Jindrichova, 1978). Chronic inflammation was observed in upper airway epithelium of welders (Werner, 1977).

Several groups of welders, in particular nonsmokers, experienced more frequent chronic rhinitis, cough, phlegm, dyspnoea, wheezing and chronic bronchitis than expected (Barhad *et al.*, 1975; Antti-Poika *et al.*, 1977; Akbarkhanzadeh, 1980; Kalliomäki *et al.*, 1982b; Keimig *et al.*, 1983; Schneider, 1983; Mur *et al.*, 1985; Cotes *et al.*, 1989). Indicators of pulmonary function, such as vital capacity and forced expired volume in 1 s, showed decrements related to welding exposures (Peters *et al.*, 1973; Barhad *et al.*, 1975; Akbarkhanzadeh, 1980; Kalliomäki *et al.*, 1982b; Cotes *et al.*, 1989). Small airway disease may be the first sign of pulmonary abnormalities in shipyard welders, as reflected by increased closing volume and closing capacity (Oxhoj *et al.*, 1979) and decreased terminal flow volumes (Kilburn *et al.*, 1985; Cotes *et al.*, 1989). One study showed a significant correlation in welders between respiratory symptoms and thoracic magnetic dust content (Näslund & Högstedt, 1982), while no such relationship was detected in another study (Stern *et al.*, 1988). (The methods used to detect magnetic dust have been reviewed (Lippmann, 1986), and there is evidence that magnetic properties are unstable in lung over long periods (Stern *et al.*, 1987).) Further, some studies indicated a minimal or no difference in prevalence rates of respiratory symptoms and pulmonary function in welders compared to control groups (Fogh *et al.*, 1969; Hayden *et al.*, 1984; McMillan & Pethybridge, 1984). Forced ventilatory capacity was decreased to similar degrees in shipyard welders, pipe-coverers and pipe-fitters, suggesting that past asbestos exposure in some groups of welders may affect pulmonary function (Peters *et al.*, 1973). [The Working Group noted that possible selection bias among long-term welders, interaction with smoking, questionable validity of control groups and poor characterization of the exposures decreased the value of some studies.]

Early reports suggested that inhalation of welding fumes may cause siderosis, a benign pneumoconiosis (Doig & McLaughlin, 1936; Enzer & Sander, 1938); small, rounded opacities (Attfield & Ross, 1978) and nonspecific reticulomicronodulation (Mur *et al.*, 1989) were seen on X-ray examination. Some authors have reported no fibrosis or related pulmonary function changes (Harding *et al.*, 1958; Morgan & Kerr, 1963) and it has been shown that the radiographic changes may be reversible (Doig & McLaughlin, 1948; Garnuszewski & Dobrzynski, 1967; Kujawska & Marek, 1979). In other cases, analysis of histology and of pulmonary function abnormalities have indicated pulmonary fibrosis of varying degrees in welders (Charr, 1953, 1956; Angervall *et al.*, 1960; Stanescu *et al.*, 1967; Slepicka *et al.*, 1970; Brun *et al.*, 1972; Irmscher *et al.*, 1975; Patel *et al.*, 1977). Although considerable accumulation of iron oxide dust was documented in these studies, the demonstration of asbestosis in shipyard welders (Selikoff *et al.*, 1980; McMillan, 1983; Kilburn *et al.*, 1985) would suggest that factors other than iron oxide, such as silica (Friede & Rachow, 1961; Meyer *et al.*, 1967; Fabre *et al.*, 1976), could contribute to the pathogenesis of pulmonary fibrosis.

The number of days lost due to sickness attributed to respiratory disease was 2.3 times higher in welders at a petrochemical plant than among other workers not exposed to welding fumes (Fawer *et al.*, 1982). In one study, absence of welders due to sickness appeared to be related primarily to smoking (McMillan, 1981).

A slight increase in serum creatinine level was seen in SS welders, which was unrelated to urinary chromium excretion; no sign of tubular damage was detected (Verschoor *et al.*, 1988), in agreement with the results of a previous study (Littorin *et al.*, 1984). No increased risk for chronic kidney disease was seen in welders (Hagberg *et al.*, 1986).

### (c)   *Effects on reproduction and prenatal toxicity*

At a fertility clinic, poor sperm quality was seen more often among male SS and other metal welders than expected, and women employed as SS welders had delayed conception (Rachootin & Olsen, 1983). Among patients examined for sperm quality at other fertility clinics, welders had a significantly increased risk of reduced sperm quality (Haneke, 1973; Mortensen, 1988).

In a study using census data over a four-year period, female welders showed a slightly greater spontaneous abortion rate than other industrial workers and other employed women, but the increase was not statistically significant; no increase was seen for the wives of welders (Hemminki & Lindbohm, 1986).

### (d)   *Genetic and related effects*

The studies described below are summarized in Appendix 1 to this volume.

Husgafvel-Pursiainen *et al.* (1982) studied the frequency of sister chromatid exchange and chromosomal aberrations in a group of 23 male MMA/SS welders and in 22 males from the office of a printing company. The groups were healthy and were controlled for smoking and previous exposure to clastogenic agents; none of the subjects had had a recent viral infection, vaccination or diagnostic radiation. The age difference between the welders (mean, 45 years) and the controls (mean, 37 years) was considered not to be relevant. All of the welders worked in poorly ventilated areas, had been exposed for at least four years, with a mean of $21 \pm 10$ (SD) years, and had had little or no exposure to other agents in their occupational history. Sampling of six workers was repeated 1.5 years later. Exposure was mainly to alkaline chromates (calcium chromate and potassium dichromate), with airborne Cr[VI] levels of 0.03-4 mg/m³, and to nickel (as poorly water-soluble alloy in iron oxide fume particles), estimated to be four to eight times lower than to chromium. Urinary levels in exposed workers were 0.2-1.55 μmol/l (10-80 μg/l) chromium and 0.05-0.15 μmol/l (3-9 μg/l) nickel. No effect of exposure was observed over control values for sister chromatid exchange ($9.7 \pm 0.3$ cell) or chromatid and chromosome-type aberrations (1.8%); no change was observed during the 1.5-year observation period. [The Working Group noted the high frequency of sister chromatid exchange in controls.] An increased frequency of sister chromatid exchange ($p < 0.01$) was observed in smokers in both exposed and unexposed groups.

No increase in the frequency of cytogenetic damage was observed in a well controlled, pair-matched (for sex, age, smoking habits, socioeconomic class, living area, drug and alcohol consumption) study of 24 MMA/SS workers from six industries (Littorin et al., 1983). None of the controls had had any exposure to SS fumes or to known mutagenic or carcinogenic agents. Workers had been exposed for seven to 41 years (mean, 19 years) to Cr[VI] and to lesser amounts of nickel and molybdenum. Exposures to chromium, calculated as time-weighted average exposures for one work day from personal air samplers, were 4-415 μg/m³ total chromium (mean, 81 μg) and 5-321 μg/m³ Cr[VI] (mean, 55 μg). Urinary chromium levels were 5-155 μmol/mol creatinine (mean, 47 μmol/mol creatinine) for exposed workers versus < 0.4-7.0 μmol/mol creatinine (mean, 1.5 μmol/mol creatinine) for controls. No increase was observed in the total number of structural chromosomal aberrations (4.1% in welders, 4.4% in controls) nor in sister chromatid exchange frequency (11/cell in welders, 12/cell in controls) nor in the incidence of micronuclei (0.78% in welders, 0.79% in controls). No effect of smoking was observed, except for some types of chromosomal aberration (structural rearrangements). [The Working Group noted the high background frequencies of sister chromatid exchange and aberrations and that samples were shipped with 16-h lags to the analysing laboratory.]

In a larger study, Koshi et al. (1984) observed increased frequencies of both sister chromatid exchange and chromosomal aberrations in workers engaged in both MMA/SS and MIG/SS welding, with exposures to chromium, nickel, manganese and iron. Sampling was done three times over three years, with 17 workers sampled in the first survey and 44 in each of the subsequent surveys. Workers were exposed for five to 20 years (mean, 12.1 years). Air sampling using personal dust samplers showed a large variation (4-174 mg dust/m³) in individual exposure. Urinary chromium levels were 3-59 μg/l (mean, 9.8 ± 9.2) for exposed workers and 3-6 μg/l (mean, 4.1 ± 1.2) for controls, who were six and seven office workers for the first and second surveys, respectively, and 20 workers in a nonchemical research station for the third. The groups were controlled for smoking, alcohol and coffee intake, and previous exposure to diagnostic radiation or clastogenic drug intake. The three surveys, which gave significantly uniform results, showed an increase in sister chromatid exchange frequency ($p < 0.01$) from 8.11 ± 1.08 in controls (n = 33) to 8.80 ± 1.61 in exposed workers (n = 105). Smoking enhanced the frequency of sister chromatid exchange in the exposed workers ($p < 0.01$) and in controls; however, the difference was not statistically significant. The frequency of aberrant metaphases increased from 3.2 in controls to 4.7 ($p < 0.01$) in exposed workers. Increased frequencies of chromatid gaps (from 2.1% to 3.5%), chromosome gaps (from 0.23% to 0.3%) and chromatid breaks (from 0.2% to 0.3%) were observed ($p < 0.01$ or $p < 0.05$).

### 3.4   Case reports and epidemiological studies of carcinogenicity to humans

(a)   *Case reports and descriptive epidemiology*

(i) *Case reports*

The most frequent cancer reported in welders has been of the respiratory system (Gobbato et al., 1980; Sheers & Coles, 1980; Bergmann, 1982), but skin cancer has also been reported (Roquet-Doffiny et al., 1977).

(ii) *Mortality and morbidity statistics*

Guralnick (1963), using vital statistics, reported on mortality among welders and flame cutters in the USA aged 20-64 in 1950. The standardized mortality ratio (SMR) for all neoplasms was 91 (182 deaths [95% confidence interval (CI), 78-105]), and that for lung, trachea and bronchial cancer was 92 (34 deaths [95% CI, 64-129]). No excess mortality was reported for cancers at other sites.

Logan (1982) analysed cancer mortality by occupation using the statistics of the UK Office of Population Censuses and Surveys. For welders, the SMR for all neoplasms was 57 in 1931 and 126 in 1971; the SMR for lung cancer was 118 in 1951 and 151 in 1971. The Registrar General (Office of Population Censuses and Surveys, 1986) reported mortality by occupation for 1979-80 and 1982-83 in the UK; the SMR for lung cancer was 146 for welders (men aged 20-64).

An excess risk for lung cancer among welders and flame cutters was reported by Milham (1983) in a proportionate mortality analysis for Washington State, USA, for 1950-79, which confirmed his previous results for 1950-71 (Milham, 1976). In 1950-71, increased mortality was found for all neoplasms (257 deaths; proportionate mortality ratio [PMR], 104 [95% CI, 92-118]), for bronchus and lung cancer (67 deaths; PMR, 137 [95% CI, 106-174]) and for urinary bladder cancer (12 deaths; PMR, 162 [95% CI, 89-300]).

Petersen and Milham (1980), using the same method, analysed mortality in the state of California, USA, for 1959-61; no excess of lung cancer was seen among welders and flame cutters.

Menck and Henderson (1976) reviewed all deaths from cancer of the trachea, bronchus and lung occurring in 1968-70 among white males aged 20-64 and all newly diagnosed lung cancer cases registered by the Los Angeles County Cancer Surveillance Program, USA, for 1972-73, in relation to the occupation and industries reported on death certificates or in hospital records. For welders, they found a SMR of 137 based on 21 deaths and 27 newly diagnosed cases [95% CI, 101-182].

Decouflé et al. (1977) analysed the information on occupation contained in hospital files of cancer patients at the Roswell Park Memorial Institute in New York, USA, and compared it to that of noncancer patients. Based on 11 cases, the relative risk (RR) for lung cancer associated with occupation as a welder and flame cutter was 0.85 (0.67 when adjusted for smoking). From the same study, Houten et al. (1977) reported a nonsignificant RR of 2.5 for stomach cancer for welders and flame cutters, based on three cases.

Gottlieb (1980) analysed the lung cancer deaths occurring in Louisiana, USA, in 1960-75 among employees in the petroleum industry. Using a case-control approach, lung cancer deaths were compared to an equal number of deaths from nonneoplastic diseases. Eight of the cases and two of the controls had been welders [odds ratio, 3.5; nonsignificant].

Morton and Treyve (1982) determined all cases of lung and pleural neoplasms admitted to all 20 hospitals in three Oregon counties during 1968-72. Comparisons were made with information on occupation according to the 1970 US census. The incidence among the occupational category of 'welders, burners, etc.', was 125.8 per $10^5$ as compared with 70.8 per $10^5$ in the male population (comparative incidence, 178).

Death certificates for lung cancer cases from Alameda County, CA, USA, between 1958 and 1962 were analysed in relation to usual occupation by Milne et al. (1983), using a case-control approach. Lung cancer deaths were compared to all other cancer deaths occurring in persons over 18 years of age. The odds ratio for welders was 1.2 (nonsignificant), based on five cases and 16 controls.

Mortality among metal workers in British Columbia, Canada, during the period 1950-78 was analysed by Gallagher and Threlfall (1983) from death certificates using a proportionate mortality approach. The PMR for lung cancer (74 deaths; PMR, 145; 95% CI, 115-183) and for Hodgkin's disease (nine deaths; PMR, 242; 95% CI, 110-460) was significantly increased in welders. The PMR for all neoplasms in this group was 114 (207 deaths; 95% CI, 99-132).

Information on occupation contained in death certificates from the state of Massachusetts, USA, between 1971 and 1973 was analysed by Dubrow and Wegman (1984). A statistically significant association was reported between welding and prostatic cancer (standardized mortality odds ratio, 256; 14 deaths).

### (b)  Cohort studies

Dunn *et al.* (1960) and Dunn and Weir (1965, 1968) assembled a group of workers employed in 14 occupations in California, USA, and followed them up for mortality. Information was collected from union files and from a self-administered questionnaire reporting a full occupational history and smoking habits for members of the cohort in 1954-57; expected figures were based on age- and smoking-specific rates for the whole cohort. In the latest extension of the follow-up, until 1962, the SMR for lung cancer among 10 234 welders and burners was 105 (49 cases [95% CI, 78-139]). [The Working Group noted that three of the 14 groups used to calculate expected numbers had been exposed to asbestos, and the follow-up of cases was incomplete.]

An industrial population from facilities in Midland, MI, USA, was followed up for mortality by Ott *et al.* (1976). The cohort was constituted of all 8171 male employees between the ages of 18 and 64 on the 1954 employees census list and was followed up through 1973. There were 1214 deaths; 861 employees (10.5%) who remained untraced were assumed to be alive. Expected figures were computed on the basis of the US white male population mortality rates. The overall SMR for welders and lead burners was 98, based on 37 deaths [95% CI, 69-135], and the SMR for all malignant neoplasms was 162, based on 12 deaths [95% CI, 84-283]. No excess was found for cancer at any particular site.

Puntoni *et al.* (1979) followed up subjects who were shipyard workers in Genoa, Italy, employed or retired in 1960, 1970 and 1975 or dismissed or retired during 1960-75. Expected numbers were computed on the basis of mortality among the male population of Genoa. Among oxyacetylene (autogenous) welders, 66 deaths were observed, giving a significantly increased overall mortality (158); four deaths from lung cancer were reported, giving a RR estimate of 125 [95% CI, 34-320]. Overall mortality among electric arc welders was not increased; three deaths from lung cancer were observed, giving a RR estimate of 160 [95% CI, 33-466]. The authors noted that the group was potentially exposed to asbestos.

All white male welders employed in 1943-73 at the Oak Ridge, TN, USA, nuclear facilities were included in a study conducted by Polednak (1981). A total of 1059 subjects were followed up until 1974 and were subdivided in two subgroups: the first (536) was constituted of welders at a facility where nickel-alloy pipes were welded; the second (523) included welders working with mild steel, aluminium and stainless-steel. Data on smoking habits were available from about 1955. US national mortality rates were used for computing expected figures. Mortality from all causes and from all cancers was slightly lower than expected in both subgroups. There was an excess of deaths from lung cancer (17 cases; SMR, 150; 95% CI, 87-240), and the excess was slightly higher in the group of other welders (ten deaths; SMR, 175; 95% CI, 84-322) than in the nickel-alloy welders (seven deaths; SMR, 124; 95% CI, 50-255).

Beaumont and Weiss (1980, 1981) followed up for mortality a cohort of 3247 welders from local 104 of the International Brotherhood of Boilermakers, Iron Ship Builders, Blacksmiths, Forgers and Helpers in Seattle, WA, USA. Subjects were included if they had had at least three years of union membership and at least one of these years between January 1950 and December 1973. Vital status was ascertained as of 1 January 1977. Fifty deaths from lung cancer were observed *versus* 37.95 expected on the basis of US national mortality rates (SMR, 132 [95% CI, 98-174]). For deaths that occurred 20 years or more after first employment, the SMR was 174 (39 cases [95% CI, 124-238]). A re-analysis of the same data by Steenland *et al.* (1986), using an internal comparison group of members of the local union who were not welders and applying two types of regression analyses, yielded similar results.

McMillan and Pethybridge (1983) investigated the mortality of a cohort of welders, boilermakers, shipwrights, painters, electrical fitters and joiners employed for at least six months between 1955 and 1974 at HM Dockyard Devonport, UK, with follow up through 1975. The proportionate mortality of welders was compared to that of the other occupational groups. The PMR for lung cancer was 104 [95% CI, 34-243] based on five deaths. Three deaths from mesothelioma were also reported among the welders. [The Working Group noted that painters were included in the cohort and that there was potential exposure to asbestos.]

Lung cancer mortality in a cohort of foundry workers was investigated by Fletcher and Ades (1984). The cohort consisted of all men hired between 1946 and 1965 in nine steel foundries in the UK and employed for at least one year. The 10 250 members of the cohort were followed up until the end of 1978 and assigned to 25 occupational categories according to information from personnel officers. Lung cancer mortality for the subcohort of welders in the fettling shop was higher than expected on the basis of mortality rates for England and Wales (eight cases; SMR, 146; 95% CI, 62-288); however, for nonwelders in the fettling shop, the SMR was [177] (58 cases).

The mortality of welders and other craftsmen employed at a shipyard in Newcastle, UK, was investigated by Newhouse *et al.* (1985). All employees hired between 1940 and 1968 were included in the study, making a total of 3489 workers, of whom 1027 were welders; these were followed up until the end of 1982. The SMRs for welders compared with the general population of England and Wales were 147 for all causes and 191 for lung cancer. However, when the Newcastle conurbation was taken as a reference, the overall SMR was 114 (195 cases; 90% CI, 100-127), and the SMR for lung cancer was 113 (26 cases; 90% CI, 80-157). In addition, one death from mesothelioma was reported for welders, indicating possible exposure to asbestos.

Becker *et al.* (1985) followed up a cohort of 1221 stainless-steel welders first exposed before 1970 who had undergone the compulsory technical examination for welders in the Federal Republic of Germany. A population of 1694 turners was followed up as a comparison cohort. Smoking histories, as reported by workplace foremen, were similar for the two groups. The overall mortality of the cohort of welders was significantly lower than that of the general population (SMR, 66; based on 77 deaths [95% CI, 52-82]). The SMR for cancer of the trachea, bronchus and lung was 95 (six cases [95% CI, 35-207]) in comparison with the general population. In comparison with turners and assuming a ten-year latency, the welders had an age-adjusted rate ratio for all cancers of 2.4 (95% CI, 1.1-5.1) and a ratio for trachea, bronchus and lung cancer of 1.7 (95% CI, 0.7-4.0). In addition, two deaths from pleural mesothelioma were reported. [The Working Group could not exclude selection bias in the assembly of the cohort; the two deaths from mesothelioma among welders suggest that they were exposed to asbestos.]

Englund *et al.* (1982) linked information from the Swedish Cancer Registry files for 1961-73 to the population census file of 1960. Welders were among the occupational groups for which the incidence of tumours of the nervous system was higher than in the general population, with a standardized incidence ratio (SIR) of 135 based on 50 cases [95% CI, 100-178].

Sjögren and Carstensen (1986) analysed the results of a linkage between the 1960 census file of male welders or gas cutters and the Swedish Cancer registry files between 1961 and 1979. Smoking data from a national survey were used to adjust incidence ratios, and the Swedish male national population was chosen as a reference. A 30% increase in the incidence of cancer of the trachea, bronchus and lung, based on 193 cases, was reported after adjustment for smoking; other sites at which excesses were observed were larynx (22 cases; RR, 1.3) and kidney (70 cases; 1.3). There was a nonsignificant increase in risk for mesothelioma (four cases; 1.5).

The possible associations between intracranial gliomas and occupation were examined by McLaughlin *et al.* (1987), linking information from the 1960 census and the Swedish cancer registry for 1961-79. Expected values were derived from national age- and sex-specific reference rates. An elevated SIR of 140 was found for welders and metal cutters, based on 46 cases [95% CI, 103-187].

Sjögren (1980) and Sjögren *et al.* (1987) studied and subsequently updated the mortality of a small cohort of 234 stainless-steel welders with high exposure to chromium in Sweden. Welders were included in the cohort only if representatives from the company stated that asbestos had not been used or had been used only occasionally and never such as to generate dust. In the extension of the study, a cohort of 208 railway track welders with low levels of exposure to chromium was also included in the design. Only welders with at least five years of employment between 1950 and 1965 were included in the study and followed up until the end of 1984. Expected deaths were calculated using national rates. Both groups were characterized by a low overall mortality (SMRs, 72 and 70, respectively). Mortality from cancer of the trachea, bronchus and lung was increased among welders with high chromium exposure (SMR, 249, based on five deaths; 95% CI, 80-581); the SMR was 33 (one death; 95% CI, 0-184) among welders with low exposure. According to Swedish measurements (Ulfvarson, 1979), stainless-steel welders are exposed on average to about 100 µg/m$^3$ Cr associated with use of coated electrodes. The level measured during railroad track (mild steel) welding was usually less than 10 µg/m$^3$ Cr (see Table 6).

A large cohort of shipyard and machine shop workers in Finland was followed up for cancer incidence by Tola *et al.* (1988). The cohort included a subset of 1689 welders who had welded mainly mild steel, with no exposure to hexavalent chromium. Only workers employed for at least one year between 1945 and 1960 were included in the study and followed up (99.7% complete) for cancer incidence from 1953 to 1981 through the Finnish Cancer Registry. Smoking habits were ascertained by a postal questionnaire sent to a one-third stratified sample of the members of the cohort or of the next-of-kin of decedents. The expected figures were based on the urban population in the same geographic area. The results did not indicate substantial differences with regard to smoking habits between the study population and the general population. Welders employed in shipyards had a SIR for lung cancer of 115 based on 27 deaths (95% CI, 76-167), and welders employed in machine shops had a SIR of 142 based on 14 deaths [95% CI, 77-237]. For neither of the groups was there an association with time since first exposure.

The International Agency for Research on Cancer has reported (IARC, 1989) the results of a large multicentre cohort study carried out on the working populations of welders employed in 135 companies located in eight European countries. The study included reanalyses of previous studies described above (Becker *et al.*, 1985; Sjögren *et al.*, 1987; Tola *et al.*, 1988) and newly assembled cohorts. The populations of the three previous studies constituted approximately one-third of the total cohort and contributed equally to the different subgroups of welders. A total of

11 092 welders were included in the analysis and followed through 1982-87, depending on the country. The completeness of follow-up was 97%. The SMR for deaths from all causes was 93, based on 1093 deaths (95% CI, 87-98). Mortality from all malignant neoplasms was increased (303 deaths; SMR, 113; 95% CI, 100-126), due mainly to a statistically significant excess of cancer of the trachea, bronchus and lung (116 deaths; SMR, 134; 95% CI, 110-160). Other sites for which excess deaths were seen were larynx (7 deaths; SMR, 148; 95% CI, 59-304), bladder (15 deaths; SMR, 191; 95% CI, 107-315), kidney (12 deaths; SMR, 139; 95% CI, 72-243) and lymphosarcoma (6 deaths; SMR, 171; 95% CI, 63-371). Subjects were assigned to one of three mutually exclusive groups: welding in shipyards, mild-steel welders and ever stainless-steel welders; the latter group also included those who had been predominantly stainless-steel welders. Lung cancer mortality was as follows: welders in shipyards (36 deaths; SMR, 126; 95% CI, 88-174); mild-steel welders (40 deaths, SMR, 178; 95% CI, 127-243); ever stainless-steel welders (39 deaths; SMR, 128; 95% CI, 91-175); and predominantly stainless-steel welders (20 deaths; SMR, 123; 95% CI, 75-190). Lung cancer mortality tended to increase with time since first exposure for mild-steel and stainless-steel welders; this pattern disappeared among mild-steel welders when broken down by duration of exposure and was most evident among predominantly stainless-steel welders, for whom a statistically significant trend was evident ($p < 0.05$): the distributions of observed:expected lung cancer deaths in the four groups of years since first exposure (0-9, 10-19, 20-29, > 30) were 2:3.11, 5:5.67, 7:5.54 and 6:1.92, respectively. Five deaths from pleural mesothelioma were reported — one in the shipyard welders, two among mild-steel welders and two among stainless-steel welders (see Table 11). The results for cancer incidence followed the same pattern as those for cancer mortality.

Howe *et al.* (1983) examined the mortality of a cohort of 43 826 male pensioners of the Canadian National Railway company in 1965-77. During this period, 17 838 deaths occurred, and cause of death was ascertained for 94.4% by computerized record linkage to the Canadian national mortality data base. The only occupational information available was on that at the time of retirement. The 4629 individuals who had been exposed to welding fumes showed excess mortality from brain tumours (ten deaths; SMR, 318; 95% CI 153-586).

Stern (1987) pooled 1789 cases of lung cancer and 146 cases of leukaemia reported in epidemiological studies of different designs, most of which are reviewed here. Compared to the expected number of cases as derived from the reviewed publications, a risk ratio of 1.4 was found for respiratory cancer and 0.92 for leukaemia. The risk ratio for acute leukemia, based on 40 cases, was also 0.92.

The risks for lung cancer in the studies described above are summarized in Table 12.

**Table 11. Risks for death from respiratory cancer[a] and from pleural mesothelioma[b] by length of employment and follow-up among subcohorts of welders[c]**

| Study group | 0–19 years since first employment | | | | | ≥20 years since first employment | | | | |
|---|---|---|---|---|---|---|---|---|---|---|
| | 1–9 years' employment | | | ≥10 years' employment | | 1–9 years' employment | | | ≥10 years' employment | |
| | Lung cancer | | Meso-thelioma | Lung cancer | Meso-thelioma | Lung cancer | | Meso-thelioma | Lung cancer | Meso-thelioma |
| | Obs | SMR | Obs | Obs | SMR | Obs | Obs | SMR | Obs | Obs | SMR | Obs |
| Shipyard welders | 10 | 264 | | 1 | 69 | | 15 | 116 | 1 | 10 | 96 | |
| Mild-steel welders | 8 | 116 | 1 | 7 | 253 | | 10 | 254 | | 15 | 173 | 1 |
| Ever stainless–steel welders | 15 | 115 | | 2 | 67 | | 9 | 145 | | 13 | 157 | 1 |
| Predominantly stainless–steel welders[d] | 5 | 85 | | 2 | 69 | 1 | 2 | 161 | | 11 | 176 | |

[a]Cancers of trachea, bronchus and lung (ICD8, 162)

[b]Additional deaths due to pleural mesothelioma (ICD8, 163), which were not included in calculation of SMR

[c]From IARC (1989)

[d]Subset of ever stainless–steel welders group who were employed in companies with at least 70% of stainless–steel activity or had at least one occupational period of stainless–steel welding only

**Table 12. Lung cancer in welders (cohort studies)[a]**

| Reference (country) | No. of cases observed | SMR, PMR or SIR | 95% CI | Comments |
|---|---|---|---|---|
| Dunn & Weir (1968) (USA) | 49 | 105 | 78–139 | |
| Puntoni et al. (1979) (Italy) | 4 | 125 | 34–320 | Autogenous welders; two sets of standard rates used (male popula- tion of Genoa and male staff of hospital) |
| | | 212 | 58–542 | |
| | 3 | 160 | 33–466 | |
| | | 254 | 52–743 | Electrical welders; two sets of stan- dard rates used |
| Polednak (1981) (USA) | 17 | 150 | 87–240 | All welders |
| | 7 | 124 | 50–255 | Welders exposed to nickel com- pounds |
| | 10 | 175 | 84–322 | Other welders |
| Beaumont & Weiss (1981) (USA) | 50 | 132 | 98–174 | |
| McMillan & Pethybridge (1983) (UK) | 5 | 104 | 34–243 | PMR for respiratory cancer (three mesotheliomas) |
| Fletcher & Ades (1984) (UK) | 8 | 146 | 62–288 | |
| Newhouse et al. (1985) (UK) | 26 | 113 | 80–157 | Shipyard welders; SMR, 191 when compared with general population of England and Wales (one meso- thelioma) |
| Becker et al. (1985) (FRG) | 6 | 95 | 35–207 | Stainless-steel welders; expected number based on national mortality statistics |
| | 6 | 1.7 | 0.7–4.0 | Cohort of turners used as controls (two mesotheliomas) (rate ratio) |
| Sjögren & Carstensen (1986) (Sweden) | 193 | 142 | 123–163 | Unadjusted SMR (four mesothelio- mas) |
| Sjögren et al. (1987) (Sweden) | 5 | 249 | 80–581 | Stainless-steel welders |
| Tola et al. (1988) (Finland) | 27 | 115 | 76–167 | Welders in shipyards (SIR) |
| | 14 | 142 | 77–237 | Welders in machine shops (SIR) |

[a]SMR, standardized mortality ratio; SIR, standardized incidence ratio; PMR, proportionate mor- tality ratio; CI, confidence interval

(c)   *Case-control studies*

Questions relating to employment as a welder or exposure to welding fumes are often included in case-control studies of cancer. In many of these studies, a long list of occupations/exposures is investigated, and any positive association found is likely to be reported; therefore, the possibility of a publication bias toward positive results must be taken into account when reviewing case-control studies.

(i)   *Lung cancer*

Breslow *et al.* (1954) conducted a case-control study of 518 histologically confirmed lung cancer patients admitted to 11 hospitals in California, USA, in 1949-52, and randomly selected matched controls who were patients of the same age, sex and race admitted to the same hospitals for a condition other than cancer or a chest disease. Interviews for occupational and smoking histories were conducted by persons who were unaware of the case or control status of the interviewee. An elevated RR was seen for welders and sheet-metal workers doing welding, based on 14 cases and two controls [odds ratio, 7.2; 95% CI, 1.9-44.3; smoking-adjusted odds ratio, 7.7].

Blot *et al.* (1978) carried out a case-control investigation among male residents of a coastal area in Georgia, USA. A total of 458 newly diagnosed cases and deaths from lung cancer were compared to 553 controls collected from hospitals or from mortality registries, and matched by vital status, sex, age, race and county of residence. Persons with bladder cancer or chronic lung disease were excluded from among the controls. The results revealed an increased risk for all employment in shipyards but not for welders and burners (RR, 0.7, based on 11 cases and 20 controls).

A similar case-control study was conducted by Blot *et al.* (1980) in coastal Virginia, USA, including 336 deaths from lung cancer and 361 controls deceased from causes other than chronic respiratory diseases in 1976. Information on smoking habits and on occupation was collected by interviewing next-of-kin. Lung cancer risk was slightly elevated among workers in the shipbuilding industry, but an analysis of 11 exposed cases and nine exposed controls showed that welders and burners were not at increased risk [RR, 0.9; 95% CI, 0.4-2.3].

A case-control study of lung cancer among residents of Florence, Italy, by Buiatti *et al.* (1985) included all 376 histologically confirmed cases of primary lung cancer admitted to the main regional hospital in 1981-83. A group of 892 hospital controls of the same sex, age, period of admission and smoking habits was identified, and the ILO classification of occupation and a list of 16 known or suspected carcinogens were used for assessing occupational history. Men who had 'ever worked' in welding had an increased risk (adjusted for smoking), based on seven cases and five controls (odds ratio, 2.8; 95% CI, 0.9-8.5).

Silverstein *et al.* (1985) identified all deaths among members of the United Automobile Workers International Union ever employed at a metal stamping plant between 1966 and 1982 in Michigan, USA. Causes of death were obtained from death certificates, and information on employment from company lists. The data were analysed in a case-control fashion, with cancer deaths as cases and noncancer deaths as controls. Employment as a maintenance welder or millwright was considered to constitute exposure to coal-tar pitch volatiles and welding fumes, and all other occupations were considered to be unexposed. The RR for lung cancer was 13.2 (95% CI, 1.1-154.9), based on three cases. [The Working Group noted that millwrights may be engaged in gas cutting and not exposed to welding fumes in the usually accepted sense.]

Kjuus *et al.* (1986) conducted a case-control study in two industrialized areas of Norway and included 136 newly diagnosed male lung cancer cases and 136 controls identified through the medical files of the main hospital during 1979-83. Forty additional cases and 40 controls were included during the last two years of the study period from another hospital. Patients with obstructive lung disease were excluded from among the controls. Potential exposure to carcinogens was specifically investigated using the Nordic Classification of Occupations, and, for the last two years of the study period, subjects were asked about past exposure to 17 chemical agents and five specific work processes. For subjects already interviewed, exposures were inferred from the available occupational history. An increased risk was found for all welders (RR, 1.9; 95% CI, 0.9-3.7; 28 cases) and for the subset of stainless-steel welders (RR, 3.3; 95% CI, 1.2-9.3; 16 cases) after adjustment for smoking. Half of the cases exposed to stainless-steel welding had also been moderately or heavily exposed to asbestos; when this was taken into consideration in a logistic regression model, risk associated with stainless-steel welding was no longer statistically significant.

Gérin *et al.* (1986) presented preliminary results of a multicancer case-control study in hospitals in the Montréal, Canada, area. Lung cancer patients were used as cases and patients with cancers at 13 other sites as controls; a group of population subjects was also included in the control group. A detailed job-exposure matrix was constructed, and each subject was categorized after direct interview and evaluation of responses by experts in industrial hygiene. Welders were at increased risk for lung cancer (RR, 2.4; 95% CI, 1.0-5.4), based on 12 cases and 20 controls. For ten welders exposed to nickel, the RR was 3.3 (95% CI, 1.2-9.2).

Schoenberg *et al.* (1987) carried out a case-control investigation of lung cancer among white males in six areas of New Jersey, USA. Cases of cancer of the lung, trachea or bronchus were histologically confirmed and ascertained through hospital pathology records, the state cancer registry and death certificates in 1980-81. Controls were matched by age, race, area of residence and (for dead cases) date of death; subjects with respiratory disease were excluded. The study population comprised 763 cases and 900 controls. Information was obtained by personal interview either directly or from next-of-kin, and information on industry and job title was coded according to the 1970 census index system. Occupation as a welder or flame cutter was reported by 38 cases and 38 controls (smoking-adjusted RR, 1.2 [95% CI, 0.8-1.9]). Welders, burners, sheet-metal workers and boilermakers employed in shipyards had a significantly increased risk (RR, 3.5; 95% CI, 1.8-6.6); for those without reported exposure to asbestos, the RR was 2.5 (95% CI, 1.1-5.5).

A population-based case-control study was conducted by Lerchen *et al.* (1987) of 506 primary lung cancer cases reported to the New Mexico (USA) Tumor Registry between 1 January 1980 and 31 December 1982 and 771 controls who were interviewed about their occupational histories and smoking habits. The age-, ethnicity- and smoking-adjusted RR for welders in all industries was 3.2 (95% CI, 1.4-7.4), based on 19 cases and ten controls. When welders ever employed in shipyards were analysed separately, the RR was lower (2.2; 95% CI, 0.5-9.1), based on six cases and three controls, than for welders elsewhere than in shipyards (RR, 3.8; 95% CI, 1.4-10.7), based on 13 cases and seven controls.

Benhamou *et al.* (1988) conducted a case-control study in France of 1260 male lung cancer cases collected in 1976-80 and 2084 hospital controls matched by age, hospital of admission and interviewer. Cases and controls were classified as either nonsmokers or smokers. The RR for welders and flame cutters after adjusting for smoking was 1.4 (95% CI, 0.79-2.9), based on 18 exposed cases and 23 exposed controls.

A nested case-control analysis of deaths due to lung cancer among civilians employed at the Portsmouth Naval Shipyard, Maine, USA, between 1952 and 1977 was conducted by Rinsky *et al.* (1988); the cohort had previously been investigated by Najarian and Colton (1978) and Rinsky *et al.* (1981). Controls without cancer were matched on date of birth, year of first employment and duration of employment. Potential exposure to asbestos and to welding by-products was estimated from the job histories. The study population comprised 405 lung cancer deaths and 1215 controls from within the cohort of shipyard workers. The RR for subjects with probable exposure to welding by-products was 1.1 (95% CI, 0.8-1.7) based on 41 cases and 111 controls. When subjects with potential exposure were also included, the RR was 1.5 (95% CI, 1.2-1.8), based on 236 exposed cases and 597 controls.

A population-based case-control study of lung cancer was conducted by Ronco *et al.* (1988) in two industrialized areas of northern Italy. All 126 deaths from lung cancer occurring among male residents in the area in 1976-80 and a random sample of 384 other deaths (excluding chronic lung conditions and smoking-related cancers) occurring in the same area during the same period were included in the study. Smoking habits and occupational information were collected from next-of-kin by interview (without knowledge of case or control status) using two lists of known and suspected occupational carcinogenic exposures. Subjects never employed in any of the occupations listed were considered to be unexposed. Logistic regression analysis adjusting for age, smoking and other occupational exposure gave a risk estimate of 2.9 (95% CI, 0.87-9.8) for welders, based on six cases.

The studies described above are summarized in Table 13.

**Table 13. Lung cancer in welders (case–control studies)[a]**

| Reference (country) | No. of cases exposed | RR | 95% CI | Comments |
|---|---|---|---|---|
| Breslow et al. (1954) (USA) | 14 | 7.2 | 1.9–44.3 | RR, 7.7 adjusted for smoking |
| Blot et al. (1978) (USA) | 11 | 0.7 | – | |
| Blot et al. (1980) (USA) | 11 | 0.9 | 0.4–2.3 | |
| Rinsky et al. (1988) (USA) | 41 | 1.1 | 0.8–1.7 | Probable welding exposure |
| | 236 | 1.5 | 1.2–1.8 | Potential welding exposure |
| Buiatti et al. (1985) (Italy) | 7 | 2.8 | 0.9–8.5 | Adjusted for smoking |
| Silverstein et al. (1985) (USA) | 3 | 13.2 | 1.1–154.9 | |
| Kjuus et al. (1986) (Norway) | 28 | 1.9 | 0.9–3.7 | All welders; adjusted for smoking |
| | 16 | 3.3 | 1.2–9.3 | Stainless–steel welders; adjusted for smoking |
| Gérin et al. (1986) (Canada) | 12 | 2.4 | 1.0–5.4 | All welders |
| | 10 | 3.3 | 1.2–9.2 | Welders exposed to nickel |
| Schoenberg et al. (1987) (USA) | 38 | 1.2 | 0.8–1.9 | Welders or flame cutters; adjusted for smoking |
| Lerchen et al. (1987) (USA) | 19 | 3.2 | 1.4–7.4 | All welders |
| | 6 | 2.2 | 0.5–9.1 | Welders employed in shipyards |
| | 13 | 3.8 | 1.4–10.7 | Welders not employed in ship- yards |
| Benhamou et al. (1988) (France) | 18 | 1.4 | 0.79–2.9 | Adjusted for smoking |
| Ronco et al. (1988) (Italy) | 6 | 2.9 | 0.87–9.8 | Adjusted for smoking |

(ii) *Cancers of the urinary organs*

Howe et al. (1980) conducted a population-based case-control study of bladder cancer occurring in Canada in 1974-76 on a total of 632 case-control pairs matched by age, sex and neighbourhood of residence. Occupational histories were collected through direct interview, and two check lists of suspected occupations and substances carcinogenic for the bladder were used to obtain information on exposure. Exposure to welding fumes resulted in a RR of 2.8 (95% CI, 1.1-8.8) based on 17/6 discordant pairs (case ever worked, control never worked/case never worked, control ever worked as welder).

A case-control investigation of the lower urinary tract was conducted by Silverman *et al.* (1983) in the Detroit, USA, area. All histologically confirmed male cases, newly diagnosed from December 1977 to November 1978 in 60 of the 61 hospitals in the area, were included in the study. In total, 303 whites with bladder cancer and 296 population-based randomly selected white controls were included in the analysis. Information on occupation was collected by interview. The RR for the combined group of welders, flame cutters and solderers was 0.6 (95% CI, 0.3-1.0), based on 18 cases and 30 controls. Similar results were found when the analysis was limited to the same category within the motor vehicle manufacturing industry (RR, 0.6; 95% CI, 0.3-1.2; based on 12 cases and 22 controls).

Claude *et al.* (1988) carried out a hospital-based, matched case-control study of cancer of the lower urinary tract in northern Federal Republic of Germany. Cases were identified in the three main hospitals of the region between 1977 and 1985. The occupations of 531 male cases and their matched controls were ascertained. The RR for welders was 1.2 (95% CI, 0.52-2.8), based on 12/10 discordant pairs.

A population-based case-control investigation of bladder cancer was conducted in Canada between 1979 and 1982 by Risch *et al.* (1988). Of the 1251 eligible individuals, 835 (67%) cases were interviewed, with the consent of their physician, and 792 (53%) of the 1483 eligible controls agreed to be interviewed. The authors pointed out that this method might have affected the representativeness of cases and controls. When the data were analysed by the 26 occupations/industries specifically investigated through the questionnaire, employment in welding activities yielded a risk estimate of 1.1 (95% CI, 0.71-1.6).

The association of renal-cell carcinoma with various potential risk factors was studied by Asal *et al.* (1988) in a case-control study of 315 cases and 313 hospital and 336 population controls in the USA. Individuals were classified by occupation only if the period of exposure was one year or longer. The odds ratio for employment as a welder in comparison with population controls was 1.2 (95% CI, 0.7-2.2), based on 29 exposed cases. Results obtained using hospital controls were similar.

### (iii) *Cancers at other sites*

A case-control study of *nasal cancer* was carried out in Denmark, Finland and Sweden by Hernberg *et al.* (1983a,b) with 287 cases identified through the national cancer registries between 1977 and 1980. A total of 167 cases (58%) were included in the study when deceased patients or nonrespondents were omitted. An equal number of controls were matched for country, sex and age at diagnosis, and both cases and controls were interviewed by telephone according to a standard protocol. The risk estimate for welding, flame-cutting and soldering was 2.8 (95% CI, 1.2-6.9) based on 17/6 discordant pairs. [See also the monographs on chromium and nickel, pp. 206 and 400-401.]

Following a report by the Danish Occupational Health Agency of a large number of cases of *laryngeal cancer* in welding workplaces, Olsen *et al.* (1984) conducted a case-control study to investigate the role of occupational exposure. All male laryngeal cancer patients newly diagnosed between 1980 and 1982 in the main five hospital departments in the country were included in the study, excluding the cases which prompted the study. For each case, four controls were selected from the same municipal person-registry in which the case was listed. The refusal rate was 4% among cases and 22% among controls, leaving 271 cases and 971 age- and sex-matched controls for the analysis. The RR related to welding, adjusted for age, alcohol and tobacco consumption, was 1.3 (95% CI, 0.9-2.0), based on 42 cases and 115 controls. The risk was highest for cancer located in the subglottic region (RR, 6.3; 95% CI, 1.8-21.6). Separate analysis for welders exposed to stainless-steel welding fumes gave a RR of 1.3 (95% CI, 0.7-2.7), based on 12 cases and 30 controls.

Stern, F.B. *et al.* (1986) carried out a case-control study of deaths due to *leukaemia* within a population of 24 545 male nuclear shipyard workers in Portsmouth, NH, USA, employed between 1952 and 1977 and who had died before 31 December 1980. Controls were selected from among other deaths, and four controls per case were matched by age, data of hire and length of employment; each control should not have died before the case. The entire occupational history of each individual was reconstructed using company files and other industrial sources. The risk estimate for ever having worked in welding was 2.3 (95% CI, 0.92-5.5) for all leukaemia and 3.8 (95% CI, 1.3-11.5) for myeloid leukaemia.

A case-control study of *chronic myeloid leukaemia* was carried out in Los Angeles County, CA, USA, by Preston-Martin and Peters (1988) between 1979 and 1985. Of the 229 eligible cases, 137 (60%) were interviewed by telephone; 130 pairs matched for age, sex and race were eventually included in the analysis. Employment as a welder yielded a crude RR of 19 [95% CI, 2.8-232.5], based on 19/1 discordant pairs.

Norell *et al.* (1986) conducted a case-control study of *pancreatic cancer* in the Stockholm-Uppsala region. Out of 120 eligible cases, 99 (83%) were included in the study. Both hospital- and population-derived controls were selected, with a response rate of 91% for the former and of 85% for the latter group. Information was collected through a self-administered questionnaire and further checked by telephone. The risk estimates for exposure to 'welding materials' were 1.7 (90% CI,

0.9-3.2), based on 13 cases and 27 hospital controls, and 2.0 (90% CI, 0.9-4.3), based on 11 population controls.

Olin *et al.* (1987) conducted a case-control study of *astrocytomas* in Sweden to investigate the possible etiological role of occupational exposures. Incident cases were identified from the two main hospitals in Stockholm and in Uppsala in 1980-81. Both hospital- and population-based controls of the same sex, age and date of diagnosis as the case were included in the study. Of the original 404 study subjects, 367 (91%) were included in the study, comprising 78 cases, 197 hospital controls and 92 population controls. Information was collected through self-administered questionnaire or filled in by the spouse. No increase in risk was reported for welding activities, with risk estimates of 0.6 (95% CI, 0.2-1.7), based on five cases and 15 hospital controls, and 0.2 (95% CI, 0.1-0.7), based on 19 population controls.

A case-control study of workers employed between 1943 and 1977 at two nuclear facilities in Oak Ridge, TN, USA, was conducted by Carpenter *et al.* (1988), in order to examine the possible association of primary *central nervous system cancers* (ICD8, 191, 192) with occupational exposure to chemicals. Job titles/departments were evaluated for potential exposure to 26 chemicals or chemical groups. Seventy-two white male and 17 white female cases were identified; four controls were selected for each case and matched on race, sex, nuclear facility where initially employed, year of birth and year of hire. The odds ratio for 33 cases ever exposed to welding fumes was 1.2 [95% CI, 0.6-2.4].

The hypothesis that childhood cases of *Wilms' tumour* might be related to parental perinatal exposures was tested by Kantor *et al.* (1979) by a case-control approach using the Connecticut (USA) Tumor Registry files for 1935-73. A total of 149 cancer-free controls were identified from health department files and matched to the 149 cases by age, sex and year of birth. Information on the occupation of the father was obtained exclusively from birth certificate files. Welder as the occupation of the father was mentioned on the birth certificates of three cases and no control (not significant).

A similar case-control study of *Wilms' tumour* was conducted by Wilkins and Sinks (1984), using the Columbus, OH, USA, Children's Hospital Tumor Registry files between 1950 and 1981. For each of 105 cases, two children were randomly selected from the Ohio birth certificate files and used as controls after matching for age, sex and race. For no case and for two controls the father's occupation at the time of birth was welder (not significant).

In a further case-control study (Bunin *et al.*, 1989), paternal occupational exposures of 88 cases of Wilms' tumour, obtained from a job-exposure matrix, were compared with those of an equal number of controls, obtained by random digital dialling and matched for date of birth. For a job cluster with exposure to aromatic and aliphatic hydrocarbons, metals and inorganic compounds, elevated crude odds ratios were seen for exposure before conception (5.3, 95% CI 1.5-28.6), during pregnancy (4.3, 95% CI, 1.2-23.7) and after pregnancy (3.3, 95% CI, 0.9-18.8). Within this cluster, the occupation of the father was welder for five cases but for only one control.

# 4. Summary of Data Reported and Evaluation

## 4.1 Exposure data

Welding has been an important industrial process since the early twentieth century and has become widespread since about 1940. A wide variety of welding techniques is used, although most welding is performed using electric arc processes — manual metal arc, metal inert gas and tungsten inert gas welding — all of which have been used for at least 40 years. Although most welding is on mild steel, about 5% is on stainless-steels; welding on stainless-steels can constitute more than 20% of welding in industrial economies. Welding of aluminium and other metals amounts to only a few per cent of the total.

The number of workers worldwide whose work involves some welding is estimated to be about three million.

Welders are exposed to a range of fumes and gases. Fume particles contain a wide variety of oxides and salts of metals and other compounds, which are produced mainly from electrodes, filler wire and flux materials. Fumes from the welding of stainless-steel and other alloys contain nickel compounds and chromium[VI] and [III]. Ozone is formed during most electric arc welding, and exposures can be high in comparison to the exposure limit, particularly during metal inert gas welding of aluminium. Oxides of nitrogen are found during manual metal arc welding and particularly during gas welding. Welders who weld painted mild steel can also be exposed to a range of organic compounds produced by pyrolysis. Welders, especially in shipyards, may also be exposed to asbestos dust.

## 4.2 Experimental carcinogenicity data

Particulates collected from stainless-steel welding fumes were tested by intratracheal instillation in hamsters and by intrabronchial implantation in rats. No treatment-related tumour was seen in rats, and single lung tumours were seen in groups of hamsters receiving manual metal arc stainless-steel welding fume. No study in which animals were exposed to welding fume by inhalation was available for evaluation.

## 4.3 Human carcinogenicity data

Two cohort studies of lung cancer mortality among persons in various occupations did not show significant increases in risk among welders. A total of three pleural mesotheliomas was reported from one of these studies. One large cohort study conducted in the UK showed an almost two-fold excess risk for lung cancer among shipyard welders, which was not confirmed when comparison was made with a local referent population. A moderately increased incidence of lung cancer was found in a large study of shipyard welders in Finland. Five studies conducted in the USA and Europe indicated an increased risk for lung cancer of about 30%.

A large European cohort study, including three cohorts reported previously, detected statistically significant increases in both the incidence of and mortality from lung cancer but demonstrated no consistent difference in cancer risk among stainless-steel welders as compared to mild-steel welders or to shipyard welders. In addition, five deaths were due to mesothelioma.

Of the 12 case-control studies on the association between lung cancer and exposure or employment as a welder, two detected no excess risk. Of the remaining ten, four showed a moderate excess, which was statistically significant in the largest study, conducted in the USA. The other six studies, of welders in various occupations, gave risk estimates exceeding a two-fold increase, which in four of the studies were statistically significant.

Four case-control studies conducted on bladder cancer — two in Canada, one in the USA and one in the Federal Republic of Germany — addressed the possible role of exposures during welding. Only one of the two from Canada reported a significantly increased risk.

Two case-control studies of leukaemia from the USA reported an elevated relative risk for myeloid leukaemia. No overall excess risk for either acute or all leukaemia was observed in a pooled analysis of data from several studies of welders.

Of the case-control studies of cancers at other sites, one on nasal cancer carried out in the Nordic countries, one on laryngeal cancer from Denmark and one on pancreatic cancer from Sweden reported elevated relative risks among welders.

## 4.4  Other relevant data

Welding fumes are retained in the lungs. Experimental studies have shown that sparingly soluble compounds may be released only slowly from the lungs. Elevated concentrations of chromium and nickel are seen in blood and urine, primarily in manual metal arc stainless-steel welders. Airway irritation and metal fume fever are the commonest acute effects of welding fumes. Studies of different groups of welders have documented an increased prevalence of pulmonary function abnormalities, in particular small airway disease, chronic bronchitis and slight abnormalities on chest X-rays, but only minimal indications of pulmonary fibrosis.

Reduced sperm quality has been reported in welders. Decreased fertility was seen in both male and female rats exposed to welding fumes; and the rate of fetal death was increased in pregnant female rats exposed to welding fumes.

One of three studies showed increased levels of sister chromatid exchange and chromosomal aberrations in peripheral blood lymphocytes of workers exposed during stainless-steel welding. The greater frequencies of sister chromatid exchanges were found in exposed workers who smoked.

In a single study, manual metal arc stainless-steel welding fumes injected intraperitoneally caused a mutagenic response in the mouse spot test. No increase in the frequency of sister chromatid exchange in peripheral blood lymphocytes or of chromosomal aberrations in lymphocytes or bone-marrow cells was observed in one study in rats after inhalation of stainless-steel or mild-steel welding fumes.

Both positive and negative results were obtained in tests for gene mutation in cultured mammalian cells exposed to stainless-steel welding fumes (manual metal arc). Stainless-steel welding fumes (manual metal arc and metal inert gas) induced transformation of mammalian cells *in vitro* in a single study. The frequencies of chromosomal aberrations and of sister chromatid exchange were increased in mammalian cells exposed *in vitro* to stainless-steel welding fumes (manual metal arc or metal inert gas). In a single study, mild-steel welding fumes (manual metal arc) increased the frequency of sister chromatid exchange but not of chromosomal aberrations in the same system. Fumes from the manual metal arc welding of mild steel or cast iron using a nickel electrode increased the frequency of sister chromatid exchange, but not of chromosomal aberrations, in mammalian cells *in vitro*.

Fumes from the manual metal arc or metal inert gas welding of stainless-steel and from manual metal arc welding of mild steel, but not the fumes from metal inert gas welding on mild steel or from mild steel welding on cast iron using a nickel electrode, were mutagenic to bacteria.

### 4.5  Evaluation[1]

There is *limited evidence* in humans for the carcinogenicity of welding fumes and gases.

There is *inadequate evidence* in experimental animals for the carcinogenicity of welding fumes.

### Overall evaluation

Welding fumes *are possibly carcinogenic to humans* (Group 2B).

---

[1]For definition of the italicized terms, see Preamble, pp. 33-37.

# 5. References

Abell, M.T. & Carlsberg, J.R. (1984) A simple reliable method for the determination of airborne hexavalent chromium. *Am. ind. Hyg. Assoc. J.*, *35*, 229-233

Akbarkhanzadeh, F. (1980) Long-term effects of welding fumes upon respiratory symptoms and pulmonary function. *Arch. environ. Health*, *22*, 337-341

Åkesson, B. & Skerfving, S. (1985) Exposure in welding of high nickel alloy. *Int. Arch. occup. environ. Health*, *56*, 111-117

American Conference of Governmental Industrial Hygienists (1988) *TLVs Threshold Limit Values and Biological Exposure Indices for 1988-1989*, Cincinnati, OH, p. 38

American Welding Society (1973) *The Welding Environment*, Miami, FL

American Welding Society (1979) *Effects of Welding on Health*, Miami, FL

Angerer, J. & Lehnert, G. (1990) Occupational chronic exposure to metals. II. Nickel exposure of stainless steel workers — biological monitoring. *Int. Arch. occup. environ. Health*, *62*, 7-10

Angerer, J., Amin, W., Heinrich-Ramm, R., Szadkowski, D. & Lehnert, G. (1987) Occupational chronic exposure to metals. I. Chromium exposure of stainless steel welders — biological monitoring. *Int. Arch. occup. environ. Health*, *59*, 503-512

Angervall, L., Hansson, G. & Röckert, H. (1960) Pulmonary siderosis in electrical welder. A note on pathological appearances. *Acta pathol. microbiol. scand.*, *49*, 373-380

Anthony, J.S., Zamel, N. & Aberman, A. (1978) Abnormalities in pulmonary function after brief exposure to toxic metal fumes. *Can. med. Assoc. J.*, *119*, 586-588

Anttila, S. (1986) Dissolution of stainless steel welding fumes in the rat lung: an X-ray microanalytical study. *Br. J. ind. Med.*, *43*, 592-596

Antti-Poika, M., Hassi, J. & Pyy, L. (1977) Respiratory diseases in arc welders. *Int. Arch. occup. environ. Health*, *40*, 225-230

Asal, N.R., Lee, E.T., Geyer, J.R., Kadamani, S., Risser, D.R. & Cherng, N. (1988) Risk factors in renal cell carcinoma. II. Medical history, occupation, multivariate analysis, and conclusions. *Cancer Detect. Prev.*, *13*, 263-279

Attfield, M.D. & Ross, D.S. (1978) Radiological abnormalities in electric-arc welders. *Br. J. ind. Med.*, *35*, 117-122

Baker, R.S.U., Arlauskas, A., Tandon, R.K., Crisp, P.T. & Ellis, J. (1986) Toxic and genotoxic action of electric-arc welding fumes on cultured mammalian cells. *J. appl. Toxicol.*, *6*, 357-362

Barfoot, K.M., Mitchell, I.V., Verheyen, F. & Babeliowsky, T. (1981) Combined PIXE and X-ray SEM studies of time-resolved deposits of welding shop aerosols. *Nucl. Instr. Methods*, *181*, 449-457

Barhad, B., Teculescu, D. & Craciun, O. (1975) Respiratory symptoms, chronic bronchitis, and ventilatory function in shipyard welders. *Int. Arch. occup. environ. Health*, *36*, 137-150

Beaumont, J.J. & Weiss, N.S. (1980) Mortality of welders, shipfitters, and other metal trades workers in boilermakers local no. 104, AFL-CIO. *Am. J. Epidemiol.*, *112*, 775-786

Beaumont, J.J. & Weiss, N.S. (1981) Lung cancer among welders. *J. occup. Med.*, *23*, 839-844

Becker, N., Claude, J. & Frentzel-Beyme, R. (1985) Cancer risk of arc welders exposed to fumes containing chromium and nickel. *Scand. J. Work Environ. Health*, *11*, 75-82

Benhamou, S., Benhamou, E. & Flamant, R. (1988) Occupational risk factors of lung cancer in a French case-control study. *Br. J. ind. Med.*, *45*, 231-233

Berg, N.O., Berlin, M., Bohgard, M., Rudell, B., Schütz, A. & Warvinge, K. (1987) Broncho-carcinogenic properties of welding and thermal spraying fumes containing chromium in the rat. *Am. J. ind. Med.*, *11*, 39-54

Bergmann, L. (1982) On a possible relation between the occupational exposure of welders and the development of bronchogenic carcinoma (Ger.). *Z. Erkrank. Atm. Org.*, *158*, 322-325

Bernacki, E.J., Parsons, G.E., Roy, B.R., Mikac-Devic, M., Kennedy, C.D. & Sunderman, F.W., Jr (1978) Urine nickel concentrations in nickel-exposed workers. *Ann. clin. Lab. Sci.*, *8*, 184-189

Beton, D.C., Andrews, G.S., Davies, H.J., Howells, L. & Smith, G.F. (1966) Acute cadmium fume poisoning. Five cases with one death from renal necrosis. *Br. J. ind. Med.*, *23*, 292-301

Biggart, N.W. & Rinehart, R.R. (1987) Comparison between aqueous-phase and gas-phase exposure protocols for determining the mutagenic potential of nitrogen dioxide and the gas fraction of welding fumes. *Mutat. Res.*, *188*, 175-184

Biggart, N.W., Rinehart, R.R. & Verfaillie, J. (1987) Evidence for the presence of mutagenic compounds other than chromium in particles from mild steel welding. *Mutat. Res.*, *188*, 55-65

Bille, M., Rosendahl, C.-H., Steen, A., Svensson, L. & Wallen, K.-A. (1976) Determination of decomposition products formed during welding on painted steel. *Svetsaren*, *2*, 6-13

Bjørnerem, H., Thomassen, L.M. & Wergeland, E. (1983) Welding asthma (Norw.). *Tidsskr. Nor. Læforen.*, *103*, 1286-1288

Blot, W.J., Harrington, J.M., Toledo, A., Hoover, R., Heath, C.W., Jr & Fraumeni, J.F., Jr (1978) Lung cancer after employment in shipyards during World War II. *New Engl. J. Med.*, *299*, 620-624

Blot, W.J., Morris, L.E., Stroube, R., Tagnon, I. & Fraumeni, J.F., Jr (1980) Lung and laryngeal cancers in relation to shipyard employment in coastal Virginia. *J. natl Cancer Inst.*, *65*, 571-575

Breslow, L., Hoaglin, L., Rasmussen, G. & Abrams, H.K. (1954) Occupations and cigarette smoking as factors in lung cancer. *Am. J. public Health*, *44*, 171-181

Brillié, J. (1990) *Soudure Electrique à l'Arc* (Electric arc welding), Paris, Ecole Supérieure de Soudure Autogène

British Standards Institution (1986) *Fume from Welding and Allied Processes: Guide to Methods for Sampling and Analysis of Particulate Matter and Gases* (BS6691 Parts 1, 2), London

Brun, J., Cassan, G., Kofman, J., Gilly, J. & Magnin, F. (1972) Conglomerate siderosis in arc welders (Fr.). *J. fr. Méd.*, *26*, 133-142

Buiatti, E., Kriebel, D., Geddes, M., Santucci, M. & Pucci, N. (1985) A case control study of lung cancer in Florence, Italy. I. Occupational risk factors. *J. Epidemiol. Community Health*, *39*, 244-250

Bunin, G.R., Nass, C.C., Kramer, S. & Meadows, A.T. (1989) Parental occupation and Wilms' tumor: results of a case-control study. *Cancer Res.*, *49*, 725-729

Caccuri, S. & Fournier, E. (1969) *On Welding* (Publication Series on Occupational Hygiene and Occupational Medicine No. 9), Luxembourg, Commission of the European Communities

Carpenter, A.V., Flanders, W.D., Frome, E.L., Tankersley, W.G. & Fry, S.A. (1988) Chemical exposures and central nervous system cancers: a case-control study among workers at two nuclear facilities. *Am. J. ind. Med.*, *13*, 351-362

Casciani, G., Ruspolini, F., Verdel, U. & Cecchetti, G. (1986) Welding fumes concentration in heavy carpentry working environment and trial to correlate same with gas and powdered fluorides. In: Stern, R.M., Berlin, A., Fletcher, A.C. & Järvisalo, J., eds, *Health Hazards and Biological Effects of Welding Gumes and Gases*, Amsterdam, Excerpta Medica, pp. 153-157

Cavalleri, A. & Minoia, C. (1985) Distribution in serum and erythrocytes and urinary elimination of chromium in workers occupationally exposed to Cr(VI) and Cr(III). (Ital.) *Med. Lav.*, *7*, 35-38

Charr, R. (1953) Respiratory disorders among welders. *J. Am. med. Assoc.*, *152*, 1520-1522

Charr, R. (1956) Pulmonary changes in welders: a report of three cases. *Ann. intern. Med.*, *44*, 806-812

Claude, J.C., Frentzel-Beyme, R.R. & Kunze, E. (1988) Occupation and risk of cancer of the lower urinary tract among men. A case-control study. *Int. J. Cancer*, *41*, 371-379

Coenen, W., Grothe, I., Kühnen, G., Pfeiffer, W. & Schenk, H. (1985) Nickel and chromate in welding fume. (Ger.) *Staub*, *45*, 546-550

Coenen, W., Grothe, I. & Kühnen, G. (1986) Exposure to welding fumes in the workplace with regard to nickel and chromates. In: Stern, R.M., Berlin, A., Fletcher, A.C. & Järvisalo, J., eds, *Health Hazards and Biological Effects of Welding Fumes and Gases*, Amsterdam, Excerpta Medica, pp. 149-152

Cotes, J.E., Feinmann, E.L., Male, V.J., Rennie, F.S. & Wickham, C.A.C. (1989) Respiratory symptoms and impairment in shipyard welders and caulker/burners. *Br. J. ind. Med.*, *46*, 292-301

Dare, P.R.M., Hewitt, P.J., Hicks, R., Van Bemst, A., Zober, A. & Fleischer, M. (1984) Barium in welding fume. *Ann. occup. Hyg.*, *28*, 445-448

Decouflé, P., Stanislawczyk, K., Houten, L., Bross, I.D.J. & Viadana, E. (1977) *A Retrospective Survey of Cancer in Relation to Occupation* (DHEW (NIOSH) Publ. No. 77-178), Cincinnati, OH, National Institute for Occupational Safety and Health

Doig, A.T. & McLaughlin, A.I.G. (1936) X-Ray appearances of the lungs of electric arc welders. *Lancet*, *i*, 771-775

Doig, A.T. & McLaughlin, A.I.G. (1948) Clearing of X-ray shadows in welders' siderosis. *Lancet*, *i*, 789-791

Dubrow, R. & Wegman, D.H. (1984) Cancer and occupation in Massachusetts: a death certificate study. *Am. J. ind. Med.*, 6, 207-230

Dunn, J.E., Jr & Weir, J.M. (1965) Cancer experience of several occupational groups followed prospectively. *Am. J. public Health*, 55, 1367-1375

Dunn, J.E., Jr & Weir, J.M. (1968) A prospective study of mortality of several occupational groups. Special emphasis on lung cancer. *Arch. environ. Health*, 17, 71-76

Dunn, J.E., Jr, Linden, G. & Breslow, L. (1960) Lung cancer mortality experience of men in certain occupations in California. *Am. J. public Health*, 50, 1475-1487

Eichhorn, F. & Oldenburg, T. (1986) Welding fumes emitted during welding of high-alloyed materials — evaluation of amount, chemical composition and morphology, including the influence of welding parameters. In: Stern, R.M., Berlin, A., Fletcher, A.C. & Järvisalo, J., eds, *Health Hazards and Biological Effects of Welding Fumes and Gases*, Amsterdam, Excerpta Medica, pp. 51-59

Emmerling, G., Zschiesche, W., Schaller, K.-H., Weltle, D., Valentin, H. & Zober, A. (1987) Quantification of external and internal exposure to total chromium and chromium VI in welding with high alloy consumables. (Ger.) In: Norpoth, K., ed., *Proceedings of the 27th Annual Assembly of the German Society of Occupational Medicine, Essen, May 6-9 1987*, Stuttgart, Gentner Verlag, pp. 497-501

Emmett, E.A., Buncher, C.R., Suskind, R.B. & Rowe, K.W., Jr (1981) Skin and eye diseases among arc welders and those exposed to welding operations. *J. occup. Med.*, 23, 85-90

Englund, A., Ekman, G. & Zabrielski, L. (1982) Occupational categories among brain tumor cases recorded in the cancer registry in Sweden. *Ann. N.Y. Acad. Sci.*, 381, 188-196

Engström, K., Engström, B. & Henriks-Eckerman, M.-L. (1988) Evaluation of exposures during the welding or flame-cutting of painted steel. *Scand. J. Work Environ. Health, 14 (Suppl. 1)*, 33-34

Enzer, N. & Sander, O.A. (1938) Chronic lung changes in electric arc welders. *J. ind. Hyg. Toxicol.*, 20, 333-350

Etienne, C.F., Hooftman, R.N., de Raat, W.K., Reuzel, P.G.J., van der Sluis, H.H. & Wilmer, J.W.G.M. (1986) *The Assessment of the Carcinogenicity of Chromium- and Nickel-containing Welding Fumes. Phase I: In vitro and In vivo Genotoxicity and Cytotoxicity Studies. Final Report* (ECSC-TNO Contract 7248/22/020), Luxembourg, Commission of the European Communities

Evans, M.J., Ingle, J., Molyneux, M.K. & Sharp, G.T.H. (1979) An occupational hygiene study of a controlled welding task using a general purpose rutile electrode. *Ann. occup. Hyg.*, 22, 1-17

Fabre, M., Marais, M., Ladouch, A., Paillas, J., Blanchon, P. & Quillard, J. (1976) Pneumoconiosis in arc welders. (Fr.) *Arch. Anat. Cytol. pathol.*, 24, 481-485

Farrants, G., Reith, A., Schüler, B. & Feren, K. (1988) A simple, direct method for the collection of particles from air samples for transmission electron microscopy and digital image analysis. *J. Microsc.*, 149, 88-93

Farrell, F.J. (1987) Angioedema and urticaria as acute and late phase reactions to zinc fume exposure, with associated metal fume fever-like symptoms. *Am. J. ind. Med.*, 12, 331-337

Fasiska, E.J., Wagenblast, H.W. & Nasta, M. (1983) *Characterization of Arc Welding Fume*, Miami, FL, American Welding Society

Fawer, R.F., Gardner, A.W. & Oakes, D. (1982) Absences attributed to respiratory diseases in welders. *Br. J. ind. Med.*, *39*, 149-152

Fletcher, A.C. & Ades, A. (1984) Lung cancer mortality in a cohort of English foundry workers. *Scand. J. Work Environ. Health*, *10*, 7-16

Fogh, A., Frost, J. & Georg, J. (1969) Respiratory symptoms and pulmonary function in welders. *Ann. occup. Hyg.*, *12*, 213-218

Fregert, S. & Övrum, P. (1963) Chromate in welding fumes with special reference to contact dermatitis. *Acta dermatovenereol.*, *43*, 119-124

Friede, E. & Rachow, D.O. (1961) Symptomatic pulmonary disease in arc welders. *Ann. intern. Med.*, *54*, 121-127

Froats, J.F.K. & Mason, P.J. (1986) Worker exposure to welding fumes and gases during hydraulic plant turbine repair. In: Stern, R.M., Berlin, A., Fletcher, A.C. & Järvisalo, J., eds, *Health Hazards and Biological Effects of Welding Gumes and Gases*, Amsterdam, Excerpta Medica, pp. 137-140

Funahashi, A., Schlueter, D.P., Pintar, K., Bemis, E.L. & Siegesmund, K.A. (1988) Welder's pneumoconiosis: tissue elemental microanalysis by energy dispersive X-ray analysis. *Br. J. ind. Med.*, *45*, 14-18

Gallagher, R.P. & Threlfall, W.J. (1983) Cancer mortality in metal workers. *Can. med. Assoc. J.*, *129*, 1191-1194

Garnuszewski, Z. & Dobrzynski, W. (1967) Regression of pulmonary radiological changes in dockyard welders after cessation or decrease of exposure to welding fumes. *Pol. med. J.*, *6*, 610-613

Gérin, M., Siemiatycki, J., Bégin, D., Kemper, H., Lakhani, R., Nadon, L. & Richardson, L. (1986) Epidemiological monitoring system for identifying carcinogens in the Montréal work environment: a progress report. (Fr.) *Trav. Santé*, *2*, S42-S46

Gobbato, F., Melato, M. & Bucconi, S. (1980) Welder's lung and possible neoplastic complications. (Ital.) *Med. Lav.*, *2*, 132-140

Gottlieb, M.S. (1980) Lung cancer and the petroleum industry in Louisiana. *J. occup. Med.*, *22*, 384-388

Grandjean, P. & Kon, S.H. (1981) Lead exposure of welders and bystanders in a ship repair yard. *Am. J. ind. Med.*, *2*, 65-70

Grandjean, P., Selikoff, I.J., Shen, S.K. & Sunderman, F.W., Jr (1980) Nickel concentrations in plasma and urine of shipyard workers. *Am. J. ind. Med.*, *1*, 181-189

Grekula, A., Peura, R. & Sivonen, S.J. (1986) Quantitative energy dispersive X-ray microanalysis of welding fumes. In: Stern, R.M., Berlin, A., Fletcher, A.C. & Järvisalo, J., eds, *Health Hazards and Biological Effects of Welding Gumes and Gases*, Amsterdam, Excerpta Medica, pp. 85-88

Grozdenko, L.A. & Kuzina, A.S. (1982) Hygienic measurement of the welding arc radiation under present industrial conditions. (Russ.) *Gig. Tr. prof. Zabol.*, *5*, 31-34

Guidotti, T.L., DeNee, P.B., Abraham, J.L. & Smith, J.R. (1978) Arc welder's pneumoconiosis: application of advanced scanning electron microscopy. *Arch. environ. Health, 33,* 117-124

Guralnick, L. (1963) *Mortality by Industry and Cause of Death Among Men 20 to 64 Years of Age: United States, 1950* (Vital Statistics Special Reports 53), Washington DC, US Department of Health, Education, and Welfare, p. 246

Gustafsson, T.E., Tossavainen, A. & Aitio, A. (1986) Scanning electron microscope studies on flame cutting and welding fumes in a steel foundry. In: Stern, R.M., Berlin, A., Fletcher, A.C. & Järvisalo, J., eds, *Health Hazards and Biological Effects of Welding Fumes and Gases,* Amsterdam, Excerpta Medica, pp. 93-97

Gustavsson, C. & Welinder, H. (1986) Stainless steel manual metal-arc welding and chromium in blood. In: Stern, R.M., Berlin, A., Fletcher, A.C. & Järvisalo, J., eds, *Health Hazards and Biological Effects of Welding Fumes and Gases,* Amsterdam, Excerpta Medica, pp. 185-188

Gylseth, B., Gundersen, N. & Langård, S. (1977) Evaluation of chromium exposure based on a simplified method for urinary chromium determination. *Scand. J. Work Environ. Health, 3,* 28-31

Hagberg, M., Lindqvist, B. & Wall, S. (1986) Exposure to welding fumes and chronic renal diseases, a negative case-referent study. *Int. Arch. occup. environ. Health, 58,* 191-195

Hallne, U. & Hallberg, B.-O. (1982) *Problems of the Work Environment due to Welding,* Part 21, *Nickel Carbonyl, Carbon Monoxide and Nitrogen Oxide Emissions from Arc Welding Cast Iron Using Nickel Containing Electrodes* (Report 1982:11), Solna, Arbetarskyddsstyrelsen

Haneke, E. (1973) Ejaculation findings in electric welders (Ger.) *Dermatol. Monatsschr., 159,* 1036-1040

Hansen, K. & Stern, R.M. (1984) Toxicity and transformation potency of nickel compounds in BHK cells *in vitro.* In: Sunderman, F.W., Jr, ed., *Nickel in the Human Environment* (IARC Scientific Publications No. 53), Lyon, IARC, pp. 193-200

Hansen, K. & Stern, R.M. (1985) Welding fumes and chromium compounds in cell transformation assays. *J. appl. Toxicol., 5,* 306-314

Harding, H.E., McLaughlin, A.I.G. & Doig, A.T. (1958) Clinical, radiographic and pathological studies of the lungs of electric-arc and oxyacetylene welders. *Lancet, ii,* 394-398

Hayden, S.P., Pincock, A.C., Hayden, J., Tyler, L.E., Cross, K.W. & Bishop, J.M. (1984) Respiratory symptoms and pulmonary function of welders in the engineering industry. *Thorax, 39,* 442-447

Hedenstedt, A., Jenssen, D., Lidesten, B.-M., Ramel, C., Rannug, U. & Stern, R.M. (1977) Mutagenicity of fume particles from stainless steel welding. *Scand. J. Work Environ. Health, 3,* 203-211

Hemminki, K. & Lindbohm, M.-L. (1986) Reproductive effects of welding fumes: experimental and epidemiological studies with special reference to chromium and nickel compounds. In: Stern, R.M., Berlin, A., Fletcher, A.C. & Järvisalo, J., eds, *Health Hazards and Biological Effects of Welding Fumes and Gases,* Amsterdam, Excerpta Medica, pp. 291-302

Hernberg, S., Collan, Y., Degerth, R., Englund, A., Engzell, U., Kuosma, E., Mutanen, P., Nordlinder, H., Sand Hansen, H., Schultz-Larsen, K., Søgaard, H. & Westerholm, P. (1983a) Nasal cancer and occupational exposures. Preliminary report of a joint Nordic case-referent study. *Scand. J. Work Environ. Health, 9,* 208-213

Hernberg, S., Westerholm, P., Schultz-Larsen, K., Degerth, R., Kuosma, E., Englund, A., Engzell, U., Sand Hansen, H. & Mutanen, P. (1983b) Nasal and sinosal cancer. Connection with occupational exposures in Denmark, Finland and Sweden. *Scand. J. Work Environ. Health, 9,* 315-326

Hewitt, P.J. & Madden, M.G. (1986) Welding process parameters and hexavalent chromium in MIG fume. *Ann. occup. Hyg., 30,* 427-434

Hicks, R., Hewitt, P.J. & Lam, H.F. (1979) An investigation of the experimental induction of hypersensitivity in the guinea pig by material containing chromium, nickel and cobalt from arc welding fumes. *Int. Arch. Allergy appl. Immunol., 59,* 265-272

Hicks, R., Al-Shamma, K.J., Lam, H.F. & Hewitt, P.J. (1983) An investigation of fibrogenic and other toxic effects of arc-welding fume particles deposited in the rat lung. *J. appl. Toxicol., 3,* 297-306

Hicks, R., Lam, H.F., Al-Shamma, K.J. & Hewitt, P.J. (1984) Pneumoconiotic effects of welding-fume particles from mild and stainless steel deposited in the lung of the rat. *Arch. Toxicol., 55,* 1-10

Hicks, R., Oshodi, R.O. & Pedrick, M.J. (1987) Cytotoxic, irritant and fibrogenic effects of metal-fume particulate materials investigated by intramuscular injection in the rat and guinea pig. *Arch. Toxicol., Suppl. 11,* 220-222

Hildebrand, H.F., Collyn-D'Hooghe, M. & Stern, R.M. (1986) Cytotoxic effects of welding fumes on human embryonic epithelial pulmonary cells in culture. In: Stern, R.M., Berlin, A., Fletcher, A.C. & Järvisalo, J., eds, *Health Hazards and Biological Effects of Welding Fumes and Gases,* Amsterdam, Excerpta Medica, pp. 319-324

Houten, L., Bross, I.D.J., Viadana, E. & Sonnesso, G. (1977) Occupational cancer in men exposed to metals. *Adv. exp. Med. Biol., 91,* 93-102

Howe, G.R., Burch, J.D., Miller, A.B., Cook, G.M., Estève, J., Morrison, B., Gordon, P., Chambers, L.W., Fodor, G. & Winsor, G.M. (1980) Tobacco use, occupation, coffee, various nutrients, and bladder cancer. *J. natl Cancer Inst., 64,* 701-713

Howe, G.R., Fraser, D., Lindsay, J., Presnal, B. & Yu, S.Z. (1983) Cancer mortality (1965-77) in relation to diesel fume and coal exposure in a cohort of retired railway workers. *J. natl Cancer Inst., 70,* 1015-1019

Husgafvel-Pursiainen, K., Kalliomäki, P.-L. & Sorsa, M. (1982) A chromosome study among stainless steel welders. *J. occup. Med., 24,* 762-766

IARC (1989) *Mortality and Cancer Incidence Follow-up on an Historical Cohort of European Welders* (Intern. tech. Rep. 89/003), Lyon

Irmscher, G., Beck, B., Ahlendorf, W., Anspach, M., Konetzke, G., Ludwig, V. & Sturm, W. (1975) Experience gained in assessing doubtful cirrhosis of the lung caused by welding fumes. (Ger.) *Z. ges. Hyg., 21,* 562-566

Järvisalo, J., Olkinuora, M., Tossavainen, A., Virtamo, M., Ristola, P. & Aitio, A. (1983) Urinary and blood manganese as indicators of manganese exposure in manual metal arc welding of mild steel. In: Brown, S.S. & Savory, J., eds, *Chemical Toxicology and Clinical Chemistry of Metals*, New York, Academic Press, pp. 123-126

Jefferson, T.B. (1988) 1987: a comeback for welding sales. *Welding Design Fabrication*, July, 51-54

Jindrichova, J. (1978) Harmful effects caused by chromium in electric welders. (Ger.) *Z. ges. Hyg.*, *24*, 86-88

Kalliomäki, P.-L., Sutinen, S., Kelhä, V., Lakomaa, E., Sortti, V. & Sutinen, S. (1979) Amount and distribution of fume contaminants in the lungs of an arc welder *post mortem*. *Br. J. ind. Med.*, *36*, 224-230

Kalliomäki, P.-L., Rahkonen, E., Vaaranen, V., Kalliomäki, K. & Aittoniemi, K. (1981) Lung-retained contaminants, urinary chromium and nickel among stainless steel welders. *Int. Arch. occup. environ. Health*, *49*, 67-75

Kalliomäki, P.-L., Kiilunen, M., Vaaranen, V., Lakomaa, E.-L., Kalliomäki, K. & Kivelä, R. (1982a) Retention of stainless steel manual metal arc welding fumes in rats. *J. Toxicol. environ. Health*, *10*, 223-232

Kalliomäki, P.-L., Kalliomäki, K., Korhonen, O., Nordman, H., Rahkonen, E. & Vaaranen, V. (1982b) Respiratory status of stainless steel and mild steel welders. *Scand. J. Work Environ. Health, Suppl. 1*, 117-121

Kalliomäki, P.-L., Junttila, M.-E., Kalliomäki, K., Lakomaa, E.-L. & Kivelä, R. (1983a) Comparison of the behavior of stainless and mild steel manual metal arc welding fumes in rat lung. *Scand. J. Work Environ. Health*, *9*, 176-180

Kalliomäki, P.-L., Junttila, M.-E., Kalliomäki, K., Lakomaa, E.-L. & Kivelä, R. (1983b) Comparison of the retention and clearance of different welding fumes in rat lungs. *Am. ind. Hyg. Assoc. J.*, *44*, 733-738

Kalliomäki, P.-L., Lakomaa, E., Kalliomäki, K., Kiilunen, M., Kivelä, R. & Vaaranen, V. (1983c) Stainless steel manual metal arc welding fumes in rats. *Br. J. ind. Med.*, *40*, 229-234

Kalliomäki, P.-L., Tuomisaari, M., Lakomaa, E.-L., Kalliomäki, K. & Kivelä, R. (1983d) Retention and clearance of stainless steel shieldgas welding fumes in rat lungs. *Am. ind. Hyg. Assoc. J.*, *44*, 649-654

Kalliomäki, P.-L., Olkinuora, M., Hyvärinen, H.-K. & Kalliomäki, K. (1984) Kinetics of nickel and chromium in rats exposed to different stainless-steel welding fumes. In: Sunderman, F.W., Jr, ed., *Nickel in the Human Environment* (IARC Scientific Publications No. 53), Lyon, IARC, pp. 385-393

Kalliomäki, P.-L., Hyvärinen, H.-K., Aitio, A., Lakomaa, E.-L. & Kalliomäki, K. (1986) Kinetics of the metal components of intratracheally instilled stainless steel welding fume suspensions in rats. *Br. J. ind. Med.*, *43*, 112-119

Kantor, A.F., McCrea Curnen, M.G., Meigs, J.W. & Flannery J.T. (1979) Occupations of fathers of patients with Wilms's tumour. *J. Epidemiol. Community Health*, *33*, 253-256

Keimig, D.G., Pomrehn, P.R. & Burmeister, L.F. (1983) Respiratory symptoms and pulmonary function in welders of mild steel: a cross-sectional study. *Am. J. ind. Med.*, *4*, 489-499

Keskinen, H., Kalliomäki, P.-L. & Alanko, K. (1980) Occupational asthma due to stainless steel welding fumes. *Clin. Allergy*, *10*, 151-159

Kilburn, K.H., Warshaw, R. & Thornton, J.C. (1985) Asbestosis, pulmonary symptoms and functional impairment in shipyard workers. *Chest*, *88*, 254-259

Kjuus, J., Skjaerven R., Langård, S., Lien, J.T. & Aamodt, T. (1986) A case-referent study of lung cancer, occupational exposures and smoking. I. Comparison of title-based and exposure-based occupational information. *Scand. J. Work Environ. Health*, *12*, 193-202

Knight, G.S., Williams, H.E.M. & Hinton, D. (1985) Elevated plasma manganese levels in welders cutting manganese steel. *N.Z. med. J.*, *98*, 870

Knudsen, I. (1980) The mammalian spot test and its use for the testing of potential carcinogenicity of welding fume particles and hexavalent chromium. *Acta pharmacol. toxicol.*, *47*, 66-70

Kobayashi, M. & Tsutsumi, S. (1986) Investigation on crystalline materials in welding fumes of covered electrodes. In: Stern, R.M., Berlin, A., Fletcher, A.C. & Järvisalo, J., eds, *Health Hazards and Biological Effects of Welding Fumes and Gases*, Amsterdam, Excerpta Medica, pp. 77-80

Koponen, M., Gustaffson, T., Kalliomäki, P.-L., Kalliomäki, K. & Moilanen, M. (1981) Grinding dusts of alloyed steel and hard metal. *Ann. occup. Hyg.*, *24*, 191-204

Koshi, K. (1979) Effects of fume particles from stainless steel welding on sister chromatid exchanges and chromosomal aberrations in cultured Chinese hamster cells. *Ind. Health*, *17*, 39-49

Koshi, K., Yagami, T. & Nakanishi, Y. (1984) Cytogenetic analysis of peripheral blood lymphocytes from stainless steel welders. *Ind. Health*, *22*, 305-318

Kujawska, A. & Marek, K. (1979) Radiological picture of pneumoconiosis in welders. (Pol.) *Med. Prac.*, *30*, 79-84

Lam, H.F., Hewitt, P.J. & Hicks, R. (1979) A study of pulmonary deposition, and the elimination of some constitutent metals from welding fume in laboratory animals. *Ann. occup. Hyg.*, *21*, 363-373

Lancaster, J.F. (1980) *Metallurgy of Welding*, 3rd ed., London, George Allen & Unwin

Lerchen, M.L., Wiggins, C.L. & Samet, J.M. (1987) Lung cancer and occupation in New Mexico. *J. natl Cancer Inst.*, *79*, 639-645

Lindberg, R.A. & Braton, N.R. (1985) *Welding and Other Joining Processes*, Boston, MA, Allyn and Bacon Inc.

Lippmann, M. (1986) Magnetopneumography as a tool for measuring lung burden of industrial aerosols. In: Stern, R.M., Berlin, A., Fletcher, A.C. & Järvisalo, J., eds, *Health Hazards and Biological Effects of Welding Fumes and Gases*, Amsterdam, Excerpta Medica, pp. 199-213

Littorin, M., Högstedt, B., Strömbäck, B., Karlsson, A., Welinder, H., Mitelman, F. & Skerfving, S. (1983) No cytogenetic effects in lymphocytes of stainless steel welders. *Scand. J. Work Environ. Health*, *9*, 259-264

Littorin, M., Welinder, H. & Hultberg, B. (1984) Kidney function in stainless steel welders. *Int. Arch. occup. environ. Health*, *53*, 279-282

Logan, W.P.D., ed. (1982) *Cancer Mortality by Occupation and Social Class 1851-1971* (IARC Scientific Publications No. 36), Lyon, IARC, pp. 239, 246

Malmqvist, K.G., Johansson, G.I., Bohgard, M. & Akselsson, K.R. (1981) Elemental concentrations in airborne particles from welding and metal spraying operations. *Nucl. Instr. Methods*, *181*, 465-471

Malmqvist, K.G., Johansson, G., Bohgard, M. & Akselsson, K.R. (1986) Process-dependent characteristics of welding fume particles. In: Stern, R.M., Berlin, A., Fletcher, A.C. & Järvisalo, J., eds, *Health Hazards and Biological Effects of Welding Fumes and Gases*, Amsterdam, Excerpta Medica, pp. 31-46

Maxild, J., Andersen, M., Kiel, P. & Stern, R.M. (1978) Mutagenicity of fume particles from metal arc welding on stainless steel in the *Salmonella*/microsome test. *Mutat. Res.*, *56*, 235-243

Mayer, A. & Salsi, S. (1980) *Etude en Laboratoire de la Pollution Chimique et du Rayonnement aux Postes de Soudage à l'Arc. Résultats des Essais Préliminaire Effectués sur 18 Couples 'Produit d'Apport — Métal Soudé' Différents* [Laboratory Study of Chemical Pollution and of Radiation at Arc Welding Stations. Results of Preliminary Tests Performed on 18 Different 'Support Material—Welded Metal' Couples] (Notes scientifiques et techniques de l'INRS No. 25), Paris, Institut National de Recherche et de Sécurité

McLaughlin, J.K., Malker, H.S.R., Blot, W.J., Malker, B.K., Stone, B.J., Weiner, J.A., Ericsson, J.L.E. & Fraumeni, J.F., Jr (1987) Occupational risks for intracranial gliomas in Sweden. *J. natl Cancer Inst.*, *78*, 253-257

McMillan, G.H.G. (1981) The health of welders in naval dockyards: welding, tobacco smoking and absence attributed to respiratory diseases. *J. Soc. occup. Med.*, *31*, 112-118

McMillan, G.H.G. (1983) The health of welders in naval dockyards. The risk of asbestos-related diseases occurring in welders. *J. occup. Med.*, *25*, 727-730

McMillan, G.H.G. & Pethybridge, R.J. (1983) The health of welders in naval dockyards: proportional mortality study of welders and two control groups. *J. Soc. occup. Med.*, *33*, 75-84

McMillan, G.H.G. & Pethybridge, R.J. (1984) A clinical, radiological and pulmonary function case-control study of 135 dockyard welders aged 45 years and over. *J. Soc. occup. Med.*, *34*, 3-23

Menck, H.R. & Henderson, B.E. (1976) Occupational differences in rates of lung cancer. *J. occup. Med.*, *18*, 797-801

Meyer, E.C., Kratzinger, S.F. & Miller, W.H. (1967) Pulmonary fibrosis in an arc welder. *Arch. environ. Health*, *15*, 462-469

Milham, S., Jr (1976) *Occupational Mortality in Washington State, 1950-1971* (DHEW (NIOSH) Publ. No. 76-175), Cincinnati, OH, National Institute for Occupational Safety and Health

Milham, S., Jr (1983) *Occupational Mortality in Washington State, 1950-1979* (DHEW (NIOSH) Publication No. 83-116), Cincinnati, National Institute for Occupational Safety and Health

Milne, K.L., Sandler, D.P., Everson, R.B. & Brown, S.M. (1983) Lung cancer and occupation in Alameda county: a death certificate case-control study. *Am. J. ind. Med.*, *4*, 565-575

Minni, E. (1986) Assessment of the use of electron spectroscopy and sputtering for studies of solid fume particles. In: Stern, R.M., Berlin, A., Fletcher, A.C. & Järvisalo, J., eds, *Health Hazards and Biological Effects of Welding Fumes and Gases*, Amsterdam, Excerpta Medica, pp. 89-92

Minni, E., Gustafsson, T.E., Koponen, M. & Kalliomäki, P.-L. (1984) A study of the chemical structure of particles in the welding fumes of mild and stainless steel. *J. Aerosol Sci.*, *15*, 57-68

Moreton, J. (1986) The case for standardization of tests for welding fume emission rates and chemical composition determination. *Ann. occup. Hyg.*, *30*, 435-444

Moreton, J., Day, S.E. & Jenkins, N. (1986) Fume emission rate measurements and fume analysis on four stainless steel welding consumables. In: Stern, R.M., Berlin, A., Fletcher, A.C. & Järvisalo, J., eds, *Health Hazards and Biological Effects of Welding Fumes and Gases*, Amsterdam, Excerpta Medica, pp. 61-64

Morgan, W.K.C. (1989) On welding, wheezing and whimsy. *Am. ind. Hyg. Assoc. J.*, *50*, 59-69

Morgan, W.K.C. & Kerr, H.D. (1963) Pathologic and physiologic studies of welders' siderosis. *Ann. intern. Med.*, *58*, 293-304

Mortensen, J.T. (1988) Risk for reduced sperm quality among metal workers, with special reference to welders. *Scand. J. Work Environ. Health*, *14*, 27-30

Morton, W.E. & Treyve, E.L. (1982) Histologic differences in occupational risks of lung cancer incidence. *Am. J. ind. Med.*, *3*, 441-457

Moss, C.E. & Murray, W.E. (1979) Optical radiation levels produced in gas welding, torch brazing and oxygen cutting. *Welding J.*, *9*, 37-46

Mur, J.M., Teculescu, D., Pham, Q.T., Gaertner, M., Massin, N., Meyer-Bisch, C., Moulin, J.J., Diebold, F., Pierre, F., Meurou-Poncelet, B. & Muller, J. (1985) Lung function and clinical findings in a cross-sectional study of arc welders. An epidemiological study. *Int. Arch. occup. environ. Health*, *57*, 1-17

Mur, J.M., Pham, Q.T., Teculescu, D., Massin, N., Meyer-Bisch, C., Moulin, J.J., Wild, P., Leonard, M., Henquel, J.C., Baudin, V., Betz, M., Fontana, J.M. & Toamain, J.P. (1989) Arc welders' respiratory health evolution over five years. *Int. Arch. occup. environ. Health*, *61*, 321-327

Mutti, A., Cavatorta, A., Pedroni, C., Borghi, A., Giaroli, C. & Franchini, I. (1979) The role of chromium accumulation in the relationship between airborne and urinary chromium in welders. *Int. Arch. occup. environ. Health*, *43*, 123-133

Mutti, A., Pedroni, C., Arfini, G., Franchini, I., Minoia, C., Micoli, G. & Baldi, C. (1984) Biological monitoring of occupational exposure to different chromium compounds at various valency states. *Int. J. environ. anal. Chem.*, *17*, 35-41

Najarian, T. & Colton, T. (1978) Mortality from leukaemia and cancer in shipyard nuclear workers. *Lancet*, *i*, 1018-1020

Näslund, P.-E. & Högstedt, P. (1982) Welding and bronchitis. *Eur. J. respir. Dis.*, *118* (*Suppl.*), 69-72

National Institute for Occupational Safety and Health (1985) *Manual of Analytical Methods*, 2nd ed., *Hexavalent Chromium* (Publ. 80-125) Vol. 6, Washington DC, US Department of Health, Education, and Welfare

National Institute for Occupational Safety and Health (1988) *Criteria for a Recommended Standard, Welding, Brazing and Thermal Cutting* (DHHS (NIOSH) Publ. No. 88-110a; PB88-231774), Cincinnati, OH

Newhouse, M.L., Oakes, D. & Woolley A.J. (1985) Mortality of welders and other craftsmen at a shipyard in NE England. *Br. J. ind. Med.*, *42*, 406-410

Niebuhr, E., Stern, R.M., Thomsen, E. & Wulf, H.-C. (1980) Relative solubility of nickel welding fume fractions and their genotoxicity in sister chromatid exchange *in vitro*. In: Brown, S.S. & Sunderman, F.W., Jr, eds, *Nickel Toxicology*, London, Academic Press, pp. 129-132

Norell, S., Ahlbom, A., Olin, R., Erwald, R., Jacobson, G., Lindberg-Navier, I. & Wiechel, K.-L. (1986) Occupational factors and pancreatic cancer. *Br. J. ind. Med.*, *43*, 775-778

Office of Population Censuses and Surveys (1986) *Occupational Mortality. The Registrar General's Decennial Supplement for Great Britain, 1979-80, 1982-83. Part 1, Commentary* (Series DS No. 6), London, Her Majesty's Stationery Office, p. 72

Oláh, L. & Tölgyessy, J. (1985) Determination of heavy metals in welder's working environment using nuclear analytical methods. *J. Radioanal. nucl. Chem.*, *93*, 43-54

Oldenburg, T. (1988) *Vergleichende Bewertung von Schweissrauchen bei Verwendung Chrom-, Nickel- oder Bariumhaltiger Schweisszusatzwerkstoffe* [Comparing Assessment of Welding Fumes from Chromium-, Nickel- and Barium-containing Consumables] (Welding tech. Res. Rep. No. 21), Düsseldorf, DVS-Verlag

Olin, R.G., Ahlbom, A., Lindberg-Navier, I., Norell, S.E. & Spännare, B. (1987) Occupational factors associated with astrocytomas: a case-control study. *Am. J. ind. Med.*, *11*, 615-625

Olsen, J., Sabroe, S. & Lajer, M. (1984) Welding and cancer of the larynx: a case-control study. *Eur. J. Cancer clin. Oncol.*, *20*, 639-643

Ott, M.G., Holder, B.B. & Langner, R.R. (1976) Determinants of mortality in an industrial population. *J. occup. Med.*, *18*, 171-177

Oxhoj, H., Bake, B., Wedel, H. & Wilhelmsen, L. (1979) Effects of electric arc welding on ventilatory lung function. *Arch. environ. Health*, *34*, 211-217

Pasanen, J.T., Gustafsson, T.E., Kalliomäki, P.-L., Tossavainen, A. & Järvisalo, J.O. (1986) Cytotoxic effects of four types of welding fumes on macrophages *in vitro*: a comparative study. *J. Toxicol. environ. Health*, *18*, 143-152

Patel, K.C., Sheth, S.M. & Kamat, S.R. (1977) Arc welder's lung. A case report. *J. postgrad. Med.*, *23*, 35-38

Pedersen, B., Thomsen, E. & Stern, R.M. (1987) Some problems in sampling, analysis and evaluation of welding fumes containing Cr(VI). *Ann. occup. Hyg.*, *31*, 325-338

Peters, J.M., Murphy, R.L.H., Ferris, B.G., Burgess, W.A., Ranadive, M.V. & Pendergrass, H.P. (1973) Pulmonary function in shipyard welders. *Arch. environ. Health*, *26*, 28-31

Petersen, G.R. & Milham, S., Jr (1980) *Occupational Mortality in the State of California 1959-61* (DHEW (NIOSH) Publ. No. 80-104), Cincinnati, OH, US Department of Health, Education and Welfare

Polednak, A.P. (1981) Mortality among welders, including a group exposed to nickel oxides. *Arch. environ. Health, 36*, 235-242

Preston-Martin, S. & Peters, J.M. (1988) Prior employment as a welder associated with the development of chronic myeloid leukaemia. *Br. J. Cancer, 58*, 105-108

Puntoni, R., Vercelli, M., Merlo, F., Valerio, F. & Santi, L. (1979) Mortality among shipyard workers in Genoa, Italy. *Ann. N.Y. Acad. Sci., 330*, 353-377

de Raat, W.K. & Bakker, G.L. (1988) Induction of sister chromatid exchanges in Chinese hamster ovary cells by fume particles from various welding processes. *Ann. occup. Hyg., 32*, 191-202

Rachootin, P. & Olsen, J. (1983) The risk of infertility and delayed conception associated with exposures in the Danish workplace. *J. occup. Med., 25*, 394-402

Rahkonen, E., Junttila, M.-L., Kalliomäki, P.L., Olkinouora, M., Koponen, M. & Kalliomäki, K. (1983) Evaluation of biological monitoring among stainless steel welders. *Int. Arch. occup. environ. Health, 52*, 243-255

Raithel, H.J., Schaller, K.H., Reith, A., Svenes, K.B. & Valentin, H. (1988) Investigations on the quantitative determination of nickel and chromium in human lung tissue. Industrial medical, toxicological, and occupational medical expertise aspects. *Int. Arch. occup. environ. Health, 60*, 55-66

Reuzel, P.G.J., Beems, R.B., de Raat, W.K. & Lohman, P.H.M. (1986) Carcinogenicity and in vitro genotoxicity of the particulate fraction of two stainles steel welding fumes. In: Stern, R.M., Berlin, A., Fletcher, A.C. & Järvisalo, J., eds, *Health Hazards and Biological Effects of Welding Fumes and Gases*, Amsterdam, Excerpta Medica, pp. 329-332

Rieke, F.E. (1969) Lead intoxication in shipbuilding and shipscrapping 1941 to 1968. *Arch. environ. Health, 19*, 521-539

Rinsky, R.A., Zumwalde, R.D., Waxweiler, R.J., Murray, W.E., Jr, Bierbaum, P.J., Landrigan, P.J., Terpilak, M. & Cox, C. (1981) Cancer mortality at a naval nuclear shipyard. *Lancet, i*, 231-235

Rinsky, R.A., Melius, J.M., Hornung, R.W., Zumwalde, R.D., Waxweiler, R.J., Landrigan, P.J., Bierbaum, P.J. & Murray, W.E., Jr (1988) Case-control study of lung cancer in civilian employees at the Portsmouth naval shipyard, Kittery, Maine. *Am. J. Epidemiol., 127*, 55-64

Risch, H.A., Burch, J.D., Miller, A.B., Hill, G.B., Steele, R. & Howe, G.R. (1988) Occupational factors and the incidence of cancer of the bladder in Canada. *Br. J. ind. Med., 45*, 361-367

Ronco, G., Ciccone, G., Mirabelli, D., Troia, B. & Vineis, P. (1988) Occupation and lung cancer in two industrialized areas of Northern Italy. *Int. J. Cancer., 41*, 354-358

Roquet-Doffiny, Y., Roquet, P. & Lachapelle, J.M. (1977) Burns, artificial actinitis and multiple epitheliomas in a cutting-welder. (Fr.) *Dermatologica, 155*, 176-179

Ross, D.S. (1974) Welders' metal fume fever. *J. Soc. occup. Med., 24*, 125-129

Sawatari, K. & Serita, F. (1986) Determination of chromium speciation in fumes prepared by a plasma metal sprayer as a model of actual welding fumes. *Ind. Health*, *24*, 51-61

Schaller, K.-H., Zober, A., Weltle, D. & Valentin, H. (1986) Kinetics of chromium in biological materials during one week of stainless steel welding. In: Stern, R.M., Berlin, A., Fletcher, A.C. & Järvisalo, J., eds, *Health Hazards and Biological Effects of Welding Fumes and Gases*, Amsterdam, Excerpta Medica, pp. 189-192

Schneider, W.D. (1983) Lung diseases in welders — a cross-sectional study. (Ger.). *Z. Erkrank. Atm.-Org.*, *161*, 279-282

Schoenberg, J.B., Stemhagen, A., Mason, T.J., Patterson, J., Bill, J. & Altman, R. (1987) Occupation and lung cancer risk among New Jersey white males. *J. natl Cancer Inst.*, *79*, 13-21

Selikoff, I.J., Nicholson, W.J. & Lilis, R. (1980) Radiological evidence of asbestos disease among ship repair workers. *Am. J. ind. Med.*, *1*, 9-22

Sheers, G. & Coles, R.M. (1980) Mesothelioma risks in a naval dockyard. *Arch. environ. Health*, *35*, 276-282

Silverman, D.T., Hoover, R.N., Albert, S. & Graff, K.M. (1983) Occupation and cancer of the lower urinary tract in Detroit. *J. natl Cancer Inst.*, *70*, 237-245

Silverstein, M., Maizlish, N., Park, R. & Mirer, F. (1985) Mortality among workers exposed to coal tar pitch volatiles and welding emissions: an exercise in epidemiologic triage. *Am. J. public Health*, *75*, 1283-1287

Sipek, L. & Smårs, E. (1986) Ozone and nitrogen oxides in gas shielded arc welding. In: Stern, R.M., Berlin, A., Fletcher, A.C. & Järvisalo, J., eds, *Health Hazards and Biological Effects of Welding Fumes and Gases*, Amsterdam, Excerpta Medica, pp. 107-110

Sjögren, B. (1980) A retrospective cohort study of mortality among stainless steel welders. *Scand. J. Work Environ. Health*, *6*, 197-200

Sjögren, B. & Carstensen, J. (1986) Cancer morbidity among Swedish welders and gas-cutters. In: Stern, R.M., Berlin, A., Fletcher, A.C. & Järvisalo, J., eds, *Health Hazards and Biological Effects of Welding Fumes and Gases*, Amsterdam, Excerpta Medica, pp. 461-463

Sjögren, B., Hedström, L. & Ulfvarson, U. (1983a) Urine chromium as an estimator of air exposure to stainless steel welding fumes. *Int. Arch. occup. environ. Health*, *51*, 347-354

Sjögren, B., Lundberg, I. & Lidums, V. (1983b) Aluminium in the blood and urine of industrially exposed workers. *Br. J. ind. Med.*, *40*, 301-304

Sjögren, B., Hedström, L. & Lindstedt, G. (1984) Urinary fluoride concentration as an estimator of welding fume exposure from basic electrodes. *Br. J. ind. Med.*, *41*, 192-196

Sjögren, B., Lidums, V., Häkansson, M. & Hedström, L. (1985) Exposure and urinary excretion of aluminum during welding. *Scand. J. Work Environ. Health*, *11*, 39-43

Sjögren, B., Gustavsson, A. & Hedström, L. (1987) Mortality in two cohorts of welders exposed to high- and low-levels of hexavalent chromium. *Scand. J. Work Environ. Health*, *13*, 247-251

Sjögren, B., Elinder, C.-G., Lidums, V. & Chang, G. (1988) Uptake and urinary excretion of aluminum among welders. *Int. Arch. occup. environ. Health*, *60*, 77-79

Skriniar, J. (1986) Technical history and future development of the welding industry. In: Stern, R.M., Berlin, A., Fletcher, A.C. & Järvisalo, J., eds, *Health Hazards and Biological Effects of Welding Fumes and Gases*, Amsterdam, Excerpta Medica, pp. 23-28

Slepicka, J., Kadlec, K., Tesar, Z., Skoda, V. & Mirejovsky, P. (1970) Contribution to the problem of pneumoconiosis in electric-welders. (Ger.) *Int. Arch. Arbeitsmed.*, 27, 257-280

Stanescu, D.C., Pilat, L., Gavrilescu, N., Teculescu, D.B. & Cristescu, I. (1967) Aspects of pulmonary mechanics in arc welders' siderosis. *Br. J. ind. Med.*, 24, 143-147

Steenland, K., Beaumont, J. & Hornung, R. (1986) The use of regression analysis in a cohort mortality study of welders. *J. chronic Dis.*, 39, 287-294

Stern, F.B., Waxweiler, R.A., Beaumont, J.J., Lee, S.T., Rinsky, R.A., Zumwalde, R.D., Halperin, W.E., Bierbaum, P.J., Landrigan, P.J. & Murray, W.E., Jr (1986) A case-control study of leukemia at a naval nuclear shipyard. *Am. J. Epidemiol.*, 123, 980-992

Stern, R.M. (1977) *A Chemical, Physical and Biological Assay of Welding Fume. Part 1. Fume Characteristics*, Copenhagen, The Danish Welding Institute

Stern, R.M. (1979) Health protection in the industry. Research at the Danish Welding Institute (Fr.) *Assoc. suisse Tech. Soudage (Basel)*, 69, 66-76

Stern, R.M. (1980a) *Process Dependent Risk of Delayed Health Effects for Welders. Risk Assessment for the Welding Industry: Part II* (Report 80.50), Copenhagen, The Danish Welding Institute

Stern, R.M. (1980b) A chemical, physical and biological assay of welding fume. In: Brown, R.C., Gormley, J.P., Chamberlin M. & Davis, R., eds, *The In Vitro Effects of Mineral Dusts*, London, Academic Press, pp. 203-209

Stern, R.M. (1982) Chromium compounds: production and occupational exposure. In: Langård, S., ed., *Biological and Environmental Aspects of Chromium*, Amsterdam, Elsevier, pp. 5-47

Stern, R.M. (1983) Occupational exposure in the welding industry: health risk assessment. In: *Health Effects of Combined Exposures to Chemicals in Work and Community Environments. Proceeding of a Course by the European Cooperation on Environmental Health Aspects of the Control of Chemicals, Lodz, Poland, 18-22 October 1982*, Copenhagen, World Health Organization, pp. 226-261

Stern, R.M. (1987) Cancer incidence among welders: possible effects of exposure to extremely low frequency electromagnetic radiation (ELF) and to welding fumes. *Environ. Health Perspect.*, 76, 221-229

Stern, R.M. & Pigott, G.H. (1983) In vitro RPM fibrogenic potential assay of welding fumes. *Environ. Health Perspect.*, 51, 231-236

Stern, R.M., Pigott, G.H. & Abraham, J.L. (1983) Fibrogenic potential of welding fumes. *J. appl. Toxicol.*, 3, 18-30

Stern, R.M., Thomsen, E. & Furst, A. (1984) Cr(VI) and other metallic mutagens in fly ash and welding fumes. *Toxicol. environ. Chem.*, 8, 95-108

Stern, R.M., Berlin, A., Fletcher, A.C. & Järvisalo, J., eds (1986) *Health Hazards and Biological Effects of Welding Fumes and Gases*, Amsterdam, Excerpta Medica

Stern, R.M., Lipka, J., Madsen, M.B., Mørup, S., Thomsen, E. & Koch, C.J.W. (1987) Instability of lung retained welding fumes: a slow active Ni and Cr compartment. In: Foa, V., Emmett, E.A., Maroni, M. & Colombi, A., eds, *Occupational and Environmental Chemical Hazards: Cellular Biochemical Indices for Monitoring Toxicity*, Chichester, Ellis Horwood, pp. 444-460

Stern, R.M., Drenck, K., Lyngenbo, O., Dirksen, H. & Groth, S. (1988) Thoracic magnetic dust content, occupational exposure, and respiratory status of shipyard welders. *Arch. environ. Health, 43*, 361-370

Stettler, L.E., Groth, D.H. & Mackay, G.R. (1977) Identification of stainless steel welding fume particulates in human lung and environmental samples using electron probe microanalysis. *Am. ind. Hyg. Assoc. J., 38*, 76-82

Stuchly, M.A. & Lecuyer, D.W. (1989) Exposure to electromagnetic fields in arc welding. *Health Phys., 56*, 297-302

Thomsen, E. & Stern, R.M. (1979) A simple analytic technique for the determination of hexavalent chromium in welding fumes and other complex matrices. *Scand. J. Work Environ. Health, 5*, 386-403

Tinkler, M.J. (1983) *Evaluation and Control of Fumes Produced During Welding*, Vol. I, *Problem Survey* (Report 000 G 156), Montréal, Canadian Electrical Association

Tola, S., Kilpiö, J., Virtamo, M. & Haapa, K. (1977) Urinary chromium as an indicator of the exposure of welders to chromium. *Scand. J. Work Environ. Health, 3*, 192-202

Tola, S., Kalliomäki, P.-L., Pukkala, E., Asp, S. & Korkala, M.-L. (1988) Incidence of cancer among welders, platers, machinists, and pipe fitters in shipyards and machine shops. *Br. J. ind. Med., 45*, 209-218

Uemitsu, N., Shimizu, Y., Hosokawa, T., Nakayoshi, H., Kobayashi, M., Minato, S., Ogawa, T. & Tsutsumi, S. (1984) Inhalation toxicity study of welding fumes: effect of single or repeated exposure in the lungs of rats. *Toxicology, 30*, 75-92

Ulfvarson, U. (1979) *Arbejdsmiljöproblem vid Svetsning* [Work environment problems in welding] (Vetenskaplig skriftserie, 1979:31), Solna, Arbetarskyddsverket

Ulfvarson, U. (1981) Survey of air contaminants from welding. *Scand. J. Work Environ. Health, 7 (Suppl. 2)*, 1-28

Ulfvarson, U. (1986) Air contaminants involved in welding in Swedish industry — sources of variation in concentrations. In: Stern, R.M., Berlin, A., Fletcher, A.C. & Järvisalo, J., eds, *Health Hazards and Biological Effects of Welding Fumes and Gases*, Amsterdam, Excerpta Medica, pp. 133-136

Ulfvarson, U., Hallne, U., Bellander, T. & Hayenhjelm, H. (1978a) *Arbejdsmiljoproblem vid Svetsning* [Work environment problems in welding] (Vetenskaplig skriftserie, 1978:6), Solna, Arbetarskyddsverket

Ulfvarson, U., Hallne, U. & Bellander, T. (1978b) *Arbejdsmiljöproblem vid Svetsning* [Work environment problems in welding] (Vetenskaplig skriftserie, 1978:8), Solna, Arbetarskyddsverket

Ulfvarson, U., Hallne, U., Bergström, B. & Hallberg, B.O. (1978c) *Arbejdsmiljöproblem vid Svetsning* [Work environment problems in welding] (Vetenskaplig skriftserie, 1978:19), Solna, Arbetarskyddsverket

Verschoor, M.A., Bragt, P.C., Herber, R.F.M., Zielhuis, R.L. & Zwennis, W.C.M. (1988) Renal function of chrome-plating workers and welders. *Int. Arch. occup. environ. Health*, *60*, 67-70

van der Wal, J.F. (1985) Exposure of welders to fumes, Cr, Ni, Cu and gases in Dutch industries. *Ann. occup. Hyg.*, *29*, 377-389

van der Wal, J.F. (1986) Further studies on the exposure of welders to fumes, chromium, nickel and gases in Dutch industries: plasma welding and cutting of stainless steel. *Ann. occup. Hyg.*, *30*, 153-161

Welinder, H., Littorin, M., Gullberg, B. & Skerfving, S. (1983) Elimination of chromium in urine after stainless steel welding. *Scand. J. Work Environ. Health*, *9*, 397-403

Werner, U. (1977) Diseases of the upper respiratory tract in welders. (Ger.) *Z. ges. Hyg.*, *23*, 731-734

White, L.R., Hunt, J., Tetley, T.D. & Richards, R.J. (1981) Biochemical and cellular effects of welding fume particles in the rat lung. *Ann. occup. Hyg.*, *24*, 93-101

White, L.R., Hunt, J., Richards, R.J. & Eik-Nes, K.B. (1982) Biochemical studies of rat lung following exposure to potassium dichromate or chromium-rich welding fume particles. *Toxicol. Lett.*, *11*, 159-163

White, L.R., Marthinsen, A.B.L., Jakobsen, K. & Eik-Nes, K.B. (1983) Response of bovine alveolar macrophages *in vitro* to welding fume particles. *Environ. Health Perspect.*, *51*, 211-215

Widgery, D. (1986) Welding — the key to better productivity. *Weld. Met. Fabr.*, March, 58, 70

Widgery, D.J. (1988) Flux-cored wire: an update. *Weld. Met. Fabr.*, April, 118-124

Wilkins, J.R., III & Sinks, T.H., Jr (1984) Paternal occupation and Wilms' tumour in offspring. *J. Epidemiol. Community Health*, *38*, 7-11

Wilkinson, J. (1988) Fabrication worldwide. *Met. Constr.*, March, 134-139

Wiseman, L.G. & Chapman, E.T. (1986) Test program to determine whether nickel carbonyl forms during the welding of nickel-containing alloys: a progress report. In: Stern, R.M., Berlin, A., Fletcher, A.C. & Järvisalo, J., eds, *Health Hazards and Biological Effects of Welding Fumes and Gases*, Amsterdam, Excerpta Medica, pp. 111-113

Zielhuis, R.L. & Wanders, S.P. (1986) Health effects and medical wastage due to combined exposure in welding. In: Stern, R.M., Berlin, A., Fletcher, A.C. & Järvisalo, J., eds, *Health Hazards and Biological Effects of Welding Fumes and Gases*, Amsterdam, Excerpta Medica, pp. 497-533

Zober, A. (1981a) Symptoms and findings in the bronchopulmonary system of electric arc welders. I. Communication: epidemiology. (Ger.) *Zbl. Bakt. Hyg. I. Abt. Orig.*, *173*, 92-119

Zober, A. (1981b) Symptoms and findings in the bronchopulmonary system of electric arc welders. II. Communication: pulmonary fibroses. (Ger.) *Zbl. Bakt. Hyg. I. Abt. Orig.*, *173*, 120-148

Zschiesche, W., Wilhelm, E., Zober, A., Schaller, K.H., Weltle, D. & Valentin, H. (1986) Manganese in stainless steel welding fumes, external exposure and biological monitoring. In: Stern, R.M., Berlin, A., Fletcher, A.C. & Järvisalo, J., eds, *Health Hazards and Biological Effects of Welding Fumes and Gases*, Amsterdam, Excerpta Medica, pp. 193-196

Zschiesche, W., Emmerling, G., Schaller, K.H. & Weltle, D. (1987) Investigation on renal impairments of high alloy steel welders. In: Foa, V., Emmett, E.A., Maroni, M. & Colombi, A., eds, *Occupational and Environmental Chemical Hazards: Cellular and Biochemical Indices for Monitoring Toxicity*, Chichester, Ellis Horwood, pp. 339-343

Zschiesche, W., Emmerling, G., Schaller, K.-H. & Weltle, D. (1989) *Arbeitsmedizinische Untersuchungen zur Toxität Löslicher Barium-verbindungen aus Schweissrauchen* [Occupational Medical Investigations on the Toxicity of Soluble Barium Compounds in Welding Fumes] (German Welding Society (DVS) Report), Düsseldorf, DVS Publishers

# SUMMARY OF FINAL EVALUATIONS

| | Degree of evidence for carcinogenicity | | Overall evaluation |
|---|---|---|---|
| | Human | Animal | |
| **Chromium and chromium compounds** | | | |
| Chromium[VI] | | | 1 |
|   Chromium[VI] compounds as encountered in the chromate production, chromate pigment production and chromium plating industries | Sufficient | | |
|   Barium chromate | | Inadequate | |
|   Calcium chromate | | Sufficient | |
|   Chromium trioxide | | Limited | |
|   Lead chromates | | Sufficient | |
|   Sodium dichromate | | Limited | |
|   Strontium chromate | | Sufficient | |
|   Zinc chromates | | Sufficient | |
| Chromium[III] compounds | Inadequate | Inadequate | 3 |
| Metallic chromium | Inadequate | Inadequate | 3 |
| **Nickel and nickel compounds** | | | |
| Nickel compounds | | | 1 |
|   Nickel salts | | Limited | |
|     Nickel sulfate | Sufficient | | |
|   Combinations of nickel oxides and sulfides encountered in the nickel refining industry | Sufficient | | |
|     Nickel monoxides | | Sufficient | |
|     Nickel trioxide | | Inadequate | |
|     Nickel sulfide, amorphous | | Inadequate | |
|     Nickel sulfides, crystalline | | Sufficient | |
|   Nickel antimonide | | Limited | |
|   Nickel arsenides | | Limited | |
|   Nickel carbonyl | | Limited | |
|   Nickel hydroxides | | Sufficient | |
|   Nickelocene | | Limited | |
|   Nickel selenides | | Limited | |
|   Nickel telluride | | Limited | |
|   Nickel titanate | | Inadequate | |
| Metallic nickel | Inadequate | Sufficient | 2B |
|   Nickel alloys | Inadequate | Limited | |
| **Welding fumes** | | | 2B |
|   Welding fumes and gases | Limited | | |
|   Welding fumes | | Inadequate | |

# APPENDIX 1

# SUMMARY TABLES OF
# GENETIC AND RELATED EFFECTS

# Summary table of genetic and related effects of chromium compounds

| | Nonmammalian systems | | | | | | | | | | Mammalian systems | | | | | | | | | | | | | | | | | | | | | | | | | | | | | | |
|---|---|---|---|---|---|---|---|---|---|---|---|---|---|---|---|---|---|---|---|---|---|---|---|---|---|---|---|---|---|---|---|---|---|---|---|---|---|---|---|---|---|
| | Prokaryotes | | | Lower eukaryotes | | | | | | | Plants | | | | Insects | | | *In vitro* | | | | | | | | | | | | | | | | | | | *In vivo* | | | | | | | |
| | | | | | | | | | | | | | | | | | Animal cells | | | | | | | | Human cells | | | | | | | | Animals | | | | | | | | Humans | | | | |
| | D | G | R | A | D | G | C | R | G | C | A | D | G | C | R | G | C | D | G | S | M | C | A | T | I | D | G | S | M | C | A | T | I | D | G | S | M | C | DL | A | D | S | M | C | A |

**Cr[III] compounds**

**Chromic chloride** [CrCl₃.6H₂O]
| − | +¹ | +¹ | | | | | | | | | | | | | | | − | − | + | − | − | | | − | − | | | | | | | | − | | | | | | | | | | |

**Chromic acetate** [Cr(CH₃COO)₃]
? | | | | | | | | | | | | | | | | | | ? | + | ? | + | | | +¹ | +¹ | | | | | | ? | +¹ | | | − | | | | | | | |

**Chromic nitrate** [Cr(NO₃)₃.9H₂O]
+ | − | | | | | | | +¹ | | | | | | | | | −¹ | − | − | | | | | +¹ | | +¹ | | | | | −¹ | | | | | | | | | | | |

**Chromic sulfate** [Cr₂(SO₄)₃-4-8H₂O]
− | − | | | | | | | | | | | | | | | | | − | ? | | | | | | | | | | | | | | | | | | | | | | |

**Chromic potassium sulfate** [CrK(SO₄)₂.2H₂O]
− | +¹ | | | | | | | | | | | | | | | | | − | + | | | | | | | | | | | | | | | | | | | | | | |

**Chromium alum** [Cr₂(SO₄)₃.K₂SO₄.H₂O]
− | | | | | | | | | | | | | | | | | | − | + | | | | | | | | | | | | | | | | | | | | | | |

**Neochromium** [Cr₂(OH)SO₄.Na₂SO₄.H₂O]
− | | | | | | | | | | | | | | | | | −¹ | +¹ | | | | | | | | | | | | | | | | | | | | | | | |

**Chromic oxide** [Cr₂O₃]
−¹ | | | | | | | | | | | | | | | | | +¹ | +¹ ? | | | | | | | | | | | | | | | | | | | | | | | |

**Chromite ore** [Cr₂O₃.Fe₂O₃.Al₂O₃.SiO₂.CaO]
[+] | | | | | | | | | | | | | | | | | | (+) | (+) | | | | | | | | | | | | | | | | | | | | | | |

**Cupric chromite** [Cr₂O₃.2CuO]
| | | | | | | | | | | | | | | | | +¹ | (+) | (+) | | | | | | | | | | | | | | | | | | | | | | |

# Chromium compounds (contd)

| Cr[VI] compounds | Prok D | G | L.euk D | R | G | Plants D | G | Ins C | R | Anim C | A | D | G | S | M | C | A | T | I | Hum D | G | S | M | C | A | T | I | An D | G | S | M | C | DL | A | Hu D | S | M | C | A |
|---|---|---|---|---|---|---|---|---|---|---|---|---|---|---|---|---|---|---|---|---|---|---|---|---|---|---|---|---|---|---|---|---|---|---|---|---|---|---|---|
| Potassium dichromate [$K_2Cr_2O_7$] | + | + | + | | +[1] | | | + | | | +[1] | + | + | + | + | | + | + | | + | + | + | + | + | | | | +[1] | +[1] | +[1] | + | + | + | +[1] | | + | + | + | +[1] |
| Sodium dichromate [$Na_2Cr_2O_7 \cdot 2H_2O$] | + | + | | | +[1] | | | | | | | +[1] | +[1] | | + | | | | | | | +[1] | | | | | | + | | | | | | | | | | | |
| Ammonium dichromate [$(NH_4)_2Cr_2O_7$] | + | | | | | | | | | | | | | | | | | | | | | | | | | | | | | | | | | | | | | | |
| Potassium chromate [$K_2CrO_4$] | + | | | | −[1] | | | | | | | + | +[1] | + | + | − | + | −[1] | ? | | + | + | + | + | | | | | +[1] | + | | | | | | | | | |
| Sodium chromate [$Na_2CrO_4$] | + | | | | | | | | | | | + | +[1] | + | + | + | + | +[1] | | | + | + | + | + | | | | + | | | | | | | | | | | |
| Ammonium chromate [$(NH_4)_2CrO_4$] | + | + | | | | | | | | | | | | | | | | | | | | | | | | | | | | | | | | | | | | | |
| Chromium trioxide [$CrO_3$] | + | + | | | ? | | | | +[1] | | | −[1] | −[1] | +[1] | + | | | | | | | +[1] | +[1] | | | | | | | | | | | | | | | | |
| Calcium chromate [$CaCrO_4$] | ? | + | | | | | | | +[1] | | +[1] | + | + | + | + | + | | + | | | +[1] | +[1] | +[1] | +[1] | | | | +[1] | − | | | | | | | | | | |
| Strontium chromate [$SrCrO_4$] | +[1] | | | | | | | | | | | | | +[1] | | | | −[1] | | | | | | | | | | | | | | | | | | | | | |
| Zinc yellow [$Zn(CrO_4)_2 \cdot Zn(OH)_2 + 10\% CrO_3$] | + | | | | | | | | | | | | | | + | +[1] | | | | | | | | | | | | | | | | | | | | | | | |
| Zinc chromate [$ZnCrO_4$] | +[1] | | | | | | | | | | | +[1] | +[1] | + | +[1] | +[1] | | +[1] | | | | | | | | | | | | | | | | | | | | | |
| Chromium orange [$PbCrO_4 \cdot PbO$] | + | | | | | | | | | | | | + | | +[1] | | | | | | | | | | | | | | | | | | | | | | | | |

## Chromium compounds (contd)

| Compound | Nonmammalian systems | | | | | | | | | | | Mammalian systems — In vitro | | | | | | | | | | | | | | | | Mammalian systems — In vivo | | | | | | | | | |
|---|---|---|---|---|---|---|---|---|---|---|---|---|---|---|---|---|---|---|---|---|---|---|---|---|---|---|---|---|---|---|---|---|---|---|---|---|
| | Prokaryotes | | Lower eukaryotes | | | Plants | | | Insects | | | Animal cells | | | | | | | Human cells | | | | | | | | | Animals | | | | | | | Humans | | |
| | D | G | D | G | R | A | D | G | C | R | G | D | G | S | M | C | A | T | D | G | S | M | C | A | T | I | D | G | S | M | C | DL | A | D | S | M |
| Molybdenum orange [PbCrO$_4$.PbSO$_4$.SiO$_2$.Al$_2$O$_3$.PbMoO$_4$] | +[1] | | | | | | | | | | | | | | | | | | | | | | | | | | | | | | | | | | | |
| Barium chromate [BaCrO$_4$] | | | | | | | | | | | | | | + | +[1] | | | | | | | | | | | | | | | | | | | | | |
| Lead chromate [PbCrO$_4$] | - | (+) | | | | | | | | | (+)[1] | -[1] | - | + | + | | + | | | | (+)[1] | +[1] | (+)[1] | | | | | | | | | | | | | |
| Chromium yellow [PbCrO$_4$.PbSO$_4$.SiO$_2$.Al$_2$O$_3$] | (+)[1] | | | | | | | | | | | | | | | | | | | | | | | | | | | | | | +[1] | | | | | |
| Chromyl chloride [Cl$_2$CrO$_2$] | + | | | | | | | | | | | | | + | +[1] | | | | | | | | | | | | | | | | | | | | | |
| **Other Cr compounds** | | | | | | | | | | | | | | | | | | | | | | | | | | | | | | | | | | | | |
| Chromous[II] chloride [CrCl$_2$] | +[1] | | | | | | | | | | | -[1] | | | -[1] | | | | | | | | | | | | | | | | | | | | | |
| Chromium[0] carbonyl [Cr(CO)$_4$] | -[1] | -[1] | | | | | | | | | | | | | | | | | | | | | | | | -[1] | | | | | | | | | | |

A, aneuploidy; C, chromosomal aberrations; D, DNA damage; DL, dominant lethal mutation; G, gene mutation; I, inhibition of intercellular communication; M, micronuclei; R, mitotic recombination and gene conversion; S, sister chromatid exchange; T, cell transformation

*In completing the table, the following symbols indicate the consensus of the Working Group with regard to the results for each endpoint:*

+ considered to be positive for the specific endpoint and level of biological complexity
+[1] considered to be positive, but only one valid study was available to the Working Group
[+] results were available only for products contaminated with traces of Cr[VI]
(+) positive when artificially solubilized in acids or alkali
- considered to be negative
-[1] considered to be negative, but only one valid study was available to the Working Group
? considered to be equivocal or inconclusive (e.g., there were contradictory results from different laboratories; there were confounding exposures; the results were equivocal)

## Summary table of genetic and related effects of nickel compounds

| | Nonmammalian systems | | | | Mammalian systems | | | |
|---|---|---|---|---|---|---|---|---|
| | Prokaryotes | Lower eukaryotes | Plants | Insects | In vivo — Animal cells | In vivo — Human cells | In vivo — Animals | Humans |
| | D G R | G A D R G C | A D G C | R G C A | D G S M C A T I | D G S M C A T I | D G S M C DL A | D S M C |
| Metallic nickel | | | | | +1 | -1 | | |
| Nickel oxides | -1 | | | | + | -1 -1 +1 | | |
| Nickel sulfide (amorphous) | | | | | - | - | | |
| Nickel sulfide (crystalline) | +1 | | | | + +1 +1 + + | + | | |
| Nickel subsulfide | +1 | | | | +1a + +1a + + | -1 +1 +1 +1 | + | |
| Nickel chloride | ? - +1 +1 | | | - | + + + + +1 | +1 +1 -1 +1 | -1 + -1 | |
| Nickel sulfate | - | | | +1 | +1a + +1 +1 + | + +1 + | - | |
| Nickel nitrate | -1 -1 | | | - | | | | |
| Nickel acetate | +1a -1 | | | | + | +1 | | |
| Nickel carbonate | | | | | | | + | |
| Nickel subselenide | | | | | +1 | | | |

## Nickel compounds (contd)

| Nonmammalian systems | | | | | | | | | | | | | | | | | | Mammalian systems | | | | | | | | | | | | | | | | | | | | | | | |
|---|---|---|---|---|---|---|---|---|---|---|---|---|---|---|---|---|---|---|---|---|---|---|---|---|---|---|---|---|---|---|---|---|---|---|---|---|---|---|---|---|
| Prokary-otes | | Lower eukaryotes | | | | | | | Plants | | | | Insects | | | In vitro | | | | | | | | | | | | | | | In vivo | | | | | | | | | | |
| | | | | | | | | | | | | | | | | Animal cells | | | | | | | Human cells | | | | | | | | Animals | | | | | | | Humans | | | |
| D | G | D | R | G | A | D | G | C | R | G | C | A | C | A | | D | G | S | M | C | A | T | D | G | S | M | C | A | T | I | D | G | S | M | C | DL | A | D | S | M | C |
| Nickelocene | | | | | | | | | | | | | | | | | | | | | | | | | | | | | | | | | | | | | | | | | |
| -i | | | | | | | | | | | | | | | | | | | | | | | | | | | | | | | | | | | | | | | | | |
| Nickel potassium cyanide | | | | | | | | | | | | | | | | | | | | | | | | | | | | | | | | | | | | | | | | | |
| | | | | | | | | | | | | | | | | | | | +i | | | | | | | | | | | | | | | | | | | | | | |

A, aneuploidy; C, chromosomal aberration; D, DNA damage; DL, dominant lethal mutation; G, gene mutation; I, inhibition of intercellular communication; M, micronuclei; R, mitotic recombination and gene conversion; S, sister chromatid exchange; T, cell transformation

*In completing the table, the following symbols indicate the consensus of the Working Group with regard to the results for each endpoint:*

+   considered to be positive for the specific endpoint and level of biological complexity
+i  considered to be positive, but only one valid study was available to the Working Group
-   considered to be negative
-i  considered to be negative, but only one valid study was available to the Working Group
?   considered to be equivocal or inconclusive (e.g., there were contradictory results from different laboratories; there were confounding exposures; the results were equivocal)

aNegative result in one study for unscheduled DNA synthesis

bNegative result in one study for gene mutation to ouabain resistance in Syrian hamster embryo cells

cNegative result in one study for differential toxicity in *Escherichia coli*

# Summary table of genetic and related effects of welding fumes

| | Nonmammalian systems | | | | | | | | | | | | | | Mammalian systems | | | | | | | | | | | | | | | | | | | | | | | | | | |
|---|---|---|---|---|---|---|---|---|---|---|---|---|---|---|---|---|---|---|---|---|---|---|---|---|---|---|---|---|---|---|---|---|---|---|---|---|---|---|---|---|
| | Prokaryotes | | | Lower eukaryotes | | | | Plants | | | Insects | | | | | | *In vitro* | | | | | | | | | | | | | | | | | *In vivo* | | | | | | | |
| | | | | | | | | | | | | | | | | | Animal cells | | | | | | | | Human cells | | | | | | | | Animals | | | | | | | Humans | | | |
| | D | G | R | D | G | R | A | D | G | A | G | C | R | G | C | A | D | G | S | M | C | A | T | I | D | G | S | M | C | A | T | D | G | S | M | C | DL | A | D | S | M | C | A |
| **Welding fumes from mild steel** | | | | | | | | | | | | | | | | | | | | | | | | | | | | | | | | | | | | | | | | | | | |
| MIG | -¹ | | | | | | | | | | | | | | | | | | -¹ | -¹ | | | | | | | | | | | | | -¹ | | | -¹ | | | | | | | |
| MMA | -¹ | + | | | | | | | | | | | | | | | | | +¹ | -¹ | | | | | | | | | | | | | -¹ | | | -¹ | | | | | | | |
| **Welding fumes from stainless steel** | | | | | | | | | | | | | | | | | | | | | | | | | | | | | | | | | | | | | | | | | | | |
| MIG | -¹ | + | | | | | | | | | | | | | | | | | + | + | | | +¹ | | | | | | | | | | -¹ | | | -¹ | | | | | | | |
| MMA | +¹ | + | | | | | | | | | | | | | | | | | + | + | | | +¹ | | | | | | | | | +¹ | -¹ | -¹ | | -¹ | | | ? | -¹ | | | ? |
| **Welding fumes from mild steel or cast iron with nickel-rich electrode** | -¹ | | | | | | | | | | | | | | | | | | -¹ | -¹ | | | | | | | | | +¹ | | | | -¹ | | | -¹ | | | | | | | |

A, aneuploidy; C, chromosomal aberrations; D, DNA damage; DL, dominant lethal mutation; G, gene mutation; I, inhibition of intercellular communication; M, micronuclei; R, mitotic recombination and gene conversion; S, sister chromatid exchange; T, cell transformation

*In completing the table, the following symbols indicate the consensus of the Working Group with regard to the results for each endpoint:*

+  considered to be positive, for the specific endpoint and level of biological complexity

+¹  considered to be positive, but only one valid study was available to the Working Group

-  considered to be negative

-¹  considered to be negative, but only one valid study was available to the Working Group

?  considered to be equivocal or inconclusive (e.g., there were contradictory results from different laboratories; there were confounding exposures; the results were equivocal)

# APPENDIX 2

# ACTIVITY PROFILES FOR
# GENETIC AND RELATED EFFECTS

# APPENDIX 2

# ACTIVITY PROFILES
# FOR GENETIC AND RELATED EFFECTS

*Methods*

The x-axis of the activity profile (Waters *et al.*, 1987, 1988) represents the bioassays in phylogenetic sequence by endpoint, and the values on the y-axis represent the logarithmically transformed lowest effective doses (LED) and highest ineffective doses (HID) tested. The term 'dose', as used in this report, does not take into consideration length of treatment or exposure and may therefore be considered synonymous with concentration. In practice, the concentrations used in all the in-vitro tests were converted to μg/ml, and those for in-vivo tests were expressed as mg/kg bw. Because dose units are plotted on a log scale, differences in molecular weights of compounds do not, in most cases, greatly influence comparisons of their activity profiles. Conventions for dose conversions are given below.

Profile-line height (the magnitude of each bar) is a function of the LED or HID, which is associated with the characteristics of each individual test system – such as population size, cell-cycle kinetics and metabolic competence. Thus, the detection limit of each test system is different, and, across a given activity profile, responses will vary substantially. No attempt is made to adjust or relate responses in one test system to those of another.

Line heights are derived as follows: for negative test results, the highest dose tested without appreciable toxicity is defined as the HID. If there was evidence of extreme toxicity, the next highest dose is used. A single dose tested with a negative result is considered to be equivalent to the HID. Similarly, for positive results, the LED is recorded. If the original data were analysed statistically by the author, the dose recorded is that at which the response was significant ($p < 0.05$). If the available data were not analysed statistically, the dose required to produce an effect is estimated as follows: when a dose-related positive response is observed with two or more doses, the lower of the doses is taken as the LED; a single dose resulting in a positive response is considered to be equivalent to the LED.

In order to accommodate both the wide range of doses encountered and positive and negative responses on a continuous scale, doses are transformed logarithmically, so that effective (LED) and ineffective (HID) doses are represented by positive and negative numbers, respectively. The response, or logarithmic dose unit (LDU$_{ij}$), for a given test system $i$ and chemical $j$ is represented by the expressions

$$LDU_{ij} = -\log_{10} (\text{dose}), \text{ for HID values; LDU} \leq 0$$

and                                                                                              (1)

$$LDU_{ij} = -\log_{10} (\text{dose x } 10^{-5}), \text{ for LED values; LDU} \geq 0.$$

These simple relationships define a dose range of 0 to –5 logarithmic units for ineffective doses (1–100 000 µg/ml or mg/kg bw) and 0 to + 8 logarithmic units for effective doses (100 000–0.001 µg/ml or mg/kg bw). A scale illustrating the LDU values is shown in Figure 1. Negative responses at doses less than 1 µg/ml (mg/kg bw) are set equal to 1. Effectively, an LED value $\geq$100 000 or an HID value $\leq$1 produces an LDU = 0; no quantitative information is gained from such extreme values. The dotted lines at the levels of log dose units 1 and –1 define a 'zone of uncertainty' in which positive results are reported at such high doses (between 10 000 and 100 000 µg/ml or mg/kg bw) or negative results are reported at such low dose levels (1 to 10 µg/ml or mg/kg bw) as to call into question the adequacy of the test.

Fig. 1. Scale of log dose units used on the y–axis of activity profiles

| Positive (µg/ml or mg/kg bw) | | Log dose units | |
|---|---|---|---|
| 0.001 | .................................... | 8 | —— |
| 0.01 | .................................... | 7 | — |
| 0.1 | .................................... | 6 | — |
| 1.0 | .................................... | 5 | — |
| 10 | .................................... | 4 | — |
| 100 | .................................... | 3 | — |
| 1000 | .................................... | 2 | — |
| 10 000 | .................................... | 1 | — |
| 100 000 | ................ 1 ............... | 0 | —— |
| | ............... 10 ............... | –1 | — |
| | ............. 100 ............... | –2 | — |
| | ............ 1000 ............. | –3 | — |
| | .......... 10 000 ............. | –4 | — |
| | ......... 100 000 ............. | –5 | —— |

Negative
(µg/ml or mg/kg bw)
LED and HID are expressed as µg/ml or mg/kg bw.

In practice, an activity profile is computer generated. A data entry programme is used to store abstracted data from published reports. A sequential file (in ASCII) is created for each compound, and a record within that file consists of the name and Chemical Abstracts Service number of the compound, a three-letter code for the test system (see below), the qualitative test result (with and without an exogenous metabolic system), dose (LED or HID), citation number and additional source information. An abbreviated citation for each publication is stored in a segment of a record accessing both the test data file and the citation file. During processing of the data file, an average of the logarithmic values of the data subset is calculated, and the length of the profile line represents this average value. All dose values are plotted for each profile line, regardless of whether results are positive or negative. Results obtained in the absence of an exogenous metabolic system are indicated by a bar (–), and results obtained in the presence of an exogenous metabolic system are indicated by an upward-directed arrow (↑). When all results for a given assay are either positive or negative, the mean of the LDU values is plotted as a solid line; when conflicting data are reported for the same assay (i.e., both positive and negative results), the majority data are shown by a solid line and the minority data by a dashed line (drawn to the extreme conflicting response). In the few cases in which the numbers of positive and negative results are equal, the solid line is drawn in the positive direction and the maximal negative response is indicated with a dashed line.

Profile lines are identified by three-letter code words representing the commonly used tests. Code words for most of the test systems in current use in genetic toxicology were defined for the US Environmental Protection Agency's GENE-TOX Program (Waters, 1979; Waters & Auletta, 1981). For IARC Monographs Supplement 6, Volume 44 and subsequent volumes, including this publication, codes were redefined in a manner that should facilitate inclusion of additional tests. If a test system is not defined precisely, a general code is used that best defines the category of the test. Naming conventions are described below.

Data listings are presented with each activity profile and include endpoint and test codes, a short test code definition, results [either with (M) or without (NM) an exogenous activation system], the associated LED or HID value and a short citation. Test codes are organized phylogenetically and by endpoint from left to right across each activity profile and from top to bottom of the corresponding data listing. Endpoints are defined as follows: A, aneuploidy; C, chromosomal aberrations; D, DNA damage; F, assays of body fluids; G, gene mutation; H, host-mediated assays; I, inhibition of intercellular communication; M, micronuclei; P, sperm morphology; R, mitotic recombination or gene conversion; S, sister chromatid exchange; and T, cell transformation.

*Dose conversions for activity profiles*

Doses are converted to µg/ml for in–vitro tests and to mg/kg bw per day for in–vivo experiments.

1.   In–vitro test systems

*(a)*   Weight/volume converts directly to µg/ml.

*(b)*   Molar (M) concentration x molecular weight = mg/ml = $10^3$ µg/ml; mM concentration x molecular weight = µg/ml.

*(c)*   Soluble solids expressed as % concentration are assumed to be in units of mass per volume (i.e., 1% = 0.01 g/ml = 10 000 µg/ml; also, 1 ppm = 1 µg/ml).

*(d)*   Liquids and gases expressed as % concentration are assumed to be given in units of volume per volume. Liquids are converted to weight per volume using the density (D) of the solution (D = g/ml). Gases are converted from volume to mass using the ideal gas law, PV = nRT. For exposure at 20–37°C at standard atmospheric pressure, 1% (v/v) = 0.4 µg/ml x molecular weight of the gas. Also, 1 ppm (v/v) = $4 \times 10^{-5}$ µg/ml x molecular weight.

*(e)*   In microbial plate tests, it is usual for the doses to be reported as weight/plate, whereas concentrations are required to enter data on the activity profile chart. While remaining cognisant of the errors involved in the process, it is assumed that a 2–ml volume of top agar is delivered to each plate and that the test substance remains in solution within it; concentrations are derived from the reported weight/plate values by dividing by this arbitrary volume. For spot tests, a 1–ml volume is used in the calculation.

*(f)*   Conversion of particulate concentrations given in µg/cm$^2$ are based on the area (A) of the dish and the volume of medium per dish; i.e., for a 100–mm dish: A = $\pi R^2$ = $\pi \times (5 \text{ cm})^2$ = 78.5 cm$^2$. If the volume of medium is 10 ml, then 78.5 cm$^2$ = 10 ml and 1 cm$^2$ = 0.13 ml.

2.   In–vitro systems using in–vivo activation

For the body fluid–urine (BF–) test, the concentration used is the dose (in mg/kg bw) of the compound administered to test animals or patients.

3.   In–vivo test systems

*(a)*   Doses are converted to mg/kg bw per day of exposure, assuming 100% absorption. Standard values are used for each sex and species of rodent, including body weight and average intake per day, as reported by Gold *et al.* (1984). For example, in a test using male mice fed 50 ppm of the agent

in the diet, the standard food intake per day is 12% of body weight, and the conversion is dose = 50 ppm × 12% = 6 mg/kg bw per day.

Standard values used for humans are: weight – males, 70 kg; females, 55 kg; surface area, 1.7 m$^2$; inhalation rate, 20 l/min for light work, 30 l/min for mild exercise.

(b)   When reported, the dose at the target site is used. For example, doses given in studies of lymphocytes of humans exposed *in vivo* are the measured blood concentrations in µg/ml.

## Codes for test systems

For specific nonmammalian test systems, the first two letters of the three–symbol code word define the test organism (e.g., SA– for *Salmonella typhimurium*, EC– for *Escherichia coli*). If the species is not known, the convention used is –S–. The third symbol may be used to define the tester strain (e.g., SA8 for *S. typhimurium* TA1538, ECW for *E. coli* WP2*uvrA*). When strain designation is not indicated, the third letter is used to define the specific genetic endpoint under investigation (e.g., —D for differential toxicity, —F for forward mutation, —G for gene conversion or genetic crossing–over, —N for aneuploidy, —R for reverse mutation, —U for unscheduled DNA synthesis). The third letter may also be used to define the general endpoint under investigation when a more complete definition is not possible or relevant (e.g., —M for mutation, —C for chromosomal aberration).

For mammalian test systems, the first letter of the three–letter code word defines the genetic endpoint under investigation: A— for aneuploidy, B— for binding, C— for chromosomal aberration, D— for DNA strand breaks, G— for gene mutation, I— for inhibition of intercellular communication, M— for micronucleus formation, R— for DNA repair, S— for sister chromatid exchange, T— for cell transformation and U— for unscheduled DNA synthesis.

For animal (i.e., non–human) test systems *in vitro*, when the cell type is not specified, the code letters –IA are used. For such assays *in vivo*, when the animal species is not specified, the code letters –VA are used. Commonly used animal species are identified by the third letter (e.g., —C for Chinese hamster, —M for mouse, —R for rat, —S for Syrian hamster).

For test systems using human cells *in vitro*, when the cell type is not specified, the code letters –IH are used. For assays on humans *in vivo*, when the cell type is not specified, the code letters –VH are used. Otherwise, the second letter specifies the cell type under investigation (e.g., –BH for bone marrow, –LH for lymphocytes).

Some other specific coding conventions used for mammalian systems are as follows: BF– for body fluids, HM– for host–mediated, —L for leucocytes or lymphocytes *in vitro* (–AL, animals; –HL, humans), –L– for leucocytes *in vivo* (–LA, animals; –LH, humans), —T for transformed cells.

Note that these are examples of major conventions used to define the assay code words. The alphabetized listing of codes must be examined to confirm a specific code word. As might be expected from the limitation to three symbols, some codes do not fit the naming conventions precisely. In a few cases, test systems are defined by first–letter code words, for example: MST, mouse spot test; SLP, mouse specific locus test, postspermatogonia; SLO, mouse specific locus test, other stages; DLM, dominant lethal test in mice; DLR, dominant lethal test in rats; MHT, mouse heritable translocation test.

The genetic activity profiles and listings that follow were prepared in collaboration with Environmental Health Research and Testing Inc. (EHRT) under contract to the US Environmental Protection Agency; EHRT also determined the doses used. The references cited in each genetic activity profile listing can be found in the list of references in the appropriate monograph.

## References

Garrett, N.E., Stack, H.F., Gross, M.R. & Waters, M.D. (1984) An analysis of the spectra of genetic activity produced by known or suspected human carcinogens. *Mutat. Res.*, *134*, 89–111

Gold, L.S., Sawyer, C.B., Magaw, R., Backman, G.M., de Veciana, M., Levinson, R., Hooper, N.K., Havender, W.R., Bernstein, L., Peto, R., Pike, M.C. & Ames, B.N. (1984) A carcinogenic potency database of the standardized results of animal bioassays. *Environ. Health Perspect.*, *58*, 9–319

Waters, M.D. (1979) *The GENE–TOX program*. In: Hsie, A.W., O'Neill, J.P. & McElheny, V.K., eds, *Mammalian Cell Mutagenesis: The Maturation of Test Systems (Banbury Report 2)*, Cold Spring Harbor, NY, CHS Press, pp. 449–467

Waters, M.D. & Auletta, A. (1981) The GENE–TOX program: genetic activity evaluation. *J. chem. Inf. comput. Sci.*, *21*, 35–38

Waters, M.D., Stack, H.F., Brady, A.L., Lohman, P.H.M., Haroun, L. & Vainio, H. (1987) Appendix 1: Activity profiles for genetic and related tests. In: *IARC Monographs on the Evaluation of the Carcinogenic Risk of Chemicals to Humans*, Suppl. 6, *Genetic and Related Effects: An Update of Selected* IARC Monographs *from Volumes 1 to 42*, Lyon, IARC, pp. 687–696

Waters, M.D., Stack, H.F., Brady, A.L., Lohman, P.H.M., Haroun, L. & Vainio, H. (1988) Use of computerized data listings and activity profiles of genetic and related effects in the review of 195 compounds. *Mutat. Res.*, *205*, 295–312

CHROMIUM OCCUPATIONAL EXPOSURE

| END POINT | TEST CODE | TEST SYSTEM | RESULTS NM M | | DOSE (LED OR HID) | REFERENCE |
|---|---|---|---|---|---|---|
| S | SLH | SCE, HUMAN LYMPHOCYTES IN VIVO | + | 0 | 0.0000 | STELLA ET AL., 1982 |
| S | SLH | SCE, HUMAN LYMPHOCYTES IN VIVO | + | 0 | 0.0000 | SARTO ET AL., 1982 |
| S | SLH | SCE, HUMAN LYMPHOCYTES IN VIVO | - | 0 | 0.0000 | NAGAYA, 1986 |
| S | SLH | SCE, HUMAN LYMPHOCYTES IN VIVO | - | 0 | 0:0000 | NAGAYA ET AL., 1989 |
| S | SLH | SCE, HUMAN LYMPHOCYTES IN VIVO | + | 0 | 0.0000 | CHOI ET AL., 1987 |
| S | SLH | SCE, HUMAN LYMPHOCYTES IN VIVO | (+) | 0 | 0.0000 | DENG ET AL., 1983 |
| C | CLH | CHROM ABERR, HUMAN LYMPHOCYTES IN VIVO | + | 0 | 0.0000 | SARTO ET AL., 1982 |
| C | CLH | CHROM ABERR, HUMAN LYMPHOCYTES IN VIVO | + | 0 | 0.0000 | DENG ET AL., 1983 |
| C | CLH | CHROM ABERR, HUMAN LYMPHOCYTES IN VIVO | + | 0 | 0.0000 | BIGALIEV ET AL., 1977b |
| C | CLH | CHROM ABERR, HUMAN LYMPHOCYTES IN VIVO[1] | ? | 0 | 0.0000 | HAMANY ET AL., 1987 |
| A | AVH | ANEUPLOIDY, HUMAN CELLS IN VIVO | + | 0 | 0.0000 | BIGALIEV ET AL., 1977b |

[1]Exposure to Cr(III); all other references are to Cr(VI) exposures.

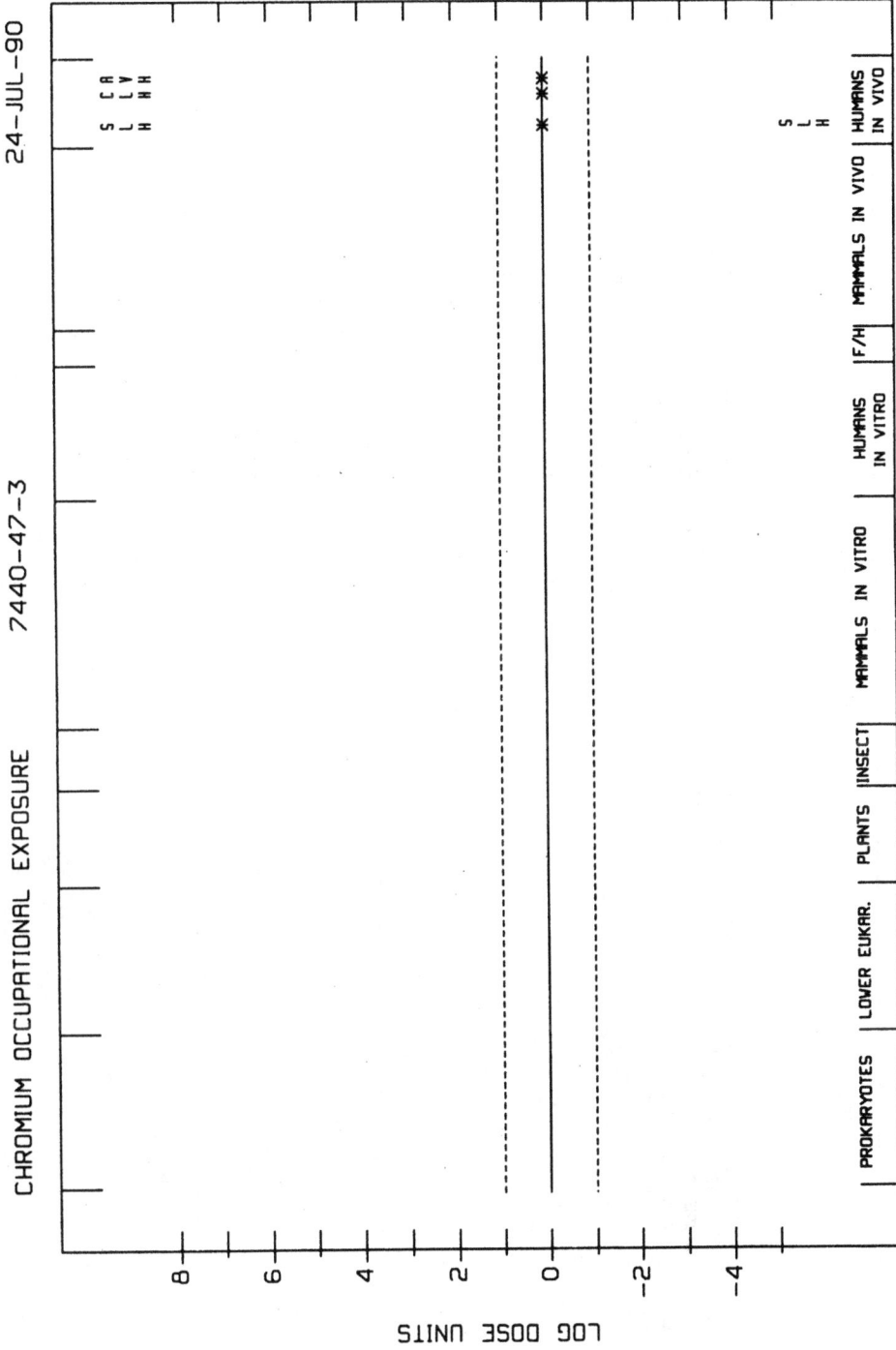

CHROMIUM OCCUPATIONAL EXPOSURE          7440-47-3          24-JUL-90

CHROMIC CHLORIDE

| END POINT | TEST CODE | TEST SYSTEM | RESULTS NN | M | DOSE[1] (LED OR HID) | REFERENCE |
|---|---|---|---|---|---|---|
| D | PRB | PROPHAGE, INDUCT/SOS/STRAND BREAKS/X-LINKS | – | 0 | 87.0000 | LLAGOSTERA ET AL., 1986 |
| D | PRB | PROPHAGE, INDUCT/SOS/STRAND BREAKS/X-LINKS | – | 0 | 26.0000 | ROSSMAN ET AL., 1984 |
| D | PRB | PROPHAGE, INDUCT/SOS/STRAND BREAKS/X-LINKS | – | 0 | 0.0520 | OLIVIER & MARZIN, 1987 |
| D | PRB | PROPHAGE, INDUCT/SOS/STRAND BREAKS/X-LINKS | – | – | 85.0000 | VENIER ET AL., 1989 |
| D | ERD | E. COLI REC, DIFFERENTIAL TOXICITY | – | 0 | 170.0000 | WARREN ET AL., 1981 |
| D | ERD | E. COLI REC, DIFFERENTIAL TOXICITY | + | – | 30.0000 | DE FLORA ET AL., 1984a |
| D | ERD | E. COLI REC, DIFFERENTIAL TOXICITY | – | 0 | 3900.0000 | YAGI & NISHIOKA, 1977 |
| D | BSD | B. SUBTILIS REC, DIFFERENTIAL TOXICITY | – | 0 | 130.0000 | NISHIOKA, 1975 |
| D | BSD | B. SUBTILIS REC, DIFFERENTIAL TOXICITY | – | 0 | 3380.0000 | NAKAMURO ET AL., 1978 |
| D | BSD | B. SUBTILIS REC, DIFFERENTIAL TOXICITY | – | 0 | 130.0000 | GENTILE ET AL., 1981 |
| D | BSD | B. SUBTILIS REC, DIFFERENTIAL TOXICITY | – | 0 | 0.0000 | MATSUI, 1980 |
| D | BRD | BACTERIA (OTHER), DIFFERENTIAL TOXICITY | – | 0 | 130.0000 | GENTILE ET AL., 1981 |
| G | SA0 | S. TYPHIMURIUM TA100, REVERSE MUTATION | – | 0 | 785.0000 | PETRILLI & DE FLORA, 1978a |
| G | SA0 | S. TYPHIMURIUM TA100, REVERSE MUTATION | – | 0 | 78.0000 | PETRILLI & DE FLORA, 1977 |
| G | SA0 | S. TYPHIMURIUM TA100, REVERSE MUTATION | – | 0 | 1.5000 | DE FLORA, 1981a |
| G | SA0 | S. TYPHIMURIUM TA100, REVERSE MUTATION | – | 0 | 5200.0000 | TSO & FUNG, 1981 |
| G | SA0 | S. TYPHIMURIUM TA100, REVERSE MUTATION | – | 0 | 14.0000 | VENIER ET AL., 1982 |
| G | SA2 | S. TYPHIMURIUM TA102, REVERSE MUTATION | – | 0 | 14.0000 | BIANCHI ET AL., 1983 |
| G | SA2 | S. TYPHIMURIUM TA102, REVERSE MUTATION | – | 0 | 0.0000 | DE FLORA ET AL., 1984b |
| G | SA5 | S. TYPHIMURIUM TA1535, REVERSE MUTATION | – | 0 | 0.0500 | MARZIN & PHI, 1985 |
| G | SA5 | S. TYPHIMURIUM TA1535, REVERSE MUTATION | – | 0 | 78.0000 | PETRILLI & DE FLORA, 1977 |
| G | SA5 | S. TYPHIMURIUM TA1535, REVERSE MUTATION | – | 0 | 1.5000 | DE FLORA, 1981a |
| G | SA5 | S. TYPHIMURIUM TA1535, REVERSE MUTATION | – | 0 | 14.0000 | BIANCHI ET AL., 1983 |
| G | SA5 | S. TYPHIMURIUM TA1535, REVERSE MUTATION | – | 0 | 14.0000 | VENIER ET AL., 1982 |
| G | SA7 | S. TYPHIMURIUM TA1537, REVERSE MUTATION | – | 0 | 130.0000 | TAMARO ET AL., 1975 |
| G | SA7 | S. TYPHIMURIUM TA1537, REVERSE MUTATION | – | – | 78.0000 | PETRILLI & DE FLORA, 1977 |
| G | SA8 | S. TYPHIMURIUM TA1538, REVERSE MUTATION | – | 0 | 1.5000 | DE FLORA, 1981a |
| G | SA8 | S. TYPHIMURIUM TA1538, REVERSE MUTATION | – | 0 | 1.5000 | DE FLORA, 1981a |
| G | SA8 | S. TYPHIMURIUM TA1538, REVERSE MUTATION | – | 0 | 14.0000 | BIANCHI ET AL., 1983 |
| G | SA8 | S. TYPHIMURIUM TA1538, REVERSE MUTATION | – | 0 | 14.0000 | VENIER ET AL., 1982 |
| G | SA8 | S. TYPHIMURIUM TA1538, REVERSE MUTATION | – | 0 | 130.0000 | TAMARO ET AL., 1975 |
| G | SA9 | S. TYPHIMURIUM TA98, REVERSE MUTATION | – | 0 | 78.0000 | PETRILLI & DE FLORA, 1977 |
| G | SA9 | S. TYPHIMURIUM TA98, REVERSE MUTATION | – | – | 1.5000 | DE FLORA, 1981a |
| G | SA9 | S. TYPHIMURIUM TA98, REVERSE MUTATION | – | 0 | 14.0000 | VENIER ET AL., 1982 |
| G | SA9 | S. TYPHIMURIUM TA98, REVERSE MUTATION | – | 0 | 14.0000 | BIANCHI ET AL., 1983 |

CHROMIC CHLORIDE

| END POINT | TEST CODE | TEST SYSTEM | RESULTS NM | M | DOSE¹ (LED OR HID) | REFERENCE |
|---|---|---|---|---|---|---|
| G | SA9 | S. TYPHIMURIUM TA98, REVERSE MUTATION | + | 0 | 0.0260 | LANGERWERF ET AL., 1985 |
| G | SAS | S. TYPHIMURIUM (OTHER), REVERSE MUTATION | - | 0 | 0.0000 | DE FLORA ET AL., 1984a |
| G | SAS | S. TYPHIMURIUM (OTHER), REVERSE MUTATION | - | 0 | 0.0000 | DE FLORA ET AL., 1984b |
| G | SAS | S. TYPHIMURIUM (OTHER), REVERSE MUTATION | + | 0 | 0.0260 | LANGERWERF ET AL., 1985 |
| G | ECF | E. COLI (EXCLUDING K12), FORWARD MUTATION | ? | 0 | 0.0000 | ZAKOUR & GLICKMAN, 1984 |
| G | ECW | E. COLI WP2 UVRA, REVERSE MUTATION | - | 0 | 0.0000 | PETRILLI & DE FLORA, 1982 |
| G | EC2 | E. COLI WP2, REVERSE MUTATION | - | 0 | 0.0000 | PETRILLI & DE FLORA, 1982 |
| R | SCG | S. CEREVISIAE, GENE CONVERSION | + | + | 4160.0000 | GALLI ET AL., 1985 |
| G | SCR | S. CEREVISIAE, REVERSE MUTATION | + | (+) | 4160.0000 | GALLI ET AL., 1985 |
| D | DIA | STRAND BREAKS/X-LINKS, ANIMAL CELLS IN VITRO | - | 0 | 10.0000 | FORNACE ET AL., 1981 |
| D | DIA | STRAND BREAKS/X-LINKS, ANIMAL CELLS IN VITRO | - | 0 | 260.0000 | BIANCHI ET AL., 1983 |
| D | UIA | UDS, OTHER ANIMAL CELLS IN VITRO | - | 0 | 16.0000 | RAFFETTO ET AL., 1977 |
| S | SIC | SCE, CHINESE HAMSTER CELLS IN VITRO | + | 0 | 50.0000 | MAJONE & RENSI, 1979 |
| S | SIC | SCE, CHINESE HAMSTER CELLS IN VITRO | - | 0 | 0.4000 | MACRAE ET AL., 1979 |
| S | SIC | SCE, CHINESE HAMSTER CELLS IN VITRO | - | 0 | 50.0000 | LEVIS & MAJONE, 1979 |
| S | SIC | SCE, CHINESE HAMSTER CELLS IN VITRO | + | 0 | 32.0000 | OHNO ET AL., 1982 |
| S | SIC | SCE, CHINESE HAMSTER CELLS IN VITRO | - | 0 | 1.0000 | KOSHI, 1979 |
| S | SIC | SCE, CHINESE HAMSTER CELLS IN VITRO | - | 0 | 50.0000 | VENIER ET AL., 1982 |
| S | SIC | SCE, CHINESE HAMSTER CELLS IN VITRO | + | 0 | 9.8000 | ELIAS ET AL., 1983 |
| S | SIC | SCE, CHINESE HAMSTER CELLS IN VITRO | - | 0 | 9.8000 | LEVIS & MAJONE, 1981 |
| S | SIC | SCE, CHINESE HAMSTER CELLS IN VITRO | - | 0 | 0.5200 | UYEKI & NISHIO, 1983 |
| S | SIC | SCE, CHINESE HAMSTER CELLS IN VITRO | - | 0 | 52.0000 | BIANCHI ET AL., 1983 |
| S | SIC | SCE, CHINESE HAMSTER CELLS IN VITRO | - | 0 | 150.0000 | BIANCHI ET AL., 1980 |
| S | SIC | SCE, CHINESE HAMSTER CELLS IN VITRO | + | 0 | 5.0000 | VENIER ET AL., 1985a |
| S | SIM | SCE, MOUSE CELLS IN VITRO | - | 0 | 52.0000 | MAJONE ET AL., 1983 |
| S | SIM | SCE, MOUSE CELLS IN VITRO | - | 0 | 52.0000 | BIANCHI ET AL., 1983 |
| S | SIS | SCE, SYRIAN HAMSTER CELLS IN VITRO | - | 0 | 52.0000 | BIANCHI ET AL., 1984 |
| C | CIC | CHROM ABERR, CHINESE HAMSTER CELLS IN VITRO | + | 0 | 50.0000 | MAJONE & RENSI, 1979 |
| C | CIC | CHROM ABERR, CHINESE HAMSTER CELLS IN VITRO | (+) | 0 | 50.0000 | LEVIS & MAJONE, 1979 |
| C | CIC | CHROM ABERR, CHINESE HAMSTER CELLS IN VITRO | + | 0 | 10.0000 | LEVIS & MAJONE, 1981 |
| C | CIC | CHROM ABERR, CHINESE HAMSTER CELLS IN VITRO | + | 0 | 0.0000 | BIANCHI ET AL., 1980 |
| C | CIM | CHROM ABERR, MOUSE CELLS IN VITRO | + | 0 | 50.0000 | VENIER ET AL., 1982 |
| C | CIS | CHROM ABERR, SYRIAN HAMSTER CELLS IN VITRO | + | 0 | 0.4000 | RAFFETTO ET AL., 1977 |
| C | CIS | CHROM ABERR, SYRIAN HAMSTER CELLS IN VITRO | - | 0 | 3.5000 | TSUDA & KATO, 1977 |
| T | TCS | CELL TRANSFORMATION, SHE, CLONAL ASSAY | - | 0 | 0.6000 | RIVEDAL & SANNER, 1981 |

CHROMIC CHLORIDE

| END POINT | TEST CODE | TEST SYSTEM | RESULTS NM M | DOSE[1] (LED OR HID) | REFERENCE |
|---|---|---|---|---|---|
| T | TCL | CELL TRANSFORMATION, OTHER CELL LINES | + 0 | 0.0400 | RAFFETTO ET AL., 1977 |
| T | TCL | CELL TRANSFORMATION, OTHER CELL LINES | - 0 | 60.0000 | BIANCHI ET AL., 1983 |
| T | TCL | CELL TRANSFORMATION, OTHER CELL LINES | - 0 | 175.0000 | HANSEN & STERN, 1985 |
| D | DIH | STRAND BREAKS/X-LINKS, HUMAN CELLS IN VITRO | - 0 | 2.6000 | MCLEAN ET AL., 1982 |
| D | DIH | STRAND BREAKS/X-LINKS, HUMAN CELLS IN VITRO | - 0 | 10.0000 | FORNACE ET AL., 1981 |
| D | UHF | UDS, HUMAN FIBROBLASTS IN VITRO | - 0 | 0.0000 | BIANCHI ET AL., 1983 |
| S | SHL | SCE, HUMAN LYMPHOCYTES IN VITRO | - 0 | 5.2000 | OGAWA ET AL., 1978 |
| S | SHL | SCE, HUMAN LYMPHOCYTES IN VITRO | - 0 | 52.0000 | STELLA ET AL., 1982 |
| C | CHL | CHROM ABERR, HUMAN LYMPHOCYTES IN VITRO | - 0 | 130.0000 | SARTO ET AL., 1980 |
| C | CHL | CHROM ABERR, HUMAN LYMPHOCYTES IN VITRO | + 0 | 0.0520 | STELLA ET AL., 1982 |
| C | CHL | CHROM ABERR, HUMAN LYMPHOCYTES IN VITRO | - 0 | 1.7000 | NAKAMURO ET AL., 1978 |
| C | CHL | CHROM ABERR, HUMAN LYMPHOCYTES IN VITRO | + 0 | 0.5000 | FRIEDMAN ET AL., 1987 |
| C | CHL | CHROM ABERR, HUMAN LYMPHOCYTES IN VITRO | + 0 | 78.5000 | KANEKO, 1976 |
| A | AIH | ANEUPLOIDY, HUMAN CELLS IN VITRO | + 0 | 5.0000 | NIJS & KIRSCH-VOLDERS, 1986 |
| D | DVA | STRAND BREAKS/X-LINKS, ANIMALS IN VIVO | - 0 | 16.0000 | TSAPAKOS ET AL., 1983b |
| D | DVA | STRAND BREAKS/X-LINKS, ANIMALS IN VIVO | - 0 | 16.0000 | CUPO & WETTERHAHN, 1985 |

[1]Doses are given as concentrations of the element, not the concentration of the compound.

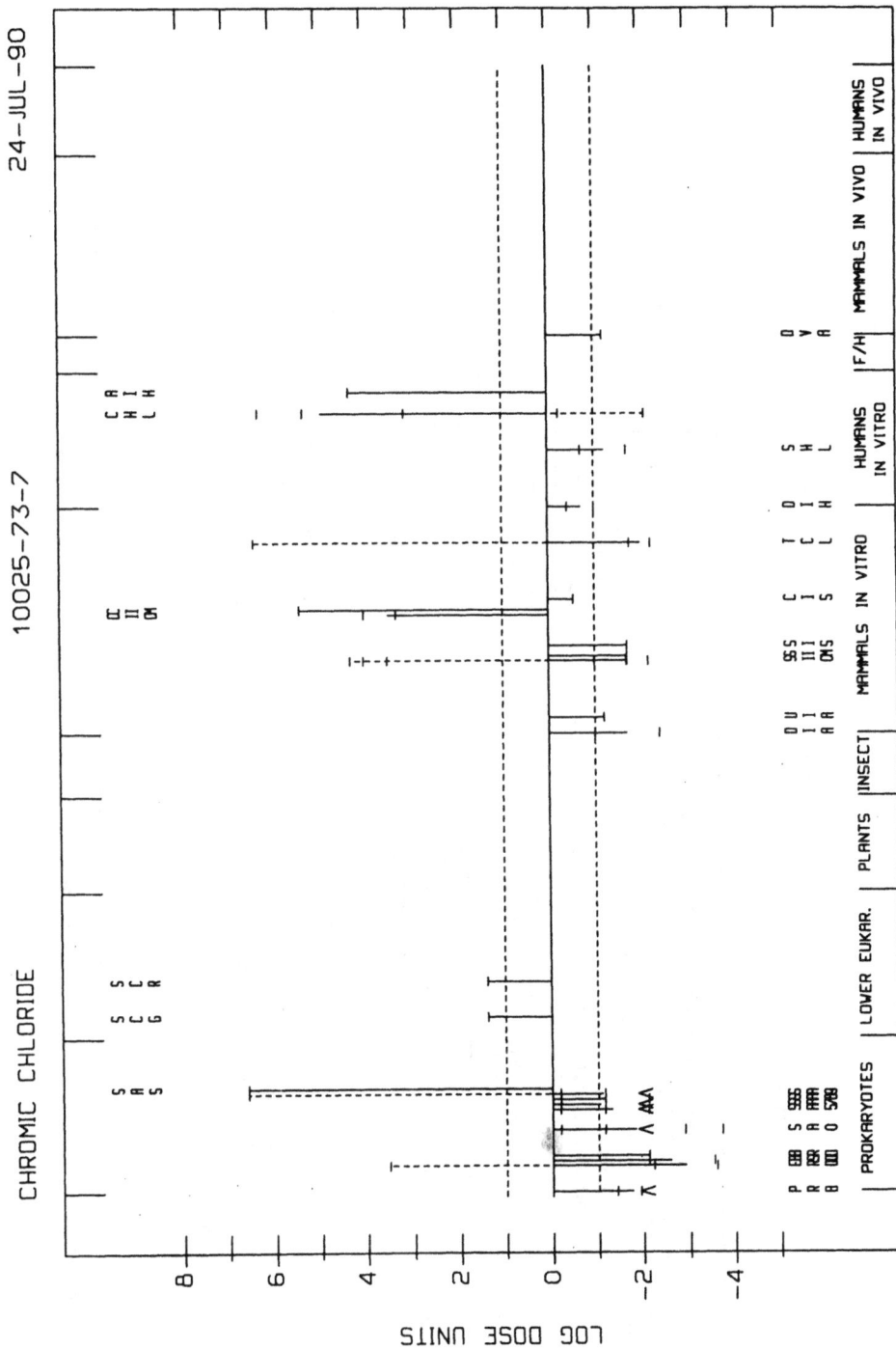

CHROMIC ACETATE

| END POINT | TEST CODE | TEST SYSTEM | RESULTS NM | M | DOSE[1] (LED OR HID) | REFERENCE |
|---|---|---|---|---|---|---|
| D | PRB | PROPHAGE, INDUCT/SOS/STRAND BREAKS/X-LINKS | − | 0 | 70.0000 | LLAGOSTERA ET AL., 1986 |
| D | PRB | PROPHAGE, INDUCT/SOS/STRAND BREAKS/X-LINKS | + | − | 75.0000 | VENIER ET AL., 1989 |
| D | ERD | E. COLI REC, DIFFERENTIAL TOXICITY | + | + | 105.0000 | DE FLORA ET AL., 1984a |
| D | BSD | B. SUBTILIS REC, DIFFERENTIAL TOXICITY | + | 0 | 170.0000 | NAKAMURO ET AL., 1978 |
| G | SA0 | S. TYPHIMURIUM TA100, REVERSE MUTATION | − | 0 | 3.6000 | DE FLORA, 1981a |
| G | SA2 | S. TYPHIMURIUM TA102, REVERSE MUTATION | + | − | 1135.0000 | BENNICELLI ET AL., 1983 |
| G | SA2 | S. TYPHIMURIUM TA102, REVERSE MUTATION | − | 0 | 570.0000 | PETRILLI ET AL., 1985 |
| G | SA2 | S. TYPHIMURIUM TA102, REVERSE MUTATION | − | 0 | 0.0000 | DE FLORA ET AL., 1984b |
| G | SA5 | S. TYPHIMURIUM TA1535, REVERSE MUTATION | − | 0 | 3.6000 | DE FLORA, 1981a |
| G | SA7 | S. TYPHIMURIUM TA1537, REVERSE MUTATION | − | 0 | 3.6000 | DE FLORA, 1981a |
| G | SA8 | S. TYPHIMURIUM TA1538, REVERSE MUTATION | − | 0 | 3.6000 | DE FLORA, 1981a |
| G | SA9 | S. TYPHIMURIUM TA98, REVERSE MUTATION | − | 0 | 3.6000 | DE FLORA, 1981a |
| G | SAS | S. TYPHIMURIUM (OTHER), REVERSE MUTATION | − | 0 | 0.0000 | DE FLORA ET AL., 1984a |
| G | SAS | S. TYPHIMURIUM (OTHER), REVERSE MUTATION | − | 0 | 0.0000 | DE FLORA ET AL., 1984b |
| G | ECW | E. COLI WP2 UVRA, REVERSE MUTATION | − | 0 | 0.0000 | PETRILLI & DE FLORA, 1982 |
| G | EC2 | E. COLI WP2, REVERSE MUTATION | − | 0 | 0.0000 | PETRILLI & DE FLORA, 1982 |
| G | ECR | E. COLI (OTHER), REVERSE MUTATION | + | 0 | 0.8000 | NAKAMURO ET AL., 1978 |
| G | GCO | MUTATION, CHO CELLS IN VITRO | − | 0 | 42.0000 | BIANCHI ET AL., 1983 |
| G | G9H | MUTATION, CHL V79 CELLS, HPRT | − | 0 | 45.0000 | NEWBOLD ET AL., 1979 |
| S | SIC | SCE, CHINESE HAMSTER CELLS IN VITRO | − | 0 | 20.0000 | LEVIS & MAJONE, 1979 |
| S | SIC | SCE, CHINESE HAMSTER CELLS IN VITRO | − | 0 | 150.0000 | BIANCHI ET AL., 1980 |
| S | SIM | SCE, MOUSE CELLS IN VITRO | + | 0 | 0.5200 | ANDERSEN, 1983 |
| C | CIC | CHROM ABERR, CHINESE HAMSTER CELLS IN VITRO | + | 0 | 5.0000 | LEVIS & MAJONE, 1979 |
| C | CIC | CHROM ABERR, CHINESE HAMSTER CELLS IN VITRO | + | 0 | 0.0000 | BIANCHI ET AL., 1980 |
| S | SHL | SCE, HUMAN LYMPHOCYTES IN VITRO | + | 0 | 5.2000 | ANDERSEN, 1983 |
| C | CHL | CHROM ABERR, HUMAN LYMPHOCYTES IN VITRO | + | 0 | 0.8000 | NAKAMURO ET AL., 1978 |

[1]Doses are given as concentrations of the element, not the concentration of the compound.

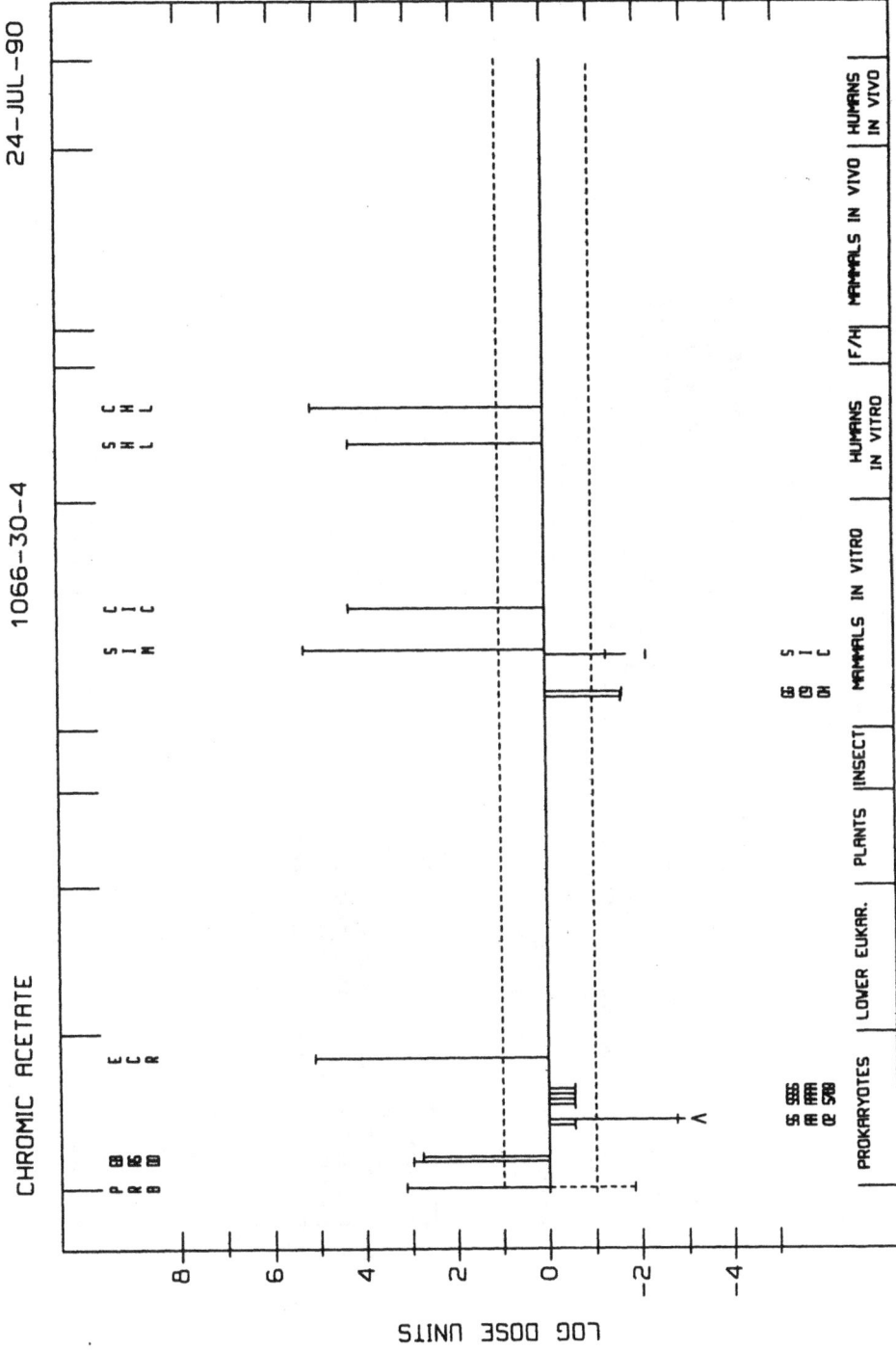

CHROMIC NITRATE

| END POINT | TEST CODE | TEST SYSTEM | RESULTS NM | M | DOSE[1] (LED OR HID) | REFERENCE |
|---|---|---|---|---|---|---|
| D | PRB | PROPHAGE, INDUCT/SOS/STRAND BREAKS/X-LINKS | - | 0 | 30.0000 | LLAGOSTERA ET AL., 1986 |
| D | PRB | PROPHAGE, INDUCT/SOS/STRAND BREAKS/X-LINKS | - | - | 19.0000 | VENIER ET AL., 1989 |
| D | ERD | E. COLI REC, DIFFERENTIAL TOXICITY | + | - | 68.0000 | DE FLORA ET AL., 1984a |
| D | BSD | B. SUBTILIS REC, DIFFERENTIAL TOXICITY | + | 0 | 83.0000 | NAKAMURO ET AL., 1978 |
| G | SA0 | S. TYPHIMURIUM TA100, REVERSE MUTATION | + | - | 875.0000 | PETRILLI & DE FLORA, 1978a |
| G | SA0 | S. TYPHIMURIUM TA100, REVERSE MUTATION | - | 0 | 1.0000 | DE FLORA, 1981a |
| G | SA0 | S. TYPHIMURIUM TA100, REVERSE MUTATION | - | - | 1500.0000 | VENIER ET AL., 1982 |
| G | SA2 | S. TYPHIMURIUM TA102, REVERSE MUTATION | - | - | 1530.0000 | BIANCHI ET AL., 1983 |
| G | SA2 | S. TYPHIMURIUM TA102, REVERSE MUTATION | - | - | 2185.0000 | BENNICELLI ET AL., 1983 |
| G | SA5 | S. TYPHIMURIUM TA1535, REVERSE MUTATION | - | 0 | 0.0000 | DE FLORA ET AL., 1984b |
| G | SA5 | S. TYPHIMURIUM TA1535, REVERSE MUTATION | - | 0 | 1.0000 | DE FLORA, 1981a |
| G | SA5 | S. TYPHIMURIUM TA1535, REVERSE MUTATION | - | - | 1500.0000 | VENIER ET AL., 1982 |
| G | SA7 | S. TYPHIMURIUM TA1537, REVERSE MUTATION | - | 0 | 130.0000 | TAMARO ET AL., 1975 |
| G | SA8 | S. TYPHIMURIUM TA1538, REVERSE MUTATION | - | 0 | 1.0000 | DE FLORA, 1981a |
| G | SA8 | S. TYPHIMURIUM TA1538, REVERSE MUTATION | - | 0 | 1.0000 | DE FLORA, 1981a |
| G | SA8 | S. TYPHIMURIUM TA1538, REVERSE MUTATION | - | - | 1500.0000 | VENIER ET AL., 1982 |
| G | SA9 | S. TYPHIMURIUM TA98, REVERSE MUTATION | - | 0 | 130.0000 | TAMARO ET AL., 1975 |
| G | SA9 | S. TYPHIMURIUM TA98, REVERSE MUTATION | - | 0 | 1.0000 | DE FLORA, 1981a |
| G | SAS | S. TYPHIMURIUM TA98, REVERSE MUTATION | - | - | 1500.0000 | VENIER ET AL., 1982 |
| G | SAS | S. TYPHIMURIUM (OTHER), REVERSE MUTATION | - | - | 0.0000 | DE FLORA ET AL., 1984a |
| G | SAS | S. TYPHIMURIUM (OTHER), REVERSE MUTATION | - | 0 | 0.0000 | DE FLORA ET AL., 1984b |
| C | VFC | VICIA FABA, CHROM ABERR | + | 0 | 0.0000 | GLASS, 1955 |
| D | DIA | STRAND BREAKS/X-LINKS, ANIMAL CELLS IN VITRO | - | 0 | 13.0000 | TSAPAKOS ET AL., 1983a |
| S | SIC | SCE, CHINESE HAMSTER CELLS IN VITRO | - | 0 | 150.0000 | LEVIS & MAJONE, 1979 |
| S | SIC | SCE, CHINESE HAMSTER CELLS IN VITRO | - | 0 | 150.0000 | BIANCHI ET AL., 1980 |
| S | SIC | SCE, CHINESE HAMSTER CELLS IN VITRO | - | 0 | 150.0000 | VENIER ET AL., 1982 |
| C | CIC | CHROM ABERR, CHINESE HAMSTER CELLS IN VITRO | - | 0 | 150.0000 | LEVIS & MAJONE, 1979 |
| C | CIC | CHROM ABERR, CHINESE HAMSTER CELLS IN VITRO | - | 0 | 150.0000 | BIANCHI ET AL., 1980 |
| C | CIC | CHROM ABERR, CHINESE HAMSTER CELLS IN VITRO | - | 0 | 150.0000 | VENIER ET AL., 1982 |
| C | CHL | CHROM ABERR, HUMAN LYMPHOCYTES IN VITRO | - | 0 | 1.7000 | NAKAMURO ET AL., 1978 |
| M | MVM | MICRONUCLEUS TEST, MICE IN VIVO | - | 0 | 110.0000 | FABRY, 1980 |

[1]Doses are given as concentrations of the element, not the concentration of the compound.

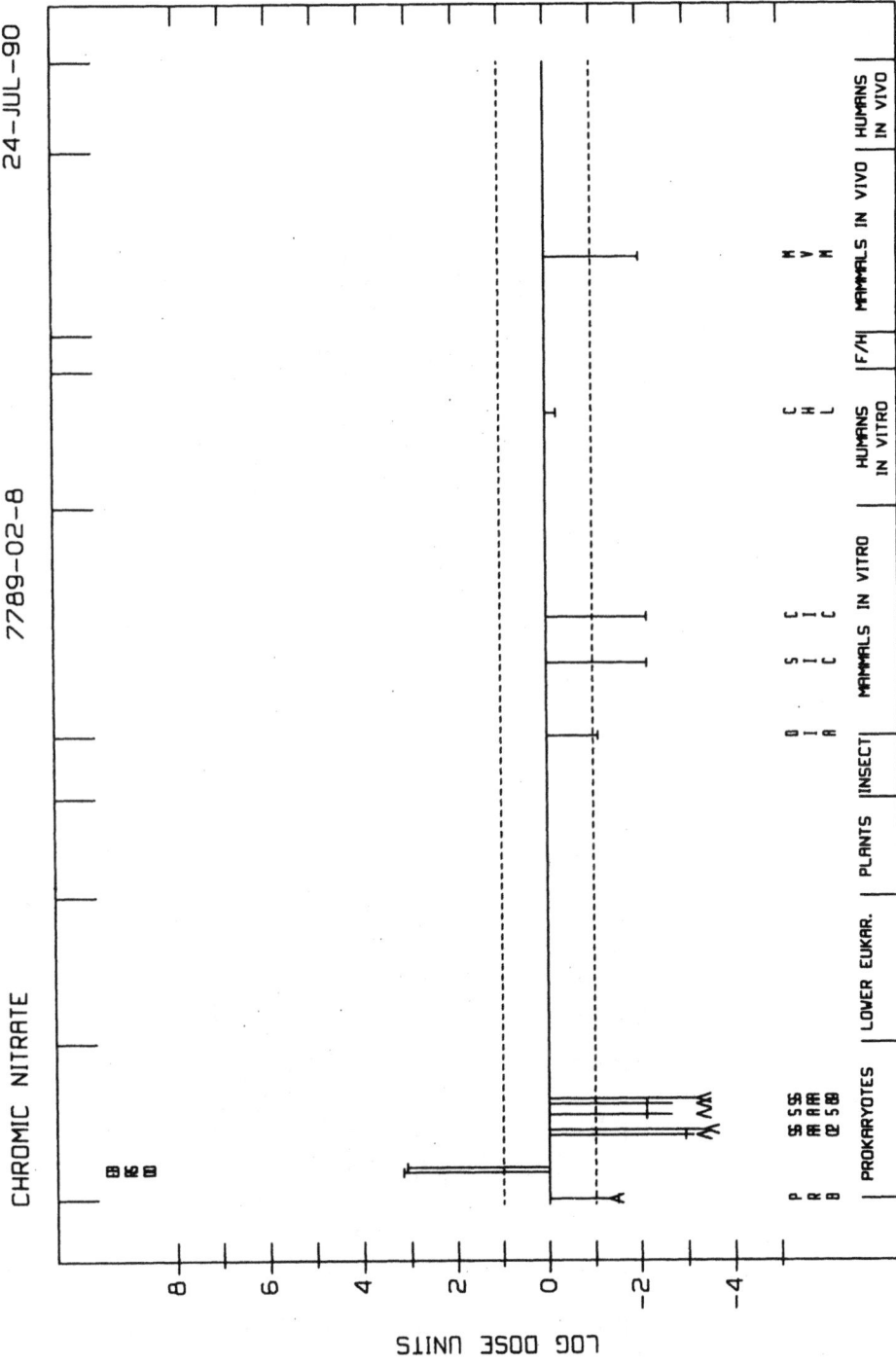

CHROMIC NITRATE    7789-02-8    24-JUL-90

CHROMIC SULPATE

| END POINT | TEST CODE | TEST SYSTEM | RESULTS NM | M | DOSE¹ (LED OR HID) | REFERENCE |
|---|---|---|---|---|---|---|
| D | BSD | B. SUBTILIS REC, DIFFERENTIAL TOXICITY | - | 0 | 260.0000 | GENTILE ET AL., 1981 |
| D | BSD | B. SUBTILIS REC, DIFFERENTIAL TOXICITY | - | 0 | 0.0000 | KADA ET AL., 1980 |
| D | BRD | BACTERIA (OTHER), DIFFERENTIAL TOXICITY | - | 0 | 260.0000 | GENTILE ET AL., 1981 |
| G | SA0 | S. TYPHIMURIUM TA100, REVERSE MUTATION | - | 0 | 0.0000 | ARLAUSKAS ET AL., 1985 |
| G | SA0 | S. TYPHIMURIUM TA100, REVERSE MUTATION | - | - | 560.0000 | LOPRIENO ET AL., 1985 |
| G | SA5 | S. TYPHIMURIUM TA1535, REVERSE MUTATION | - | 0 | 0.0000 | ARLAUSKAS ET AL., 1985 |
| G | SA5 | S. TYPHIMURIUM TA1535, REVERSE MUTATION | - | - | 560.0000 | LOPRIENO ET AL., 1985 |
| G | SA7 | S. TYPHIMURIUM TA1537, REVERSE MUTATION | - | 0 | 0.0000 | ARLAUSKAS ET AL., 1985 |
| G | SA7 | S. TYPHIMURIUM TA1537, REVERSE MUTATION | - | - | 560.0000 | LOPRIENO ET AL., 1985 |
| G | SA8 | S. TYPHIMURIUM TA1538, REVERSE MUTATION | - | 0 | 0.0000 | ARLAUSKAS ET AL., 1985 |
| G | SA8 | S. TYPHIMURIUM TA1538, REVERSE MUTATION | - | - | 560.0000 | LOPRIENO ET AL., 1985 |
| G | SA9 | S. TYPHIMURIUM TA98, REVERSE MUTATION | - | 0 | 0.0000 | ARLAUSKAS ET AL., 1985 |
| G | SA9 | S. TYPHIMURIUM TA98, REVERSE MUTATION | - | - | 560.0000 | LOPRIENO ET AL., 1985 |
| G | ECR | E. COLI (OTHER), REVERSE MUTATION | - | 0 | 0.0000 | ARLAUSKAS ET AL., 1985 |
| S | SIC | SCE, CHINESE HAMSTER CELLS IN VITRO | - | 0 | 6.0000 | OHNO ET AL., 1982 |
| S | SIC | SCE, CHINESE HAMSTER CELLS IN VITRO | - | 0 | 34.0000 | LEVIS & MAJONE, 1981 |
| S | SIC | SCE, CHINESE HAMSTER CELLS IN VITRO | - | 0 | 0.2200 | LOPRIENO ET AL., 1985 |
| C | CIC | CHROM ABERR, CHINESE HAMSTER CELLS IN VITRO | + | 0 | 5.6000 | LEVIS & MAJONE, 1981 |
| C | CIC | CHROM ABERR, CHINESE HAMSTER CELLS IN VITRO | + | 0 | 10.0000 | ROSSNER ET AL., 1981 |
| C | CIS | CHROM ABERR, SYRIAN HAMSTER CELLS IN VITRO | - | 0 | 3.5000 | TSUDA & KATO, 1977 |
| C | CIT | CHROM ABERR, TRANSFORMED CELLS IN VITRO | - | 0 | 104.0000 | UMEDA & NISHIMURA, 1979 |

¹Doses are given as concentrations of the element, not the concentration of the compound.

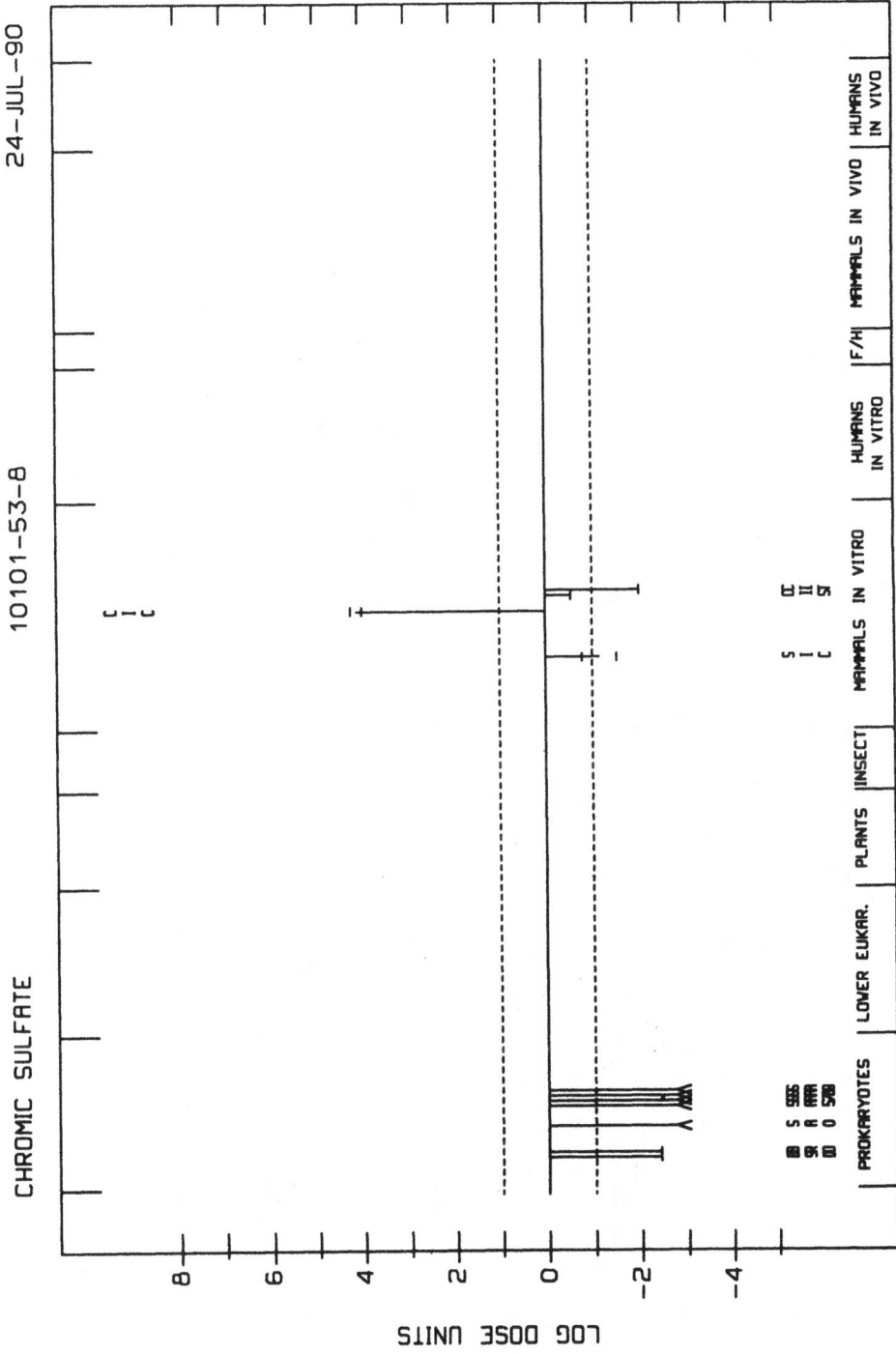

CHROMIC SULFATE

10101-53-8

24-JUL-90

LOG DOSE UNITS

CHROMIC POTASSIUM SULFATE

| END POINT | TEST CODE | TEST SYSTEM | RESULTS NN | RESULTS M | DOSE[1] (LED OR HID) | REFERENCE |
|---|---|---|---|---|---|---|
| D | PRB | PROPHAGE, INDUCT/SOS/STRAND BREAKS/X-LINKS | - | 0 | 4.0000 | DE FLORA ET AL., 1985a |
| D | PRB | PROPHAGE, INDUCT/SOS/STRAND BREAKS/X-LINKS | - | - | 17.0000 | VENIER ET AL., 1989 |
| D | ERD | E. COLI REC, DIFFERENTIAL TOXICITY | + | - | 65.0000 | DE FLORA ET AL., 1984a |
| D | BSD | B. SUBTILIS REC, DIFFERENTIAL TOXICITY | - | 0 | 130.0000 | GENTILE ET AL., 1981 |
| D | BSD | B. SUBTILIS REC, DIFFERENTIAL TOXICITY | - | 0 | 0.0000 | KADA ET AL., 1980 |
| D | BRD | BACTERIA (OTHER), DIFFERENTIAL TOXICITY | - | 0 | 130.0000 | GENTILE ET AL., 1981 |
| G | SA0 | S. TYPHIMURIUM TA100, REVERSE MUTATION | - | - | 400.0000 | PETRILLI & DE FLORA, 1978a |
| G | SA0 | S. TYPHIMURIUM TA100, REVERSE MUTATION | - | - | 42.0000 | PETRILLI & DE FLORA, 1977 |
| G | SA0 | S. TYPHIMURIUM TA100, REVERSE MUTATION | - | 0 | 0.8000 | DE FLORA, 1981a |
| G | SA2 | S. TYPHIMURIUM TA102, REVERSE MUTATION | - | - | 1042.0000 | BENNICELLI ET AL., 1983 |
| G | SA2 | S. TYPHIMURIUM TA102, REVERSE MUTATION | - | 0 | 0.0000 | DE FLORA ET AL., 1984b |
| G | SA5 | S. TYPHIMURIUM TA1535, REVERSE MUTATION | - | 0 | 42.0000 | PETRILLI & DE FLORA, 1977 |
| G | SA5 | S. TYPHIMURIUM TA1535, REVERSE MUTATION | - | - | 0.8000 | DE FLORA, 1981a |
| G | SA7 | S. TYPHIMURIUM TA1537, REVERSE MUTATION | - | 0 | 42.0000 | PETRILLI & DE FLORA, 1977 |
| G | SA7 | S. TYPHIMURIUM TA1537, REVERSE MUTATION | - | - | 0.8000 | DE FLORA, 1981a |
| G | SA8 | S. TYPHIMURIUM TA1538, REVERSE MUTATION | - | - | 0.8000 | DE FLORA, 1981a |
| G | SA9 | S. TYPHIMURIUM TA98, REVERSE MUTATION | - | 0 | 42.0000 | PETRILLI & DE FLORA, 1977 |
| G | SA9 | S. TYPHIMURIUM TA98, REVERSE MUTATION | - | - | 0.8000 | DE FLORA, 1981a |
| G | SA9 | S. TYPHIMURIUM TA98, REVERSE MUTATION | - | 0 | 1.3000 | LANGERWERF ET AL., 1985 |
| G | SAS | S. TYPHIMURIUM (OTHER), REVERSE MUTATION | - | 0 | 0.0000 | DE FLORA ET AL., 1984a |
| G | SAS | S. TYPHIMURIUM (OTHER), REVERSE MUTATION | - | 0 | 1.3000 | LANGERWERF ET AL., 1985 |
| G | SAS | S. TYPHIMURIUM (OTHER), REVERSE MUTATION | - | 0 | 0.0000 | DE FLORA ET AL., 1984b |
| D | PLU | PLANTS, UDS | + | 0 | 104.0000 | JACKSON & LINSKENS, 1982 |
| S | SIC | SCE, CHINESE HAMSTER CELLS IN VITRO | - | 0 | 150.0000 | LEVIS & MAJONE, 1979 |
| S | SIC | SCE, CHINESE HAMSTER CELLS IN VITRO | - | 0 | 150.0000 | BIANCHI ET AL., 1980 |
| C | CIC | CHROM ABERR, CHINESE HAMSTER CELLS IN VITRO | + | 0 | 150.0000 | LEVIS & MAJONE, 1979 |
| C | CIC | CHROM ABERR, CHINESE HAMSTER CELLS IN VITRO | + | 0 | 0.0000 | BIANCHI ET AL., 1980 |

[1]Doses are given as concentrations of the element, not the concentration of the compound.

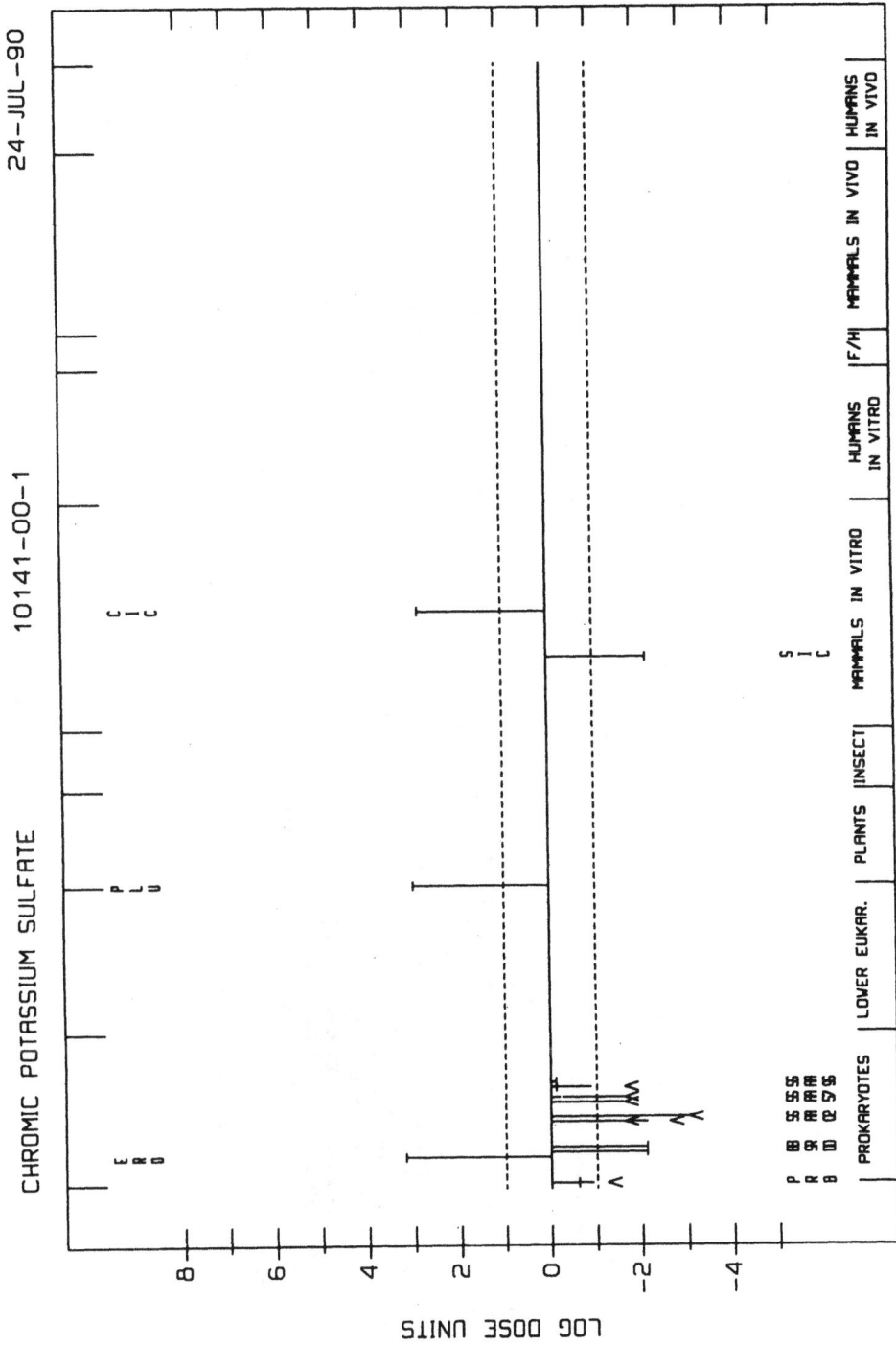

CHROMIC POTASSIUM SULFATE    10141-00-1    24-JUL-90

CHROMIUM ALUM

| END POINT | TEST CODE | TEST SYSTEM | RESULTS NM M | DOSE[1] (LED OR HID) | REFERENCE |
|---|---|---|---|---|---|
| G | SA0 | S. TYPHIMURIUM TA100, REVERSE MUTATION | − 0 | 712.0000 | PETRILLI & DE FLORA, 1978a |
| G | SA0 | S. TYPHIMURIUM TA100, REVERSE MUTATION | − 0 | 5.5000 | DE FLORA, 1981a |
| G | SA0 | S. TYPHIMURIUM TA100, REVERSE MUTATION | − 0 | 340.0000 | VENIER ET AL., 1982 |
| G | SA5 | S. TYPHIMURIUM TA1535, REVERSE MUTATION | − 0 | 5.5000 | DE FLORA, 1981a |
| G | SA5 | S. TYPHIMURIUM TA1535, REVERSE MUTATION | − 0 | 340.0000 | VENIER ET AL., 1982 |
| G | SA7 | S. TYPHIMURIUM TA1537, REVERSE MUTATION | − 0 | 5.5000 | DE FLORA, 1981a |
| G | SA8 | S. TYPHIMURIUM TA1538, REVERSE MUTATION | − 0 | 5.5000 | DE FLORA, 1981a |
| G | SA8 | S. TYPHIMURIUM TA1538, REVERSE MUTATION | − 0 | 340.0000 | VENIER ET AL., 1982 |
| G | SA9 | S. TYPHIMURIUM TA98, REVERSE MUTATION | − 0 | 5.5000 | DE FLORA, 1981a |
| G | SA9 | S. TYPHIMURIUM TA98, REVERSE MUTATION | − 0 | 340.0000 | VENIER ET AL., 1982 |
| S | SIC | SCE, CHINESE HAMSTER CELLS IN VITRO[2] | + 0 | 0.1800 | VENIER ET AL., 1982 |
| S | SIC | SCE, CHINESE HAMSTER CELLS IN VITRO | − 0 | 27.0000 | LEVIS & MAJONE, 1981 |
| C | CIC | CHROM ABERR, CHINESE HAMSTER CELLS IN VITRO | + 0 | 4.5000 | LEVIS & MAJONE, 1981 |
| C | CIC | CHROM ABERR, CHINESE HAMSTER CELLS IN VITRO[2] | + 0 | 0.1800 | VENIER ET AL., 1982 |

[1]Doses are given as concentrations of the element, not the concentration of the compound.
[2]Contaminated with traces of Cr[VI]

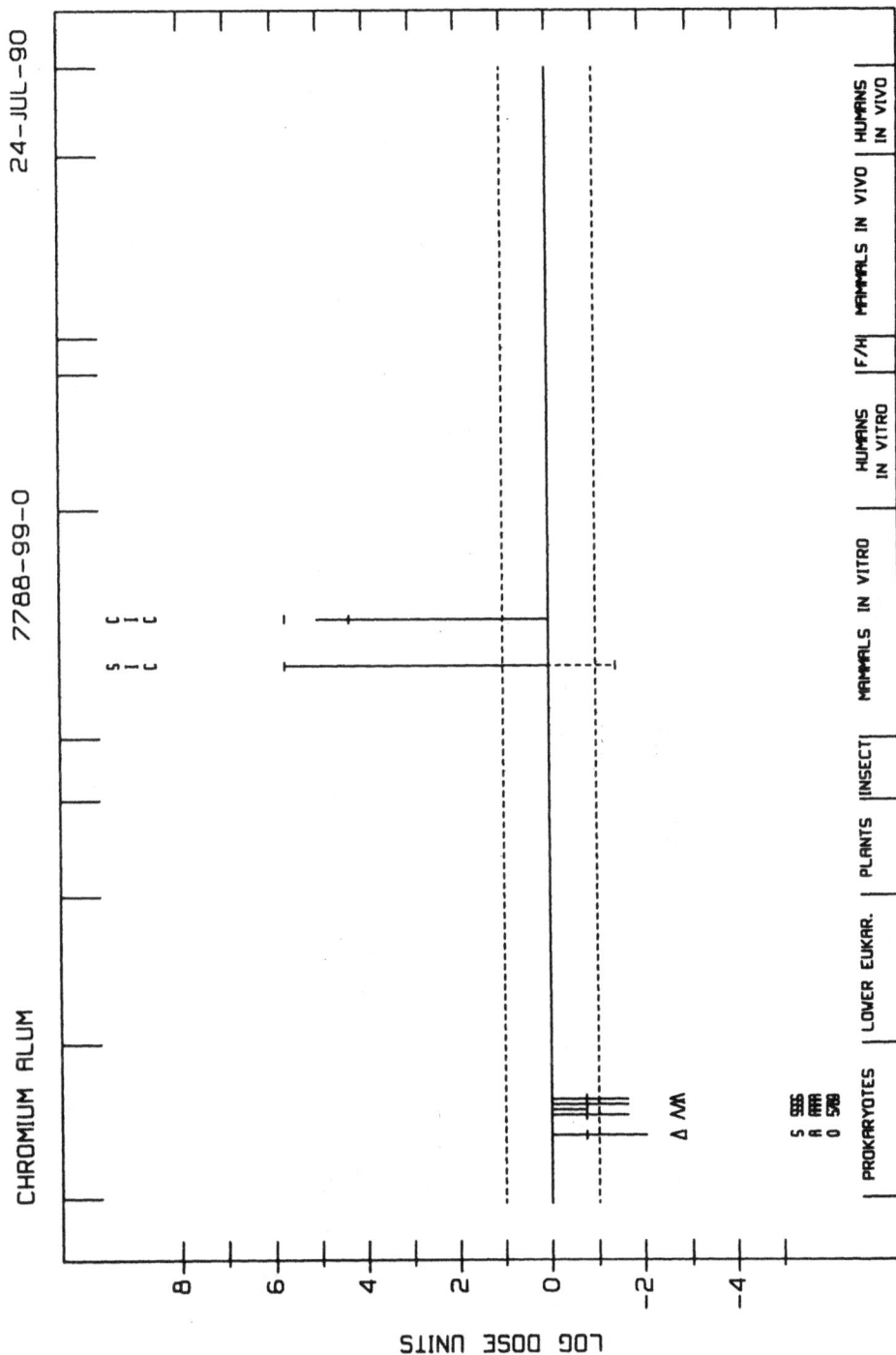

CHROMIUM ALUM            7788-99-0            24-JUL-90

LOG DOSE UNITS

PROKARYOTES | LOWER EUKAR. | PLANTS | INSECT | MAMMALS IN VITRO | HUMANS IN VITRO | F/H | MAMMALS IN VIVO | HUMANS IN VIVO

NEOCHROMIUM (CHROMIC SULFATE, BASIC)

| END POINT | TEST CODE | TEST SYSTEM | RESULTS NM M | DOSE[1] (LED OR HID) | REFERENCE |
|---|---|---|---|---|---|
| G | SA0 | S. TYPHIMURIUM TA100, REVERSE MUTATION | − 0 | 640.0000 | PETRILLI & DE FLORA, 1978a |
| G | SA0 | S. TYPHIMURIUM TA100, REVERSE MUTATION | − 0 | 2.6000 | DE FLORA, 1981a |
| G | SA5 | S. TYPHIMURIUM TA1535, REVERSE MUTATION | − 0 | 2.6000 | DE FLORA, 1981a |
| G | SA7 | S. TYPHIMURIUM TA1537, REVERSE MUTATION | − 0 | 2.6000 | DE FLORA, 1981a |
| G | SA8 | S. TYPHIMURIUM TA1538, REVERSE MUTATION | − 0 | 2.6000 | DE FLORA, 1981a |
| G | SA9 | S. TYPHIMURIUM TA98, REVERSE MUTATION | − 0 | 2.6000 | DE FLORA, 1981a |
| S | SIC | SCE, CHINESE HAMSTER CELLS IN VITRO | − 0 | 24.0000 | LEVIS & MAJONE, 1981 |
| C | CIC | CHROM ABERR, CHINESE HAMSTER CELLS IN VITRO | + 0 | 0.8000 | LEVIS & MAJONE, 1981 |

[1]Doses are given as concentrations of the element, not the concentration of the compound.

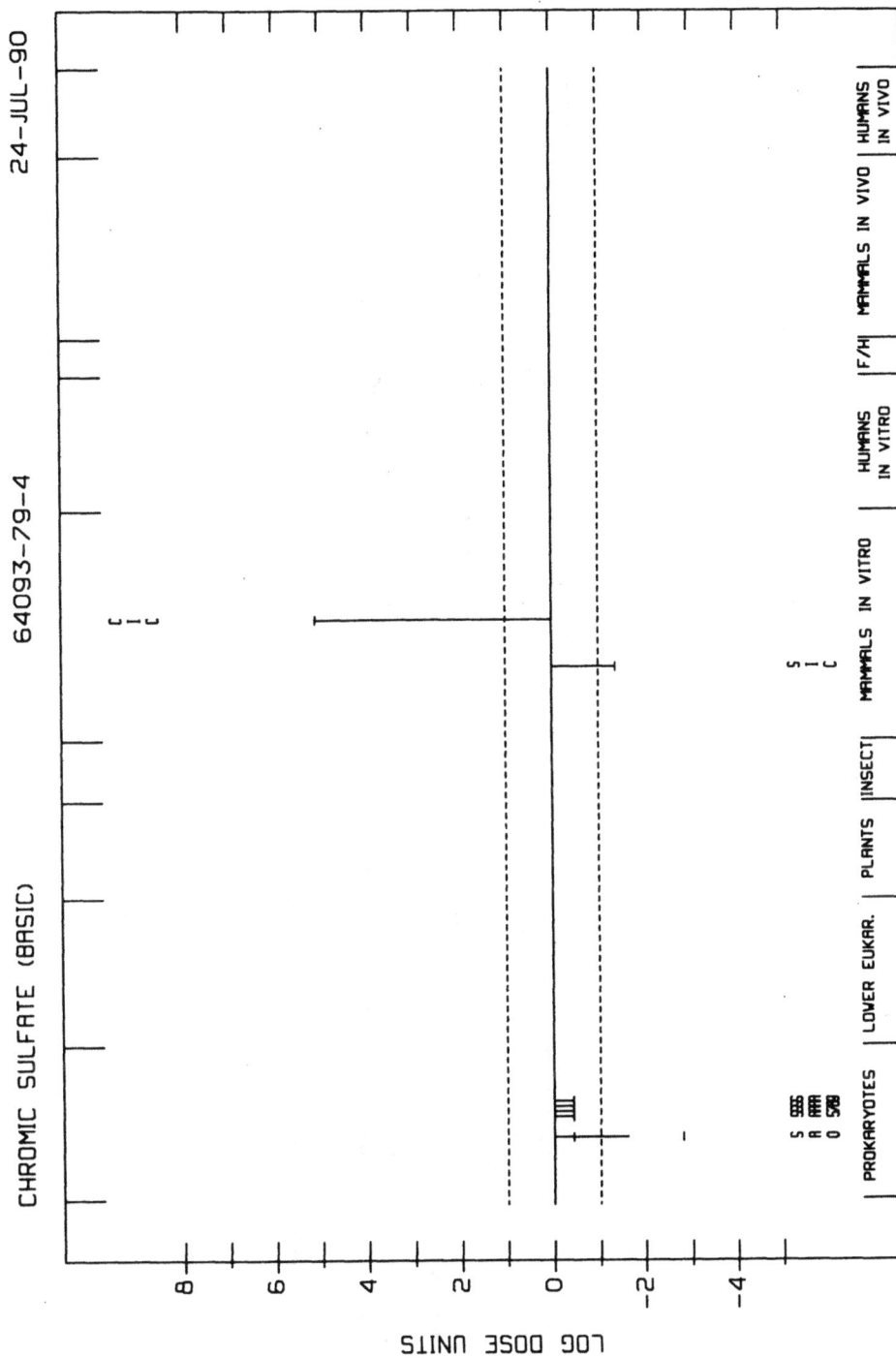

CHROMIC SULFATE (BASIC)   64093-79-4   24-JUL-90

CHROMIC OXIDE

| END POINT | TEST CODE | TEST SYSTEM | RESULTS NW M | DOSE[1] (LED OR HID) | REFERENCE |
|---|---|---|---|---|---|
| D | ERD | E. COLI REC, DIFFERENTIAL TOXICITY | − 0 | 3760.0000 | YAGI & NISHIOKA, 1977 |
| G | G9H | MUTATION, CHL V79 CELLS, HPRT | + 0 | 10.0000 | ELIAS ET AL., 1986 |
| S | SIC | SCE, CHINESE HAMSTER CELLS IN VITRO | + 0 | 34.0000 | ELIAS ET AL., 1983 |
| S | SIM | SCE, MOUSE CELLS IN VITRO | − 0 | 104.0000 | ANDERSEN, 1983 |
| T | TCL | CELL TRANSFORMATION, OTHER CELL LINES | − 0 | 274.0000 | HANSEN & STERN, 1985 |

[1]Doses are given as concentrations of the element, not the concentration of the compound.

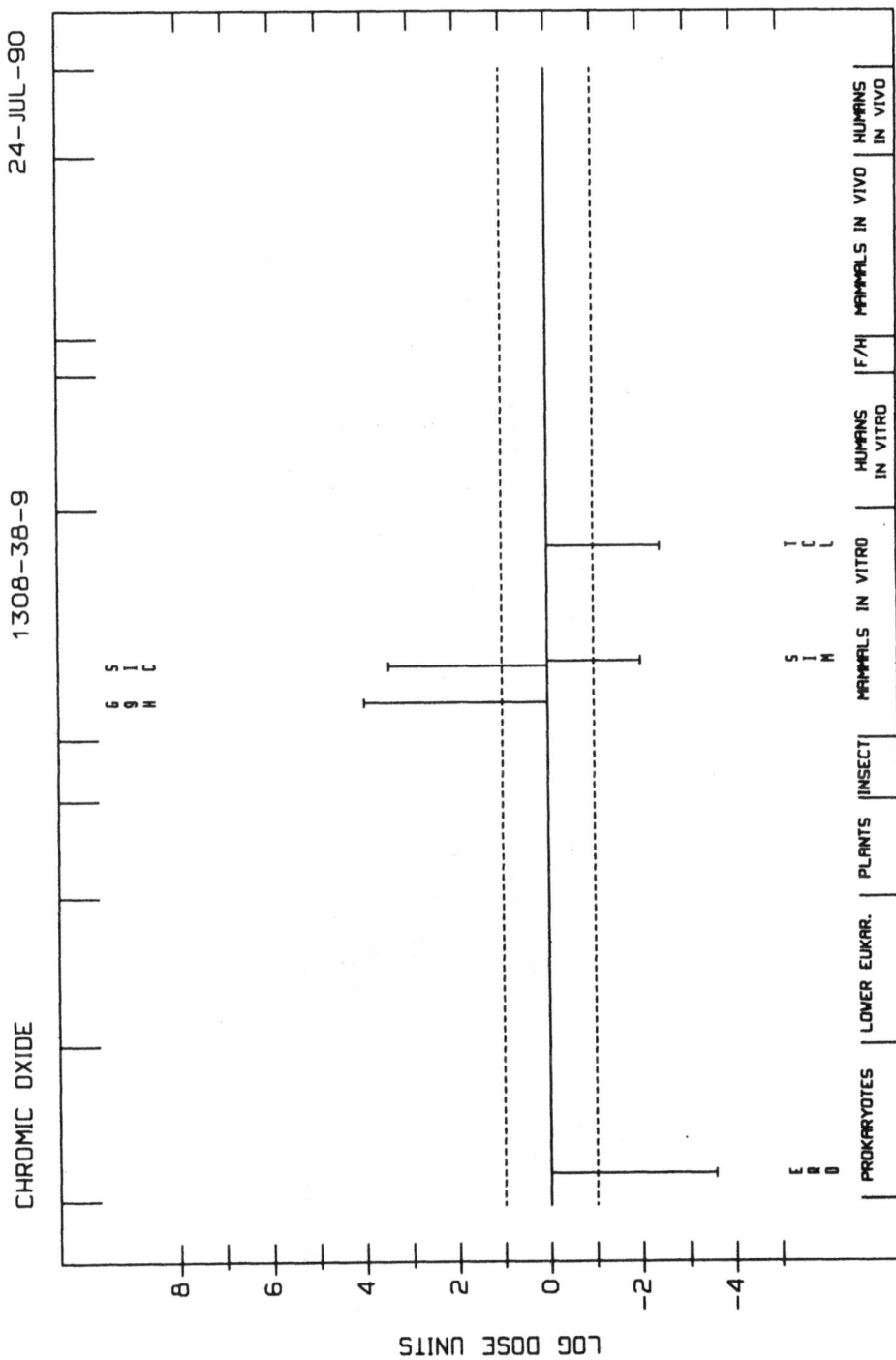

CHROMIC OXIDE

1308-38-9

24-JUL-90

LOG DOSE UNITS

PROKARYOTES | LOWER EUKAR. | PLANTS | INSECT | MAMMALS IN VITRO | HUMANS IN VITRO | F/H | MAMMALS IN VIVO | HUMANS IN VIVO

CHROMITE ORE

| END POINT | TEST CODE | TEST SYSTEM | RESULTS NM M | DOSE[1] (LED OR HID) | REFERENCE |
|---|---|---|---|---|---|
| G | SA0 | S. TYPHIMURIUM TA100, REVERSE MUTATION[2] | + 0 | 390.0000 | PETRILLI & DE FLORA, 1978a |
| G | SA0 | S. TYPHIMURIUM TA100, REVERSE MUTATION[2] | + 0 | 390.0000 | DE FLORA, 1981a |
| G | SA0 | S. TYPHIMURIUM TA100, REVERSE MUTATION[2] | + + | 1000.0000 | VENIER ET AL., 1982 |
| G | SA0 | S. TYPHIMURIUM TA100, REVERSE MUTATION[2] | + (+) | 196:0000 | BIANCHI ET AL., 1983 |
| G | SA5 | S. TYPHIMURIUM TA1535, REVERSE MUTATION[2] | - 0 | 390.0000 | DE FLORA, 1981a |
| G | SA7 | S. TYPHIMURIUM TA1537, REVERSE MUTATION[2] | - 0 | 390.0000 | DE FLORA, 1981a |
| G | SA8 | S. TYPHIMURIUM TA1538, REVERSE MUTATION[2] | - 0 | 390.0000 | DE FLORA, 1981a |
| G | SA9 | S. TYPHIMURIUM TA98, REVERSE MUTATION[2] | - 0 | 390.0000 | DE FLORA, 1981a |
| S | SIC | SCE, CHINESE HAMSTER CELLS IN VITRO[2] | + 0 | 1.9000 | VENIER ET AL., 1982 |
| S | SIC | SCE, CHINESE HAMSTER CELLS IN VITRO[2] | + 0 | 1.0000 | LEVIS & MAJONE, 1981 |
| C | CIC | CHROM ABERR, CHINESE HAMSTER CELLS IN VITRO[2] | + 0 | 1.0000 | LEVIS & MAJONE, 1981 |
| C | CIC | CHROM ABERR, CHINESE HAMSTER CELLS IN VITRO[2] | + 0 | 1.9000 | VENIER ET AL., 1982 |

[1]Doses are given as concentrations of the element, not the concentration of the compound.
[2]Contaminated with traces of Cr(VI)

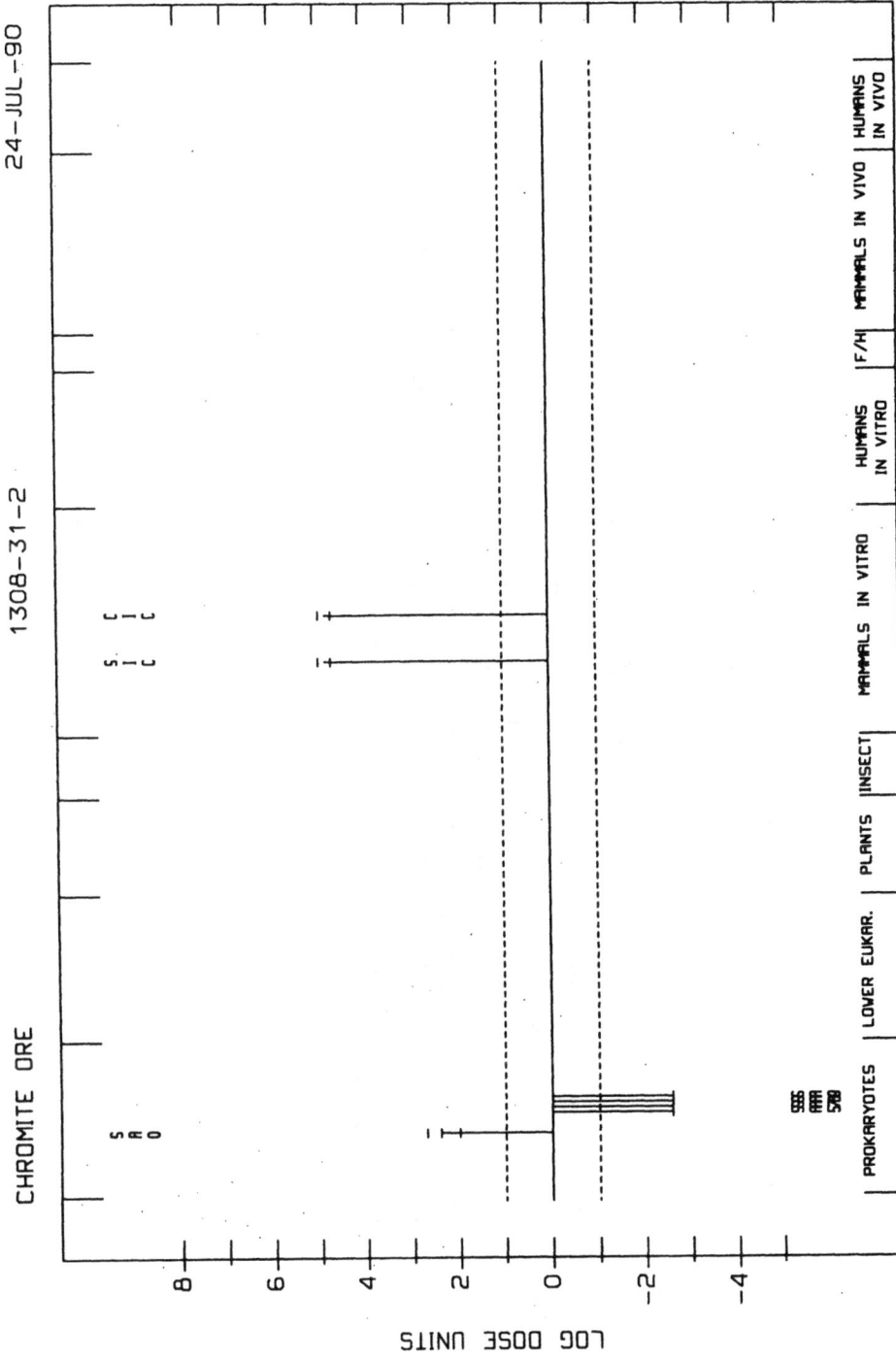

CUPRIC CHROMITE

| END POINT | TEST CODE | TEST SYSTEM | RESULTS NM M | DOSE[1] (LED OR HID) | REFERENCE |
|---|---|---|---|---|---|
| D | DIA | STRAND BREAKS/X-LINKS, ANIMAL CELLS IN VITRO | + 0 | 52.0000 | WEDRYCHOWSKI ET AL., 1986a |

[1]Doses are given as concentrations of the element, not the concentration of the compound.

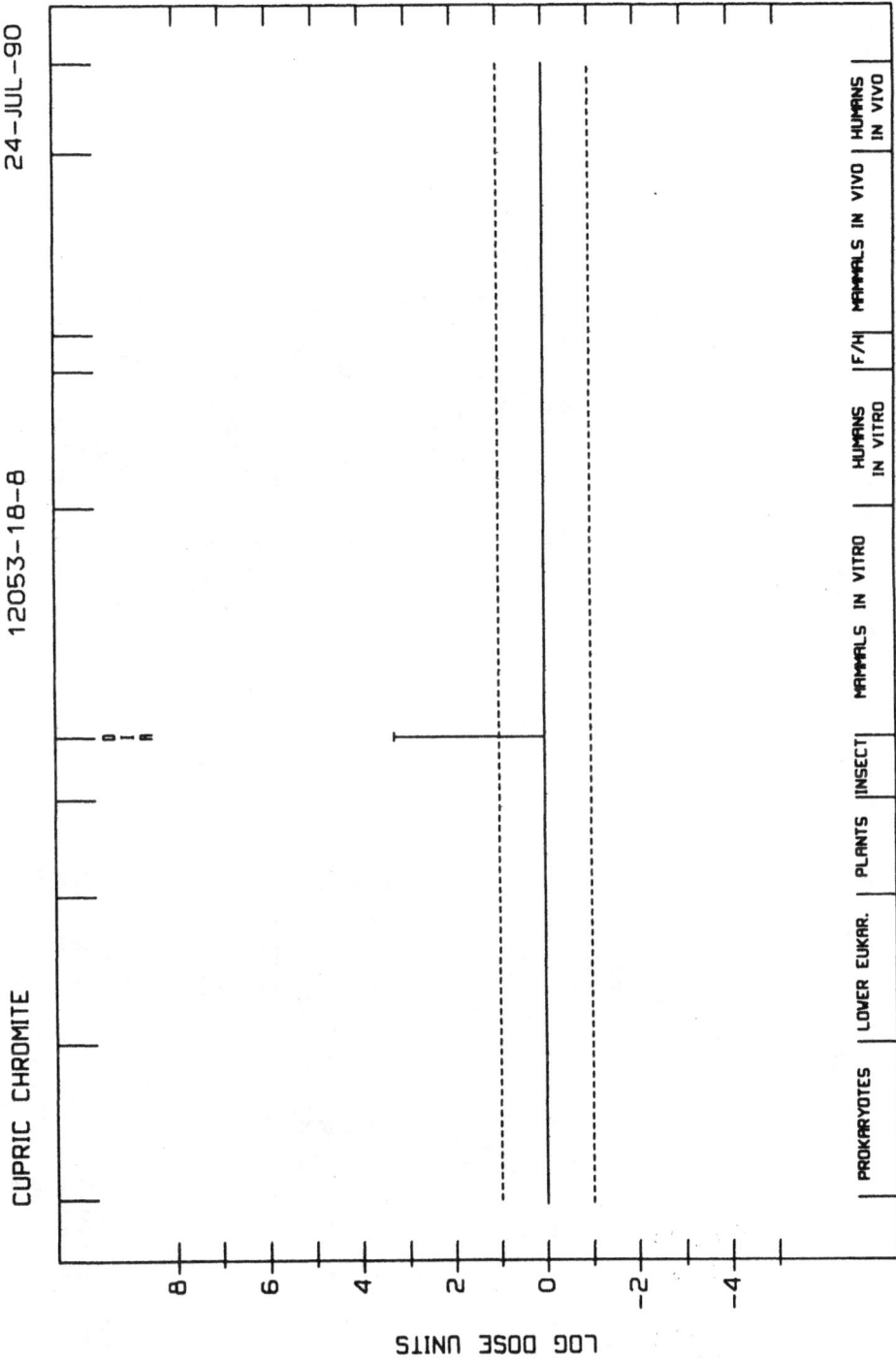

CUPRIC CHROMITE 12053-18-8 24-JUL-90

LOG DOSE UNITS

PROKARYOTES | LOWER EUKAR. | PLANTS | INSECT | MAMMALS IN VITRO | HUMANS IN VITRO | F/H | MAMMALS IN VIVO | HUMANS IN VIVO

POTASSIUM DICHROMATE

| END POINT | TEST CODE | TEST SYSTEM | RESULTS NM | M | DOSE[1] (LED OR HID) | REFERENCE |
|---|---|---|---|---|---|---|
| D | PRB | PROPHAGE, INDUCT/SOS/STRAND BREAKS/X-LINKS | + | 0 | 3.5000 | LLAGOSTERA ET AL., 1986 |
| D | PRB | PROPHAGE, INDUCT/SOS/STRAND BREAKS/X-LINKS | + | (+) | 0.1000 | OLIVIER & MARZIN, 1987 |
| D | PRB | PROPHAGE, INDUCT/SOS/STRAND BREAKS/X-LINKS | + | (+) | 12.0000 | VENIER ET AL., 1989 |
| D | PRB | PROPHAGE, INDUCT/SOS/STRAND BREAKS/X-LINKS | (+) | 0 | 76.0000 | NAKAMURA ET AL., 1987 |
| D | ECB | E. COLI, STRAND BREAKS/X-LINKS/REPAIR | + | 0 | 90.0000 | KALININA & MINSETTOVA, 1983b |
| D | ERD | E. COLI REC, DIFFERENTIAL TOXICITY | + | 0 | 17685.0000 | YAGI & NISHIOKA, 1977 |
| D | BSD | B. SUBTILIS REC, DIFFERENTIAL TOXICITY | + | 0 | 26.0000 | NISHIOKA, 1975 |
| D | BSD | B. SUBTILIS REC, DIFFERENTIAL TOXICITY | + | 0 | 166.0000 | NAKAMURO ET AL., 1978 |
| D | BSD | B. SUBTILIS REC, DIFFERENTIAL TOXICITY | + | 0 | 26.0000 | KADA ET AL., 1980 |
| D | BSD | B. SUBTILIS REC, DIFFERENTIAL TOXICITY | + | 0 | 260.0000 | GENTILE ET AL., 1981 |
| D | BSD | B. SUBTILIS REC, DIFFERENTIAL TOXICITY | + | 0 | 1.0000 | MATSUI, 1980 |
| D | BRD | BACTERIA (OTHER), DIFFERENTIAL TOXICITY | + | 0 | 260.0000 | GENTILE ET AL., 1981 |
| G | SA0 | S. TYPHIMURIUM TA100, REVERSE MUTATION | + | 0 | 4.4000 | BIANCHI ET AL., 1983 |
| G | SA0 | S. TYPHIMURIUM TA100, REVERSE MUTATION | + | 0 | 1.7500 | VENIER ET AL., 1982 |
| G | SA0 | S. TYPHIMURIUM TA100, REVERSE MUTATION | – | 0 | 0.0000 | KANEMATSU ET AL., 1980 |
| G | SA0 | S. TYPHIMURIUM TA100, REVERSE MUTATION | + | (+) | 1.7500 | LOPRIENO ET AL., 1985 |
| G | SA2 | S. TYPHIMURIUM TA102, REVERSE MUTATION | + | 0 | 2.8000 | GAVA ET AL., 1989b |
| G | SA5 | S. TYPHIMURIUM TA1535, REVERSE MUTATION | + | 0 | 0.0006 | MARZIN & PHI, 1985 |
| G | SA5 | S. TYPHIMURIUM TA1535, REVERSE MUTATION | – | 0 | 7.0000 | BIANCHI ET AL., 1983 |
| G | SA5 | S. TYPHIMURIUM TA1535, REVERSE MUTATION | – | 0 | 7.0000 | VENIER ET AL., 1982 |
| G | SA5 | S. TYPHIMURIUM TA1535, REVERSE MUTATION | – | 0 | 0.0000 | KANEMATSU ET AL., 1980 |
| G | SA5 | S. TYPHIMURIUM TA1535, REVERSE MUTATION | – | 0 | 7.0000 | LOPRIENO ET AL., 1985 |
| G | SA7 | S. TYPHIMURIUM TA1537, REVERSE MUTATION | + | 0 | 1.3000 | TAMARO ET AL., 1975 |
| G | SA7 | S. TYPHIMURIUM TA1537, REVERSE MUTATION | – | 0 | 0.0000 | KANEMATSU ET AL., 1980 |
| G | SA8 | S. TYPHIMURIUM TA1538, REVERSE MUTATION | – | 0 | 7.0000 | LOPRIENO ET AL., 1985 |
| G | SA8 | S. TYPHIMURIUM TA1538, REVERSE MUTATION | + | 0 | 1.8000 | BIANCHI ET AL., 1983 |
| G | SA8 | S. TYPHIMURIUM TA1538, REVERSE MUTATION | – | 0 | 7.0000 | VENIER ET AL., 1982 |
| G | SA8 | S. TYPHIMURIUM TA1538, REVERSE MUTATION | – | 0 | 0.0000 | KANEMATSU ET AL., 1980 |
| G | SA8 | S. TYPHIMURIUM TA1538, REVERSE MUTATION | – | 0 | 7.0000 | LOPRIENO ET AL., 1985 |
| G | SA9 | S. TYPHIMURIUM TA98, REVERSE MUTATION | (+) | 0 | 1.3000 | TAMARO ET AL., 1975 |
| G | SA9 | S. TYPHIMURIUM TA98, REVERSE MUTATION | (+) | 0 | 1.8000 | BIANCHI ET AL., 1983 |
| G | SA9 | S. TYPHIMURIUM TA98, REVERSE MUTATION | – | 0 | 1.7500 | VENIER ET AL., 1982 |
| G | SA9 | S. TYPHIMURIUM TA98, REVERSE MUTATION | – | 0 | 0.0000 | KANEMATSU ET AL., 1980 |
| G | SA9 | S. TYPHIMURIUM TA98, REVERSE MUTATION | + | (+) | 1.7500 | LOPRIENO ET AL., 1985 |
| G | SAS | S. TYPHIMURIUM (OTHER), REVERSE MUTATION | + | 0 | 3.5000 | GAVA ET AL., 1989b |

POTASSIUM DICHROMATE

| END POINT | TEST CODE | TEST SYSTEM | RESULTS NM | M | DOSE[1] (LED OR HID) | REFERENCE |
|---|---|---|---|---|---|---|
| G | ECF | E. COLI (EXCLUDING K12), FORWARD MUTATION | + | 0 | 0.0000 | ZAKOUR & GLICKMAN, 1984 |
| G | ECF | E. COLI (EXCLUDING K12), FORWARD MUTATION | + | 0 | 624.0000 | HAYES ET AL., 1984 |
| G | ECK | E. COLI K12, FORWARD OR REVERSE MUTATION | + | 0 | 177.0000 | KALININA & MINSEITOVA, 1983b |
| G | ECW | E. COLI WP2 UVRA, REVERSE MUTATION | + | 0 | 125.0000 | NISHIOKA, 1975 |
| G | ECW | E. COLI WP2 UVRA, REVERSE MUTATION | + | 0 | 0.5000 | VENITT & BOSWORTH, 1983 |
| G | ECW | E. COLI WP2 UVRA, REVERSE MUTATION | + | 0 | 3.5000 | VENIER ET AL., 1987 |
| G | EC2 | E. COLI WP2, REVERSE MUTATION | + | 0 | 125.0000 | NISHIOKA, 1975 |
| G | EC2 | E. COLI WP2, REVERSE MUTATION | + | 0 | 0.0000 | KANEMATSU ET AL., 1980 |
| G | ECR | E. COLI (OTHER), REVERSE MUTATION | + | 0 | 16.0000 | NAKAMURO ET AL., 1978 |
| R | SCG | S. CEREVISIAE, GENE CONVERSION | + | + | 260.0000 | GALLI ET AL., 1985 |
| R | SCG | S. CEREVISIAE, GENE CONVERSION | + | 0 | 0.0000 | SINGH, 1983 |
| R | SCG | S. CEREVISIAE, GENE CONVERSION | + | 0 | 21.0000 | KHARAB & SINGH, 1985 |
| R | SZG | S. POMBE, GENE CONVERSION | + | 0 | 10.4000 | BONATTI ET AL., 1976 |
| G | SCF | S. CEREVISIAE, FORWARD MUTATION | - | 0 | 1000.0000 | KHARAB & SINGH, 1987 |
| G | SCR | S. CEREVISIAE, REVERSE MUTATION | + | 0 | 104.0000 | GALLI ET AL., 1985 |
| G | SCR | S. CEREVISIAE, REVERSE MUTATION | + | 0 | 0.0000 | SINGH, 1983 |
| G | SCR | S. CEREVISIAE, REVERSE MUTATION | + | 0 | 21.0000 | KHARAB & SINGH, 1985 |
| G | SZF | S. POMBE, FORWARD MUTATION | + | 0 | 10.4000 | BONATTI ET AL., 1976 |
| A | SCN | S. CEREVISIAE, ANEUPLOIDY | + | 0 | 7.2000 | SORA ET AL., 1986 |
| G | DMX | D. MELANOGASTER, SEX-LINKED RECESSIVES | + | 0 | 106.0000 | RODRIGUEZ-ARNAIZ & MOLINA-MARTINEZ, 1986 |
| G | DMX | D. MELANOGASTER, SEX-LINKED RECESSIVES | + | 0 | 5.2000 | GAVA ET AL., 1989b |
| A | DMN | D. MELANOGASTER, ANEUPLOIDY | + | 0 | 140.0000 | RODRIGUEZ-ARNAIZ & MOLINA-MARTINEZ, 1986 |
| D | DIA | STRAND BREAKS/X-LINKS, ANIMAL CELLS IN VITRO | + | 0 | 52.0000 | WEDRYCHOWSKI ET AL., 1986a |
| D | DIA | STRAND BREAKS/X-LINKS, ANIMAL CELLS IN VITRO | + | 0 | 20.0000 | FORNACE ET AL., 1981 |
| D | DIA | STRAND BREAKS/X-LINKS, ANIMAL CELLS IN VITRO | - | 0 | 52.0000 | BIANCHI ET AL., 1983 |
| D | DIA | STRAND BREAKS/X-LINKS, ANIMAL CELLS IN VITRO | + | 0 | 1.3000 | HAMILTON-KOCH ET AL., 1986 |
| D | UIA | UDS, OTHER ANIMAL CELLS IN VITRO | + | 0 | 0.1500 | RAFFETTO ET AL., 1977 |
| G | GCO | MUTATION, CHO CELLS IN VITRO | + | 0 | 0.0350 | PASCHIN ET AL., 1983 |
| G | G9H | MUTATION, CHL V79 CELLS, HPRT | + | 0 | 0.0400 | PASCHIN & KOZACHENKO, 1982 |
| G | G9H | MUTATION, CHL V79 CELLS, HPRT | + | 0 | 0.0400 | PASCHIN ET AL., 1983 |
| G | G9H | MUTATION, CHL V79 CELLS, HPRT | + | 0 | 0.0400 | PASCHIN ET AL., 1981 |
| G | G9H | MUTATION, CHL V79 CELLS, HPRT | + | 0 | 0.1800 | NEWBOLD ET AL., 1979 |
| G | G9H | MUTATION, CHL V79 CELLS, HPRT | + | 0 | 11.0000 | RAINALDI ET AL., 1982 |
| G | G9H | MUTATION, CHL V79 CELLS, HPRT | + | 0 | 0.7000 | BIANCHI ET AL., 1983 |
| G | G9H | MUTATION, CHL V79 CELLS, HPRT | + | 0 | 0.2600 | CELOTTI ET AL., 1987 |

POTASSIUM DICHROMATE

| END POINT | TEST CODE | TEST SYSTEM | RESULTS NN M | DOSE¹ (LED OR HID) | REFERENCE |
|---|---|---|---|---|---|
| G | G9H | MUTATION, CHL V79 CELLS, HPRT | + 0 | 5.2000 | HARTWIG & BEYERSMANN, 1987 |
| G | G9O | MUTATION, CHL V79 CELLS, OUABAIN | + 0 | 6.0000 | RAINALDI ET AL., 1982 |
| G | G5T | MUTATION, L5178Y CELLS, TK LOCUS | + 0 | 1.0000 | OBERLY ET AL., 1982 |
| S | SIC | SCE, CHINESE HAMSTER CELLS IN VITRO | + 0 | 0.8000 | OHNO ET AL., 1982 |
| S | SIC | SCE, CHINESE HAMSTER CELLS IN VITRO | + 0 | 0.1000 | VENIER ET AL., 1982 |
| S | SIC | SCE, CHINESE HAMSTER CELLS IN VITRO | + 0 | 0.1000 | MAJONE ET AL., 1982 |
| S | SIC | SCE, CHINESE HAMSTER CELLS IN VITRO | + 0 | 0.1000 | LEVIS & MAJONE, 1981 |
| S | SIC | SCE, CHINESE HAMSTER CELLS IN VITRO | + 0 | 0.1000 | BIANCHI ET AL., 1983 |
| S | SIC | SCE, CHINESE HAMSTER CELLS IN VITRO | + 0 | 1.0000 | UYEKI & NISHIO, 1983 |
| S | SIC | SCE, CHINESE HAMSTER CELLS IN VITRO | + 0 | 0.1000 | LEVIS & MAJONE, 1979 |
| S | SIC | SCE, CHINESE HAMSTER CELLS IN VITRO | + 0 | 0.0000 | BIANCHI ET AL., 1980 |
| S | SIC | SCE, CHINESE HAMSTER CELLS IN VITRO | + 0 | 0.1000 | MAJONE & LEVIS, 1979 |
| S | SIC | SCE, CHINESE HAMSTER CELLS IN VITRO | + 0 | 0.0100 | MONTALDI ET AL., 1987b |
| S | SIC | SCE, CHINESE HAMSTER CELLS IN VITRO | + 0 | 0.0400 | LOPRIENO ET AL., 1985 |
| S | SIC | SCE, CHINESE HAMSTER CELLS IN VITRO | + 0 | 6.0000 | RAINALDI ET AL., 1982 |
| S | SIM | SCE, MOUSE CELLS IN VITRO | + 0 | 0.1000 | MAJONE ET AL., 1983 |
| S | SIM | SCE, MOUSE CELLS IN VITRO | + 0 | 0.1000 | BIANCHI ET AL., 1983 |
| S | SIM | SCE, MOUSE CELLS IN VITRO | + 0 | 0.1000 | ANDERSEN, 1983 |
| S | SIM | SCE, MOUSE CELLS IN VITRO | + 0 | 0.1000 | IIJIMA ET AL., 1983 |
| S | SIS | SCE, SYRIAN HAMSTER CELLS IN VITRO | + 0 | 2.0000 | BIANCHI ET AL., 1984 |
| C | CIC | CHROM ABERR, CHINESE HAMSTER CELLS IN VITRO | + 0 | 0.1000 | LEVIS & MAJONE, 1979 |
| C | CIC | CHROM ABERR, CHINESE HAMSTER CELLS IN VITRO | + 0 | 0.1000 | VENIER ET AL., 1982 |
| C | CIC | CHROM ABERR, CHINESE HAMSTER CELLS IN VITRO | + 0 | 0.1000 | LEVIS & MAJONE, 1981 |
| C | CIC | CHROM ABERR, CHINESE HAMSTER CELLS IN VITRO | + 0 | 0.0000 | BIANCHI ET AL., 1980 |
| C | CIC | CHROM ABERR, CHINESE HAMSTER CELLS IN VITRO | + 0 | 0.1000 | MAJONE & LEVIS, 1979 |
| C | CIC | CHROM ABERR, CHINESE HAMSTER CELLS IN VITRO | + 0 | 0.1800 | NEWBOLD & LEVIS, 1979 |
| C | CIM | CHROM ABERR, MOUSE CELLS IN VITRO | + 0 | 0.0150 | RAFFETTO ET AL., 1977 |
| C | CIR | CHROM ABERR, RAT CELLS IN VITRO | + 0 | 0.7000 | NEWTON & LILLY, 1986 |
| C | CIS | CHROM ABERR, SYRIAN HAMSTER CELLS IN VITRO | + 0 | 0.0400 | TSUDA & KATO, 1977 |
| C | CIT | CHROM ABERR, TRANSFORMED CELLS IN VITRO | + 0 | 0.0350 | UMEDA & NISHIMURA, 1979 |
| C | CIA | CHROM ABERR, OTHER ANIMAL CELLS IN VITRO | + 0 | 0.1500 | BIGALIEV ET AL., 1977a |
| T | TCM | CELL TRANSFORMATION, C3H10T1/2 CELLS | - 0 | 0.5000 | PATIERNO ET AL., 1988 |
| T | TCS | CELL TRANSFORMATION, SHE, CLONAL ASSAY | + 0 | 0.0400 | TSUDA & KATO, 1977 |
| T | TCS | CELL TRANSFORMATION, SHE, CLONAL ASSAY | + 0 | 0.1000 | HANSEN & STERN, 1985 |

POTASSIUM DICHROMATE

| END POINT | TEST CODE | TEST SYSTEM | RESULTS NM | M | DOSE[1] (LED OR HID) | REFERENCE |
|---|---|---|---|---|---|---|
| T | TCL | CELL TRANSFORMATION, OTHER CELL LINES | + | 0 | 0.0150 | RAFFETTO ET AL., 1977 |
| T | TCL | CELL TRANSFORMATION, OTHER CELL LINES | + | 0 | 1.8000 | BIANCHI ET AL., 1983 |
| T | TCL | CELL TRANSFORMATION, OTHER CELL LINES | + | 0 | 2.6000 | HANSEN & STERN, 1985 |
| T | TCL | CELL TRANSFORMATION, OTHER CELL LINES | + | 0 | 5.2000 | LANFRANCHI ET AL., 1988 |
| D | DIH | STRAND BREAKS/X-LINKS, HUMAN CELLS IN VITRO | + | 0 | 0.1200 | SNYDER, 1988 |
| D | DIH | STRAND BREAKS/X-LINKS, HUMAN CELLS IN VITRO | + | 0 | 5.2000 | MCLEAN ET AL., 1982 |
| D | DIH | STRAND BREAKS/X-LINKS, HUMAN CELLS IN VITRO | + | 0 | 0.5200 | HAMILTON-KOCH ET AL., 1986 |
| D | UHF | UDS, HUMAN FIBROBLASTS IN VITRO | - | 0 | 104.0000 | BIANCHI ET AL., 1983 |
| D | UHF | UDS, HUMAN FIBROBLASTS IN VITRO | - | 0 | 104.0000 | BIANCHI ET AL., 1982b |
| S | SHF | SCE, HUMAN FIBROBLASTS IN VITRO | + | 0 | 0.0100 | MACRAE ET AL., 1979 |
| S | SHL | SCE, HUMAN LYMPHOCYTES IN VITRO | + | 0 | 0.0180 | GOMEZ-ARROYO ET AL., 1981 |
| S | SHL | SCE, HUMAN LYMPHOCYTES IN VITRO | + | 0 | 0.0025 | STELLA ET AL., 1982 |
| S | SHL | SCE, HUMAN LYMPHOCYTES IN VITRO | + | 0 | 0.1000 | OGAWA ET AL., 1978 |
| S | SHL | SCE, HUMAN LYMPHOCYTES IN VITRO | + | 0 | 1.0000 | ANDERSEN, 1983 |
| C | CHL | CHROM ABERR, HUMAN LYMPHOCYTES IN VITRO | + | 0 | 0.0520 | NAKAMURO ET AL., 1978 |
| C | CHL | CHROM ABERR, HUMAN LYMPHOCYTES IN VITRO | + | 0 | 0.0010 | STELLA ET AL., 1982 |
| G | MST | MOUSE SPOT TEST | + | 0 | 3.5000 | KNUDSON, 1980 |
| S | SVA | SCE, ANIMALS IN VIVO | + | 0 | 3.5000 | KATHS, 1981 |
| M | MVM | MICRONUCLEUS TEST, MICE IN VIVO | + | 0 | 18.0000 | FABRY, 1980 |
| M | MVM | MICRONUCLEUS TEST, MICE IN VIVO | + | 0 | 0.3500 | PASCHIN & TOROPZEV, 1982 |
| M | MVC | MICRONUCLEUS TEST, HAMSTERS IN VIVO | + | 0 | 7.0000 | KATHS, 1981 |
| C | CBA | CHROM ABERR, ANIMAL BONE MARROW IN VIVO | - | 0 | 0.7000 | PASCHIN ET AL., 1981 |
| C | CBA | CHROM ABERR, ANIMAL BONE MARROW IN VIVO | + | 0 | 6.0000 | NEWTON & LILLY, 1986 |
| C | CBA | CHROM ABERR, ANIMAL BONE MARROW IN VIVO | + | 0 | 1.0000 | BIGALIEV ET AL., 1977b |
| A | AVA | ANEUPLOIDY, ANIMAL CELLS IN VIVO | + | 0 | 1.0000 | BIGALIEV ET AL., 1977b |
| C | CLA | CHROM ABERR, ANIMAL LEUCOCYTES IN VIVO | + | 0 | 7.0000 | NEWTON & LILLY, 1986 |
| C | DLM | DOMINANT LETHAL TEST, MICE | + | 0 | 0.7000 | PASCHIN ET AL., 1982 |
| C | DLM | DOMINANT LETHAL TEST, MICE | - | 0 | 0.5300 | PASCHIN ET AL., 1981 |

[1]Doses are given as concentrations of the element, not the concentration of the compound.

POTASSIUM DICHROMATE                    7778-50-9                    24-JUL-90

LOG DOSE UNITS

SODIUM DICHROMATE

| END POINT | TEST CODE | TEST SYSTEM | RESULTS NM | M | DOSE[1] (LED OR HID) | REFERENCE |
|---|---|---|---|---|---|---|
| D | PRB | PROPHAGE, INDUCT/SOS/STRAND BREAKS/X-LINKS | + | 0 | 2.0000 | DE FLORA ET AL., 1985a |
| D | ERD | E. COLI REC, DIFFERENTIAL TOXICITY | + | 0 | 0.0000 | PETRILLI & DE FLORA, 1982 |
| D | ERD | E. COLI REC, DIFFERENTIAL TOXICITY | + | + | 35.0000 | DE FLORA ET AL., 1984a |
| D | BSD | B. SUBTILIS REC, DIFFERENTIAL TOXICITY | + | 0 | 130.0000 | GENTILE ET AL., 1981 |
| D | BRD | BACTERIA (OTHER), DIFFERENTIAL TOXICITY | + | 0 | 130.0000 | GENTILE ET AL., 1981 |
| G | SA0 | S. TYPHIMURIUM TA100, REVERSE MUTATION | + | + | 9.0000 | PETRILLI & DE FLORA, 1977 |
| G | SA0 | S. TYPHIMURIUM TA100, REVERSE MUTATION | + | - | 3.5000 | PETRILLI & DE FLORA, 1978b |
| G | SA0 | S. TYPHIMURIUM TA100, REVERSE MUTATION | + | - | 1.3000 | DE FLORA, 1981a |
| G | SA0 | S. TYPHIMURIUM TA100, REVERSE MUTATION | + | 0 | 3.5000 | BENNICELLI ET AL., 1983 |
| G | SA0 | S. TYPHIMURIUM TA100, REVERSE MUTATION | + | (+) | 3.5000 | DE FLORA, 1978 |
| G | SA0 | S. TYPHIMURIUM TA100, REVERSE MUTATION | + | 0 | 7.0000 | DE FLORA & BOIDO, 1980 |
| G | SA0 | S. TYPHIMURIUM TA100, REVERSE MUTATION | + | (+) | 3.5000 | DE FLORA, 1981b |
| G | SA0 | S. TYPHIMURIUM TA100, REVERSE MUTATION | + | + | 4.5000 | PETRILLI & DE FLORA, 1982 |
| G | SA0 | S. TYPHIMURIUM TA100, REVERSE MUTATION | + | 0 | 0.9000 | PEDERSEN ET AL., 1983 |
| G | SA0 | S. TYPHIMURIUM TA100, REVERSE MUTATION | + | 0 | 3.5000 | PETRILLI ET AL., 1985 |
| G | SA0 | S. TYPHIMURIUM TA100, REVERSE MUTATION | + | (+) | 10.0000 | DE FLORA ET AL., 1985b |
| G | SA0 | S. TYPHIMURIUM TA100, REVERSE MUTATION | + | (+) | 5.0000 | DE FLORA ET AL., 1985c |
| G | SA0 | S. TYPHIMURIUM TA100, REVERSE MUTATION | + | - | 5.0000 | PETRILLI ET AL., 1986b |
| G | SA0 | S. TYPHIMURIUM TA100, REVERSE MUTATION | + | + | 7.0000 | PETRILLI ET AL., 1980 |
| G | SA0 | S. TYPHIMURIUM TA100, REVERSE MUTATION | + | 0 | 5.0000 | PETRUZZELLI ET AL., 1989 |
| G | SA0 | S. TYPHIMURIUM TA100, REVERSE MUTATION | + | 0 | 5.0000 | DE FLORA ET AL., 1989b |
| G | SA0 | S. TYPHIMURIUM TA100, REVERSE MUTATION | + | (+) | 6.0000 | DE FLORA ET AL., 1987b |
| G | SA0 | S. TYPHIMURIUM TA100, REVERSE MUTATION | + | - | 5.2500 | DE FLORA ET AL., 1989c |
| G | SA0 | S. TYPHIMURIUM TA100, REVERSE MUTATION | + | (+) | 5.0000 | DE FLORA ET AL., 1987d |
| G | SA0 | S. TYPHIMURIUM TA100, REVERSE MUTATION | + | + | 3.5000 | BENNICELLI ET AL., 1983 |
| G | SA2 | S. TYPHIMURIUM TA102, REVERSE MUTATION | + | 0 | 0.0000 | DE FLORA ET AL., 1984b |
| G | SA2 | S. TYPHIMURIUM TA102, REVERSE MUTATION | + | 0 | 9.0000 | DE FLORA ET AL., 1984c |
| G | SA2 | S. TYPHIMURIUM TA102, REVERSE MUTATION | + | 0 | 5.7000 | PETRILLI ET AL., 1985 |
| G | SA2 | S. TYPHIMURIUM TA102, REVERSE MUTATION | + | 0 | 70.0000 | DE FLORA ET AL., 1985a |
| G | SA2 | S. TYPHIMURIUM TA102, REVERSE MUTATION | + | (+) | 10.0000 | DE FLORA ET AL., 1985b |
| G | SA2 | S. TYPHIMURIUM TA102, REVERSE MUTATION | + | - | 5.0000 | PETRILLI ET AL., 1986b |
| G | SA5 | S. TYPHIMURIUM TA1535, REVERSE MUTATION | - | 0 | 10.0000 | DE FLORA ET AL., 1987a |
| G | SA5 | S. TYPHIMURIUM TA1535, REVERSE MUTATION | - | 0 | 1.3000 | DE FLORA, 1981a |
| G | SA5 | S. TYPHIMURIUM TA1535, REVERSE MUTATION | - | - | 0.0000 | PETRILLI & DE FLORA, 1978b |

SODIUM DICHROMATE

| END POINT | TEST CODE | TEST SYSTEM | RESULTS NM | M | DOSE[1] (LED OR HID) | REFERENCE |
|---|---|---|---|---|---|---|
| G | SA5 | S. TYPHIMURIUM TA1535, REVERSE MUTATION | - | - | 35.0000 | PETRILLI & DE FLORA, 1977 |
| G | SA5 | S. TYPHIMURIUM TA1535, REVERSE MUTATION | - | 0 | 9.0000 | BENNICELLI ET AL., 1983 |
| G | SA5 | S. TYPHIMURIUM TA1535, REVERSE MUTATION | - | 0 | 9.0000 | PETRILLI & DE FLORA, 1982 |
| G | SA7 | S. TYPHIMURIUM TA1537, REVERSE MUTATION | + | - | 9.0000 | PETRILLI & DE FLORA, 1977 |
| G | SA7 | S. TYPHIMURIUM TA1537, REVERSE MUTATION | (+) | 0 | 0.0000 | PETRILLI & DE FLORA, 1978b |
| G | SA7 | S. TYPHIMURIUM TA1537, REVERSE MUTATION | (+) | 0 | 1.3000 | DE FLORA, 1981a |
| G | SA7 | S. TYPHIMURIUM TA1537, REVERSE MUTATION | (+) | 0 | 9.0000 | BENNICELLI ET AL., 1983 |
| G | SA8 | S. TYPHIMURIUM TA1538, REVERSE MUTATION | - | 0 | 9.0000 | PETRILLI & DE FLORA, 1982 |
| G | SA8 | S. TYPHIMURIUM TA1538, REVERSE MUTATION | (+) | 0 | 1.3000 | DE FLORA, 1981a |
| G | SA8 | S. TYPHIMURIUM TA1538, REVERSE MUTATION | (+) | 0 | 9.0000 | BENNICELLI ET AL., 1983 |
| G | SA9 | S. TYPHIMURIUM TA98, REVERSE MUTATION | - | - | 9.0000 | PETRILLI & DE FLORA, 1982 |
| G | SA9 | S. TYPHIMURIUM TA98, REVERSE MUTATION | (+) | 0 | 0.0000 | PETRILLI & DE FLORA, 1978b |
| G | SA9 | S. TYPHIMURIUM TA98, REVERSE MUTATION | + | 0 | 9.0000 | PETRILLI & DE FLORA, 1977 |
| G | SA9 | S. TYPHIMURIUM TA98, REVERSE MUTATION | (+) | 0 | 1.3000 | DE FLORA, 1981a |
| G | SA9 | S. TYPHIMURIUM TA98, REVERSE MUTATION | (+) | 0 | 3.5000 | BENNICELLI ET AL., 1983 |
| G | SAS | S. TYPHIMURIUM (OTHER), REVERSE MUTATION | + | 0 | 9.0000 | PETRILLI & DE FLORA, 1982 |
| G | SAS | S. TYPHIMURIUM (OTHER), REVERSE MUTATION | + | 0 | 0.0000 | DE FLORA ET AL., 1984a |
| G | SAS | S. TYPHIMURIUM (OTHER), REVERSE MUTATION | + | 0 | 3.5000 | PETRILLI & DE FLORA, 1982 |
| G | SAS | S. TYPHIMURIUM (OTHER), REVERSE MUTATION | + | 0 | 0.0000 | DE FLORA ET AL., 1984b |
| G | SAS | S. TYPHIMURIUM (OTHER), REVERSE MUTATION | + | 0 | 5.2500 | BENNICELLI ET AL., 1983 |
| G | ECW | E. COLI WP2 UVRA, REVERSE MUTATION | + | 0 | 7.0000 | PETRILLI & DE FLORA, 1982 |
| G | EC2 | E. COLI WP2, REVERSE MUTATION | + | 0 | 9.0000 | PETRILLI & DE FLORA, 1982 |
| D | DMM | D. MELANOGASTER, SOMATIC MUTAT/RECOMB | + | 0 | 244.0000 | RASMUSON, 1985 |
| D | DIA | STRAND BREAKS/X-LINKS, ANIMAL CELLS IN VITRO | + | 0 | 3.1000 | SINA ET AL., 1983 |
| S | SIC | SCE, CHINESE HAMSTER CELLS IN VITRO | + | 0 | 0.1000 | LEVIS & MAJONE, 1979 |
| S | SIC | SCE, CHINESE HAMSTER CELLS IN VITRO | + | 0 | 0.0300 | ELIAS ET AL., 1983 |
| S | SIC | SCE, CHINESE HAMSTER CELLS IN VITRO | + | 0 | 0.1000 | MAJONE & LEVIS, 1979 |
| S | SIC | SCE, CHINESE HAMSTER CELLS IN VITRO | + | 0 | 0.0000 | BIANCHI ET AL., 1980 |
| C | CIC | CHROM ABERR, CHINESE HAMSTER CELLS IN VITRO | + | 0 | 0.1000 | LEVIS & MAJONE, 1979 |
| C | CIC | CHROM ABERR, CHINESE HAMSTER CELLS IN VITRO | + | 0 | 0.1000 | MAJONE & LEVIS, 1979 |

SODIUM DICHROMATE

| END POINT | TEST CODE | TEST SYSTEM | RESULTS NM M | DOSE[1] (LED OR HID) | REFERENCE |
|---|---|---|---|---|---|
| C | CIC | CHROM ABERR, CHINESE HAMSTER CELLS IN VITRO | + 0 | 0.0000 | BIANCHI ET AL., 1980 |
| C | CHL | CHROM ABERR, HUMAN LYMPHOCYTES IN VITRO | + 0 | 0.2000 | SARTO ET AL., 1980 |
| D | DVA | STRAND BREAKS/X-LINKS, ANIMALS IN VIVO | + 0 | 20.0000 | TSAPAKOS ET AL., 1981 |
| D | DVA | STRAND BREAKS/X-LINKS, ANIMALS IN VIVO | + 0 | 20.0000 | TSAPAKOS ET AL., 1983a |
| C | FSC | FISH, CHROM ABERR | + 0 | 1.0000 | KRISHNAJA & REGE, 1982 |

[1]Doses are given as concentrations of the element, not the concentration of the compound.

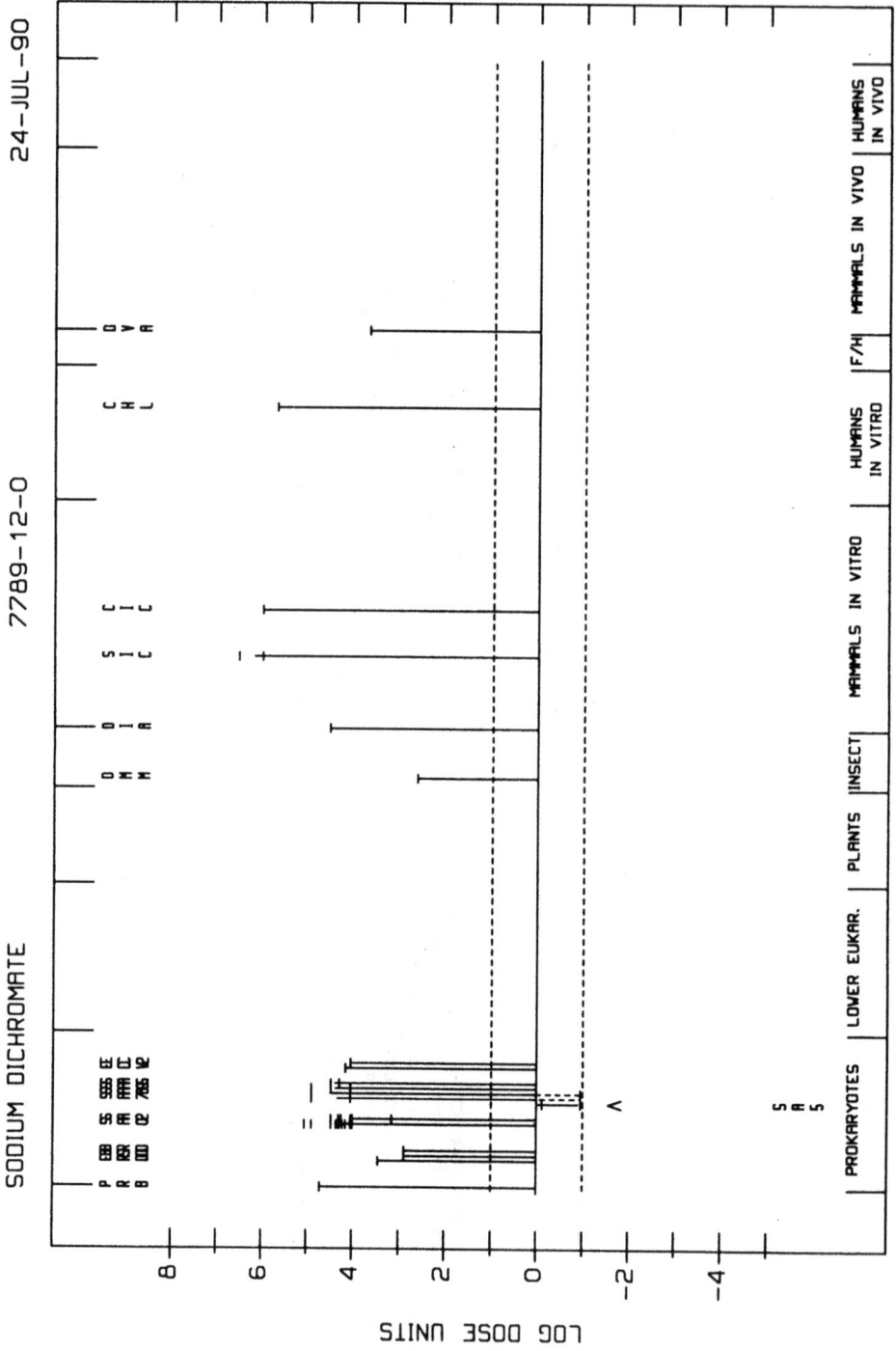

AMMONIUM DICHROMATE

| END POINT | TEST CODE | TEST SYSTEM | RESULTS NM M | DOSE[1] (LED OR HID) | REFERENCE |
|---|---|---|---|---|---|
| D | ERD | E. COLI REC, DIFFERENTIAL TOXICITY | + 0 | 5200.0000 | YAGI & NISHIOKA, 1977 |
| D | BSD | B. SUBTILIS REC, DIFFERENTIAL TOXICITY | + 0 | 260.0000 | GENTILE ET AL., 1981 |
| D | BRD | BACTERIA (OTHER), DIFFERENTIAL TOXICITY | + 0 | 260.0000 | GENTILE ET AL., 1981 |

[1]Doses are given as concentrations of the element, not the concentration of the compound.

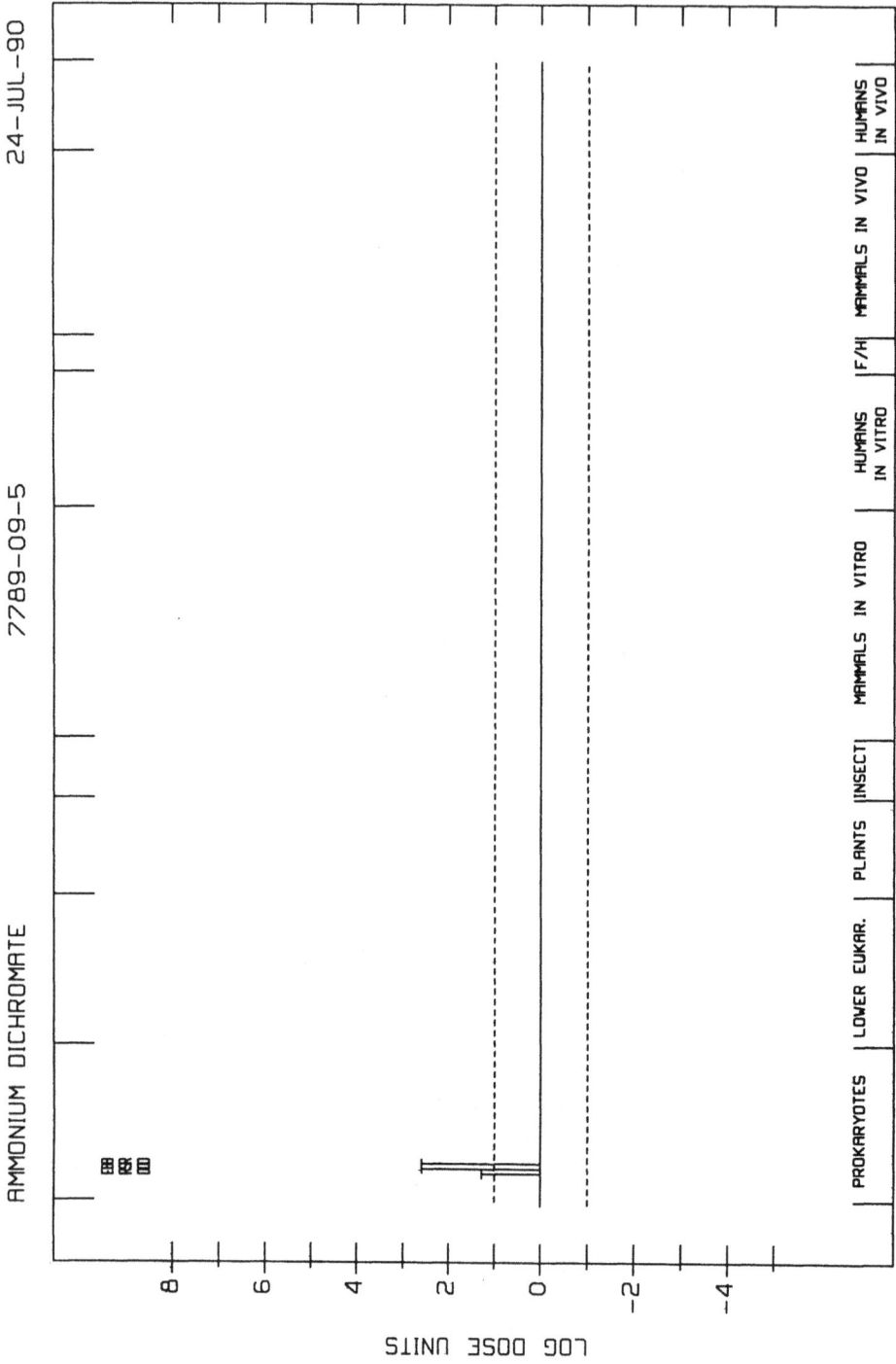

AMMONIUM DICHROMATE          7789-09-5          24-JUL-90

POTASSIUM CHROMATE

| END POINT | TEST CODE | TEST SYSTEM | RESULTS NM | M | DOSE[1] (LED OR HID) | REFERENCE |
|---|---|---|---|---|---|---|
| D | PRB | PROPHAGE, INDUCT/SOS/STRAND BREAKS/X-LINKS | + | 0 | 0.2000 | ROSSMAN ET AL., 1984 |
| D | PRB | PROPHAGE, INDUCT/SOS/STRAND BREAKS/X-LINKS | + | 0 | 13.0000 | LLAGOSTERA ET AL., 1986 |
| D | PRB | PROPHAGE, INDUCT/SOS/STRAND BREAKS/X-LINKS | + | (+) | 0.3000 | OLIVIER & MARZIN, 1987 |
| D | PRB | PROPHAGE, INDUCT/SOS/STRAND BREAKS/X-LINKS | + | (+) | 18.0000 | VENIER ET AL., 1989 |
| D | ERD | E. COLI REC, DIFFERENTIAL TOXICITY | + | + | 40.0000 | DE FLORA ET AL., 1984a |
| D | ERD | E. COLI REC, DIFFERENTIAL TOXICITY | + | | 5360.0000 | YAGI & NISHIOKA, 1977 |
| D | BSD | B. SUBTILIS REC, DIFFERENTIAL TOXICITY | + | 0 | 130.0000 | NISHIOKA, 1975 |
| D | BSD | B. SUBTILIS REC, DIFFERENTIAL TOXICITY | + | 0 | 52.0000 | NAKAMURO ET AL., 1978 |
| D | BSD | B. SUBTILIS REC, DIFFERENTIAL TOXICITY | + | 0 | 13.0000 | KADA ET AL., 1980 |
| G | SA0 | S. TYPHIMURIUM TA100, REVERSE MUTATION | + | - | 5.4000 | PETRILLI & DE FLORA, 1978b |
| G | SA0 | S. TYPHIMURIUM TA100, REVERSE MUTATION | + | 0 | 2.0000 | DE FLORA, 1981a |
| G | SA0 | S. TYPHIMURIUM TA100, REVERSE MUTATION | + | (+) | 1300.0000 | BEYERSMANN ET AL., 1984 |
| G | SA0 | S. TYPHIMURIUM TA100, REVERSE MUTATION | + | 0 | 0.2000 | BAKER ET AL., 1984 |
| G | SA0 | S. TYPHIMURIUM TA100, REVERSE MUTATION | + | 0 | 0.2400 | ARLAUSKAS ET AL., 1985 |
| G | SA0 | S. TYPHIMURIUM TA100, REVERSE MUTATION | + | 0 | 0.0100 | LANGERWERF ET AL., 1985 |
| G | SA2 | S. TYPHIMURIUM TA102, REVERSE MUTATION | + | 0 | 0.0007 | MARZIN & PHI, 1985 |
| G | SA5 | S. TYPHIMURIUM TA1535, REVERSE MUTATION | - | 0 | 2.0000 | DE FLORA, 1981a |
| G | SA5 | S. TYPHIMURIUM TA1535, REVERSE MUTATION | - | - | 11.0000 | PETRILLI & DE FLORA, 1978b |
| G | SA5 | S. TYPHIMURIUM TA1535, REVERSE MUTATION | (+) | 0 | 5.0000 | TAMARO ET AL., 1975 |
| G | SA7 | S. TYPHIMURIUM TA1537, REVERSE MUTATION | + | - | 5.4000 | PETRILLI & DE FLORA, 1978b |
| G | SA7 | S. TYPHIMURIUM TA1537, REVERSE MUTATION | (+) | 0 | 2.0000 | DE FLORA, 1981a |
| G | SA7 | S. TYPHIMURIUM TA1537, REVERSE MUTATION | + | 0 | 0.0000 | ARLAUSKAS ET AL., 1985 |
| G | SA8 | S. TYPHIMURIUM TA1538, REVERSE MUTATION | (+) | 0 | 2.0000 | DE FLORA, 1981a |
| G | SA8 | S. TYPHIMURIUM TA1538, REVERSE MUTATION | (+) | 0 | 2.5000 | TAMARO ET AL., 1975 |
| G | SA9 | S. TYPHIMURIUM TA98, REVERSE MUTATION | + | - | 5.4000 | PETRILLI & DE FLORA, 1978b |
| G | SA9 | S. TYPHIMURIUM TA98, REVERSE MUTATION | (+) | 0 | 2.0000 | DE FLORA, 1981a |
| G | SA9 | S. TYPHIMURIUM TA98, REVERSE MUTATION | + | 0 | 0.0100 | ARLAUSKAS ET AL., 1985 |
| G | SA9 | S. TYPHIMURIUM TA98, REVERSE MUTATION | - | 0 | 0.0000 | LANGERWERF ET AL., 1985 |
| G | SAS | S. TYPHIMURIUM (OTHER), REVERSE MUTATION | + | 0 | 0.0000 | DE FLORA ET AL., 1984a |
| G | SAS | S. TYPHIMURIUM (OTHER), REVERSE MUTATION | + | 0 | 0.0050 | LANGERWERF ET AL., 1985 |
| G | ECF | E. COLI (EXCLUDING K12), FORWARD MUTATION | - | - | 0.3600 | LA VELLE, 1986a |
| G | ECW | E. COLI WP2 UVRA, REVERSE MUTATION | + | 0 | 0.0025 | VENITT & LEVY, 1974 |
| G | EC2 | E. COLI WP2, REVERSE MUTATION | + | 0 | 0.1300 | GREEN ET AL., 1976 |
| G | EC2 | E. COLI WP2, REVERSE MUTATION | + | 0 | 0.0025 | VENITT & LEVY, 1974 |
| G | ECR | E. COLI (OTHER), REVERSE MUTATION | + | 0 | 0.0025 | VENITT & LEVY, 1974 |

POTASSIUM CHROMATE

| END POINT | TEST CODE | TEST SYSTEM | RESULTS NM M | DOSE[1] (LED OR HID) | REFERENCE |
|---|---|---|---|---|---|
| G | ECR | E. COLI (OTHER), REVERSE MUTATION | + 0 | 0.6500 | ARLAUSKAS ET AL., 1985 |
| G | ECR | E. COLI (OTHER), REVERSE MUTATION | + 0 | 8.0000 | NAKAMURO ET AL., 1978 |
| M | TSI | TRADESCANTIA SPECIES, MICRONUCLEI | - 0 | 5200.0000 | MA ET AL., 1984 |
| D | DIA | STRAND BREAKS/X-LINKS, ANIMAL CELLS IN VITRO | + 0 | 1.3000 | FORNACE ET AL., 1981 |
| D | DIA | STRAND BREAKS/X-LINKS, ANIMAL CELLS IN VITRO | + 0 | 1.7000 | MILLER & COSTA, 1988 |
| D | DIA | STRAND BREAKS/X-LINKS, ANIMAL CELLS IN VITRO | + 0 | 10.0000 | WEDRYCHOWSKI ET AL., 1986b |
| G | G5T | MUTATION, L5178Y CELLS, TK LOCUS | + 0 | 1.0000 | OBERLY ET AL., 1982 |
| S | SIC | SCE, CHINESE HAMSTER CELLS IN VITRO | + 0 | 0.1500 | MAJONE & RENSI, 1979 |
| S | SIC | SCE, CHINESE HAMSTER CELLS IN VITRO | + 0 | 0.0400 | MACRAE ET AL., 1979 |
| S | SIC | SCE, CHINESE HAMSTER CELLS IN VITRO | + 0 | 0.2500 | LEVIS & MAJONE, 1979 |
| S | SIC | SCE, CHINESE HAMSTER CELLS IN VITRO | + 0 | 0.8000 | OHNO ET AL., 1982 |
| S | SIC | SCE, CHINESE HAMSTER CELLS IN VITRO | + 0 | 0.0300 | ELIAS ET AL., 1983 |
| S | SIC | SCE, CHINESE HAMSTER CELLS IN VITRO | + 0 | 0.0500 | MAJONE ET AL., 1982 |
| S | SIC | SCE, CHINESE HAMSTER CELLS IN VITRO | + 0 | 0.0000 | BIANCHI ET AL., 1980 |
| S | SIC | SCE, CHINESE HAMSTER CELLS IN VITRO | + 0 | 0.1300 | PRICE-JONES ET AL., 1980 |
| C | CIC | CHROM ABERR, CHINESE HAMSTER CELLS IN VITRO | + 0 | 0.2500 | LEVIS & MAJONE, 1979 |
| C | CIC | CHROM ABERR, CHINESE HAMSTER CELLS IN VITRO | + 0 | 0.1500 | MAJONE & RENSI, 1979 |
| C | CIC | CHROM ABERR, CHINESE HAMSTER CELLS IN VITRO | + 0 | 0.0000 | BIANCHI ET AL., 1980 |
| C | CIC | CHROM ABERR, CHINESE HAMSTER CELLS IN VITRO | + 0 | 0.3000 | KOSHI & IWASAKI, 1983 |
| A | AIA | ANEUPLOIDY, ANIMAL CELLS IN VITRO | - 0 | 0.1300 | PRICE-JONES ET AL., 1980 |
| C | CIT | CHROM ABERR, TRANSFORMED CELLS IN VITRO | + 0 | 0.1700 | UMEDA & NISHIMURA, 1979 |
| T | TCS | CELL TRANSFORMATION, SHE, CLONAL ASSAY | - 0 | 0.1400 | RIVEDAL & SANNER, 1981 |
| T | T7S | CELL TRANSFORMATION, SA7/SHE CELLS | + 0 | 0.3000 | CASTO ET AL., 1979 |
| D | DIH | STRAND BREAKS/X-LINKS, HUMAN CELLS IN VITRO | + 0 | 26.0000 | WHITING ET AL., 1979 |
| D | DIH | STRAND BREAKS/X-LINKS, HUMAN CELLS IN VITRO | + 0 | 2.7000 | FORNACE, 1982 |
| D | DIH | STRAND BREAKS/X-LINKS, HUMAN CELLS IN VITRO | + 0 | 1.3000 | FORNACE ET AL., 1981 |
| D | UHF | UDS, HUMAN FIBROBLASTS IN VITRO | + 0 | 0.0500 | WHITING ET AL., 1979 |
| S | SHF | SCE, HUMAN FIBROBLASTS IN VITRO | + 0 | 0.0050 | MACRAE ET AL., 1979 |
| S | SHL | SCE, HUMAN LYMPHOCYTES IN VITRO | + 0 | 2.0000 | DOUGLAS ET AL., 1980 |
| C | CHF | CHROM ABERR, HUMAN FIBROBLASTS IN VITRO | + 0 | 0.0400 | MACRAE ET AL., 1979 |
| C | CHL | CHROM ABERR, HUMAN LYMPHOCYTES IN VITRO | + 0 | 2.0000 | NAKAMURO ET AL., 1978 |
| C | CHL | CHROM ABERR, HUMAN LYMPHOCYTES IN VITRO | + 0 | 1.0000 | DOUGLAS ET AL., 1980 |
| S | SVA | SCE, ANIMALS IN VIVO | + 0 | 2.7000 | KATHS, 1981 |
| M | MVM | MICRONUCLEUS TEST, MICE IN VIVO | + 0 | 6.5000 | WILD, 1978 |

POTASSIUM CHROMATE

| END POINT | TEST CODE | TEST SYSTEM | RESULTS NM M | DOSE[1] (LED OR HID) | REFERENCE |
|---|---|---|---|---|---|
| M | MVM | MICRONUCLEUS TEST, MICE IN VIVO | + 0 | 50.0000 | HAYASHI ET AL., 1982 |
| M | MVM | MICRONUCLEUS TEST, MICE IN VIVO | + 0 | 8.0000 | COLLABORATIVE STUDY GROUP, 1986 |
| M | MVM | MICRONUCLEUS TEST, MICE IN VIVO | + 0 | 8.0000 | COLLABORATIVE STUDY GROUP, 1988 |
| M | MVC | MICRONUCLEUS TEST, HAMSTERS IN VIVO | + 0 | 10.0000 | KATHS, 1981 |

[1]Doses are given as concentrations of the element, not the concentration of the compound.

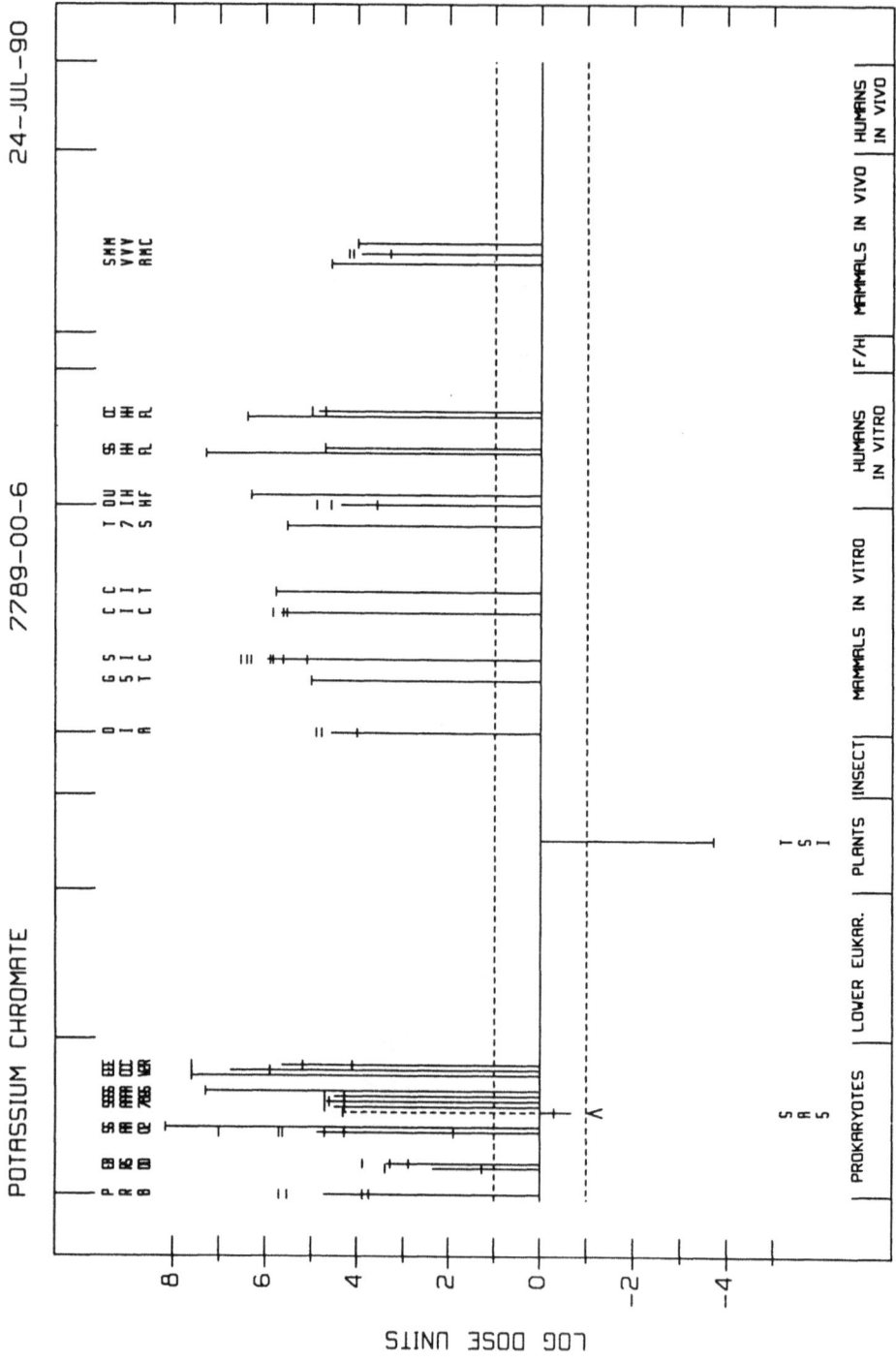

SODIUM CHROMATE

| END POINT | TEST CODE | TEST SYSTEM | RESULTS NM M | DOSE[1] (LED OR HID) | REFERENCE |
|---|---|---|---|---|---|
| D | BSD | B. SUBTILIS REC, DIFFERENTIAL TOXICITY | + 0 | 130.0000 | GENTILE ET AL., 1981 |
| D | BRD | BACTERIA (OTHER), DIFFERENTIAL TOXICITY | + 0 | 130.0000 | GENTILE ET AL., 1981 |
| G | SAO | S. TYPHIMURIUM TA100, REVERSE MUTATION | + + | 6.0000 | LOPRIENO ET AL., 1985 |
| G | ECW | E. COLI WP2 UVRA, REVERSE MUTATION | + 0 | 250:0000 | VENITT & LEVY, 1974 |
| G | EC2 | E. COLI WP2, REVERSE MUTATION | + 0 | 0.0025 | VENITT & LEVY, 1974 |
| G | ECR | E. COLI (OTHER), REVERSE MUTATION | + 0 | 26.0000 | MOHN & ELLENBERGER, 1977 |
| D | DIA | STRAND BREAKS/X-LINKS, ANIMAL CELLS IN VITRO | + 0 | 2.6000 | SUGIYAMA ET AL., 1987 |
| D | DIA | STRAND BREAKS/X-LINKS, ANIMAL CELLS IN VITRO | + 0 | 2.6000 | SUGIYAMA ET AL., 1988 |
| G | GIA | MUTATION, OTHER ANIMAL CELLS IN VITRO | + 0 | 0.0160 | BIGGART & MURPHY, 1988 |
| S | SIC | SCE, CHINESE HAMSTER CELLS IN VITRO | + 0 | 0.2500 | LEVIS & MAJONE, 1979 |
| S | SIC | SCE, CHINESE HAMSTER CELLS IN VITRO | + 0 | 0.0000 | BIANCHI ET AL., 1980 |
| S | SIC | SCE, CHINESE HAMSTER CELLS IN VITRO | + 0 | 0.0300 | ELIAS ET AL., 1983 |
| C | CIC | CHROM ABERR, CHINESE HAMSTER CELLS IN VITRO | + 0 | 0.2500 | LEVIS & MAJONE, 1979 |
| C | CIC | CHROM ABERR, CHINESE HAMSTER CELLS IN VITRO | + 0 | 0.0000 | BIANCHI ET AL., 1980 |
| T | TCS | CELL TRANSFORMATION, SHE, CLONAL ASSAY | + 0 | 0.1000 | DIPAOLO & CASTO, 1979 |
| A | AIH | ANEUPLOIDY, HUMAN CELLS IN VITRO | + 0 | 0.5000 | NIJS & KIRSCH-VOLDERS, 1986 |

[1]Doses are given as concentrations of the element, not the concentration of the compound.

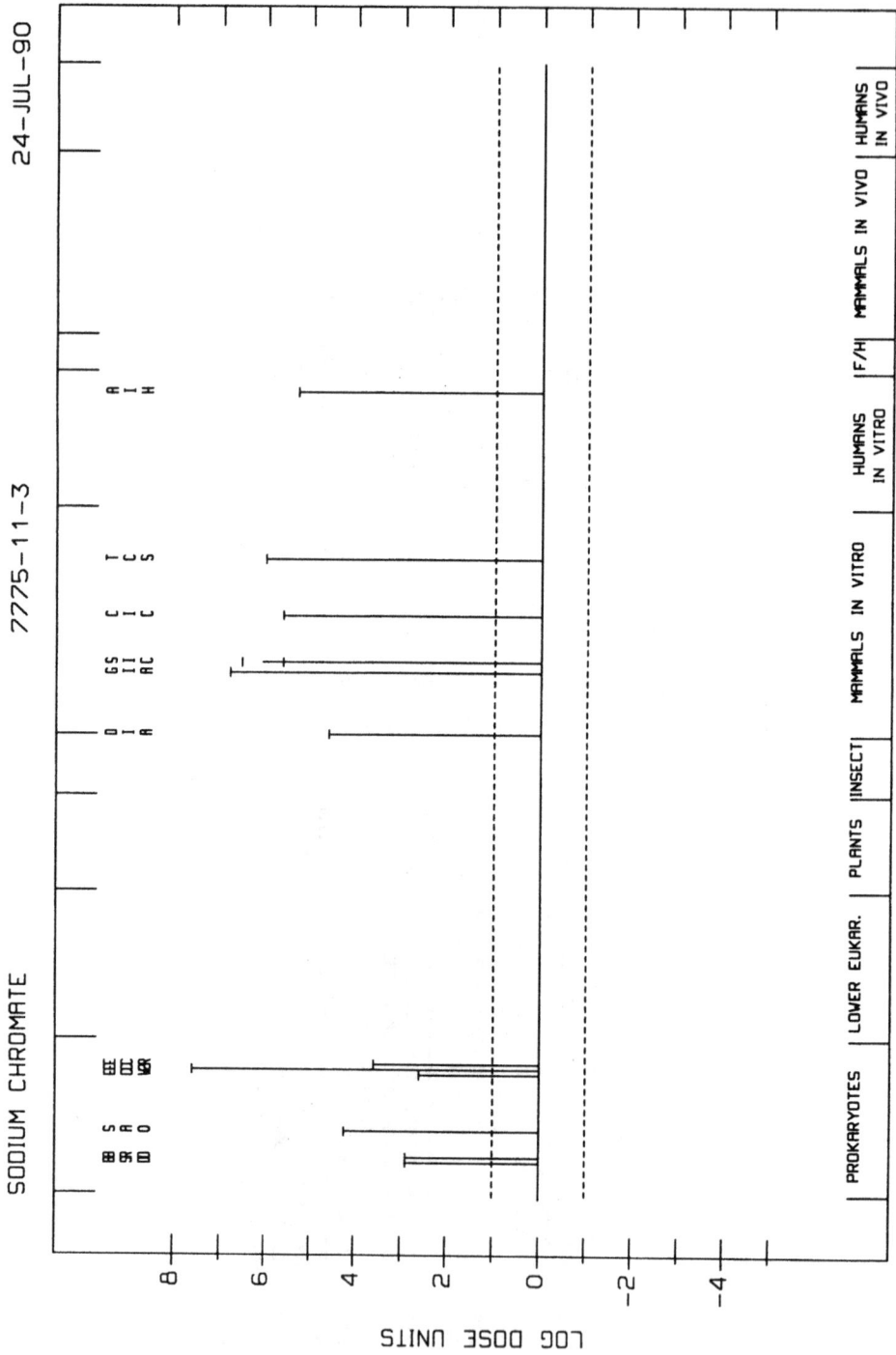

AMMONIUM CHROMATE

| END POINT | TEST CODE | TEST SYSTEM | RESULTS NM M | | DOSE[1] (LED OR HID) | REFERENCE |
|---|---|---|---|---|---|---|
| D | ERD | E. COLI REC, DIFFERENTIAL TOXICITY | + | + | 38.0000 | DE FLORA ET AL., 1984a |
| G | SA0 | S. TYPHIMURIUM TA100, REVERSE MUTATION | + | 0 | 0.0150 | DE FLORA, 1981a |
| G | SA0 | S. TYPHIMURIUM TA100, REVERSE MUTATION | + | (+) | 6.0000 | DE FLORA ET AL., 1987c |
| G | SA5 | S. TYPHIMURIUM TA1535, REVERSE MUTATION | – | 0 | 0:0150 | DE FLORA, 1981a |
| G | SA7 | S. TYPHIMURIUM TA1537, REVERSE MUTATION | (+) | 0 | 0.0150 | DE FLORA, 1981a |
| G | SA8 | S. TYPHIMURIUM TA1538, REVERSE MUTATION | (+) | 0 | 0.0150 | DE FLORA, 1981a |
| G | SA9 | S. TYPHIMURIUM TA98, REVERSE MUTATION | (+) | 0 | 0.0150 | DE FLORA, 1981a |
| G | SAS | S. TYPHIMURIUM (OTHER), REVERSE MUTATION | + | 0 | 0.0000 | DE FLORA ET AL., 1984a |

[1]Doses are given as concentrations of the element, not the concentration of the compound.

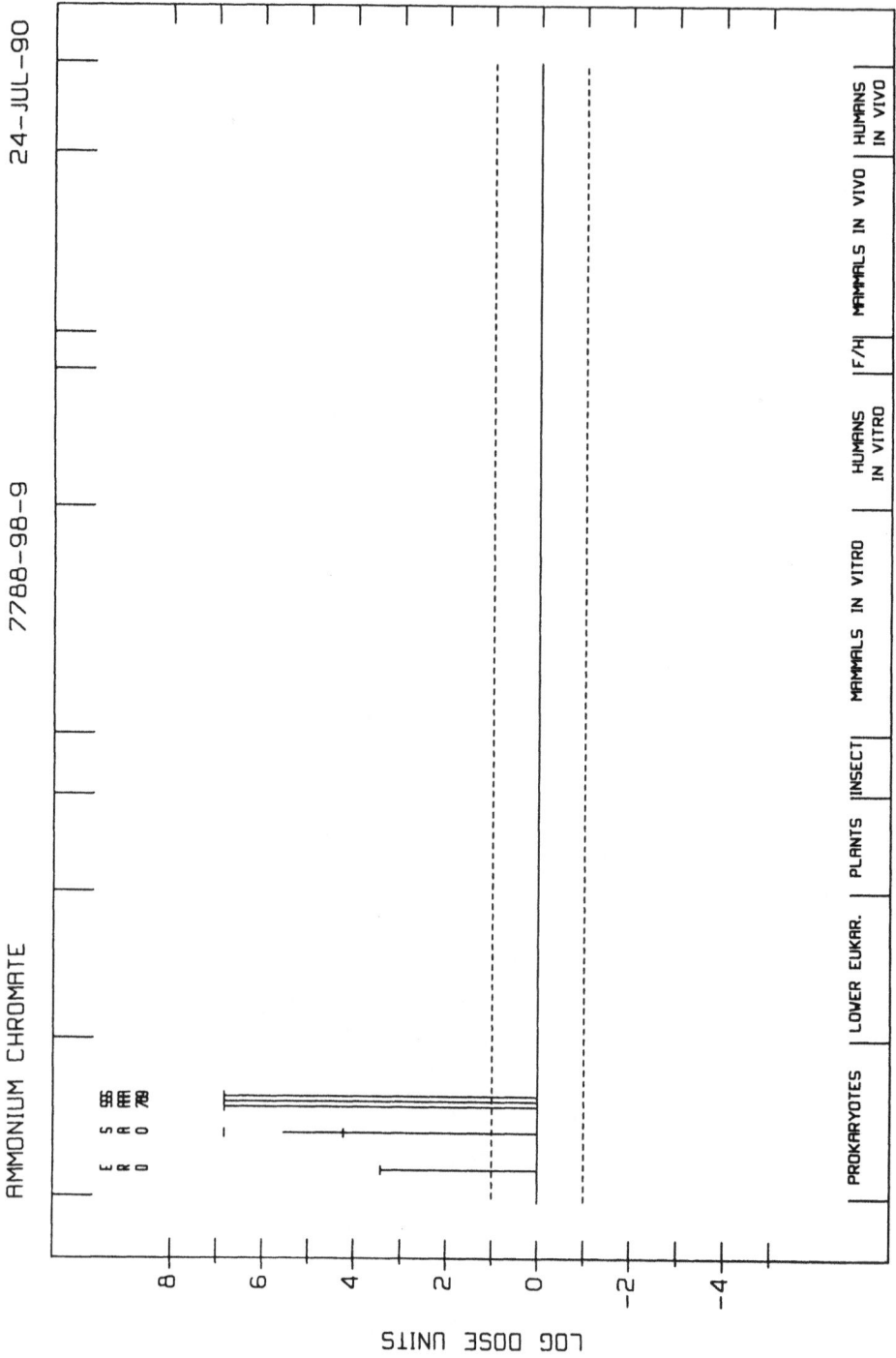

AMMONIUM CHROMATE                    7788-98-9                    24-JUL-90

CHROMIUM TRIOXIDE

| END POINT | TEST CODE | TEST SYSTEM | RESULTS NM | M | DOSE[1] (LED OR HID) | REFERENCE |
|---|---|---|---|---|---|---|
| D | PRB | PROPHAGE, INDUCT/SOS/STRAND BREAKS/X-LINKS | + | 0 | 26.0000 | LLAGOSTERA ET AL., 1986 |
| D | ERD | E. COLI REC, DIFFERENTIAL TOXICITY | + | + | 50.0000 | DE FLORA ET AL., 1984a |
| D | BSD | B. SUBTILIS REC, DIFFERENTIAL TOXICITY | + | 0 | 83.0000 | NAKAMURO ET AL., 1978 |
| D | BSD | B. SUBTILIS REC, DIFFERENTIAL TOXICITY | + | 0 | 26.0000 | KADA ET AL., 1980 |
| D | BSD | B. SUBTILIS REC, DIFFERENTIAL TOXICITY | + | 0 | 130.0000 | GENTILE ET AL., 1981 |
| D | BRD | BACTERIA (OTHER), DIFFERENTIAL TOXICITY | + | 0 | 130.0000 | GENTILE ET AL., 1981 |
| G | SAF | S. TYPHIMURIUM, FORWARD MUTATION | + | + | 0.0200 | RUIZ-RUBIO ET AL., 1985 |
| G | SA0 | S. TYPHIMURIUM TA100, REVERSE MUTATION | + | (+) | 3.2500 | PETRILLI & DE FLORA, 1977 |
| G | SA0 | S. TYPHIMURIUM TA100, REVERSE MUTATION | + | 0 | 3.9000 | NESTMANN ET AL., 1979 |
| G | SA0 | S. TYPHIMURIUM TA100, REVERSE MUTATION | + | 0 | 0.0100 | DE FLORA, 1981a |
| G | SA0 | S. TYPHIMURIUM TA100, REVERSE MUTATION | + | 0 | 52.0000 | TSO & FUNG, 1981 |
| G | SA0 | S. TYPHIMURIUM TA100, REVERSE MUTATION | + | (+) | 5.2000 | DE FLORA ET AL., 1987c |
| G | SA2 | S. TYPHIMURIUM TA102, REVERSE MUTATION | + | 0 | 2.6000 | BENNICELLI ET AL., 1983 |
| G | SA2 | S. TYPHIMURIUM TA102, REVERSE MUTATION | + | 0 | 2.5000 | PETRILLI ET AL., 1985 |
| G | SA5 | S. TYPHIMURIUM TA1535, REVERSE MUTATION | - | 0 | 0.0100 | DE FLORA, 1981a |
| G | SA5 | S. TYPHIMURIUM TA1535, REVERSE MUTATION | - | - | 52.0000 | PETRILLI & DE FLORA, 1977 |
| G | SA7 | S. TYPHIMURIUM TA1537, REVERSE MUTATION | - | + | 13.0000 | PETRILLI & DE FLORA, 1977 |
| G | SA7 | S. TYPHIMURIUM TA1537, REVERSE MUTATION | (+) | 0 | 0.0100 | DE FLORA, 1981a |
| G | SA8 | S. TYPHIMURIUM TA1538, REVERSE MUTATION | (+) | 0 | 0.0100 | DE FLORA, 1981a |
| G | SA9 | S. TYPHIMURIUM TA98, REVERSE MUTATION | + | + | 3.2500 | PETRILLI & DE FLORA, 1977 |
| G | SA9 | S. TYPHIMURIUM TA98, REVERSE MUTATION | (+) | + | 3.9000 | NESTMANN ET AL., 1979 |
| G | SA9 | S. TYPHIMURIUM TA98, REVERSE MUTATION | (+) | 0 | 0.0100 | DE FLORA, 1981a |
| G | SAS | S. TYPHIMURIUM (OTHER), REVERSE MUTATION | + | 0 | 0.0000 | DE FLORA ET AL., 1984a |
| G | ECW | E. COLI WP2 UVRA, REVERSE MUTATION | + | 0 | 0.2500 | NESTMANN ET AL., 1979 |
| G | EC2 | E. COLI WP2, REVERSE MUTATION | - | 0 | 0.0000 | KANEMATSU ET AL., 1980 |
| R | SCG | S. CEREVISIAE, GENE CONVERSION | - | 0 | 52.0000 | FUKUNAGA ET AL., 1982 |
| G | SCR | S. CEREVISIAE, REVERSE MUTATION | - | 0 | 52.0000 | FUKUNAGA ET AL., 1982 |
| M | TSI | TRADESCANTIA SPECIES, MICRONUCLEI | - | 0 | 26.0000 | MA ET AL., 1984 |
| M | TSI | TRADESCANTIA SPECIES, MICRONUCLEI | + | 0 | 5.0000 | ZHANG ET AL., 1984 |
| G | DMX | D. MELANOGASTER, SEX-LINKED RECESSIVES | + | 0 | 52.0000 | RODRIGUEZ-ARNAIZ & MOLINA-MARTINEZ, 1986 |
| A | DMN | D. MELANOGASTER, ANEUPLOIDY | - | 0 | 156.0000 | RODRIGUEZ-ARNAIZ & MOLINA-MARTINEZ, 1986 |
| D | DIA | STRAND BREAKS/X-LINKS, ANIMAL CELLS IN VITRO | + | 0 | 52.0000 | WEDRYCHOWSKI ET AL., 1986a |
| S | SIC | SCE, CHINESE HAMSTER CELLS IN VITRO | + | 0 | 0.1000 | LEVIS & MAJONE, 1979 |
| S | SIC | SCE, CHINESE HAMSTER CELLS IN VITRO | + | 0 | 0.0400 | KOSHI, 1979 |
| S | SIC | SCE, CHINESE HAMSTER CELLS IN VITRO | + | 0 | 0.3200 | OHNO ET AL., 1982 |

CHROMIUM TRIOXIDE

| END POINT | TEST CODE | TEST SYSTEM | RESULTS NM M | DOSE[1] (LED OR HID) | REFERENCE |
|---|---|---|---|---|---|
| S | SIC | SCE, CHINESE HAMSTER CELLS IN VITRO | + 0 | 0.0000 | BIANCHI ET AL., 1980 |
| C | CIC | CHROM ABERR, CHINESE HAMSTER CELLS IN VITRO | + 0 | 0.1000 | LEVIS & MAJONE, 1979 |
| C | CIC | CHROM ABERR, CHINESE HAMSTER CELLS IN VITRO | + 0 | 0.1000 | KOSHI, 1979 |
| C | CIC | CHROM ABERR, CHINESE HAMSTER CELLS IN VITRO | + 0 | 0.0000 | BIANCHI ET AL., 1980 |
| C | CIS | CHROM ABERR, SYRIAN HAMSTER CELLS IN VITRO | + 0 | 0.0400 | TSUDA & KATO, 1977 |
| C | CIT | CHROM ABERR, TRANSFORMED CELLS IN VITRO | + 0 | 0.0500 | UMEDA & NISHIMURA, 1979 |
| S | SHL | SCE, HUMAN LYMPHOCYTES IN VITRO | + 0 | 0.0170 | GOMEZ-ARROYO ET AL., 1981 |
| C | CIH | CHROM ABERR, OTHER HUMAN CELLS IN VITRO | + 0 | 1.0000 | KANEKO, 1976 |

[1]Doses are given as concentrations of the element, not the concentration of the compound.

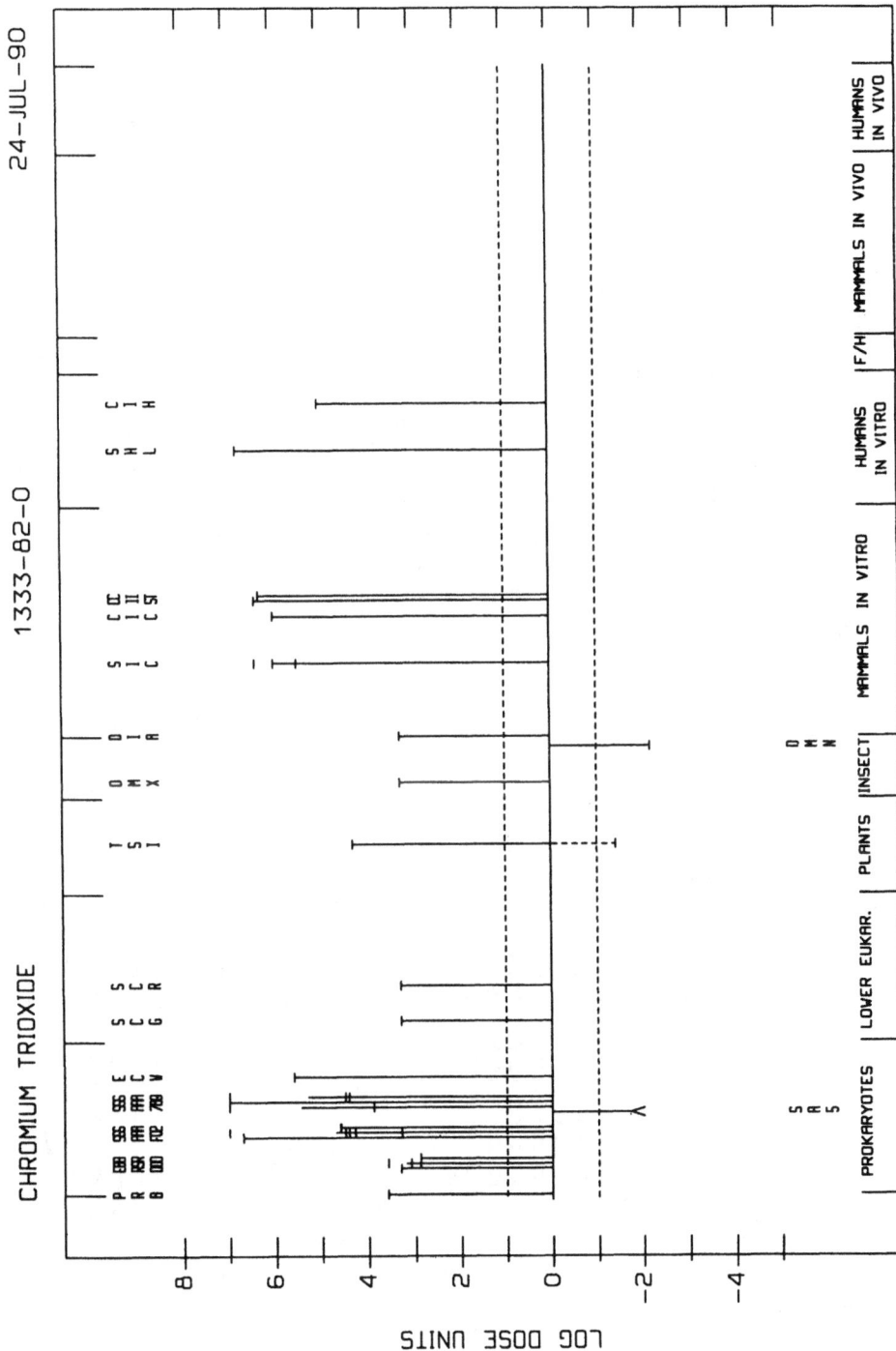

CALCIUM CHROMATE

| END POINT | TEST CODE | TEST SYSTEM | RESULTS NM | RESULTS M | DOSE[1] (LED OR HID) | REFERENCE |
|---|---|---|---|---|---|---|
| D | PRB | PROPHAGE, INDUCT/SOS/STRAND BREAKS/X-LINKS | − | − | 32.0000 | BRAMS ET AL., 1987 |
| D | ERD | E. COLI REC, DIFFERENTIAL TOXICITY | + | + | 83.0000 | DE FLORA ET AL., 1984a |
| G | SA0 | S. TYPHIMURIUM TA100, REVERSE MUTATION | + | (+) | 6.0000 | HAWORTH ET AL., 1983 |
| G | SA0 | S. TYPHIMURIUM TA100, REVERSE MUTATION | + | + | 8.0000 | PETRILLI & DE FLORA, 1977 |
| G | SA0 | S. TYPHIMURIUM TA100, REVERSE MUTATION | + | 0 | 0.0075 | DE FLORA, 1981a |
| G | SA0 | S. TYPHIMURIUM TA100, REVERSE MUTATION | + | − | 3.3000 | VENIER ET AL., 1985b |
| G | SA0 | S. TYPHIMURIUM TA100, REVERSE MUTATION | + | + | 17.0000 | DUNKEL ET AL., 1984 |
| G | SA0 | S. TYPHIMURIUM TA100, REVERSE MUTATION | + | (+) | 12.0000 | DE FLORA ET AL., 1987c |
| G | SA2 | S. TYPHIMURIUM TA102, REVERSE MUTATION | + | (+) | 3.3000 | BENNICELLI ET AL., 1983 |
| G | SA2 | S. TYPHIMURIUM TA102, REVERSE MUTATION | + | 0 | 8.0000 | PETRILLI ET AL., 1985 |
| G | SA5 | S. TYPHIMURIUM TA1535, REVERSE MUTATION | − | − | 33.0000 | PETRILLI & DE FLORA, 1977 |
| G | SA5 | S. TYPHIMURIUM TA1535, REVERSE MUTATION | − | 0 | 0.0075 | DE FLORA, 1981a |
| G | SA5 | S. TYPHIMURIUM TA1535, REVERSE MUTATION | − | − | 6.0000 | HAWORTH ET AL., 1983 |
| G | SA5 | S. TYPHIMURIUM TA1535, REVERSE MUTATION | − | − | 17.0000 | DUNKEL ET AL., 1984 |
| G | SA7 | S. TYPHIMURIUM TA1537, REVERSE MUTATION | − | − | 6.0000 | HAWORTH ET AL., 1983 |
| G | SA7 | S. TYPHIMURIUM TA1537, REVERSE MUTATION | + | + | 8.0000 | PETRILLI & DE FLORA, 1977 |
| G | SA7 | S. TYPHIMURIUM TA1537, REVERSE MUTATION | (+) | 0 | 0.0075 | DE FLORA, 1981a |
| G | SA7 | S. TYPHIMURIUM TA1537, REVERSE MUTATION | − | − | 17.0000 | DUNKEL ET AL., 1984 |
| G | SA8 | S. TYPHIMURIUM TA1538, REVERSE MUTATION | (+) | 0 | 0.0075 | DE FLORA, 1981a |
| G | SA8 | S. TYPHIMURIUM TA1538, REVERSE MUTATION | − | 0 | 17.0000 | DUNKEL ET AL., 1984 |
| G | SA9 | S. TYPHIMURIUM TA98, REVERSE MUTATION | + | (+) | 3.0000 | HAWORTH ET AL., 1983 |
| G | SA9 | S. TYPHIMURIUM TA98, REVERSE MUTATION | + | + | 8.0000 | PETRILLI & DE FLORA, 1977 |
| G | SA9 | S. TYPHIMURIUM TA98, REVERSE MUTATION | (+) | 0 | 0.0075 | DE FLORA, 1981a |
| G | SA9 | S. TYPHIMURIUM TA98, REVERSE MUTATION | − | ? | 17.0000 | DUNKEL ET AL., 1984 |
| G | SAS | S. TYPHIMURIUM (OTHER), REVERSE MUTATION | + | 0 | 0.0000 | DE FLORA ET AL., 1984a |
| G | ECF | E. COLI (EXCLUDING K12), FORWARD MUTATION | − | 0 | 0.0000 | CORBETT ET AL., 1970 |
| G | ECW | E. COLI WP2 UVRA, REVERSE MUTATION | + | + | 33.0000 | DUNKEL ET AL., 1984 |
| G | EC2 | E. COLI WP2, REVERSE MUTATION | + | 0 | 55.0000 | VENITT & LEVY, 1974 |
| G | SCF | S. CEREVISIAE, FORWARD MUTATION | + | 0 | 0.0025 | EGILSSON ET AL., 1979 |
| C | DMC | D. MELANOGASTER, CHROM ABERR | + | 0 | 50.0000 | ZIMMERING, 1983 |
| A | DMN | D. MELANOGASTER, ANEUPLOIDY | + | 0 | 167.0000 | ZIMMERING, 1983 |
| D | DIA | STRAND BREAKS/X-LINKS, ANIMAL CELLS IN VITRO | + | 0 | 167.0000 | ROBISON ET AL., 1982 |
| D | DIA | STRAND BREAKS/X-LINKS, ANIMAL CELLS IN VITRO | + | 0 | 1.3000 | ROBISON ET AL., 1984 |
| D | DIA | STRAND BREAKS/X-LINKS, ANIMAL CELLS IN VITRO | + | 0 | 5.0000 | CANTONI & COSTA, 1984 |
| D | DIA | STRAND BREAKS/X-LINKS, ANIMAL CELLS IN VITRO | + | 0 | 0.0080 | CHRISTIE ET AL., 1984 |

CALCIUM CHROMATE

| END POINT | TEST CODE | TEST SYSTEM | RESULTS NM | M | DOSE[1] (LED OR HID) | REFERENCE |
|---|---|---|---|---|---|---|
| D | DIA | STRAND BREAKS/X-LINKS, ANIMAL CELLS IN VITRO | + | 0 | 1.0500 | SUGIYAMA ET AL., 1986b |
| D | RIA | OTHER DNA REPAIR, ANIMAL CELLS IN VITRO | + | 0 | 1.0000 | ROBISON ET AL., 1984 |
| G | GCO | MUTATION, CHO CELLS IN VITRO | + | 0 | 3.0000 | PATIERNO ET AL., 1988 |
| G | G5T | MUTATION, L5178Y CELLS, TK LOCUS | + | + | 0.4000 | MCGREGOR ET AL., 1987 |
| G | G5T | MUTATION, L5178Y CELLS, TK LOCUS | + | + | 0.8000 | MYHR & CASPARY, 1988 |
| G | GIA | MUTATION, OTHER ANIMAL CELLS IN VITRO | - | 0 | 6.0000 | PATIERNO ET AL., 1988 |
| S | SIC | SCE, CHINESE HAMSTER CELLS IN VITRO | + | 0 | 0.0520 | SEN & COSTA, 1986 |
| S | SIC | SCE, CHINESE HAMSTER CELLS IN VITRO | + | 0 | 0.0400 | VENIER ET AL., 1985b |
| C | CIC | CHROM ABERR, CHINESE HAMSTER CELLS IN VITRO | + | 0 | 0.5000 | LEVIS & MAJONE, 1979 |
| C | CIC | CHROM ABERR, CHINESE HAMSTER CELLS IN VITRO | + | 0 | 1.3000 | SEN ET AL., 1987 |
| C | CIC | CHROM ABERR, CHINESE HAMSTER CELLS IN VITRO | + | 0 | 0.5000 | KOSHI & IWASAKI, 1983 |
| C | CIM | CHROM ABERR, MOUSE CELLS IN VITRO | + | 0 | 0.2600 | SEN ET AL., 1987 |
| T | TBM | CELL TRANSFORMATION, BALB/C3T3 CELLS | + | 0 | 0.0300 | DUNKEL ET AL., 1981 |
| T | TCM | CELL TRANSFORMATION, C3H10T1/2 CELLS | - | 0 | 2.5000 | PATIERNO ET AL., 1988 |
| T | TCS | CELL TRANSFORMATION, SHE, CLONAL ASSAY | + | 0 | 0.1700 | DUNKEL ET AL., 1981 |
| T | TCL | CELL TRANSFORMATION, OTHER CELL LINES | + | 0 | 0.0800 | FRADKIN ET AL., 1975 |
| T | TCL | CELL TRANSFORMATION, OTHER CELL LINES | + | 0 | 2.2000 | BIANCHI ET AL., 1983 |
| T | TCL | CELL TRANSFORMATION, OTHER CELL LINES | + | 0 | 2.5000 | HANSEN & STERN, 1985 |
| T | TCL | CELL TRANSFORMATION, OTHER CELL LINES | + | 0 | 6.5000 | LANFRANCHI ET AL., 1988 |
| T | TRR | CELL TRANSFORMATION, RLV/FISCHER RAT | + | 0 | 0.0200 | DUNKEL ET AL., 1981 |
| T | TRR | CELL TRANSFORMATION, RLV/FISCHER RAT | + | 0 | 0.0300 | TRAUL ET AL., 1981 |
| T | T7S | CELL TRANSFORMATION, SA7/SHE CELLS | + | 0 | 0.3000 | CASTO ET AL., 1979 |
| D | DIH | STRAND BREAKS/X-LINKS, HUMAN CELLS IN VITRO | + | 0 | 1.0500 | SUGIYAMA ET AL., 1986b |
| S | SHL | SCE, HUMAN LYMPHOCYTES IN VITRO | + | 0 | 0.0030 | GOMEZ-ARROYO ET AL., 1981 |
| A | AIH | ANEUPLOIDY, HUMAN CELLS IN VITRO | + | 0 | 0.5000 | NIJS & KIRSCH-VOLDERS, 1986 |
| S | SVA | SCE, ANIMALS IN VIVO | + | 0 | 3.3000 | KATHS, 1981 |
| M | MVM | MICRONUCLEUS TEST, MICE IN VIVO | - | 0 | 50.0000 | FABRY, 1980 |
| M | MVC | MICRONUCLEUS TEST, HAMSTERS IN VIVO | - | 0 | 13.3000 | KATHS, 1981 |

[1]Doses are given as concentrations of the element, not the concentration of the compound.

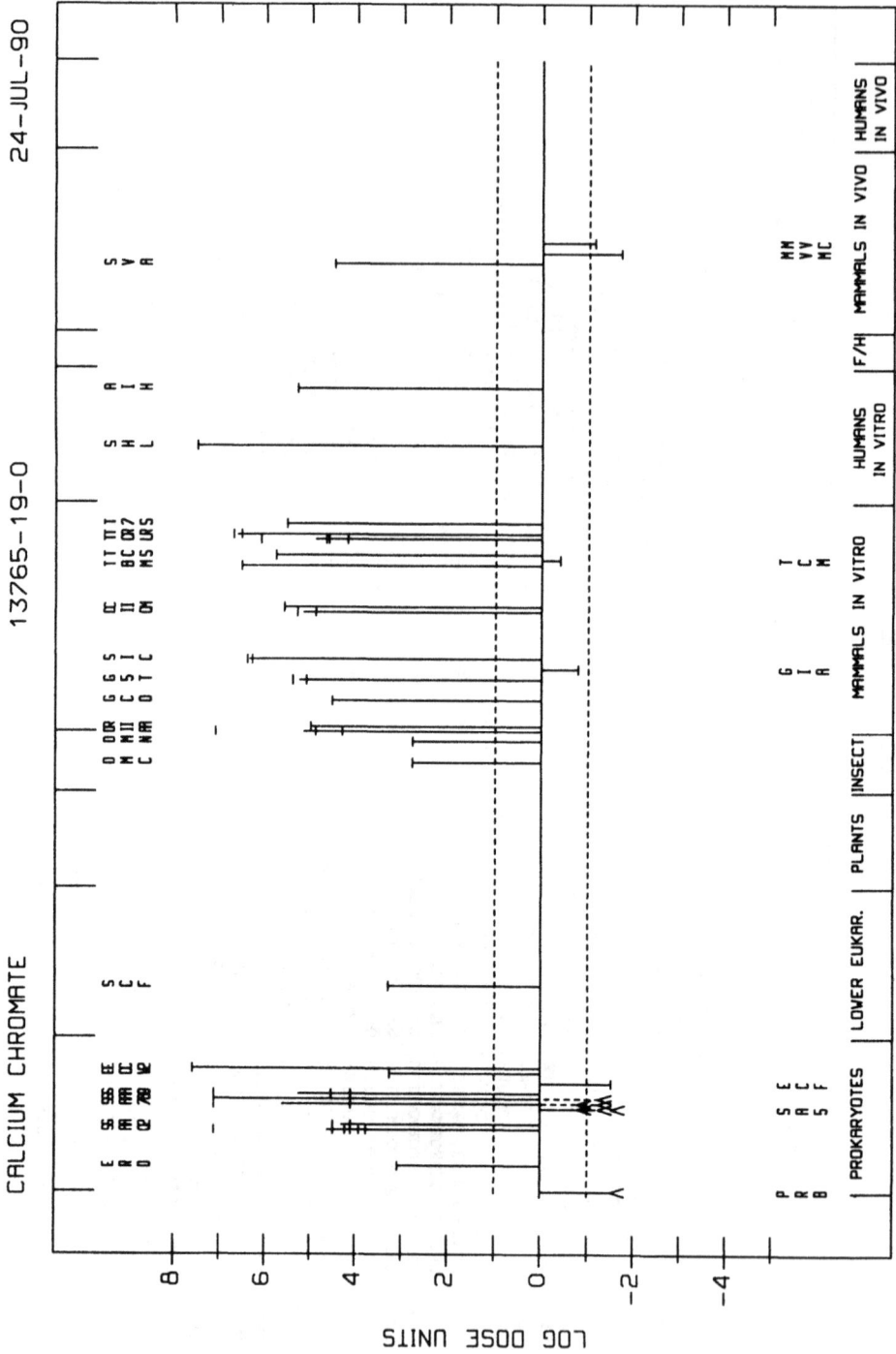

STRONTIUM CHROMATE

| END POINT | TEST CODE | TEST SYSTEM | RESULTS NM M | DOSE[1] (LED OR HID) | REFERENCE |
|---|---|---|---|---|---|
| G | SAO | S. TYPHIMURIUM TA100, REVERSE MUTATION | + − | 2.5000 | VENIER ET AL., 1985b |
| S | SIC | SCE, CHINESE HAMSTER CELLS IN VITRO | + 0 | 0.0250 | VENIER ET AL., 1985b |
| T | TCM | CELL TRANSFORMATION, C3H10T1/2 CELLS | − 0 | 1.0000 | PATIERNO ET AL., 1988 |

[1]Doses are given as concentrations of the element, not the concentration of the compound.

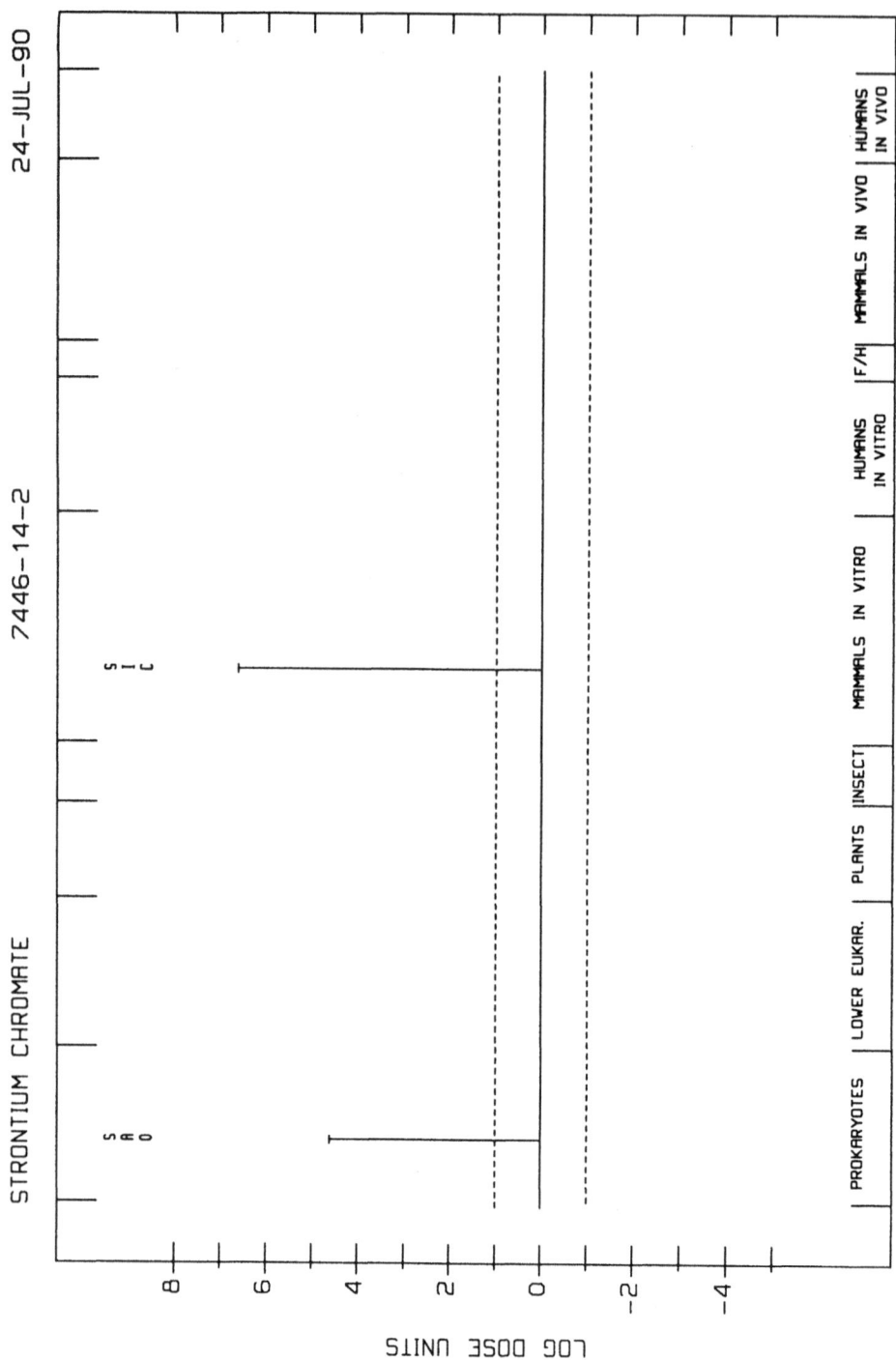

STRONTIUM CHROMATE                    7446-14-2                    24-JUL-90

LOG DOSE UNITS

PROKARYOTES | LOWER EUKAR. | PLANTS | INSECT | MAMMALS IN VITRO | HUMANS IN VITRO | F/H | MAMMALS IN VIVO | HUMANS IN VIVO

ZINC YELLOW

| END POINT | TEST CODE | TEST SYSTEM | RESULTS NM | M | DOSE[1] (LED OR HID) | REFERENCE |
|---|---|---|---|---|---|---|
| G | SA0 | S. TYPHIMURIUM TA100, REVERSE MUTATION | + | — | 0.0000 | PETRILLI & DE FLORA, 1978b |
| G | SA0 | S. TYPHIMURIUM TA100, REVERSE MUTATION | + | 0 | 0.0300 | DE FLORA, 1981a |
| G | SA5 | S. TYPHIMURIUM TA1535, REVERSE MUTATION | — | 0 | 0.0300 | DE FLORA, 1981a |
| G | SA5 | S. TYPHIMURIUM TA1535, REVERSE MUTATION | — | — | 0.0000 | PETRILLI & DE FLORA, 1978b |
| G | SA7 | S. TYPHIMURIUM TA1537, REVERSE MUTATION | (+) | — | 0.0000 | PETRILLI & DE FLORA, 1978b |
| G | SA7 | S. TYPHIMURIUM TA1537, REVERSE MUTATION | + | 0 | 0.0300 | DE FLORA, 1981a |
| G | SA8 | S. TYPHIMURIUM TA1538, REVERSE MUTATION | + | 0 | 0.0300 | DE FLORA, 1981a |
| G | SA9 | S. TYPHIMURIUM TA98, REVERSE MUTATION | (+) | — | 0.0000 | PETRILLI & DE FLORA, 1978b |
| G | SA9 | S. TYPHIMURIUM TA98, REVERSE MUTATION | + | 0 | 0.0300 | DE FLORA, 1981a |
| S | SIC | SCE, CHINESE HAMSTER CELLS IN VITRO | + | 0 | 0.8000 | LEVIS & MAJONE, 1981 |
| S | SIC | SCE, CHINESE HAMSTER CELLS IN VITRO | + | 0 | 0.0200 | VENIER ET AL., 1985b |
| C | CIC | CHROM ABERR, CHINESE HAMSTER CELLS IN VITRO | + | 0 | 0.8000 | LEVIS & MAJONE, 1981 |

[1]Doses are given as concentrations of the element, not the concentration of the compound.

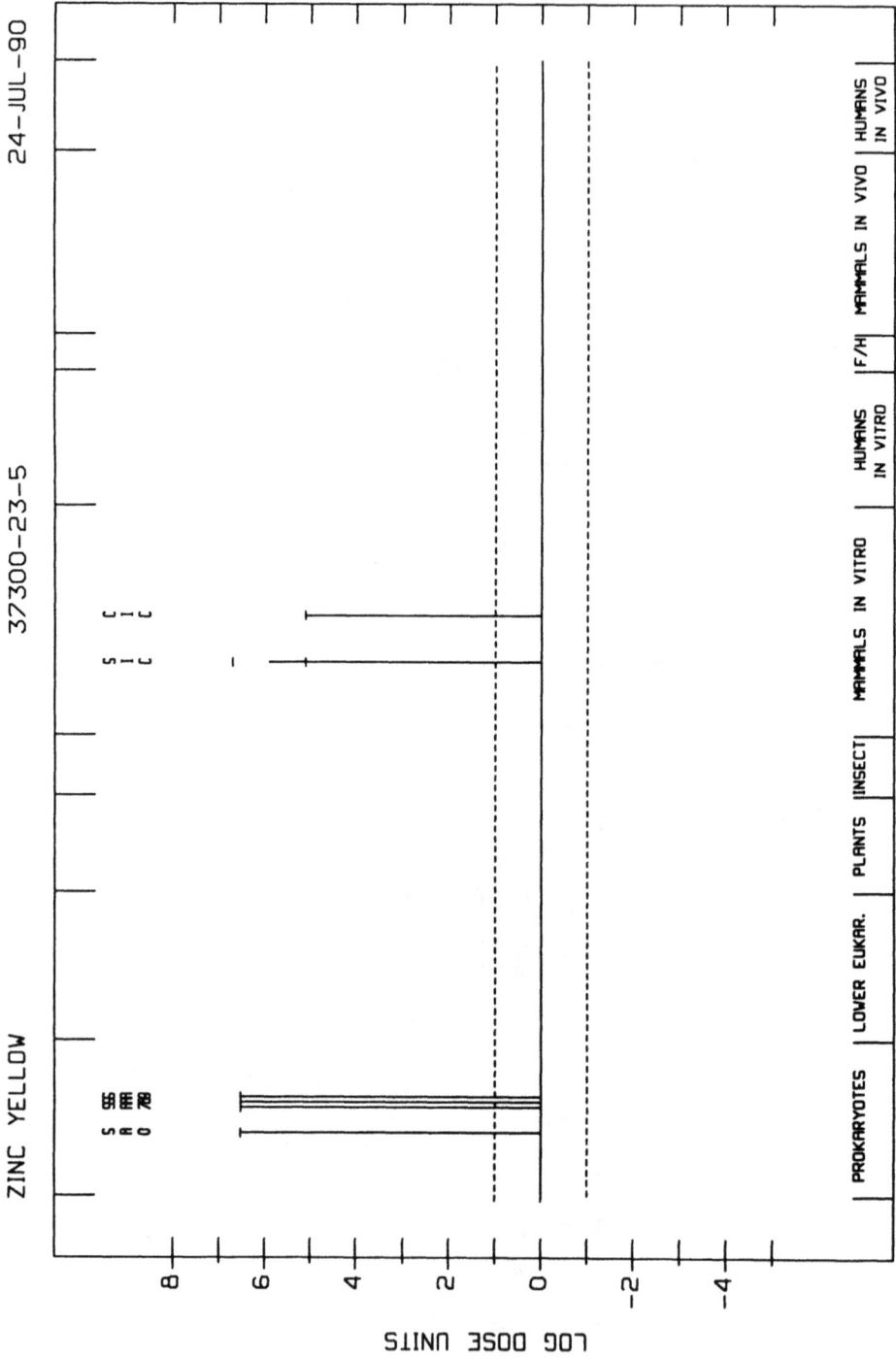

ZINC YELLOW

37300-23-5

24-JUL-90

LOG DOSE UNITS

ZINC CHROMATE

| END POINT | TEST CODE | TEST SYSTEM | RESULTS NM M | DOSE[1] (LED OR HID) | REFERENCE |
|---|---|---|---|---|---|
| G | SA0 | S. TYPHIMURIUM TA100, REVERSE MUTATION | + (+) | 3.0000 | VENIER ET AL., 1985b |
| G | G9H | MUTATION, CHL V79 CELLS, HPRT | + 0 | 1.1500 | NEWBOLD ET AL., 1979 |
| S | SIC | SCE, CHINESE HAMSTER CELLS IN VITRO | + 0 | 0.0300 | VENIER ET AL., 1985b |
| C | CIC | CHROM ABERR, CHINESE HAMSTER CELLS IN VITRO | + 0 | 0.3000 | KOSHI & IWASAKI, 1983 |
| T | TCL | CELL TRANSFORMATION, OTHER CELL LINES | + 0 | 3.1000 | HANSEN & STERN, 1985 |
| T | T7S | CELL TRANSFORMATION, SA7/SHE CELLS | + 0 | 0.1300 | CASTO ET AL., 1979 |

[1]Doses are given as concentrations of the element, not the concentration of the compound.

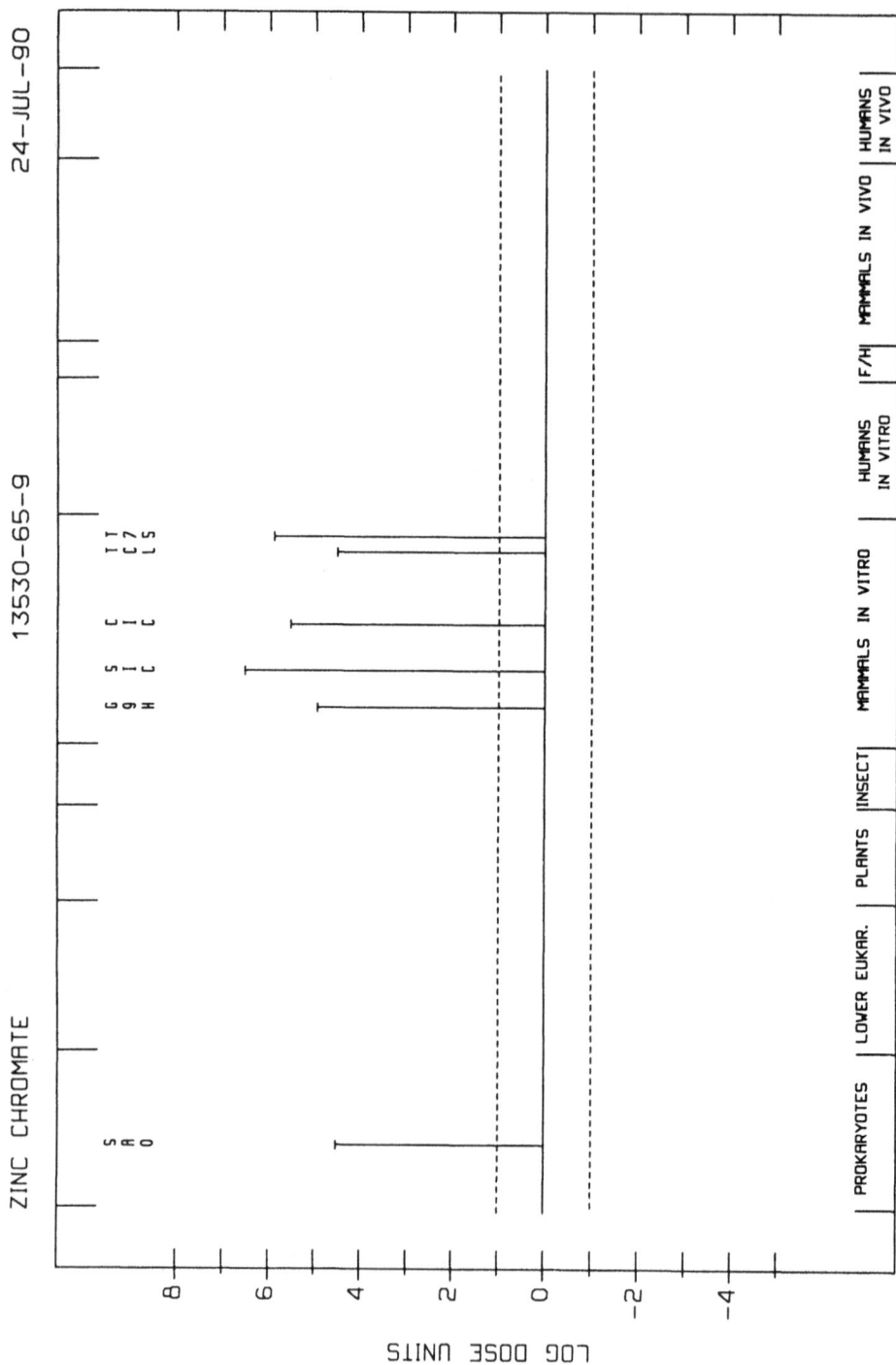

ZINC CHROMATE

13530-65-9

24-JUL-90

CHROMIUM ORANGE

| END POINT | TEST CODE | TEST SYSTEM | RESULTS NM | M | DOSE[1] (LED OR HID) | REFERENCE |
|---|---|---|---|---|---|---|
| G | SA0 | S. TYPHIMURIUM TA100, REVERSE MUTATION | + | - | 0.0000 | PETRILLI & DE FLORA, 1978b |
| G | SA0 | S. TYPHIMURIUM TA100, REVERSE MUTATION | + | 0 | 190.0000 | DE FLORA, 1981a |
| G | SA0 | S. TYPHIMURIUM TA100, REVERSE MUTATION[2] | + | 0 | 0.0000 | DE FLORA, 1981a |
| G | SA0 | S. TYPHIMURIUM TA100, REVERSE MUTATION[2] | - | - | 7.6000 | VENIER ET AL., 1985b |
| G | SA0 | S. TYPHIMURIUM TA100, REVERSE MUTATION[2] | + | - | 0.9500 | VENIER ET AL., 1985b |
| G | SA0 | S. TYPHIMURIUM TA100, REVERSE MUTATION | - | - | 38.0000 | LOPRIENO ET AL., 1985 |
| G | SA5 | S. TYPHIMURIUM TA1535, REVERSE MUTATION | - | - | 38.0000 | LOPRIENO ET AL., 1985 |
| G | SA5 | S. TYPHIMURIUM TA1535, REVERSE MUTATION | - | 0 | 190.0000 | DE FLORA, 1981a |
| G | SA5 | S. TYPHIMURIUM TA1535, REVERSE MUTATION[2] | + | 0 | 0.0000 | DE FLORA, 1981a |
| G | SA7 | S. TYPHIMURIUM TA1537, REVERSE MUTATION | - | - | 38.0000 | LOPRIENO ET AL., 1985 |
| G | SA7 | S. TYPHIMURIUM TA1537, REVERSE MUTATION | - | 0 | 190.0000 | DE FLORA, 1981a |
| G | SA7 | S. TYPHIMURIUM TA1537, REVERSE MUTATION[2] | + | 0 | 0.0000 | DE FLORA, 1981a |
| G | SA8 | S. TYPHIMURIUM TA1538, REVERSE MUTATION[2] | - | - | 38.0000 | LOPRIENO ET AL., 1985 |
| G | SA8 | S. TYPHIMURIUM TA1538, REVERSE MUTATION | - | 0 | 190.0000 | DE FLORA, 1981a |
| G | SA8 | S. TYPHIMURIUM TA1538, REVERSE MUTATION[2] | + | 0 | 0.0000 | DE FLORA, 1981a |
| G | SA9 | S. TYPHIMURIUM TA98, REVERSE MUTATION | - | - | 38.0000 | LOPRIENO ET AL., 1985 |
| G | SA9 | S. TYPHIMURIUM TA98, REVERSE MUTATION | - | 0 | 190.0000 | DE FLORA, 1981a |
| G | SA9 | S. TYPHIMURIUM TA98, REVERSE MUTATION[2] | + | 0 | 0.0000 | DE FLORA, 1981a |
| S | SIC | SCE, CHINESE HAMSTER CELLS IN VITRO | + | 0 | 0.5000 | LEVIS & MAJONE, 1981 |
| S | SIC | SCE, CHINESE HAMSTER CELLS IN VITRO[2] | + | 0 | 0.1000 | LEVIS & MAJONE, 1981 |
| S | SIC | SCE, CHINESE HAMSTER CELLS IN VITRO | + | 0 | 0.1000 | LOPRIENO ET AL., 1985 |
| C | CIC | CHROM ABERR, CHINESE HAMSTER CELLS IN VITRO | + | 0 | 0.5000 | LEVIS & MAJONE, 1981 |
| C | CIC | CHROM ABERR, CHINESE HAMSTER CELLS IN VITRO[2] | + | 0 | 0.1000 | LEVIS & MAJONE, 1981 |

[1]Doses are given as concentrations of the element, not the concentration of the compound.
[2]Dissolved in NaOH

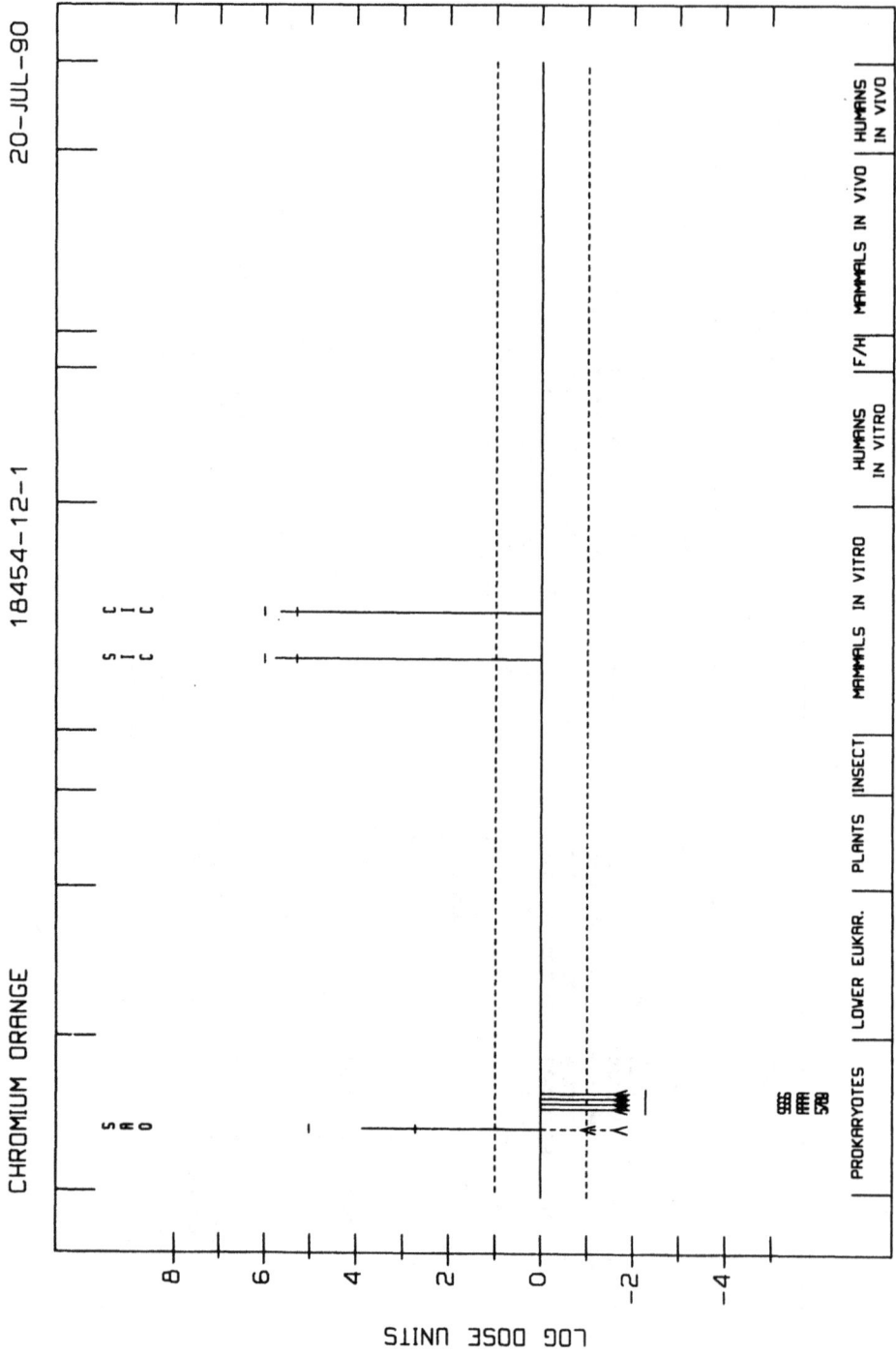

CHROMIUM ORANGE                18454-12-1                20-JUL-90

LOG DOSE UNITS

MOLYBDENUM ORANGE

| END POINT | TEST CODE | TEST SYSTEM | RESULTS NM | M | DOSE¹ (LED OR HID) | REFERENCE |
|---|---|---|---|---|---|---|
| G | SA0 | S. TYPHIMURIUM TA100, REVERSE MUTATION | + | 0 | 90.0000 | DE FLORA, 1981a |
| G | SA0 | S. TYPHIMURIUM TA100, REVERSE MUTATION[2] | + | 0 | 0.0000 | DE FLORA, 1981a |
| G | SA5 | S. TYPHIMURIUM TA1535, REVERSE MUTATION | - | 0 | 90.0000 | DE FLORA, 1981a |
| G | SA5 | S. TYPHIMURIUM TA1535, REVERSE MUTATION[2] | + | 0 | 0.0000 | DE FLORA, 1981a |
| G | SA7 | S. TYPHIMURIUM TA1537, REVERSE MUTATION | + | 0 | 90.0000 | DE FLORA, 1981a |
| G | SA7 | S. TYPHIMURIUM TA1537, REVERSE MUTATION[2] | - | 0 | 0.0000 | DE FLORA, 1981a |
| G | SA8 | S. TYPHIMURIUM TA1538, REVERSE MUTATION | + | 0 | 90.0000 | DE FLORA, 1981a |
| G | SA8 | S. TYPHIMURIUM TA1538, REVERSE MUTATION[2] | - | 0 | 0.0000 | DE FLORA, 1981a |
| G | SA9 | S. TYPHIMURIUM TA98, REVERSE MUTATION | + | 0 | 90.0000 | DE FLORA, 1981a |
| G | SA9 | S. TYPHIMURIUM TA98, REVERSE MUTATION[2] | + | 0 | 0.0000 | DE FLORA, 1981a |
| S | SIC | SCE, CHINESE HAMSTER CELLS IN VITRO | + | 0 | 0.2000 | LEVIS & MAJONE, 1981 |
| S | SIC | SCE, CHINESE HAMSTER CELLS IN VITRO[2] | + | 0 | 0.1000 | LEVIS & MAJONE, 1981 |
| S | SIC | SCE, CHINESE HAMSTER CELLS IN VITRO | + | 0 | 0.0070 | VENIER ET AL., 1985b |
| C | CIC | CHROM ABERR, CHINESE HAMSTER CELLS IN VITRO | + | 0 | 0.2000 | LEVIS & MAJONE, 1981 |
| C | CIC | CHROM ABERR, CHINESE HAMSTER CELLS IN VITRO[2] | + | 0 | 0.1000 | LEVIS & MAJONE, 1981 |

[1]Doses are given as concentrations of the element, not the concentration of the compound.
[2]Dissolved in NaOH

MOLYBDENUM ORANGE                    12709-98-7                    20-JUL-90

LOG DOSE UNITS

BARIUM CHROMATE

| END POINT | TEST CODE | TEST SYSTEM | RESULTS NM M | DOSE[1] (LED OR HID) | REFERENCE |
|---|---|---|---|---|---|
| G | SA0 | S. TYPHIMURIUM TA100, REVERSE MUTATION | – – | 66.0000 | VENIER ET AL., 1985b |
| G | SA0 | S. TYPHIMURIUM TA100, REVERSE MUTATION[2] | – – | 66.0000 | VENIER ET AL., 1985b |
| S | SIC | SCE, CHINESE HAMSTER CELLS IN VITRO | + 0 | 0.0230 | VENIER ET AL., 1985b |

[1]Doses are given as concentrations of the element, not the concentration of the compound.
[2]Dissolved in NaOH

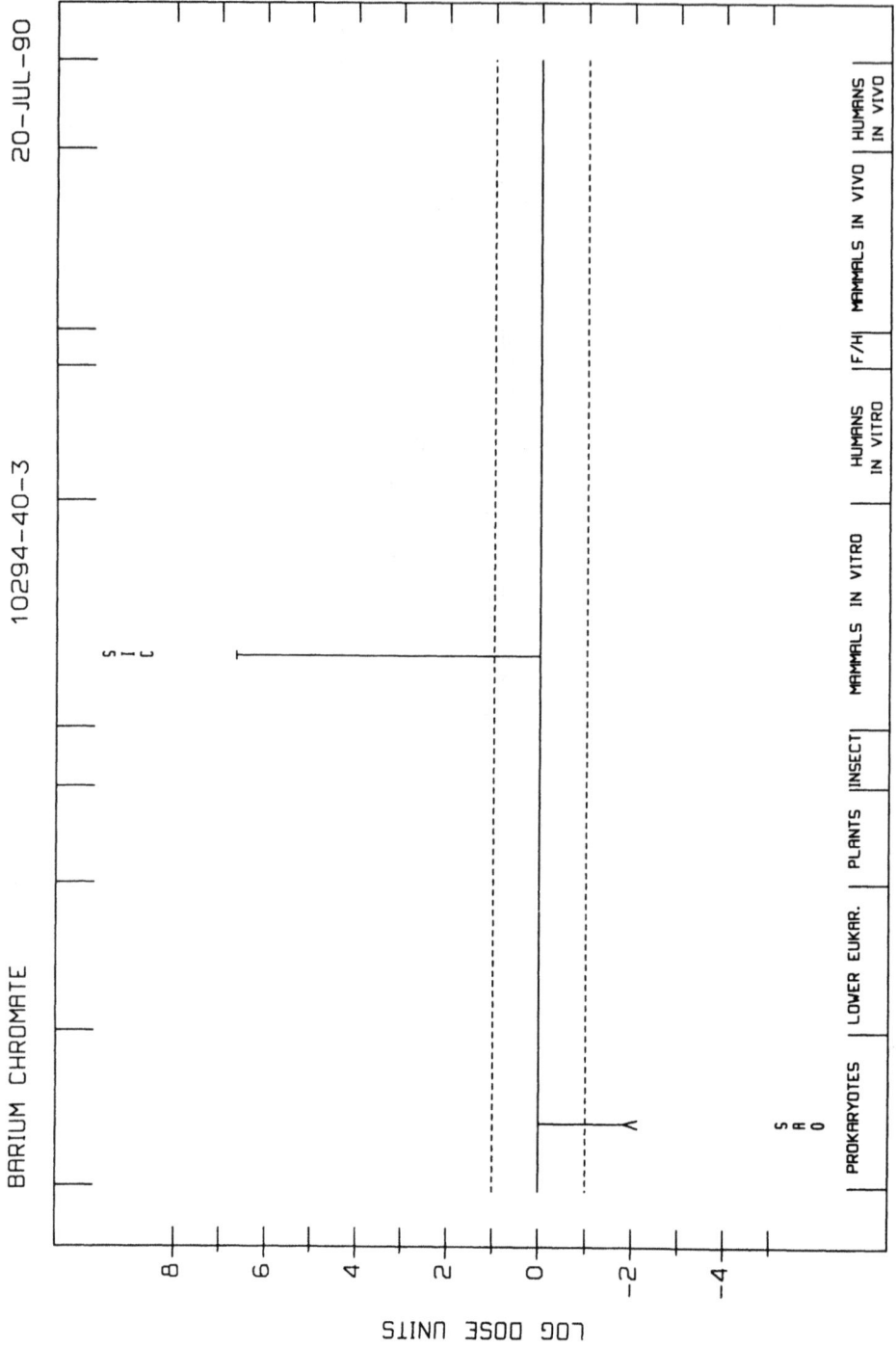

BARIUM CHROMATE

10294-40-3

20-JUL-90

LOG DOSE UNITS

LEAD CHROMATE

| END POINT | TEST CODE | TEST SYSTEM | RESULTS NM | RESULTS M | DOSE[1] (LED OR HID) | REFERENCE |
|---|---|---|---|---|---|---|
| D | PRB | PROPHAGE, INDUCT/SOS/STRAND BREAKS/X-LINKS | – | – | 275.0000 | VENIER ET AL., 1989 |
| D | ECD | E. COLI POL A, DIFFERENTIAL TOX (SPOT)[3] | – | 0 | 25.0000 | NESTMANN ET AL., 1979 |
| D | ECD | E. COLI POL A, DIFFERENTIAL TOX (SPOT) | – | 0 | 8.0000 | VENIER ET AL., 1987 |
| D | ECL | E. COLI POL A, DIFFERENTIAL TOX (LIQUID) | – | 0 | 0.0000 | VENIER ET AL., 1987 |
| G | SA0 | S. TYPHIMURIUM TA100, REVERSE MUTATION[2] | + | 0 | 32.0000 | NESTMANN ET AL., 1979 |
| G | SA0 | S. TYPHIMURIUM TA100, REVERSE MUTATION | – | 0 | 13.0000 | LOPRIENO ET AL., 1985 |
| G | SA0 | S. TYPHIMURIUM TA100, REVERSE MUTATION | – | – | 13.0000 | VENIER ET AL., 1985b |
| G | SA0 | S. TYPHIMURIUM TA100, REVERSE MUTATION[3] | + | + | 1.6000 | VENIER ET AL., 1985b |
| G | SA2 | S. TYPHIMURIUM TA102, REVERSE MUTATION | – | 0 | 1030.0000 | DE FLORA ET AL., 1985a |
| G | SA5 | S. TYPHIMURIUM TA1535, REVERSE MUTATION | – | – | 64.0000 | NESTMANN ET AL., 1979 |
| G | SA7 | S. TYPHIMURIUM TA1537, REVERSE MUTATION[2] | + | + | 32.0000 | NESTMANN ET AL., 1979 |
| G | SA8 | S. TYPHIMURIUM TA1538, REVERSE MUTATION[2] | + | + | 16.0000 | NESTMANN ET AL., 1979 |
| G | SA9 | S. TYPHIMURIUM TA98, REVERSE MUTATION[2] | + | + | 32.0000 | NESTMANN ET AL., 1979 |
| G | ECK | E. COLI K12, FORWARD OR REVERSE MUTATION[3] | + | 0 | 16.0000 | NESTMANN ET AL., 1979 |
| G | ECW | E. COLI WP2 UVRA, REVERSE MUTATION[3] | + | 0 | 0.2500 | NESTMANN ET AL., 1979 |
| R | SCG | S. CEREVISIAE, GENE CONVERSION[2] | + | (+) | 10.0000 | NESTMANN ET AL., 1979 |
| G | DMX | D. MELANOGASTER, SEX-LINKED RECESSIVES | + | 0 | 0.0600 | COSTA ET AL., 1988 |
| G | DMX | D. MELANOGASTER, SEX-LINKED RECESSIVES[3] | (+) | 0 | 0.0600 | COSTA ET AL., 1988 |
| D | DIA | STRAND BREAKS/X-LINKS, ANIMAL CELLS IN VITRO[3] | – | 0 | 5.0000 | DOUGLAS ET AL., 1980 |
| G | GCO | MUTATION, CHO CELLS IN VITRO | – | 0 | 5.0000 | PATIERNO ET AL., 1988 |
| G | G9H | MUTATION, CHL V79 CELLS, HPRT | – | 0 | 1.6000 | NEWBOLD ET AL., 1979 |
| G | G9H | MUTATION, CHL V79 CELLS, HPRT | – | 0 | 5.0000 | CELOTTI ET AL., 1987 |
| G | GIA | MUTATION, OTHER ANIMAL CELLS IN VITRO | – | 0 | 5.0000 | PATIERNO ET AL., 1988 |
| S | SIC | SCE, CHINESE HAMSTER CELLS IN VITRO | + | 0 | 0.0200 | LOPRIENO ET AL., 1985 |
| S | SIC | SCE, CHINESE HAMSTER CELLS IN VITRO | + | 0 | 0.0520 | MONTALDI ET AL., 1987b |
| C | CIC | CHROM ABERR, CHINESE HAMSTER CELLS IN VITRO | + | 0 | 5.2000 | MONTALDI ET AL., 1987b |
| C | CIC | CHROM ABERR, CHINESE HAMSTER CELLS IN VITRO | + | 0 | 0.0800 | KOSHI & IWASAKI, 1983 |
| T | TCM | CELL TRANSFORMATION, C3H10T1/2 CELLS | + | 0 | 1.3000 | PATIERNO ET AL., 1988 |
| T | TCL | CELL TRANSFORMATION, OTHER CELL LINES | + | 0 | 32.0000 | HANSEN & STERN, 1985 |

LEAD CHROMATE

| END POINT | TEST CODE | TEST SYSTEM | RESULTS NM M | DOSE[1] (LED OR HID) | REFERENCE |
|---|---|---|---|---|---|
| T | T7S | CELL TRANSFORMATION, SA7/SHE CELLS | + 0 | 2.0000 | CASTO ET AL., 1979 |
| S | SHL | SCE, HUMAN LYMPHOCYTES IN VITRO[3] | + 0 | 0.0250 | DOUGLAS ET AL., 1980 |
| M | MIH | MICRONUCLEUS TEST, HUMAN CELLS IN VITRO | + 0 | 0.5200 | MONTALDI ET AL., 1987b |
| C | CHL | CHROM ABERR, HUMAN LYMPHOCYTES IN VITRO[3] | + 0 | 0.7000 | DOUGLAS ET AL., 1980 |
| M | MVM | MICRONUCLEUS TEST, MICE IN VIVO | + 0 | 160.8880 | WATANABE ET AL., 1985 |

[1]Doses are given as concentrations of the element, not the concentration of the compound.
[2]Dissolved in HCl
[3]Dissolved in NaOH

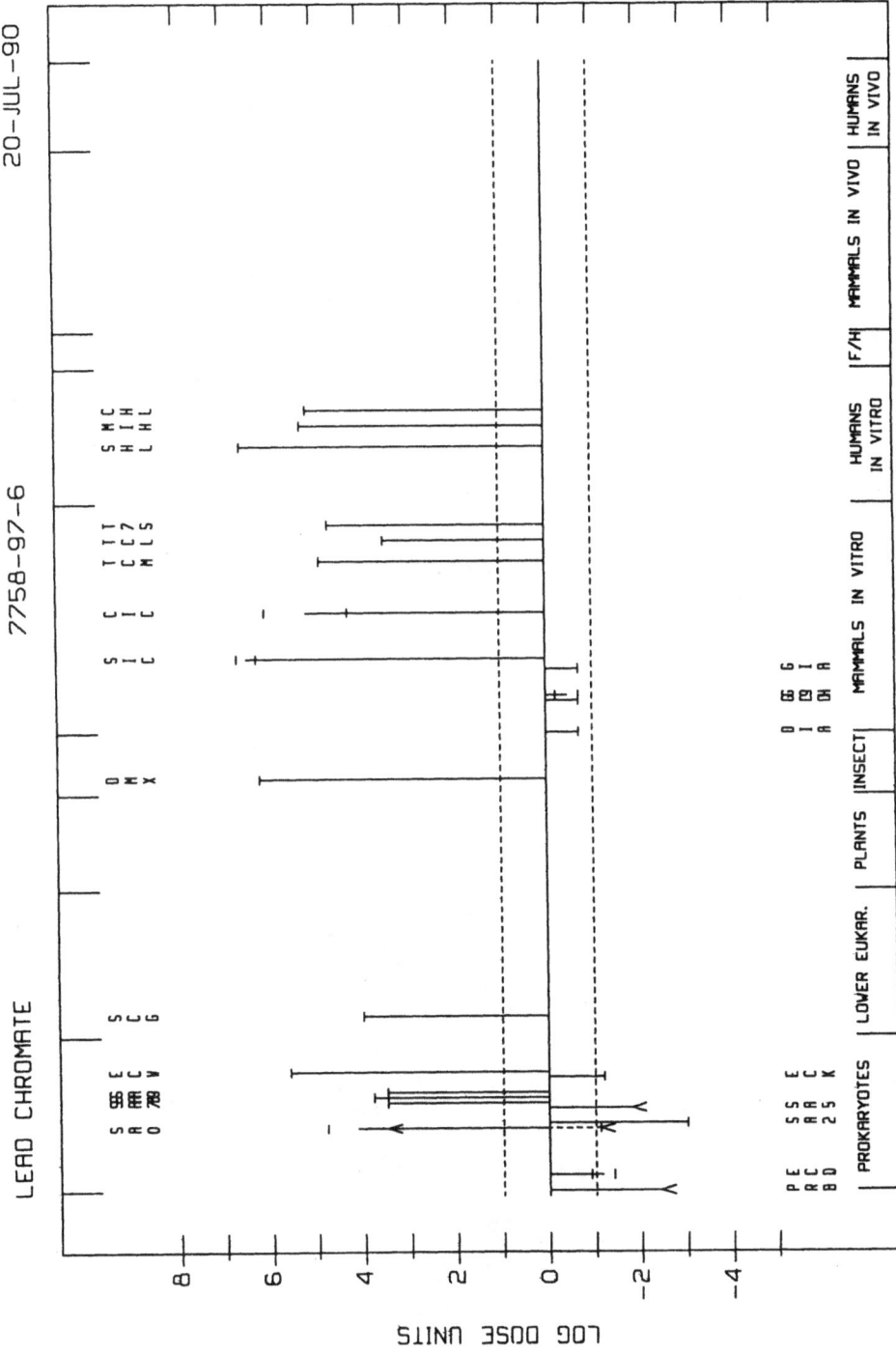

CHROMIUM YELLOW

| END POINT | TEST CODE | TEST SYSTEM | RESULTS NM M | DOSE[1] (LED OR HID) | REFERENCE |
|---|---|---|---|---|---|
| G | SA0 | S. TYPHIMURIUM TA100, REVERSE MUTATION | − 0 | 0.0000 | DE FLORA, 1981a |
| G | SA0 | S. TYPHIMURIUM TA100, REVERSE MUTATION[2] | + 0 | 0.0000 | DE FLORA, 1981a |
| G | SA5 | S. TYPHIMURIUM TA1535, REVERSE MUTATION | − 0 | 0.0000 | DE FLORA, 1981a |
| G | SA5 | S. TYPHIMURIUM TA1535, REVERSE MUTATION[2] | + 0 | 0.0000 | DE FLORA, 1981a |
| G | SA7 | S. TYPHIMURIUM TA1537, REVERSE MUTATION | − 0 | 0.0000 | DE FLORA, 1981a |
| G | SA7 | S. TYPHIMURIUM TA1537, REVERSE MUTATION[2] | + 0 | 0.0000 | DE FLORA, 1981a |
| G | SA8 | S. TYPHIMURIUM TA1538, REVERSE MUTATION | − 0 | 0.0000 | DE FLORA, 1981a |
| G | SA8 | S. TYPHIMURIUM TA1538, REVERSE MUTATION[2] | + 0 | 0.0000 | DE FLORA, 1981a |
| G | SA9 | S. TYPHIMURIUM TA98, REVERSE MUTATION | − 0 | 0.0000 | DE FLORA, 1981a |
| G | SA9 | S. TYPHIMURIUM TA98, REVERSE MUTATION[2] | + 0 | 0.0000 | DE FLORA, 1981a |
| S | SIC | SCE, CHINESE HAMSTER CELLS IN VITRO | + 0 | 0.3000 | LEVIS & MAJONE, 1981 |
| S | SIC | SCE, CHINESE HAMSTER CELLS IN VITRO[2] | + 0 | 0.1000 | LEVIS & MAJONE, 1981 |
| S | SIC | SCE, CHINESE HAMSTER CELLS IN VITRO | + 0 | 0.0050 | VENIER ET AL., 1985b |
| C | CIC | CHROM ABERR, CHINESE HAMSTER CELLS IN VITRO | + 0 | 0.3000 | LEVIS & MAJONE, 1981 |
| C | CIC | CHROM ABERR, CHINESE HAMSTER CELLS IN VITRO[2] | + 0 | 0.1000 | LEVIS & MAJONE, 1981 |

[1]Doses are given as concentrations of the element, not the concentration of the compound.
[2]Dissolved in NaOH

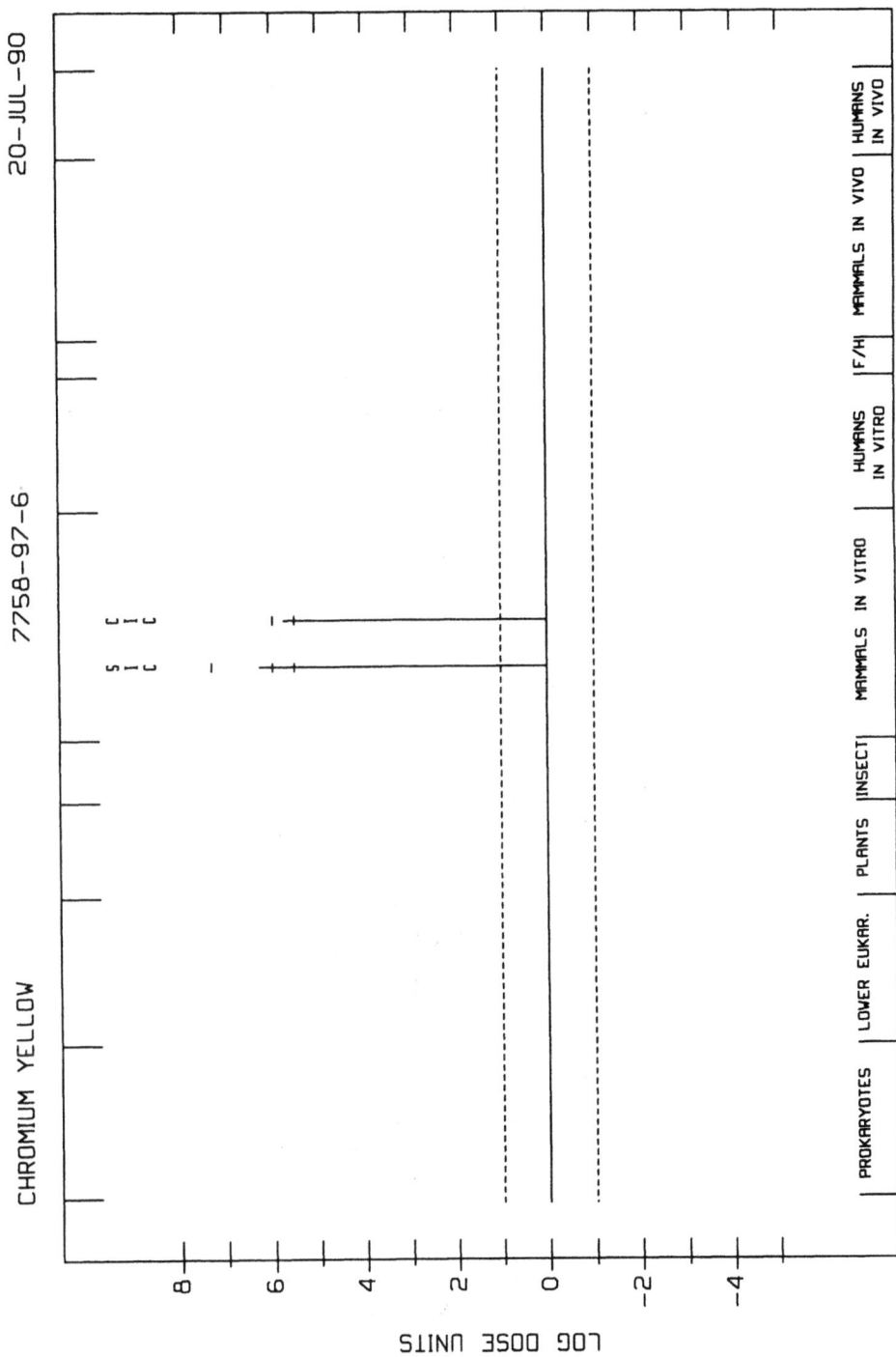

CHROMIUM YELLOW          7758-97-6          20-JUL-90

CHROMYL CHLORIDE

| END POINT | TEST CODE | TEST SYSTEM | RESULTS NM M | DOSE[1] (LED OR HID) | REFERENCE |
|---|---|---|---|---|---|
| G | SA0 | S. TYPHIMURIUM TA100, REVERSE MUTATION | + 0 | 0.0200 | DE FLORA, 1981a |
| G | SA0 | S. TYPHIMURIUM TA100, REVERSE MUTATION | + + | 17.0000 | DE FLORA ET AL., 1980 |
| G | SA5 | S. TYPHIMURIUM TA1535, REVERSE MUTATION | - 0 | 0.0200 | DE FLORA, 1981a |
| G | SA7 | S. TYPHIMURIUM TA1537, REVERSE MUTATION | + 0 | 0:0200 | DE FLORA, 1981a |
| G | SA8 | S. TYPHIMURIUM TA1538, REVERSE MUTATION | + 0 | 0.0200 | DE FLORA, 1981a |
| G | SA9 | S. TYPHIMURIUM TA98, REVERSE MUTATION | + 0 | 0.0200 | DE FLORA, 1981a |

[1]Doses are given as concentrations of the element, not the concentration of the compound.

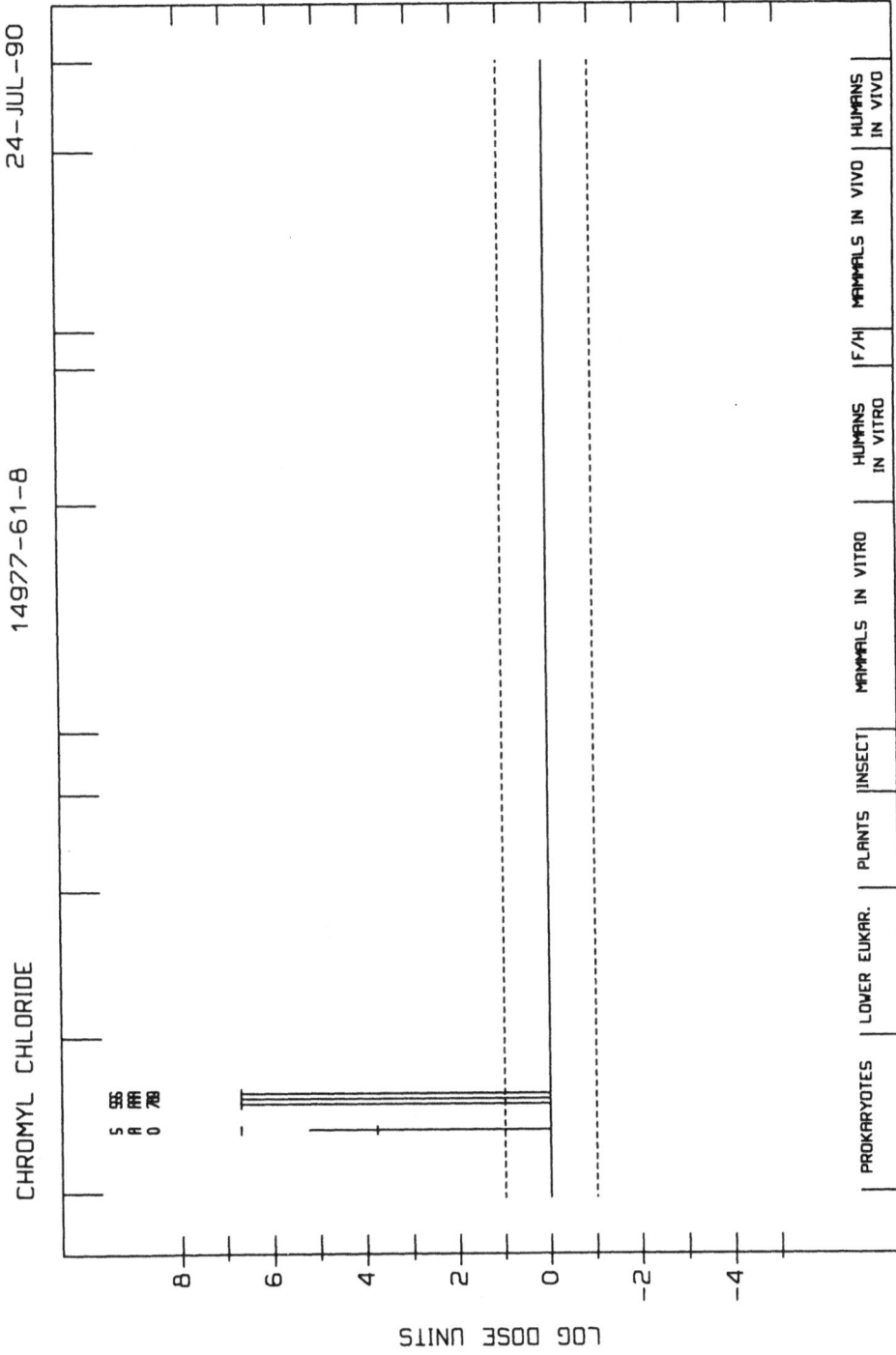

CHROMYL CHLORIDE   14977-61-8   24-JUL-90

LOG DOSE UNITS

PROKARYOTES | LOWER EUKAR. | PLANTS | INSECT | MAMMALS IN VITRO | HUMANS IN VITRO | F/H | MAMMALS IN VIVO | HUMANS IN VIVO

CHROMOUS CHLORIDE

| END POINT | TEST CODE | TEST SYSTEM | RESULTS NM M | DOSE[1] (LED OR HID) | REFERENCE |
|-----------|-----------|-------------|--------------|----------------------|-----------|
| D | DIA | STRAND BREAKS/X-LINKS, ANIMAL CELLS IN VITRO | – 0 | 52.0000 | WEDRYCHOWSKI ET AL., 1986a |
| C | CIS | CHROM ABERR, SYRIAN HAMSTER CELLS IN VITRO | – 0 | 3.5000 | TSUDA & KATO, 1977 |
| A | AIH | ANEUPLOIDY, HUMAN CELLS IN VITRO | – 0 | 0.0050 | NIJS & KIRSCH-VOLDERS, 1986 |

[1]Doses are given as concentrations of the element, not the concentration of the compound.

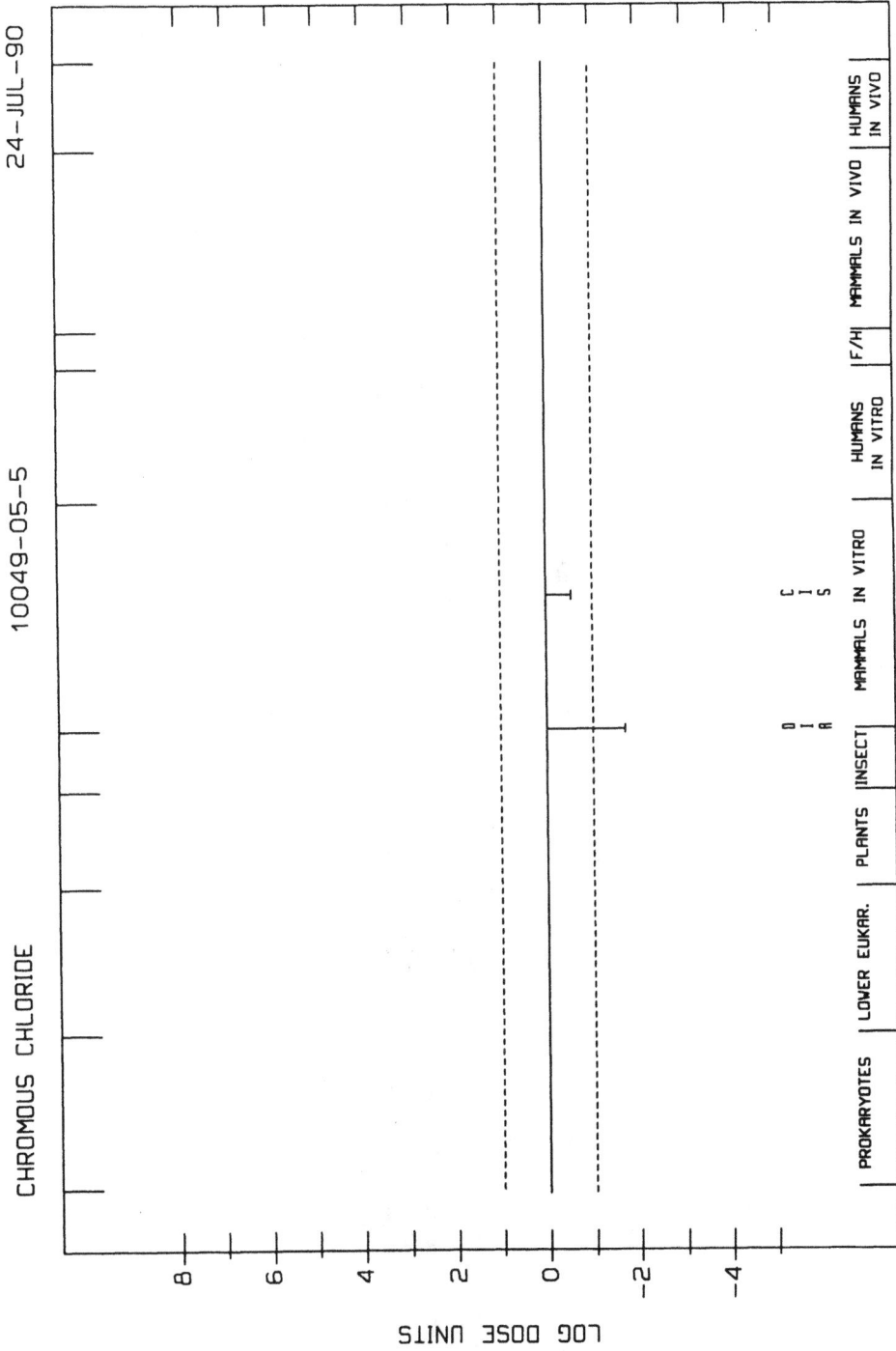

CHROMOUS CHLORIDE    10049-05-5    24-JUL-90

LOG DOSE UNITS

PROKARYOTES | LOWER EUKAR. | PLANTS | INSECT | MAMMALS IN VITRO | HUMANS IN VITRO | F/H | MAMMALS IN VIVO | HUMANS IN VIVO

CHROMIUM CARBONYL

| END POINT | TEST CODE | TEST SYSTEM | RESULTS NM M | DOSE[1] (LED OR HID) | REFERENCE |
|---|---|---|---|---|---|
| D | ERD | E. COLI REC, DIFFERENTIAL TOXICITY | – – | 370.0000 | DE FLORA ET AL., 1984a |
| G | SA0 | S. TYPHIMURIUM TA100, REVERSE MUTATION | – 0 | 0.2000 | DE FLORA, 1981a |
| G | SA5 | S. TYPHIMURIUM TA1535, REVERSE MUTATION | – 0 | 0.2000 | DE FLORA, 1981a |
| G | SA7 | S. TYPHIMURIUM TA1537, REVERSE MUTATION | – 0 | 0.2000 | DE FLORA, 1981a |
| G | SA8 | S. TYPHIMURIUM TA1538, REVERSE MUTATION | – 0 | 0.2000 | DE FLORA, 1981a |
| G | SA9 | S. TYPHIMURIUM TA98, REVERSE MUTATION | – 0 | 0.2000 | DE FLORA, 1981a |
| G | SAS | S. TYPHIMURIUM (OTHER), REVERSE MUTATION | – 0 | 0.0000 | DE FLORA ET AL., 1984a |

[1]Doses are given as concentrations of the element, not the concentration of the compound.

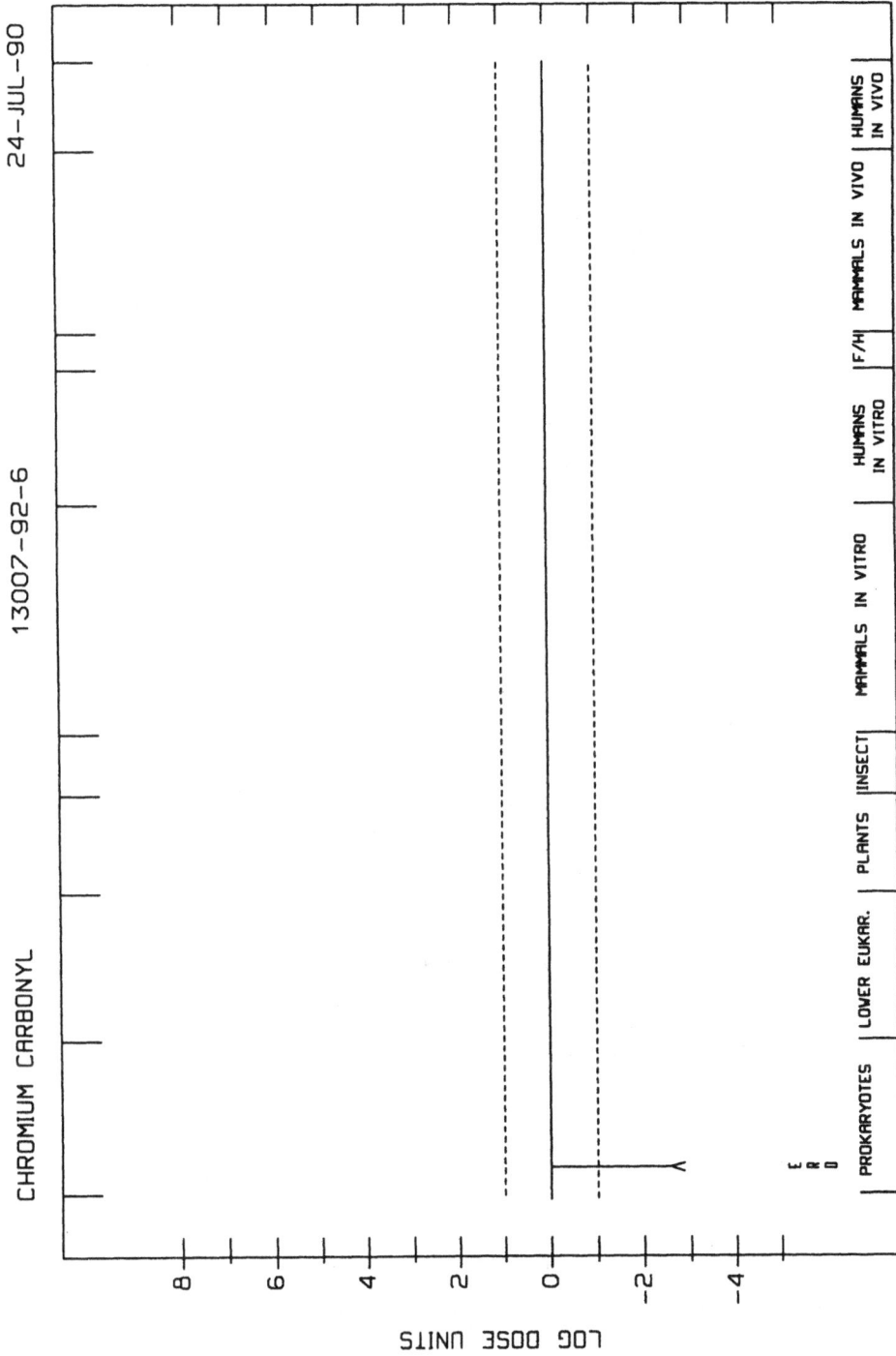

CHROMIUM CARBONYL                    13007-92-6                    24-JUL-90

LOG DOSE UNITS

NICKEL OCCUPATIONAL EXPOSURE

| END POINT | TEST CODE | TEST SYSTEM | RESULTS NM | M | DOSE (LED OR HID) | REFERENCE |
|---|---|---|---|---|---|---|
| S | SLH | SCE, HUMAN LYMPHOCYTES IN VIVO | - | 0 | 0.1400 | WAKSVIK ET AL., 1984[1] |
| S | SLH | SCE, HUMAN LYMPHOCYTES IN VIVO | - | 0 | 0.0680 | WAKSVIK & BOYSEN, 1982[2] |
| S | SLH | SCE, HUMAN LYMPHOCYTES IN VIVO | - | 0 | 0.0280 | WAKSVIK & BOYSEN, 1982[3] |
| S | SLH | SCE, HUMAN LYMPHOCYTES IN VIVO | (+) | 0 | -0.0140 | DENG ET AL., 1983[4] |
| S | SLH | SCE, HUMAN LYMPHOCYTES IN VIVO | - | 0 | 0.0000 | DECHENG ET AL., 1987[5] |
| C | CLH | CHROM ABERR, HUMAN LYMPHOCYTES IN VIVO | + | 0 | 0.1400 | WAKSVIK ET AL., 1984[1] |
| C | CLH | CHROM ABERR, HUMAN LYMPHOCYTES IN VIVO | + | 0 | 0.0680 | WAKSVIK & BOYSEN, 1982[2] |
| C | CLH | CHROM ABERR, HUMAN LYMPHOCYTES IN VIVO | + | 0 | 0.0280 | WAKSVIK & BOYSEN, 1982[3] |
| C | CLH | CHROM ABERR, HUMAN LYMPHOCYTES IN VIVO | + | 0 | 0.0140 | DENG ET AL., 1983[4] |
| C | CLH | CHROM ABERR, HUMAN LYMPHOCYTES IN VIVO | - | 0 | 0.0000 | DECHENG ET AL., 1987[5] |

[1] $NiO$ and $Ni_3S_2/NiCl_2$, $NiSO_4$ (crushing, roasting, smelting and/or electrolysis)

[2] $NiO$ and $Ni_3S_2$ (crushing, roasting, smelting)

[3] $NiCl_2$ and $NiSO_4$ (electrolysis)

[4] $Ni$ and chromium (electroplating)

[5] $Ni(CO)_4$ (production of nickel carbonyl)

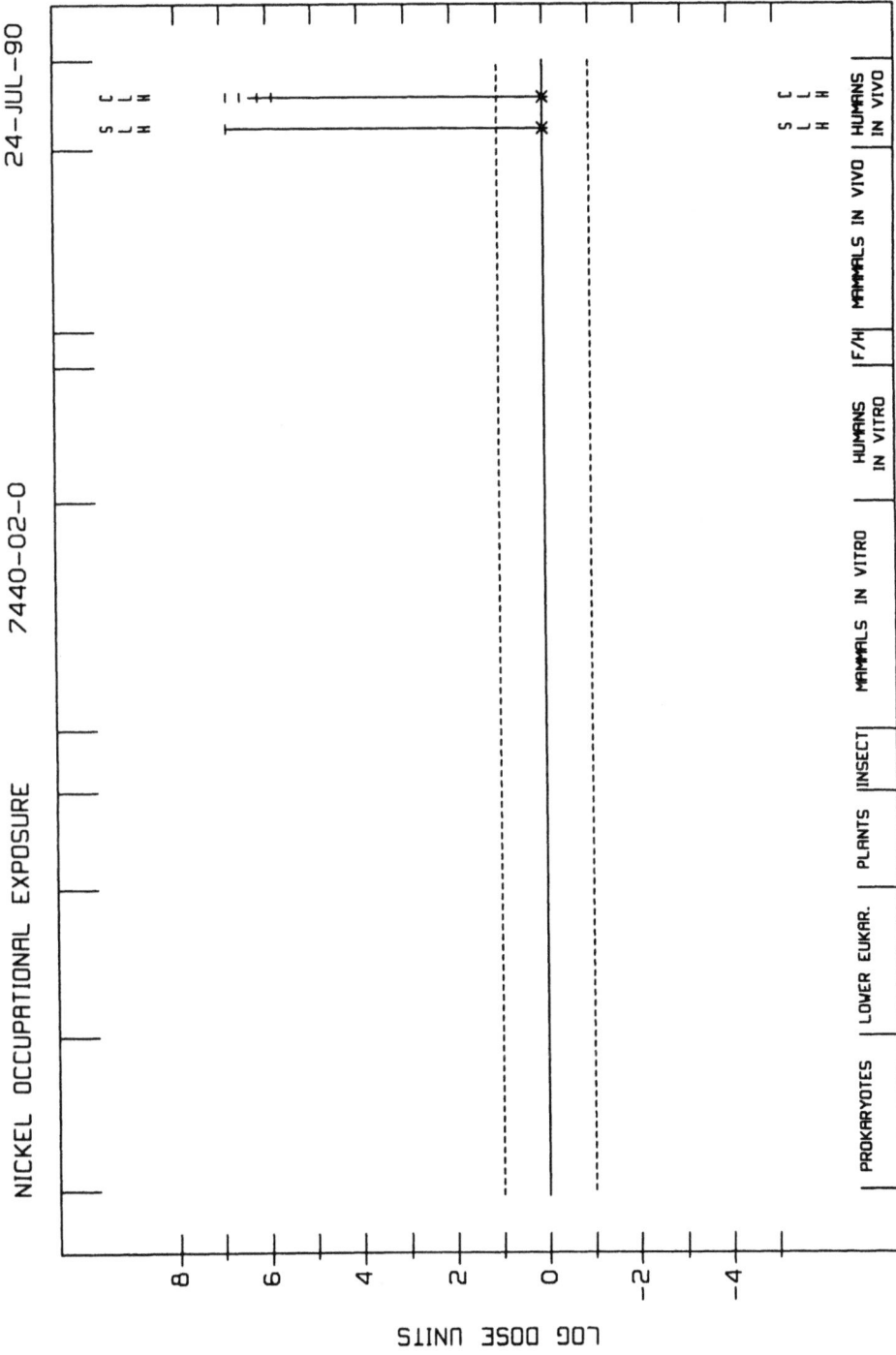

NICKEL OCCUPATIONAL EXPOSURE    7440-02-0    24-JUL-90

METALLIC NICKEL

| END POINT | TEST CODE | TEST SYSTEM | RESULTS NM M | DOSE[1] (LED OR HID) | REFERENCE |
|---|---|---|---|---|---|
| T | TCS | CELL TRANSFORMATION, SHE, CLONAL ASSAY | + 0 | 20.0000 | COSTA ET AL., 1981b |
| T | TCL | CELL TRANSFORMATION, OTHER CELL LINES | + 0 | 200.0000 | HANSEN & STERN, 1984 |
| C | CHL | CHROM ABERR, HUMAN LYMPHOCYTES IN VITRO | - 0 | 0.0000 | PATON & ALLISON, 1972 |

[1]Doses are given as concentrations of the element, not the concentration of the compound.

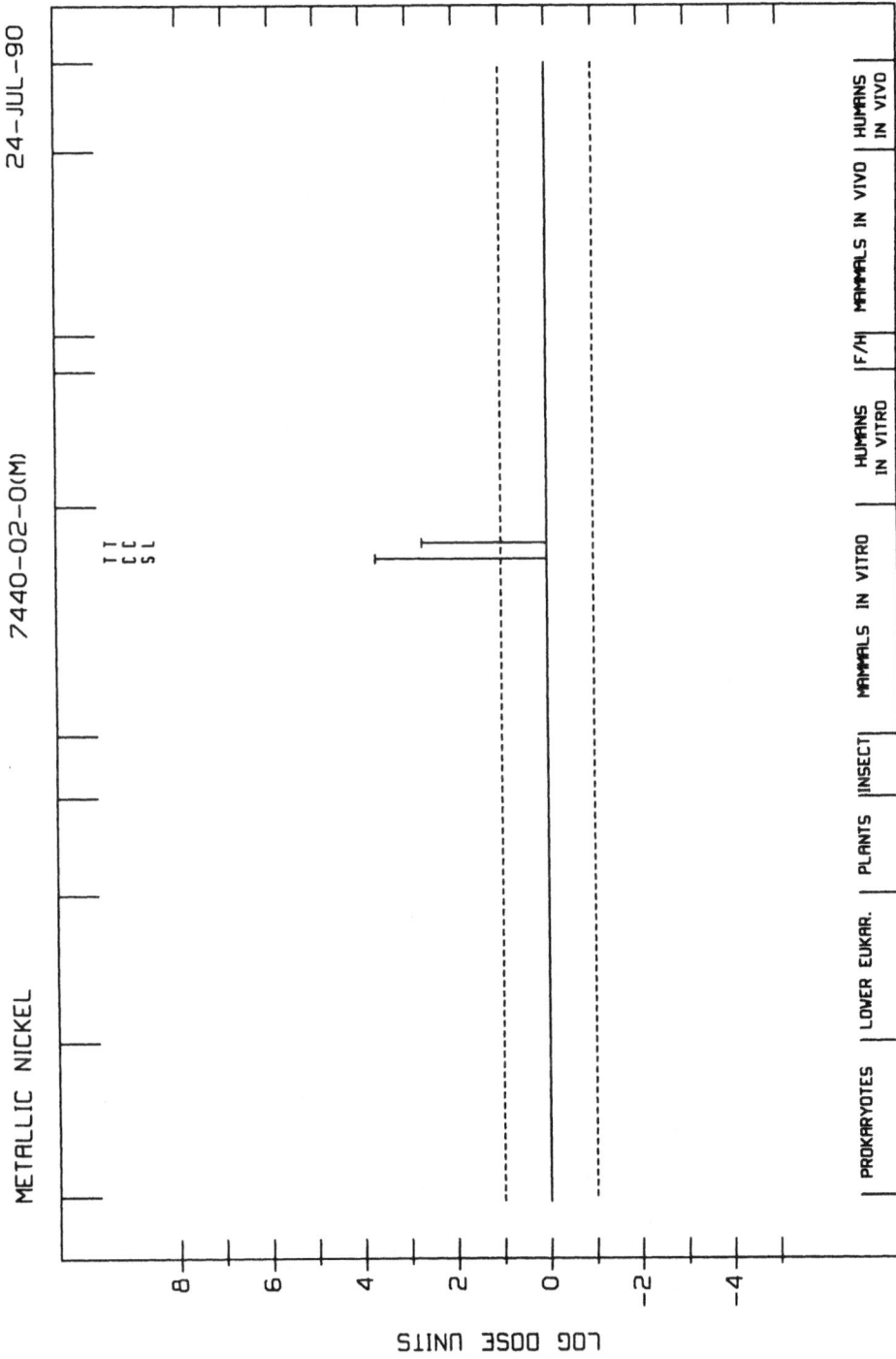

NICKEL OXIDES

| END POINT | TEST CODE | TEST SYSTEM | RESULTS NM M | DOSE[1] (LED OR HID) | REFERENCE |
|---|---|---|---|---|---|
| D | BSD | B. SUBTILIS REC, DIFFERENTIAL TOXICITY[2] | – 0 | 1475.0000 | KANEMATSU ET AL., 1980 |
| D | BSD | B. SUBTILIS REC, DIFFERENTIAL TOXICITY[3] | – 0 | 2950.0000 | KANEMATSU ET AL., 1980 |
| T | TCS | CELL TRANSFORMATION, SHE, CLONAL ASSAY[2] | + 0 | 16.0000 | COSTA ET AL., 1981b |
| T | TCS | CELL TRANSFORMATION, SHE, CLONAL ASSAY[3] | + 0 | 14.0000 | COSTA ET AL., 1981b |
| T | TCS | CELL TRANSFORMATION, SHE, CLONAL ASSAY[3] | + 0 | 7.9000 | SUNDERMAN ET AL., 1987 |
| T | TCL | CELL TRANSFORMATION, OTHER CELL LINES[2] | + 0 | 30.0000 | HANSEN & STERN, 1983 |
| T | TCL | CELL TRANSFORMATION, OTHER CELL LINES[3] | + 0 | 4.0000 | HANSEN & STERN, 1983 |
| C | CHL | CHROM ABERR, HUMAN LYMPHOCYTES IN VITRO[3] | – 0 | 0.0000 | PATON & ALLISON, 1972 |
| T | TIH | CELL TRANSFORMATION, HUMAN CELLS IN VITRO[3] | + 0 | 3.0000 | BIEDERMANN & LANDOLPH, 1987 |

[1]Doses are given as concentrations of the element, not the concentration of the compound.
[2]Nickel trioxide
[3]Nickel monoxide

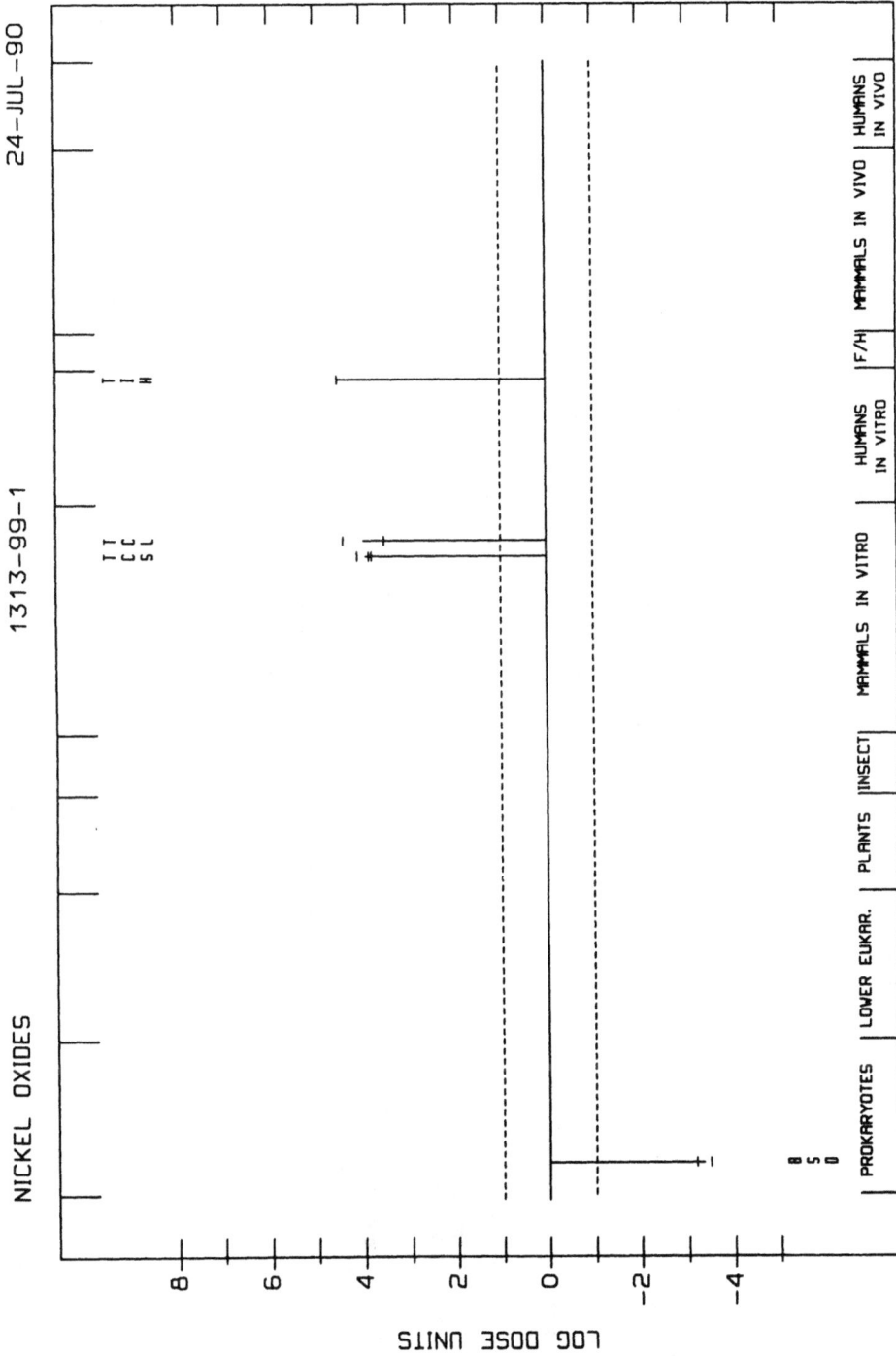

NICKEL SULFIDES (AMORPH.)

| END POINT | TEST CODE | TEST SYSTEM | RESULTS NM M | DOSE[1] (LED OR HID) | REFERENCE |
|---|---|---|---|---|---|
| D | DIA | STRAND BREAKS/X-LINKS, ANIMAL CELLS IN VITRO | – 0 | 6.5000 | COSTA ET AL., 1982 |
| D | RIA | OTHER DNA REPAIR, ANIMAL CELLS IN VITRO | – 0 | 6.5000 | ROBISON ET AL., 1983 |
| G | GCO | MUTATION, CHO CELLS IN VITRO | (+) 0 | 1.0000 | COSTA ET AL., 1980 |
| T | TCS | CELL TRANSFORMATION, SHE, CLONAL ASSAY | – 0 | 3.2500 | COSTA ET AL., 1979 |
| T | TCS | CELL TRANSFORMATION, SHE, CLONAL ASSAY | – 0 | 6.5000 | COSTA & MOLLENHAUER, 1980a |
| T | TCS | CELL TRANSFORMATION, SHE, CLONAL ASSAY | – 0 | 6.5000 | COSTA ET AL., 1982 |

[1]Doses are given as concentrations of the element, not the concentration of the compound.

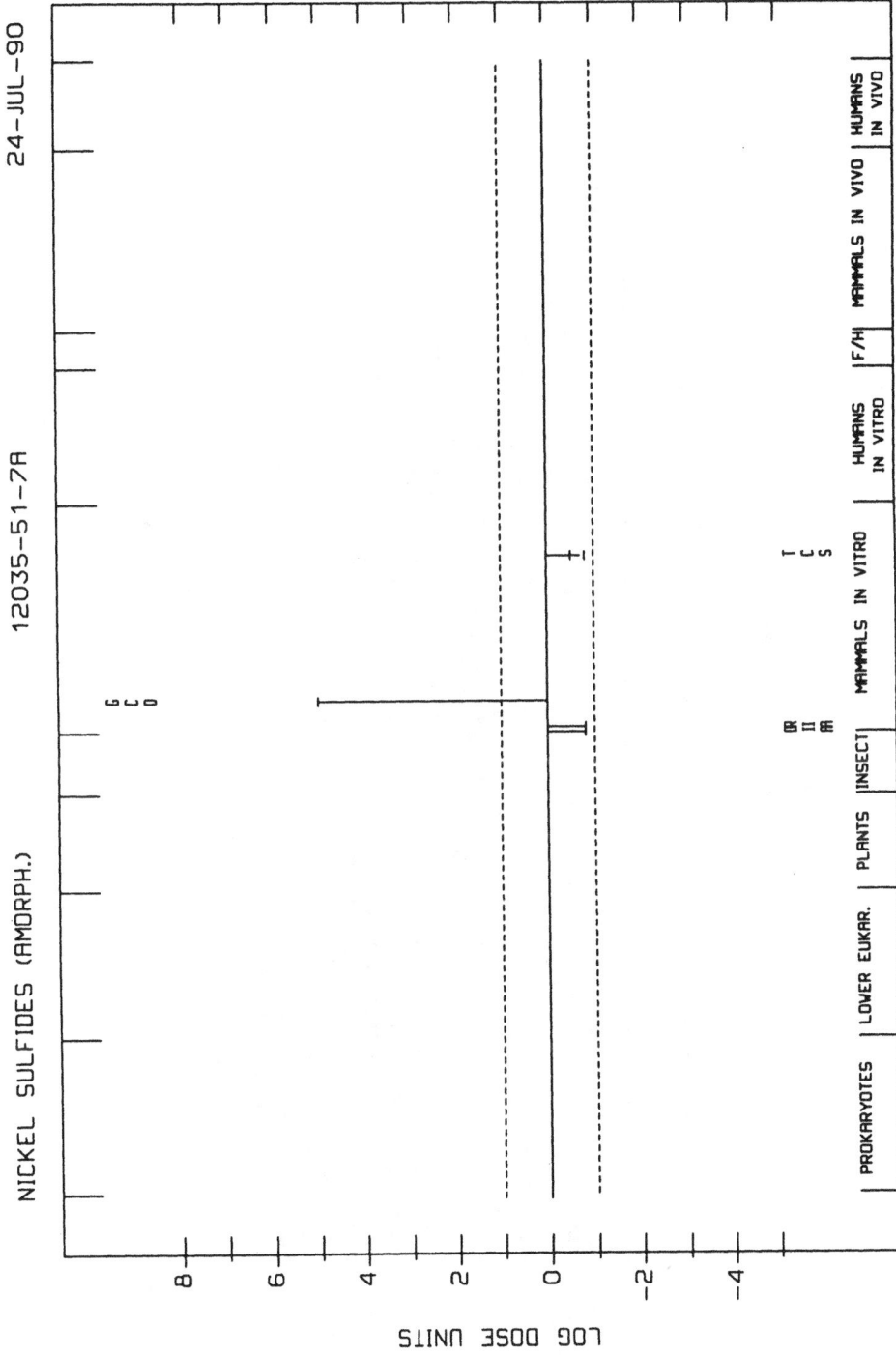

NICKEL SULFIDES (AMORPH.)        12035-51-7A        24-JUL-90

NICKEL SULFIDES (CRYST.)

| END POINT | TEST CODE | TEST SYSTEM | RESULTS NM M | DOSE[1] (LED OR HID) | REFERENCE |
|---|---|---|---|---|---|
| C | PSC | PARAMECIUM SPECIES, CHROM ABERR | + 0 | 0.3000 | SMITH-SONNEBORN ET AL., 1983 |
| D | DIA | STRAND BREAKS/X-LINKS, ANIMAL CELLS IN VITRO | (+) 0 | 114.0000 | SINA ET AL., 1983 |
| D | DIA | STRAND BREAKS/X-LINKS, ANIMAL CELLS IN VITRO | + 0 | 6.5000 | COSTA ET AL., 1982 |
| D | DIA | STRAND BREAKS/X-LINKS, ANIMAL CELLS IN VITRO | + 0 | 0.6500 | ROBISON & COSTA, 1982 |
| D | DIA | STRAND BREAKS/X-LINKS, ANIMAL CELLS IN VITRO | + 0 | 6.5000 | PATIERNO & COSTA, 1985 |
| D | DIA | STRAND BREAKS/X-LINKS, ANIMAL CELLS IN VITRO | + 0 | 7.3000 | ROBINSON ET AL., 1982 |
| D | RIA | OTHER DNA REPAIR, ANIMAL CELLS IN VITRO | + 0 | 0.6500 | ROBINSON ET AL., 1983 |
| G | G9H | MUTATION, CHL V79 CELLS, HPRT | + 0 | 4.9000 | CHRISTIE ET AL., 1990 |
| S | SIC | SCE, CHINESE HAMSTER CELLS IN VITRO | + 0 | 0.6500 | SEN & COSTA, 1986 |
| C | CIC | CHROM ABERR, CHINESE HAMSTER CELLS IN VITRO | + 0 | 3.2000 | SEN & COSTA, 1985 |
| C | CIM | CHROM ABERR, MOUSE CELLS IN VITRO | + 0 | 1.6000 | SEN ET AL., 1987 |
| C | CIT | CHROM ABERR, TRANSFORMED CELLS IN VITRO | + 0 | 38.0000 | UMEDA & NISHIMURA, 1979 |
| C | CIT | CHROM ABERR, TRANSFORMED CELLS IN VITRO | + 0 | 24.0000 | NISHIMURA & UMEDA, 1979 |
| T | TCS | CELL TRANSFORMATION, SHE, CLONAL ASSAY | + 0 | 6.5000 | COSTA ET AL., 1982 |
| T | TCS | CELL TRANSFORMATION, SHE, CLONAL ASSAY | + 0 | 3.2500 | COSTA & MOLLENHAUER, 1980c |
| C | CVA | CHROM ABERR, OTHER ANIMAL CELLS IN VIVO | + 0 | 250.0000 | CHRISTIE ET AL., 1988 |

[1]Doses are given as concentrations of the element, not the contration of the compound.

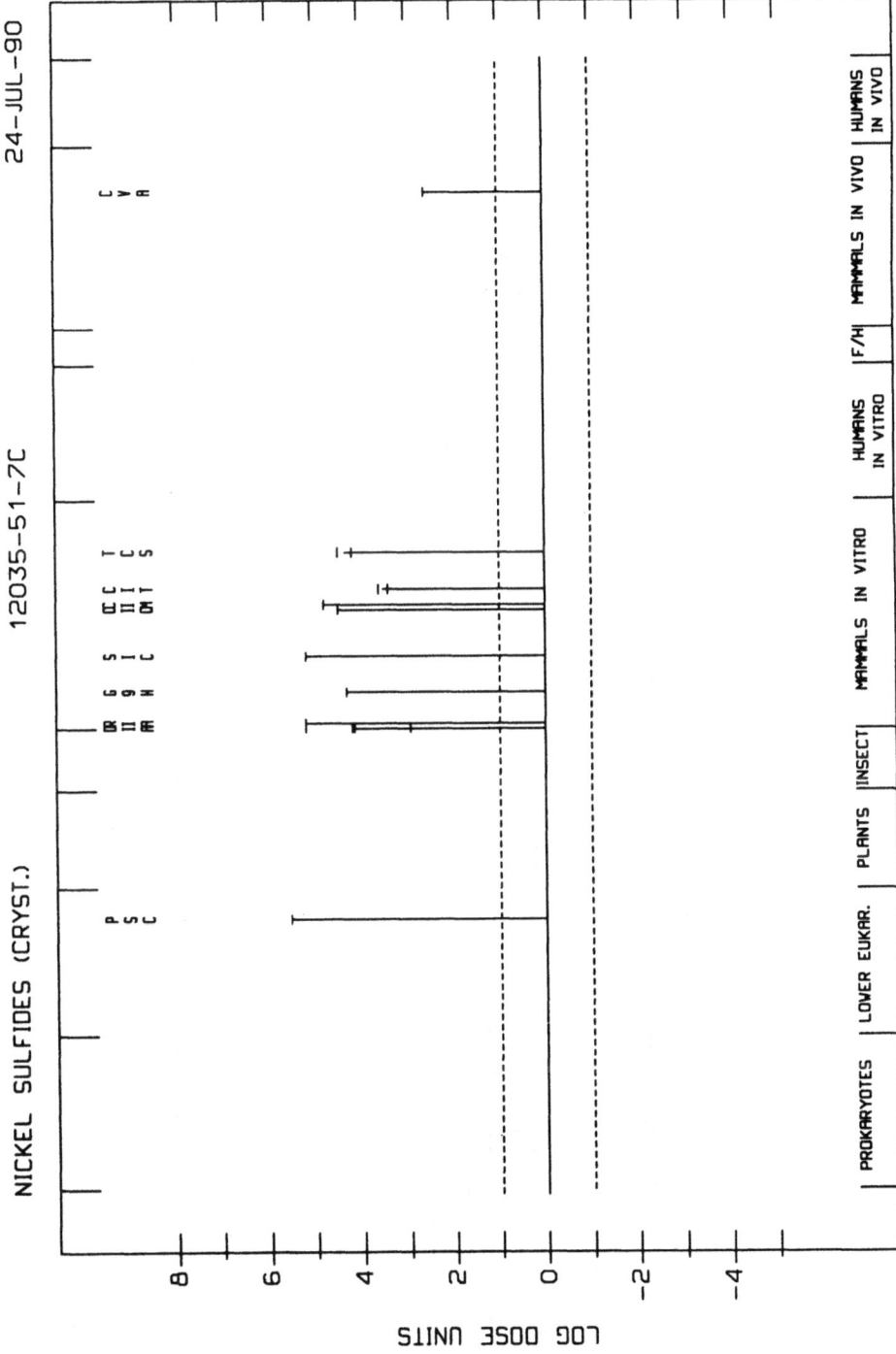

NICKEL SULFIDES (CRYST.)            12035-51-7C            24-JUL-90

NICKEL SUBSULFIDES

| END POINT | TEST CODE | TEST SYSTEM | RESULTS NN | M | DOSE[1] (LED OR HID) | REFERENCE |
|---|---|---|---|---|---|---|
| C | PSC | PARAMECIUM SPECIES, CHROM ABERR | + | 0 | 0.4000 | SMITH-SONNEBORN ET AL., 1983 |
| D | RIA | OTHER DNA REPAIR, ANIMAL CELLS IN VITRO | + | 0 | 7.3000 | ROBISON ET AL., 1983 |
| D | URP | UDS, RAT PRIMARY HEPATOCYTES | – | 0 | 20.0000 | SWIERENGA & MCLEAN, 1985 |
| G | GCO | MUTATION, CHO CELLS IN VITRO | (+) | 0 | 1.1000 | COSTA ET AL., 1980 |
| G | GIA | MUTATION, OTHER ANIMAL CELLS IN VITRO | + | 0 | 3.7000 | SWIERENGA & MCLEAN, 1985 |
| T | TCM | CELL TRANSFORMATION, C3H10T1/2 CELLS | + | 0 | 0.0007 | SAXHOLM ET AL., 1981 |
| T | TCS | CELL TRANSFORMATION, SHE, CLONAL ASSAY | + | 0 | 0.7300 | DIPAOLO & CASTO, 1979 |
| T | TCS | CELL TRANSFORMATION, SHE, CLONAL ASSAY | + | 0 | 0.0730 | COSTA ET AL., 1979 |
| T | TCS | CELL TRANSFORMATION, SHE, CLONAL ASSAY | + | 0 | 0.7300 | COSTA & MOLLENHAUER, 1980a |
| T | TCS | CELL TRANSFORMATION, SHE, CLONAL ASSAY | + | 0 | 3.7000 | COSTA & MOLLENHAUER, 1980c |
| T | TCL | CELL TRANSFORMATION, OTHER CELL LINES | + | 0 | 3.7000 | HANSEN & STERN, 1983 |
| T | TCL | CELL TRANSFORMATION, OTHER CELL LINES | – | 0 | 1.8000 | SWIERENGA ET AL., 1989 |
| G | GIH | MUTATION, HUMAN CELLS IN VITRO | + | 0 | 0.6000 | BIEDERMANN & LANDOLPH, 1987 |
| S | SHL | SCE, HUMAN LYMPHOCYTES IN VITRO | + | 0 | 0.7300 | SAXHOLM ET AL., 1981 |
| T | TIH | CELL TRANSFORMATION, HUMAN CELLS IN VITRO | + | 0 | 0.6000 | BIEDERMANN & LANDOLPH, 1987 |

[1]Doses are given as concentrations of the element, not the concentration of the compound.

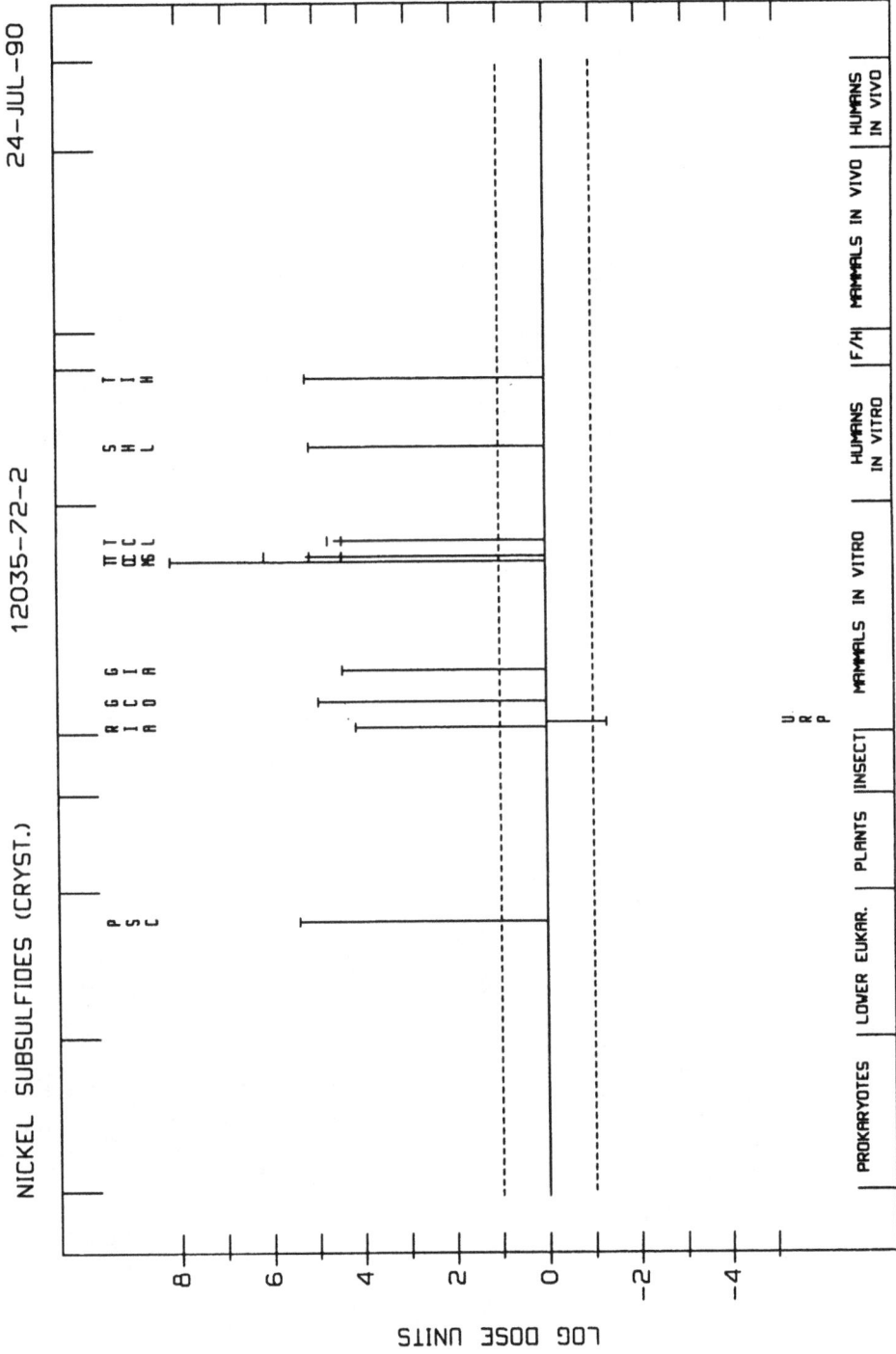

NICKEL CHLORIDE

| END POINT | TEST CODE | TEST SYSTEM | RESULTS NM | M | DOSE[1] (LED OR HID) | REFERENCE |
|---|---|---|---|---|---|---|
| D | ERD | E. COLI REC, DIFFERENTIAL TOXICITY | – | – | 567.0000 | DE FLORA ET AL., 1984a |
| D | ERD | E. COLI REC, DIFFERENTIAL TOXICITY | + | 0 | 90.0000 | TWEATS ET AL., 1981 |
| D | ERD | E. COLI REC, DIFFERENTIAL TOXICITY | – | 0 | 0.0100 | DUBINS & LA VELLE, 1986 |
| D | BSD | B. SUBTILIS REC, DIFFERENTIAL TOXICITY | – | 0 | 1475.0000 | KANEMATSU ET AL., 1980 |
| D | BSD | B. SUBTILIS REC, DIFFERENTIAL TOXICITY | – | 0 | 147.5000 | NISHIOKA, 1975 |
| G | SA0 | S. TYPHIMURIUM TA100, REVERSE MUTATION | – | 0 | 587.0000 | TSO & FUNG, 1981 |
| G | SA0 | S. TYPHIMURIUM TA100, REVERSE MUTATION | – | 0 | 0.0000 | ARLAUSKAS ET AL., 1985 |
| G | SA0 | S. TYPHIMURIUM TA100, REVERSE MUTATION | – | 0 | 0.0000 | DE FLORA ET AL., 1984a |
| G | SA2 | S. TYPHIMURIUM TA102, REVERSE MUTATION | – | – | 590.0000 | BIGGART & COSTA, 1986 |
| G | SA5 | S. TYPHIMURIUM TA1535, REVERSE MUTATION | – | 0 | 0.0000 | ARLAUSKAS ET AL., 1985 |
| G | SA5 | S. TYPHIMURIUM TA1535, REVERSE MUTATION | – | 0 | 118.0000 | BIGGART & COSTA, 1986 |
| G | SA5 | S. TYPHIMURIUM TA1535, REVERSE MUTATION | – | 0 | 0.0000 | DE FLORA ET AL., 1984a |
| G | SA7 | S. TYPHIMURIUM TA1537, REVERSE MUTATION | – | 0 | 0.0000 | ARLAUSKAS ET AL., 1985 |
| G | SA7 | S. TYPHIMURIUM TA1537, REVERSE MUTATION | – | 0 | 0.0000 | DE FLORA ET AL., 1984a |
| G | SA8 | S. TYPHIMURIUM TA1538, REVERSE MUTATION | – | 0 | 0.0000 | ARLAUSKAS ET AL., 1985 |
| G | SA8 | S. TYPHIMURIUM TA1538, REVERSE MUTATION | – | 0 | 118.0000 | BIGGART & COSTA, 1986 |
| G | SA8 | S. TYPHIMURIUM TA1538, REVERSE MUTATION | – | 0 | 0.0000 | DE FLORA ET AL., 1984a |
| G | SA9 | S. TYPHIMURIUM TA98, REVERSE MUTATION | – | 0 | 0.0000 | ARLAUSKAS ET AL., 1985 |
| G | SA9 | S. TYPHIMURIUM TA98, REVERSE MUTATION | – | 0 | 0.0000 | DE FLORA ET AL., 1984a |
| G | SAS | S. TYPHIMURIUM (OTHER), REVERSE MUTATION | – | 0 | 590.0000 | TSO & FUNG, 1981 |
| G | SAS | S. TYPHIMURIUM (OTHER), REVERSE MUTATION | – | 0 | 118.0000 | BIGGART & COSTA, 1986 |
| G | SAS | S. TYPHIMURIUM (OTHER), REVERSE MUTATION | – | 0 | 0.0000 | DE FLORA ET AL., 1984a |
| G | EC2 | E. COLI WP2, REVERSE MUTATION | – | 0 | 4.5000 | GREEN ET AL., 1976 |
| R | SCG | S. CEREVISIAE, GENE CONVERSION | + | 0 | 176.0000 | FUKUNAGA ET AL., 1982 |
| R | SCR | S. CEREVISIAE, REVERSE MUTATION | + | 0 | 1535.0000 | EGILSSON ET AL., 1979 |
| G | DMM | D. MELANOGASTER, SOMATIC MUTAT/RECOMB | – | 0 | 12.0000 | RASMUSON, 1985 |
| G | DMX | D. MELANOGASTER, SEX-LINKED RECESSIVES | – | 0 | 248.0000 | VOGEL, 1976 |
| D | DIA | STRAND BREAKS/X-LINKS, ANIMAL CELLS IN VITRO | + | 0 | 0.4500 | ROBISON & COSTA, 1982 |
| D | DIA | STRAND BREAKS/X-LINKS, ANIMAL CELLS IN VITRO | + | 0 | 150.0000 | PATIERNO & COSTA, 1985 |
| D | DIA | STRAND BREAKS/X-LINKS, ANIMAL CELLS IN VITRO | + | 0 | 5.9000 | ROBISON ET AL., 1982 |
| D | DIA | STRAND BREAKS/X-LINKS, ANIMAL CELLS IN VITRO | + | 0 | 59.0000 | ROBISON ET AL., 1984 |
| D | RIA | OTHER DNA REPAIR, ANIMAL CELLS IN VITRO | + | 0 | 5.9000 | ROBISON ET AL., 1983 |
| G | GCO | MUTATION, CHO CELLS IN VITRO | (+) | 0 | 0.0000 | HSIE ET AL., 1979 |
| G | G9H | MUTATION, CHL V79 CELLS, HPRT | (+) | 0 | 23.0000 | MIYAKI ET AL., 1979 |
| G | G9E | MUTATION, CHL V79 CELLS, HPRT | + | 0 | 29.5000 | HARTWIG & BEYERSMANN, 1989 |

NICKEL CHLORIDE

| END POINT | TEST CODE | TEST SYSTEM | RESULTS NM M | DOSE[1] (LED OR HID) | REFERENCE |
|---|---|---|---|---|---|
| G | G5T | MUTATION, L5178Y CELLS, TK LOCUS | + 0 | 10.0000 | AMACHER & PAILLET, 1980 |
| G | GIA | MUTATION, OTHER ANIMAL CELLS IN VITRO | + 0 | 2.4000 | BIGGART & MURPHY, 1988 |
| G | GIA | MUTATION, OTHER ANIMAL CELLS IN VITRO | + 0 | 45.0000 | SWIERENGA & MCLEAN, 1985 |
| S | SIC | SCE, CHINESE HAMSTER CELLS IN VITRO | + 0 | 8.0000 | OHNO ET AL., 1982 |
| S | SIC | SCE, CHINESE HAMSTER CELLS IN VITRO | + 0 | 0.6000 | SEN & COSTA, 1986 |
| S | SIC | SCE, CHINESE HAMSTER CELLS IN VITRO | + 0 | 17.7000 | HARTWIG & BEYERSMANN, 1989 |
| C | CIC | CHROM ABERR, CHINESE HAMSTER CELLS IN VITRO | + 0 | 0.6000 | SEN & COSTA, 1985 |
| C | CIC | CHROM ABERR, CHINESE HAMSTER CELLS IN VITRO | + 0 | 6.0000 | SEN ET AL., 1987 |
| C | CIT | CHROM ABERR, TRANSFORMED CELLS IN VITRO | (+) 0 | 38.0000 | UMEDA & NISHIMURA, 1979 |
| C | CIT | CHROM ABERR, TRANSFORMED CELLS IN VITRO | + 0 | 35.0000 | NISHIMURA & UMEDA, 1979 |
| T | TCS | CELL TRANSFORMATION, SHE, CLONAL ASSAY | + 0 | 2.2500 | ZHANG & BARRETT, 1988 |
| D | DIH | STRAND BREAKS/X-LINKS, HUMAN CELLS IN VITRO | ? 0 | 3.0000 | MCLEAN ET AL., 1982 |
| S | SHL | SCE, HUMAN LYMPHOCYTES IN VITRO | + 0 | 0.6000 | NEWMAN ET AL., 1982 |
| H | HMM | HOST-MEDIATED ASSAY, MICROBIAL CELLS | - 0 | 23.0000 | BUSELMAIER ET AL., 1972 |
| M | MVM | MICRONUCLEUS TEST, MICE IN VIVO | - 0 | 11.000 | DEKNUDT & LEONARD, 1982 |
| C | CBA | CHROM ABERR, ANIMAL BONE MARROW IN VIVO | + 0 | 2.3000 | CHORVATOVICOVA, 1983 |
| C | CBA | CHROM ABERR, ANIMAL BONE MARROW IN VIVO | + 0 | 2.7000 | MOHARTY, 1987 |
| C | DLM | DOMINANT LETHAL TEST, MICE | - 0 | 46.0000 | DEKNUDT & LEONARD, 1982 |

[1]Doses are given as concentrations of the element, not the concentration of the compound.

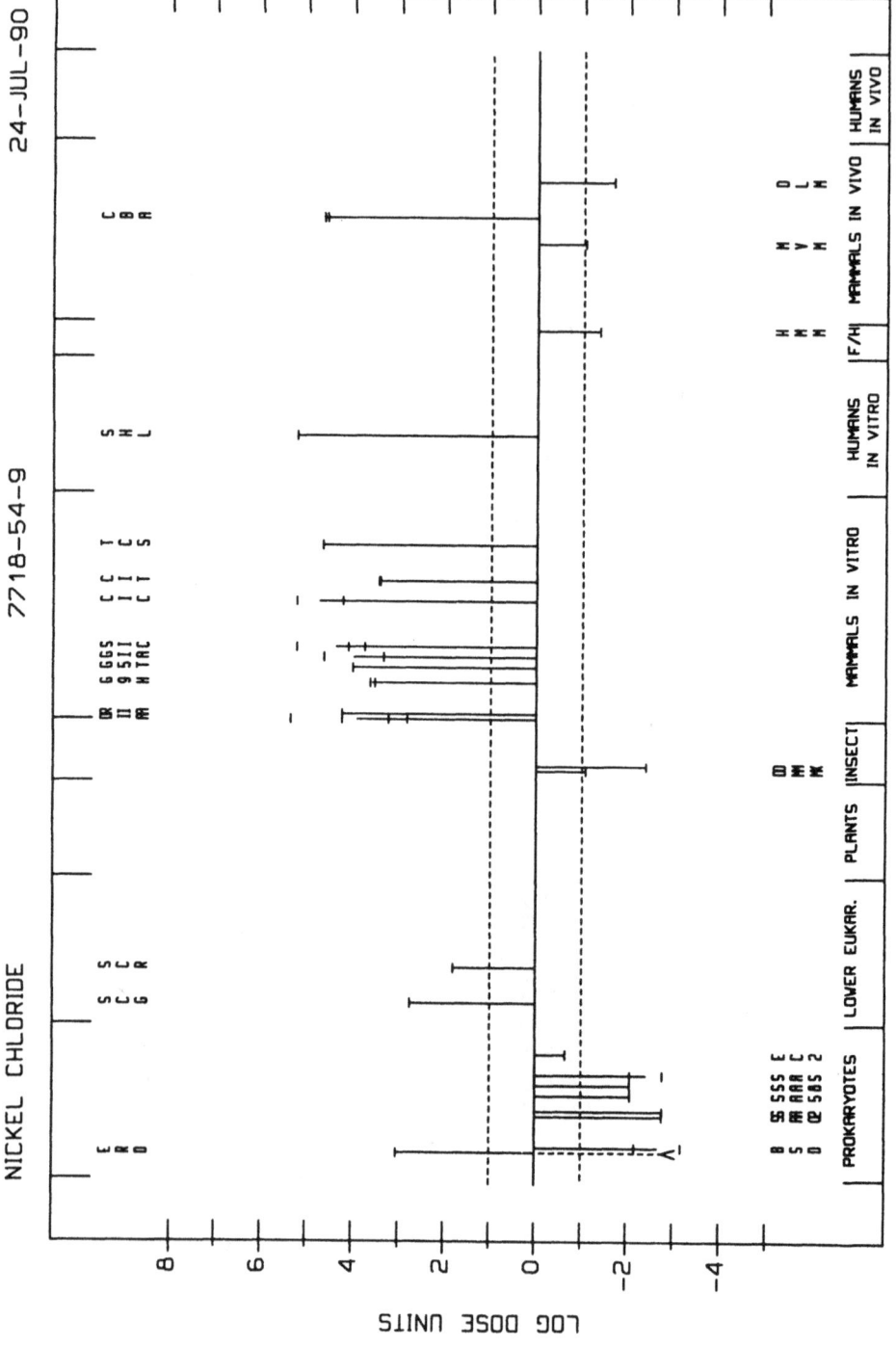

NICKEL SULFATE

| END POINT | TEST CODE | TEST SYSTEM | RESULTS NM M | | DOSE[1] (LED OR HID) | REFERENCE |
|---|---|---|---|---|---|---|
| G | BPF | BACTERIOPHAGE, FORWARD MUTATION | – | 0 | 114.0000 | CORBETT ET AL., 1970 |
| G | SAO | S. TYPHIMURIUM TA100, REVERSE MUTATION | – | 0 | 0.0000 | ARLAUSKAS ET AL., 1985 |
| G | SA5 | S. TYPHIMURIUM TA1535, REVERSE MUTATION | – | 0 | 0.0000 | ARLAUSKAS ET AL., 1985 |
| G | SA7 | S. TYPHIMURIUM TA1537, REVERSE MUTATION | – | 0 | 0.0000 | ARLAUSKAS ET AL., 1985 |
| G | SA8 | S. TYPHIMURIUM TA1538, REVERSE MUTATION | – | 0 | 0.0000 | ARLAUSKAS ET AL., 1985 |
| G | SA9 | S. TYPHIMURIUM TA98, REVERSE MUTATION | – | 0 | 0.0000 | ARLAUSKAS ET AL., 1985 |
| G | EC2 | E. COLI WP2, REVERSE MUTATION | – | 0 | 0.0000 | ARLAUSKAS ET AL., 1985 |
| G | DMX | D. MELANOGASTER, SEX-LINKED RECESSIVES | + | 0 | 45.0000 | RODRIGUEZ-ARNAIZ & RAMOS, 1986 |
| A | DMN | D. MELANOGASTER, ANEUPLOIDY | (+) | 0 | 90.0000 | RODRIGUEZ-ARNAIZ & RAMOS, 1986 |
| G | GIA | MUTATION, OTHER ANIMAL CELLS IN VITRO | – | 0 | 1.0000 | RIVEDAL & SANNER, 1980 |
| G | GIA | MUTATION, OTHER ANIMAL CELLS IN VITRO | (+) | 0 | 6.0000 | CHRISTIE ET AL., 1990 |
| S | SIC | SCE, CHINESE HAMSTER CELLS IN VITRO | + | 0 | 0.1700 | DENG & QU, 1981 |
| S | SIC | SCE, CHINESE HAMSTER CELLS IN VITRO | + | 0 | 8.0000 | OHNO ET AL., 1982 |
| S | SIM | SCE, MOUSE CELLS IN VITRO | + | 0 | 6.0000 | ANDERSEN, 1983 |
| S | SIS | SCE, SYRIAN HAMSTER CELLS IN VITRO | + | 0 | 0.2000 | LARRAMENDY ET AL., 1981 |
| S | SIA | SCE, OTHER ANIMAL CELLS IN VITRO | (+) | 0 | 6.0000 | ANDERSEN, 1983 |
| C | CIS | CHROM ABERR, SYRIAN HAMSTER CELLS IN VITRO | + | 0 | 1.0000 | LARRAMENDY ET AL., 1981 |
| T | TCS | CELL TRANSFORMATION, SHE, CLONAL ASSAY | + | 0 | 4.5000 | RIVEDAL & SANNER, 1980 |
| T | TCS | CELL TRANSFORMATION, SHE, CLONAL ASSAY | + | 0 | 9.0000 | PIENTA ET AL., 1977 |
| T | TCS | CELL TRANSFORMATION, SHE, CLONAL ASSAY | + | 0 | 1.0000 | DIPAOLO & CASTO, 1979 |
| T | TCS | CELL TRANSFORMATION, SHE, CLONAL ASSAY | + | 0 | 1.9000 | ZHANG & BARRETT, 1988 |
| T | TEV | CELL TRANSFORMATION, OTHER VIRAL SYSTEMS | + | 0 | 4.0000 | WILSON & KHOOBYARIAN, 1982 |
| D | DIH | STRAND BREAKS/X-LINKS, HUMAN CELLS IN VITRO | – | 0 | 56.0000 | FORNACE, 1982 |
| S | SHL | SCE, HUMAN LYMPHOCYTES IN VITRO | + | 0 | 1.4000 | WULF, 1980 |
| S | SHL | SCE, HUMAN LYMPHOCYTES IN VITRO | + | 0 | 0.6000 | LARRAMENDY ET AL., 1981 |
| S | SHL | SCE, HUMAN LYMPHOCYTES IN VITRO | + | 0 | 0.1000 | DENG & QU, 1981 |
| S | SHL | SCE, HUMAN LYMPHOCYTES IN VITRO | + | 0 | 0.6000 | ANDERSEN, 1983 |
| C | CHL | CHROM ABERR, HUMAN LYMPHOCYTES IN VITRO | + | 0 | 1.0000 | LARRAMENDY ET AL., 1981 |
| T | TIH | CELL TRANSFORMATION, HUMAN CELLS IN VITRO | + | 0 | 4.0000 | LECHNER ET AL., 1984 |
| T | TIH | CELL TRANSFORMATION, HUMAN CELLS IN VITRO | + | 0 | 0.6000 | BIEDERMANN & LANDOLPH, 1987 |
| C | CBA | CHROM ABERR, ANIMAL BONE MARROW IN VIVO | – | 0 | 1.3000 | MATHUR ET AL., 1978 |
| C | CCC | CHROM ABERR, SPERMATOCYTES | – | 0 | 1.3000 | MATHUR ET AL., 1978 |
| I | ICR | INHIBIT CELL COMMUNICATION, ANIMAL CELLS | + | 0 | 60.0000 | MIKI ET AL., 1987 |

[1]Doses are given as concentrations of the element, not the concentration of the compound.

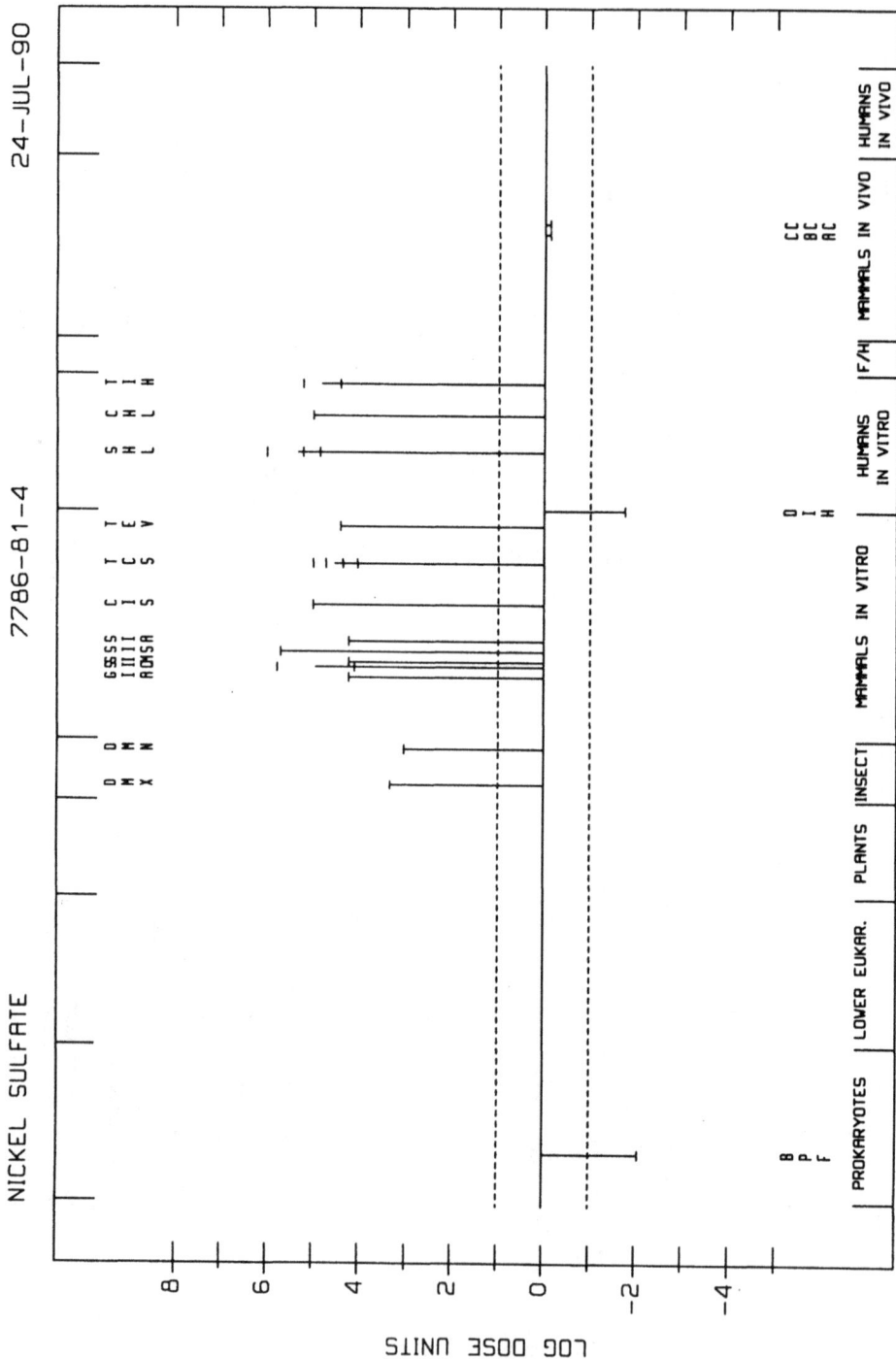

NICKEL SULFATE                    7786-81-4                    24-JUL-90

NICKEL NITRATE

| END POINT | TEST CODE | TEST SYSTEM | RESULTS NM M | DOSE[1] (LED OR HID) | REFERENCE |
|---|---|---|---|---|---|
| D | ERD | E. COLI REC, DIFFERENTIAL TOXICITY | – – | 605.0000 | DE FLORA ET AL., 1984a |
| G | SA0 | S. TYPHIMURIUM TA100, REVERSE MUTATION | – – | 0.0000 | DE FLORA ET AL., 1984a |
| G | SA5 | S. TYPHIMURIUM TA1535, REVERSE MUTATION | – – | 0.0000 | DE FLORA ET AL., 1984a |
| G | SA7 | S. TYPHIMURIUM TA1537, REVERSE MUTATION | – – | 0.0000 | DE FLORA ET AL., 1984a |
| G | SA8 | S. TYPHIMURIUM TA1538, REVERSE MUTATION | – – | 0.0000 | DE FLORA ET AL., 1984a |
| G | SA9 | S. TYPHIMURIUM TA98, REVERSE MUTATION | – – | 0.0000 | DE FLORA ET AL., 1984a |
| G | SAS | S. TYPHIMURIUM (OTHER), REVERSE MUTATION | – – | 0.0000 | DE FLORA ET AL., 1984a |
| G | DMM | D. MELANOGASTER, SOMATIC MUTAT/RECOMB | – 0 | 8.2500 | RASMUSON, 1985 |
| G | DMX | D. MELANOGASTER, SEX-LINKED RECESSIVES | – 0 | 8.2500 | RASMUSON, 1985 |
| G | DMX | D. MELANOGASTER, SEX-LINKED RECESSIVES | – 0 | 407.0000 | VOGEL, 1976 |
| M | MVM | MICRONUCLEUS TEST, MICE IN VIVO | – 0 | 18.0000 | DEKNUDT & LEONARD, 1982 |
| C | DLM | DOMINANT LETHAL TEST, MICE | – 0 | 37.0000 | DEKNUDT & LEONARD, 1982 |
| C | DLM | DOMINANT LETHAL TEST, MICE | – 0 | 18.0000 | JAQUET & MAYENCE, 1982 |

[1]Doses are given as concentrations of the element, not the concentration of the compound.

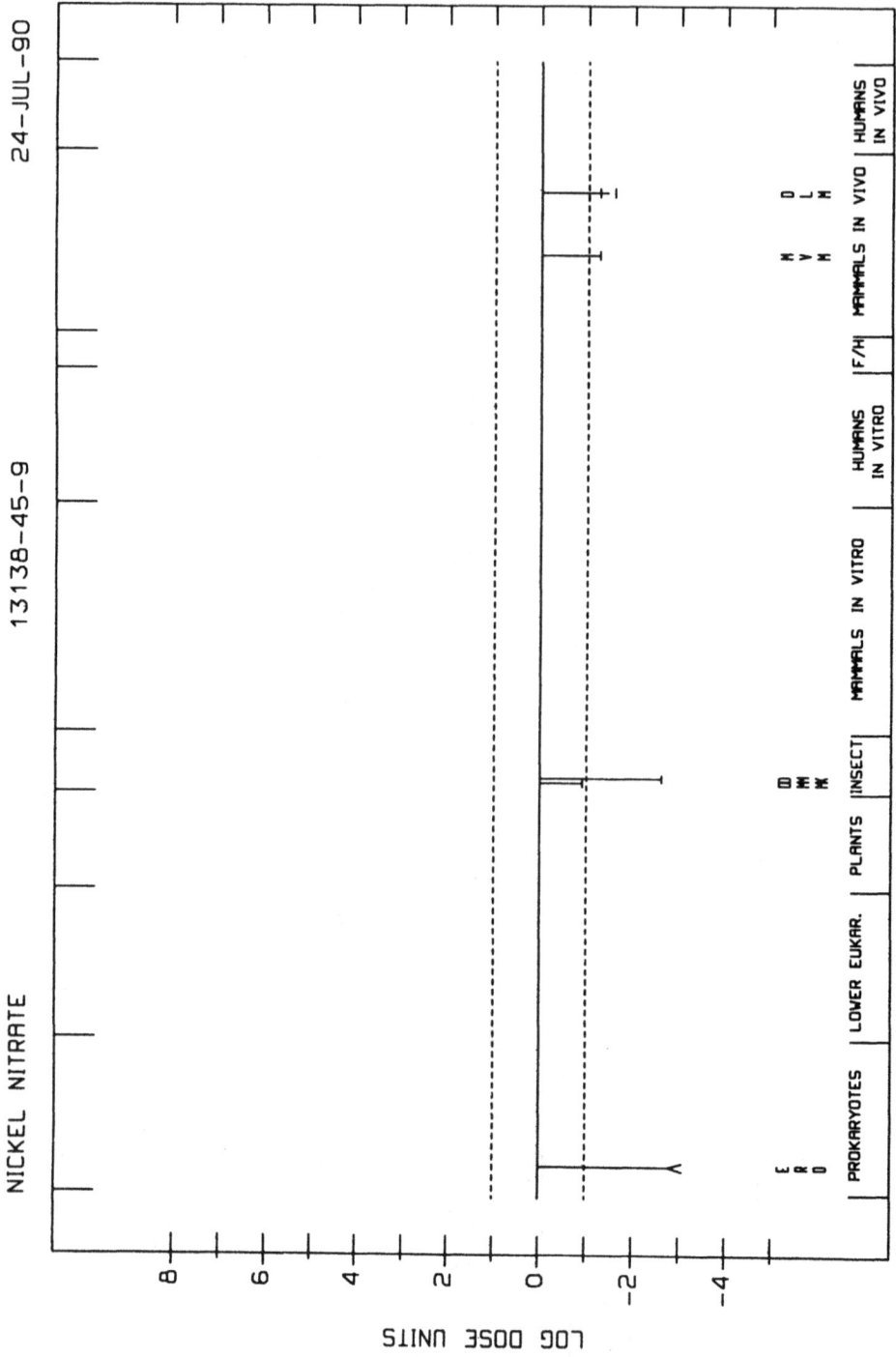

NICKEL NITRATE                13138-45-9                24-JUL-90

LOG DOSE UNITS

NICKEL ACETATE

| END POINT | TEST CODE | TEST SYSTEM | RESULTS NM | M | DOSE[1] (LED OR HID) | REFERENCE |
|---|---|---|---|---|---|---|
| D | PRB | PROPHAGE, INDUCT/SOS/STRAND BREAKS/X-LINKS | (+) | 0 | 9.4000 | ROSSMAN ET AL., 1984 |
| D | ERD | E. COLI REC, DIFFERENTIAL TOXICITY | - | - | 417.0000 | DE FLORA ET AL., 1984a |
| G | SA0 | S. TYPHIMURIUM TA100, REVERSE MUTATION | - | - | 0.0000 | DE FLORA ET AL., 1984a |
| G | SA5 | S. TYPHIMURIUM TA1535, REVERSE MUTATION | - | - | 0.0000 | DE FLORA ET AL., 1984a |
| G | SA7 | S. TYPHIMURIUM TA1537, REVERSE MUTATION | - | - | 0.0000 | DE FLORA ET AL., 1984a |
| G | SA8 | S. TYPHIMURIUM TA1538, REVERSE MUTATION | - | - | 0.0000 | DE FLORA ET AL., 1984a |
| G | SA9 | S. TYPHIMURIUM TA98, REVERSE MUTATION | - | - | 0.0000 | DE FLORA ET AL., 1984a |
| G | SAS | S. TYPHIMURIUM (OTHER), REVERSE MUTATION | - | - | 0.0000 | DE FLORA ET AL., 1984a |
| C | CIT | CHROM ABERR, TRANSFORMED CELLS IN VITRO | + | 0 | 38.0000 | UMEDA & NISHIMURA, 1979 |
| C | CIT | CHROM ABERR, TRANSFORMED CELLS IN VITRO | + | 0 | 35.0000 | NISHIMURA & UMEDA, 1979 |
| T | TCL | CELL TRANSFORMATION, OTHER CELL LINES | + | 0 | 33.0000 | HANSEN & STERN, 1983 |
| T | TIH | CELL TRANSFORMATION, HUMAN CELLS IN VITRO | + | 0 | 0.6000 | BIEDERMANN & LANDOLPH, 1987 |

[1]Doses are given as concentrations of the element, not the concentration of the compound.

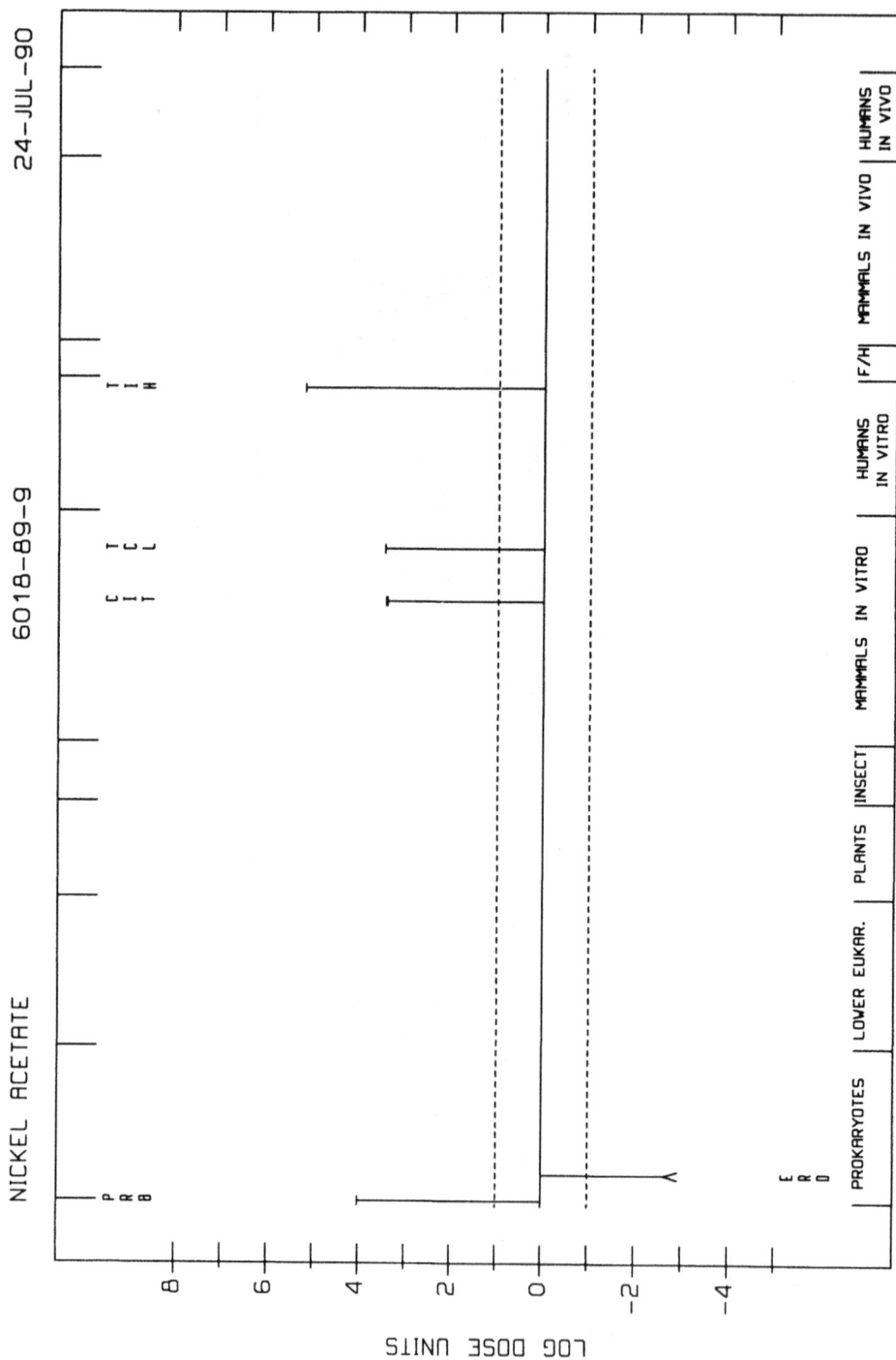

NICKEL ACETATE                6018-89-9                24-JUL-90

NICKEL (OTHER COMPOUNDS)

| END POINT | TEST CODE | TEST SYSTEM | RESULTS NM | M | DOSE[1] (LED OR HID) | REFERENCE |
|---|---|---|---|---|---|---|
| G | SA0 | S. TYPHIMURIUM TA100, REVERSE MUTATION | - | - | 50.0000 | HAWORTH ET AL., 1983[2] |
| G | SA5 | S. TYPHIMURIUM TA1535, REVERSE MUTATION | - | - | 50.0000 | HAWORTH ET AL., 1983[2] |
| G | SA7 | S. TYPHIMURIUM TA1537, REVERSE MUTATION | - | - | 50.0000 | HAWORTH ET AL., 1983[2] |
| G | SA9 | S. TYPHIMURIUM TA98, REVERSE MUTATION | - | - | 167:0000 | HAWORTH ET AL., 1983[2] |
| C | CIT | CHROM ABERR, TRANSFORMED CELLS IN VITRO | + | 0 | 12.0000 | NISHIMURA & UMEDA, 1979[3] |
| T | TCS | CELL TRANSFORMATION, SHE, CLONAL ASSAY | + | 0 | 2.6000 | COSTA & MOLLENHAUER, 1980c[4] |
| D | DVA | STRAND BREAKS/X-LINKS, ANIMALS IN VIVO | + | 0 | 5.0000 | CICCARELLI & WETTERHAHN, 1982[5] |
| D | DVA | STRAND BREAKS/X-LINKS, ANIMALS IN VIVO | + | 0 | 7.5000 | CICCARELLI ET AL., 1981[5] |

[1] Doses are given as concentrations of the element, not the concentration of the compound.
[2] Nickelocene
[3] Nickel potassium cyanide
[4] Nickel subselenide (crystalline)
[5] Nickel carbonate

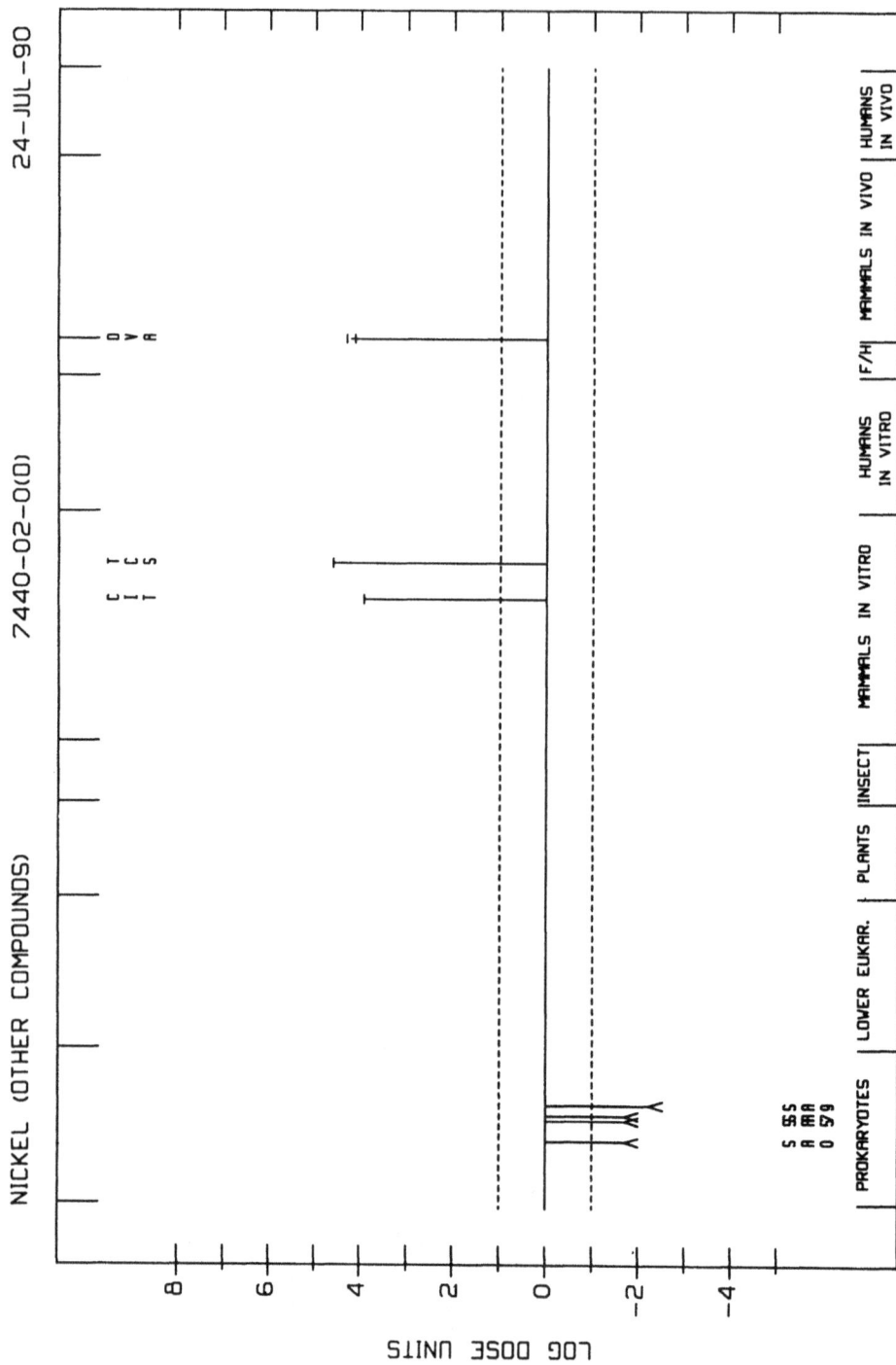

NICKEL (OTHER COMPOUNDS)        7440-02-0(0)        24-JUL-90

LOG DOSE UNITS

MILD STEEL WELDING (METAL INERT GAS)

| END POINT | TEST CODE | TEST SYSTEM | RESULTS NM M | DOSE (LED OR HID) | REFERENCE |
|---|---|---|---|---|---|
| D | ECD | E. COLI POL A, DIFFERENTIAL TOX (SPOT) | – – | 0.0000 | HEDENSTEDT ET AL., 1977 |
| G | SA0 | S. TYPHIMURIUM TA100, REVERSE MUTATION | – – | 0.0000 | HEDENSTEDT ET AL., 1977 |
| G | SA0 | S. TYPHIMURIUM TA100, REVERSE MUTATION | – – | 4000.0000 | MAXILD ET AL., 1978 |
| G | SA0 | S. TYPHIMURIUM TA100, REVERSE MUTATION | – – | 10000.0000 | ETIENNE ET AL., 1986 |
| G | SA2 | S. TYPHIMURIUM TA102, REVERSE MUTATION | – – | 10000.0000 | ETIENNE ET AL., 1986 |
| G | SA9 | S. TYPHIMURIUM TA98, REVERSE MUTATION | – – | 4000.0000 | MAXILD ET AL., 1978 |
| G | SA9 | S. TYPHIMURIUM TA98, REVERSE MUTATION | – – | 10000.0000 | ETIENNE ET AL., 1986 |
| G | SAS | S. TYPHIMURIUM (OTHER), REVERSE MUTATION | – – | 10000.0000 | ETIENNE ET AL., 1986 |
| S | SIC | SCE, CHINESE HAMSTER CELLS IN VITRO | – 0 | 750.0000 | DE RAAT & BAKKER, 1988 |
| C | CIC | CHROM ABERR, CHINESE HAMSTER CELLS IN VITRO | – 0 | 1000.0000 | ETIENNE ET AL., 1986 |
| T | TCL | CELL TRANSFORMATION, OTHER CELL LINES | – 0 | 600.0000 | HANSEN & STERN, 1985 |
| S | SVA | SCE, ANIMALS IN VIVO | – 0 | 26.0000 | ETIENNE ET AL., 1986 |
| C | CBA | CHROM ABERR, ANIMAL BONE MARROW IN VIVO | – 0 | 26.0000 | ETIENNE ET AL., 1986 |
| C | CLA | CHROM ABERR, ANIMAL LEUCOCYTES IN VIVO | – 0 | 26.0000 | ETIENNE ET AL., 1986 |

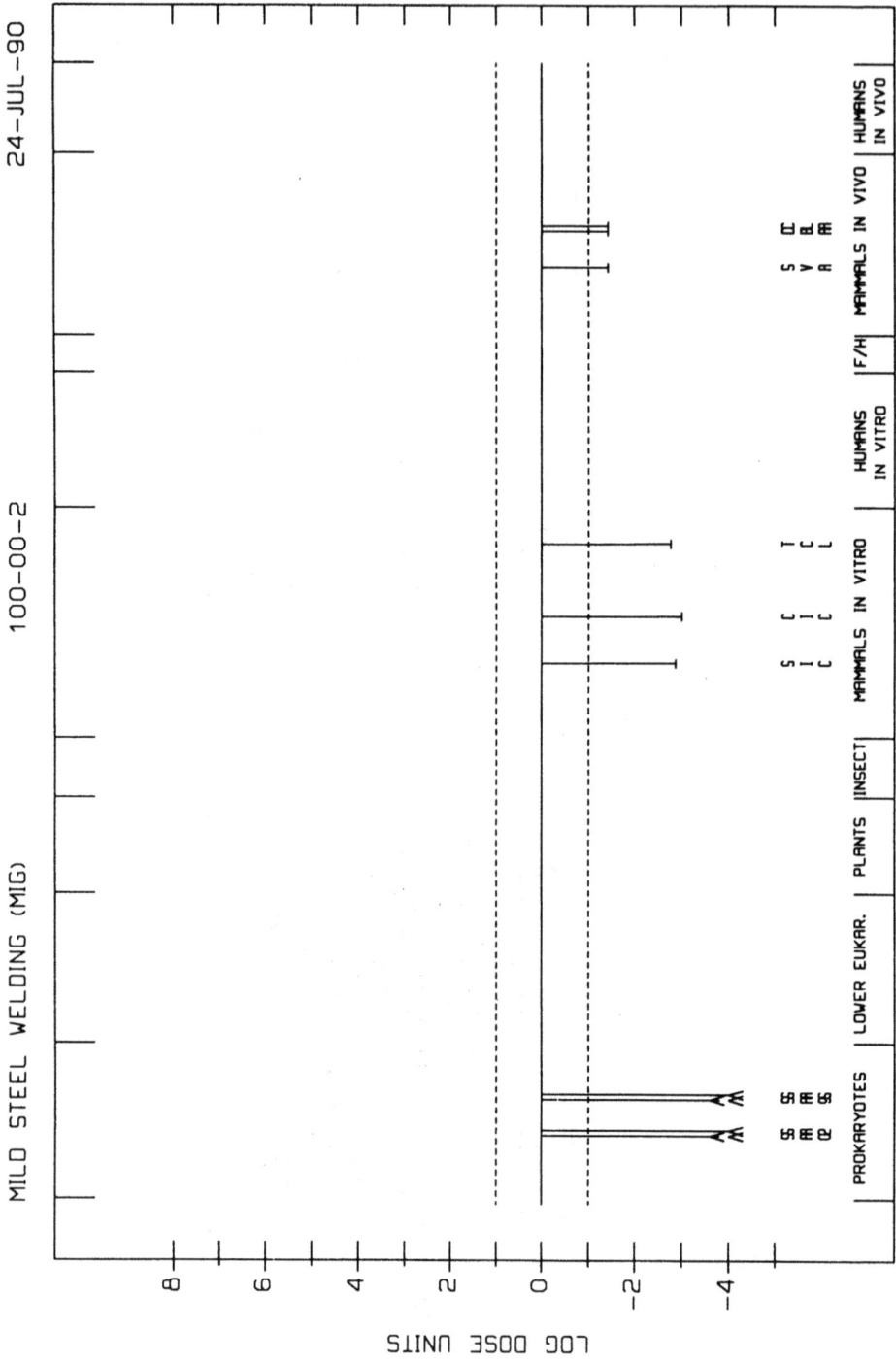

MILD STEEL WELDING (MIG)

24-JUL-90

100-00-2

LOG DOSE UNITS

MILD STEEL WELDING (MANUAL METAL ARC)

| END POINT | TEST CODE | TEST SYSTEM | RESULTS NM M | DOSE (LED OR HID) | REFERENCE |
|---|---|---|---|---|---|
| D | ECD | E. COLI POL A, DIFFERENTIAL TOX (SPOT) | - - | 0.0000 | HEDENSTEDT ET AL., 1977 |
| G | SA0 | S. TYPHIMURIUM TA100, REVERSE MUTATION | - - | 0.0000 | HEDENSTEDT ET AL., 1977 |
| G | SA0 | S. TYPHIMURIUM TA100, REVERSE MUTATION | - - | 4000.0000 | MAXILD ET AL., 1978 |
| G | SA0 | S. TYPHIMURIUM TA100, REVERSE MUTATION | - - | 10000.-0000 | ETIENNE ET AL., 1986 |
| G | SA2 | S. TYPHIMURIUM TA102, REVERSE MUTATION | - - | 10000.0000 | ETIENNE ET AL., 1986 |
| G | SA5 | S. TYPHIMURIUM TA1535, REVERSE MUTATION[1] | + 0 | 0.0000 | BIGGART & RINEHART, 1987 |
| G | SA8 | S. TYPHIMURIUM TA1538, REVERSE MUTATION[2] | (+) 0 | 0.0000 | BIGGART & RINEHART, 1987 |
| G | SA8 | S. TYPHIMURIUM TA1538, REVERSE MUTATION | + + | 50.0000 | BIGGART ET AL., 1987 |
| G | SA9 | S. TYPHIMURIUM TA98, REVERSE MUTATION | - - | 4000.0000 | MAXILD ET AL., 1978 |
| G | SA9 | S. TYPHIMURIUM TA98, REVERSE MUTATION | - - | 10000.0000 | ETIENNE ET AL., 1986 |
| G | SAS | S. TYPHIMURIUM (OTHER), REVERSE MUTATION | - 0 | 10000.0000 | ETIENNE ET AL., 1986 |
| G | GCO | MUTATION, CHO CELLS IN VITRO | + + | 300.0000 | DE RAAT & BAKKER, 1988 |
| S | SIC | SCE, CHINESE HAMSTER CELLS IN VITRO | + 0 | 300.0000 | DE RAAT & BAKKER, 1988 |
| C | CIC | CHROM ABERR, CHINESE HAMSTER CELLS IN VITRO | - 0 | 32.0000 | ETIENNE ET AL., 1986 |
| T | TCL | CELL TRANSFORMATION, OTHER CELL LINES | - 0 | 600.0000 | HANSEN & STERN, 1985 |
| S | SVA | SCE, ANIMALS IN VIVO | - 0 | 39.0000 | ETIENNE ET AL., 1986 |
| C | CBA | CHROM ABERR, ANIMAL BONE MARROW IN VIVO | - 0 | 39.0000 | ETIENNE ET AL., 1986 |
| C | CLA | CHROM ABERR, ANIMAL LEUCOCYTES IN VIVO | - 0 | 39.0000 | ETIENNE ET AL., 1986 |

[1]Gaseous phase only
[2]Particulates only

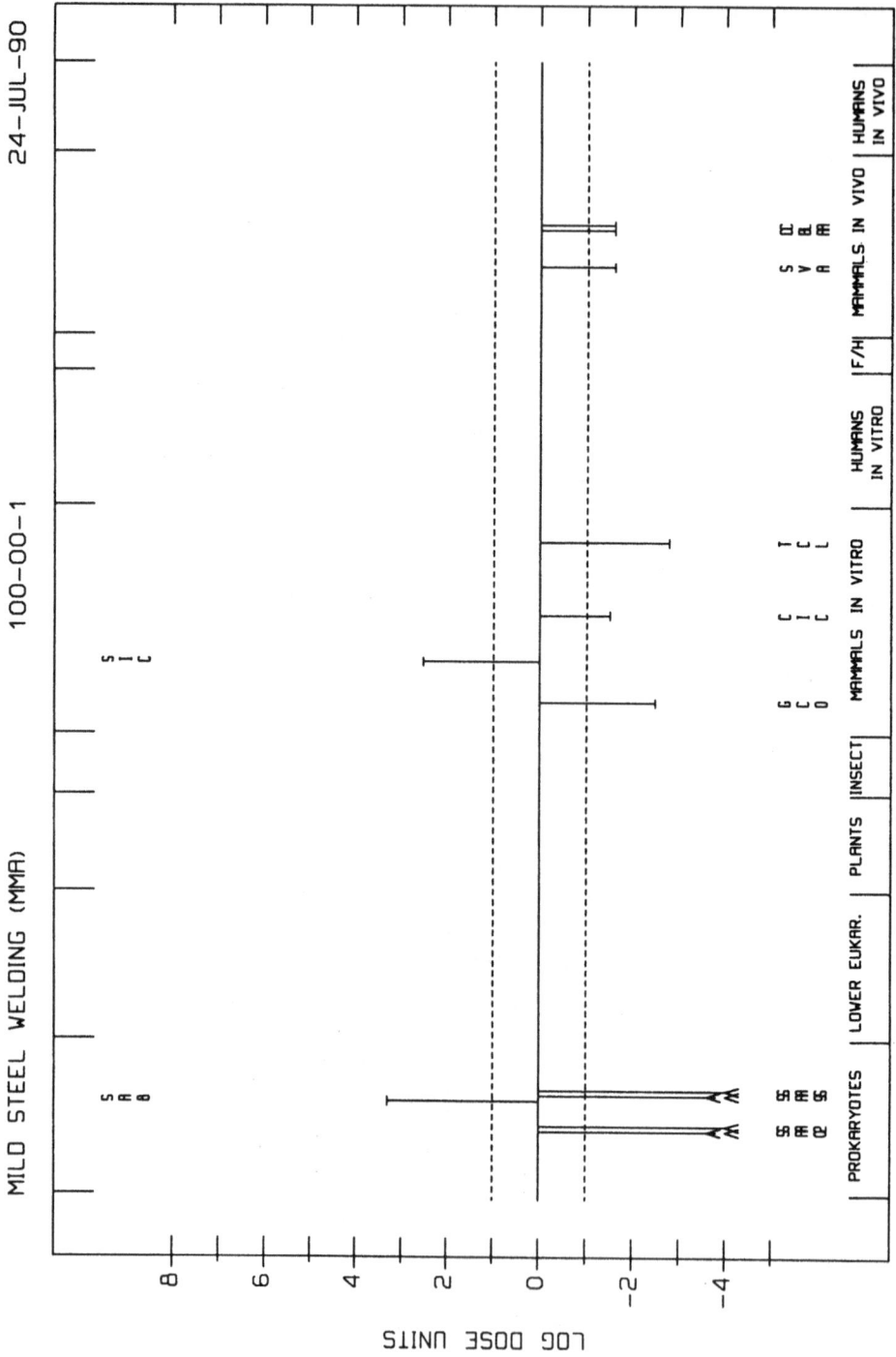

MILD STEEL WELDING (MMA)

100-00-1        24-JUL-90

LOG DOSE UNITS

STAINLESS STEEL WELDING (METAL INERT GAS)

| END POINT | TEST CODE | TEST SYSTEM | RESULTS NM | M | DOSE (LED OR HID) | REFERENCE |
|---|---|---|---|---|---|---|
| D | ECD | E. COLI POL A, DIFFERENTIAL TOX (SPOT) | - | - | 0.0000 | HEDENSTEDT ET AL., 1977 |
| G | SAO | S. TYPHIMURIUM TA100, REVERSE MUTATION | (+) | - | 500.0000 | HEDENSTEDT ET AL., 1977 |
| G | SAO | S. TYPHIMURIUM TA100, REVERSE MUTATION | + | - | 1000.0000 | MAXILD ET AL., 1978 |
| G | SAO | S. TYPHIMURIUM TA100, REVERSE MUTATION | (+) | - | 7500.0000 | ETIENNE ET AL., 1986 |
| G | SA2 | S. TYPHIMURIUM TA102, REVERSE MUTATION | + | + | 5000.0000 | ETIENNE ET AL., 1986 |
| G | SA9 | S. TYPHIMURIUM TA98, REVERSE MUTATION | (+) | (+) | 500.0000 | MAXILD ET AL., 1978 |
| G | SA9 | S. TYPHIMURIUM TA98, REVERSE MUTATION | (+) | - | 10000.0000 | ETIENNE ET AL., 1986 |
| G | SAS | S. TYPHIMURIUM (OTHER), REVERSE MUTATION | (+) | - | 7500.0000 | ETIENNE ET AL., 1986 |
| S | SIC | SCE, CHINESE HAMSTER CELLS IN VITRO | + | 0 | 200.0000 | DE RATT & BAKKER, 1988 |
| S | SIC | SCE, CHINESE HAMSTER CELLS IN VITRO | + | 0 | 50.0000 | KOSHI, 1979 |
| C | CIC | CHROM ABERR, CHINESE HAMSTER CELLS IN VITRO | + | 0 | 50.0000 | KOSHI, 1979 |
| C | CIC | CHROM ABERR, CHINESE HAMSTER CELLS IN VITRO | + | 0 | 320.0000 | ETIENNE ET AL., 1986 |
| T | TFS | CELL TRANSFORMATION, SHE, FOCUS ASSAY | + | 0 | 18.0000 | HANSEN & STERN, 1985 |
| T | TCL | CELL TRANSFORMATION, OTHER CELL LINES | + | 0 | 400.0000 | HANSEN & STERN, 1985 |
| S | SVA | SCE, ANIMALS IN VIVO | - | 0 | 31.0000 | ETIENNE ET AL., 1986 |
| C | CBA | CHROM ABERR, ANIMAL BONE MARROW IN VIVO | - | 0 | 31.0000 | ETIENNE ET AL., 1986 |
| C | CLA | CHROM ABERR, ANIMAL LEUCOCYTES IN VIVO[1] | - | 0 | 31.0000 | ETIENNE ET AL., 1986 |
| S | SLH | SCE, HUMAN LYMPHOCYTES IN VIVO[1] | (+) | 0 | 0.0000 | KOSHI ET AL., 1984 |
| C | CLH | CHROM ABERR, HUMAN LYMPHOCYTES IN VIVO[1] | (+) | 0 | 0.0000 | KOSHI ET AL., 1984 |

[1]Exposure also to Manual Metal Arc

STAINLESS STEEL WELDING (MIG)          100-00-5          24-JUL-90

LOG DOSE UNITS

STAINLESS STEEL WELDING (MANUAL METAL ARC)

| END POINT | TEST CODE | TEST SYSTEM | RESULTS NM | RESULTS M | DOSE (LED OR HID) | REFERENCE |
|---|---|---|---|---|---|---|
| D | ECD | E. COLI POL A, DIFFERENTIAL TOX (SPOT) | + | + | 0.0000 | HEDENSTEDT ET AL., 1977 |
| G | SAO | S. TYPHIMURIUM TA100, REVERSE MUTATION | + | - | 100.0000 | HEDENSTEDT ET AL., 1977 |
| G | SAO | S. TYPHIMURIUM TA100, REVERSE MUTATION | + | + | 100.0000 | MAXILD ET AL., 1978 |
| G | SAO | S. TYPHIMURIUM TA100, REVERSE MUTATION | + | + | 250.0000 | ETIENNE ET AL., 1986 |
| G | SA2 | S. TYPHIMURIUM TA102, REVERSE MUTATION | + | - | 50.0000 | ETIENNE ET AL., 1986 |
| G | SA9 | S. TYPHIMURIUM TA98, REVERSE MUTATION | + | + | 100.0000 | HEDENSTEDT ET AL., 1977 |
| G | SA9 | S. TYPHIMURIUM TA98, REVERSE MUTATION | + | - | 100.0000 | MAXILD ET AL., 1978 |
| G | SA9 | S. TYPHIMURIUM TA98, REVERSE MUTATION | + | + | 125.0000 | ETIENNE ET AL., 1986 |
| G | SAS | S. TYPHIMURIUM (OTHER), REVERSE MUTATION | ? | + | 125.0000 | ETIENNE ET AL., 1986 |
| G | GCO | MUTATION, CHO CELLS IN VITRO | ? | 0 | 10.0000 | ETIENNE ET AL., 1986 |
| G | G9H | MUTATION, CHL V79 CELLS, HPRT | + | 0 | 10.0000 | HEDENSTEDT ET AL., 1977 |
| G | G9H | MUTATION, CHL V79 CELLS, HPRT | + | 0 | 3.0000 | ETIENNE ET AL., 1986 |
| S | SIC | SCE, CHINESE HAMSTER CELLS IN VITRO | + | 0 | 3.5000 | DE RAIT & BAKKER, 1988 |
| S | SIC | SCE, CHINESE HAMSTER CELLS IN VITRO | + | 0 | 0.7000 | BAKER ET AL., 1986 |
| S | SIC | SCE, CHINESE HAMSTER CELLS IN VITRO | + | 0 | 1.0000 | KOSHI, 1979 |
| C | CIC | CHROM ABERR, CHINESE HAMSTER CELLS IN VITRO | + | 0 | 1.0000 | KOSHI, 1979 |
| C | CIC | CHROM ABERR, CHINESE HAMSTER CELLS IN VITRO | + | 0 | 0.3200 | ETIENNE ET AL., 1986 |
| T | TFS | CELL TRANSFORMATION, SHE, FOCUS ASSAY | + | 0 | 5.0000 | HANSEN & STERN, 1985 |
| T | TCL | CELL TRANSFORMATION, OTHER CELL LINES | + | 0 | 50.0000 | HANSEN & STERN, 1985 |
| G | MST | MOUSE SPOT TEST | + | 0 | 100.0000 | KNUDSON, 1980 |
| S | SVA | SCE, ANIMALS IN VIVO | - | 0 | 18.0000 | ETIENNE ET AL., 1986 |
| C | CBA | CHROM ABERR, ANIMAL BONE MARROW IN VIVO | - | 0 | 18.0000 | ETIENNE ET AL., 1986 |
| C | CLA | CHROM ABERR, ANIMAL LEUCOCYTES IN VIVO | - | 0 | 18.0000 | ETIENNE ET AL., 1986 |
| S | SLH | SCE, HUMAN LYMPHOCYTES IN VIVO | (+) | 0 | 0.0000 | HUSGAFVEL-PURSIANEN ET AL., 1982 |
| S | SLH | SCE, HUMAN LYMPHOCYTES IN VIVO | - | 0 | 0.0000 | LITTORIN ET AL., 1983 |
| S | SLH | SCE, HUMAN LYMPHOCYTES IN VIVO[1] | - | 0 | 0.0000 | KOSHI ET AL., 1984 |
| M | MVH | MICRONUCLEUS TEST, HUMAN CELLS IN VIVO | - | 0 | 0.0000 | HUSGAFVEL-PURSIANEN ET AL., 1982 |
| C | CLH | CHROM ABERR, HUMAN LYMPHOCYTES IN VIVO | - | 0 | 0.0000 | LITTORIN ET AL., 1983 |
| C | CLH | CHROM ABERR, HUMAN LYMPHOCYTES IN VIVO | - | 0 | 0.0000 | LITTORIN ET AL., 1983 |
| C | CLH | CHROM ABERR, HUMAN LYMPHOCYTES IN VIVO[1] | (+) | 0 | 0.0000 | KOSHI ET AL., 1984 |

[1] Exposure also to Metal Inert Gas

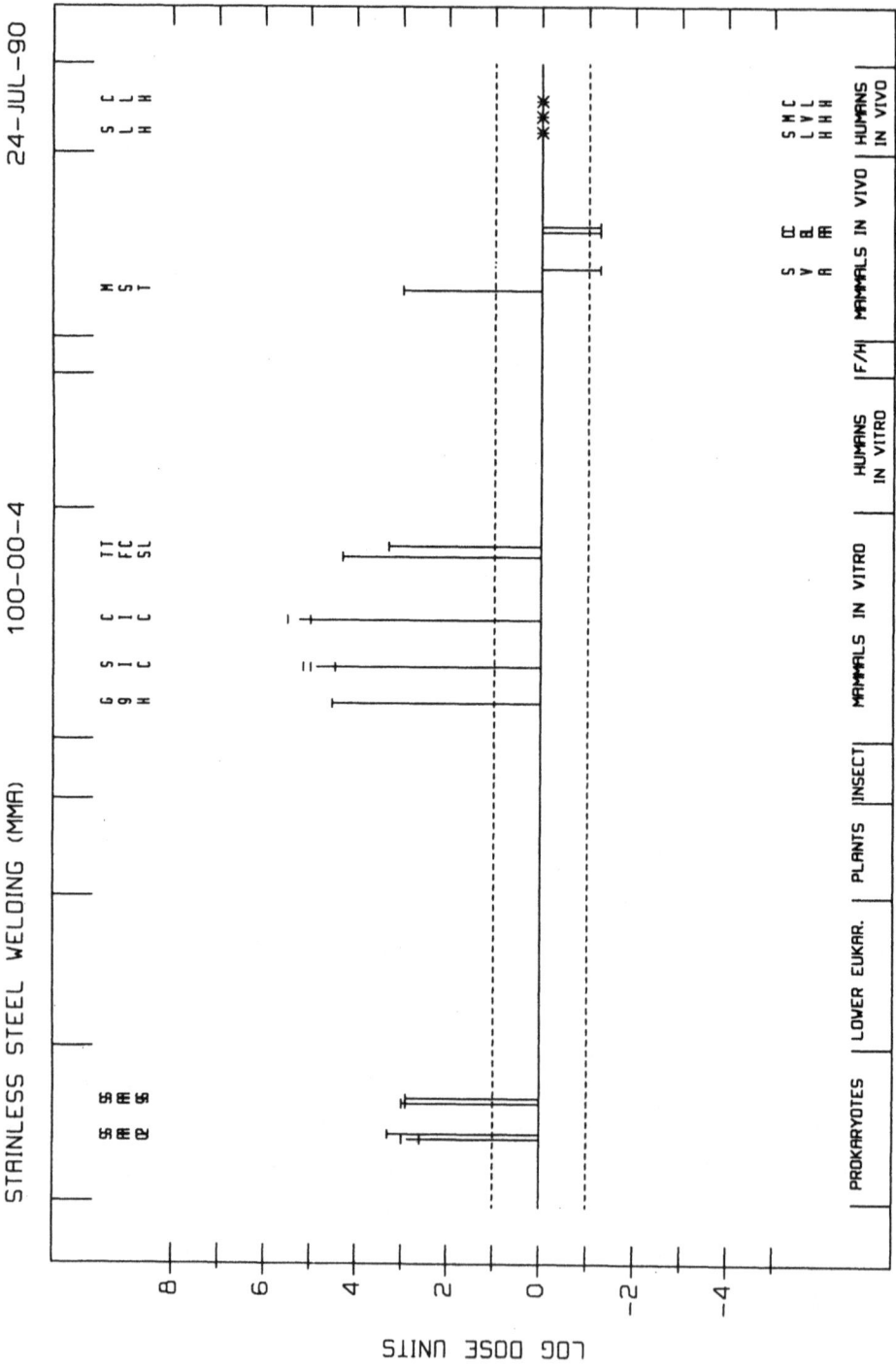

STAINLESS STEEL WELDING (MMA)          100-00-4          24-JUL-90

LOG DOSE UNITS

MILD STEEL & CAST IRON WELDING WITH NICKEL-RICH ELECTRODES

| END POINT | TEST CODE | TEST SYSTEM | RESULTS NM M | DOSE (LED OR HID) | REFERENCE |
|---|---|---|---|---|---|
| G | SA0 | S. TYPHIMURIUM TA100, REVERSE MUTATION | - - | 10000.0000 | ETIENNE ET AL., 1986 |
| G | SA2 | S. TYPHIMURIUM TA102, REVERSE MUTATION | - - | 10000.0000 | ETIENNE ET AL., 1986 |
| G | SA9 | S. TYPHIMURIUM TA98, REVERSE MUTATION | - - | 10000.0000 | ETIENNE ET AL., 1986 |
| G | SAS | S. TYPHIMURIUM (OTHER), REVERSE MUTATION | - - | 10000.0000 | ETIENNE ET AL., 1986 |
| G | GCO | MUTATION, CHO CELLS IN VITRO | - 0 | 100.0000 | ETIENNE ET AL., 1986 |
| C | CIC | CHROM ABERR, CHINESE HAMSTER CELLS IN VITRO | - 0 | 320.0000 | ETIENNE ET AL., 1986 |
| T | TCL | CELL TRANSFORMATION, OTHER CELL LINES | + 0 | 100.0000 | HANSEN & STERN, 1984 |
| S | SIH | SCE, OTHER HUMAN CELLS IN VITRO | + 0 | 0.0000 | NIEBUHR ET AL., 1980 |
| S | SVA | SCE, ANIMALS IN VIVO | - 0 | 10.0000 | ETIENNE ET AL., 1986 |
| C | CBA | CHROM ABERR, ANIMAL BONE MARROW IN VIVO | - 0 | 10.0000 | ETIENNE ET AL., 1986 |
| C | CLA | CHROM ABERR, ANIMAL LEUCOCYTES IN VIVO | - 0 | 10.0000 | ETIENNE ET AL., 1986 |

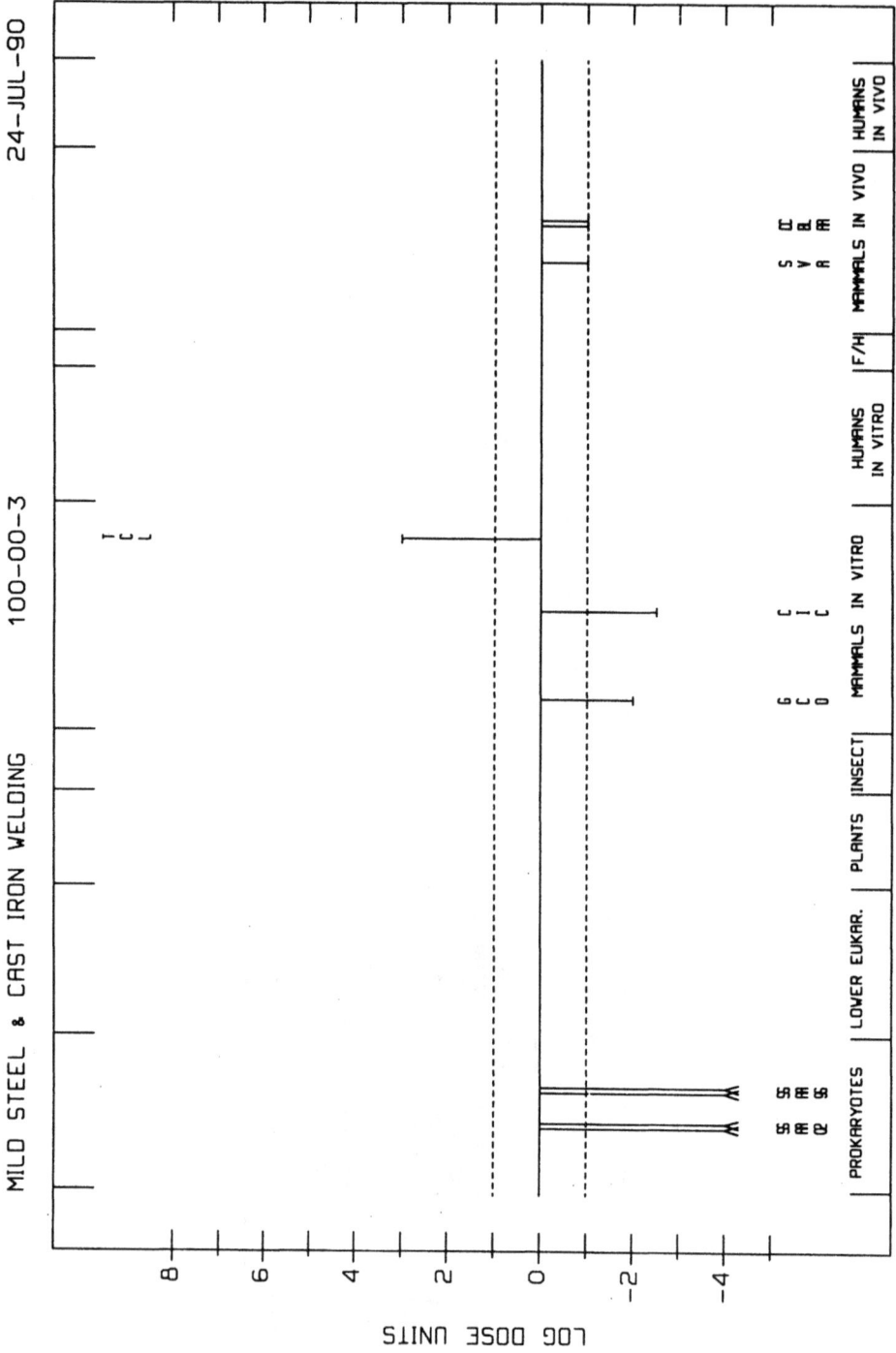

MILD STEEL & CAST IRON WELDING

100-00-3

24-JUL-90

LOG DOSE UNITS

# CUMULATIVE CROSS INDEX TO *IARC MONOGRAPHS ON THE EVALUATION OF CARCINOGENIC RISKS TO HUMANS*

The volume, page and year are given. References to corrigenda are given in parentheses.

## A

| | |
|---|---|
| A-α–C | *40*, 245 (1986); *Suppl. 7*, 56 (1987) |
| Acetaldehyde | *36*, 101 (1985) (*corr. 42*, 263); *Suppl. 7*, 77 (1987) |
| Acetaldehyde formylmethylhydrazone (*see* Gyromitrin) | |
| Acetamide | *7*, 197 (1974); *Suppl. 7*, 389 (1987) |
| Acridine orange | *16*, 145 (1978); *Suppl. 7*, 56 (1987) |
| Acriflavinium chloride | *13*, 31 (1977); *Suppl. 7*, 56 (1987) |
| Acrolein | *19*, 479 (1979); *36*,133 (1985); *Suppl. 7*, 78 (1987); |
| Acrylamide | *39*, 41 (1986); *Suppl. 7*, 56 (1987) |
| Acrylic acid | *19*, 47 (1979); *Suppl. 7*, 56 (1987) |
| Acrylic fibres | *19*, 86 (1979); *Suppl. 7*, 56 (1987) |
| Acrylonitrile | *19*, 73 (1979); *Suppl. 7*, 79 (1987) |
| Acrylonitrile-butadiene-styrene copolymers | *19*, 91 (1979); *Suppl. 7*, 56 (1987) |
| Actinolite (*see* Asbestos) | |
| Actinomycins | *10*, 29 (1976) (*corr. 42*, 255); *Suppl. 7*, 80 (1987) |
| Adriamycin | *10*, 43 (1976); *Suppl. 7*, 82 (1987) |
| AF–2 | *31*, 47 (1983); *Suppl. 7*, 56 (1987) |
| Aflatoxins | *1*, 145 (1972) (*corr. 42*, 251); *10*, 51 (1976); *Suppl. 7*, 83 (1987) |
| Aflatoxin $B_1$ (*see* Aflatoxins) | |
| Aflatoxin $B_2$ (*see* Aflatoxins) | |
| Aflatoxin $G_1$ (*see* Aflatoxins) | |
| Aflatoxin $G_2$ (*see* Aflatoxins) | |
| Aflatoxin $M_1$ (*see* Aflatoxins) | |
| Agaritine | *31*, 63 (1983); *Suppl. 7*, 56 (1987) |
| Alcohol drinking | *44* |

Aldrin                                                    *5*, 25 (1974); *Suppl. 7*, 88 (1987)
Allyl chloride                                            *36*, 39 (1985); *Suppl. 7*, 56 (1987)
Allyl isothiocyanate                                     *36*, 55 (1985); *Suppl. 7*, 56 (1987)
Allyl isovalerate                                        *36*, 69 (1985); *Suppl. 7*, 56 (1987)
Aluminium production                                     *34*, 37 (1984); *Suppl. 7*, 89 (1987)
Amaranth                                                 *8*, 41 (1975); *Suppl. 7*, 56 (1987)
5-Aminoacenaphthene                                     *16*, 243 (1978); *Suppl. 7*, 56 (1987)
2-Aminoanthraquinone                                    *27*, 191 (1982); *Suppl. 7*, 56 (1987)
*para*-Aminoazobenzene                                  *8*, 53 (1975); *Suppl. 7*, 390 (1987)
*ortho*-Aminoazotoluene                                 *8*, 61 (1975) (*corr. 42*, 254); Suppl..
                                                         7, 56 (1987)

*para*-Aminobenzoic acid                                *16*, 249 (1978); *Suppl. 7*, 56 (1987)
4-Aminobiphenyl                                          *1*, 74 (1972) (*corr. 42*, 251); Suppl.
                                                         7, 91 (1987)

2-Amino-3,4-dimethylimidazo[4,5-*f*]quinoline (*see* MeIQ)
2-Amino-3,8-dimethylimidazo[4,5-*f*]quinoxaline (*see* MeIQx)
3-Amino-1,4-dimethyl-5*H*-pyrido[4,3-*b*]indole (*see* Trp-P-1)
2-Aminodipyrido[1,2-*a*:3′,2′-*d*]imidazole (*see* Glu-P-2)
1-Amino-2-methylanthraquinone                           *27*, 199 (1982); *Suppl. 7*, 57 (1987)
2-Amino-3-methylimidazo[4,5-*f*]quinoline (*see* IQ)
2-Amino-6-methyldipyrido[1,2-*a*:3′,2′-*d*]-imidazole (*see* Glu-P-1)
2-Amino-3-methyl-9*H*-pyrido[2,3-*b*]indole (*see* MeA-α-C)
3-Amino-1-methyl-5*H*-pyrido[4,3-*b*]indole (*see* Trp-P-2)
2-Amino-5-(5-nitro-2-furyl)-1,3,4-thiadiazole           *7*, 143 (1974); *Suppl. 7*, 57 (1987)
4-Amino-2-nitrophenol                                   *16*, 43 (1978); *Suppl.7*, 57 (1987)
2-Amino-5-nitrothiazole                                 *31*, 71 (1983); *Suppl. 7*, 57 (1987)
2-Amino-9*H*-pyrido[2,3-*b*]indole [*see* A-α-C)
11-Aminoundecanoic acid                                 *39*, 239 (1986); *Suppl. 7*, 57 (1987)
Amitrole                                                 *7*, 31 (1974); *41*, 293 (1986)
                                                         *Suppl. 7*, 92 (1987)

Ammonium potassium selenide (*see* Selenium and selenium
   compounds)
Amorphous silica (*see also* Silica)                    *Suppl. 7*, 341 (1987)
Amosite (*see* Asbestos)
Anabolic steroids (*see* Androgenic (anabolic) steroids)
Anaesthetics, volatile                                  *11*, 285 (1976); *Suppl. 7*, 93 (1987)
Analgesic mixtures containing phenacetin (*see also* Phenacetin)  *Suppl. 7*, 310 (1987)
Androgenic (anabolic) steroids                          *Suppl. 7*, 96 (1987)
Angelicin and some synthetic derivatives (*see also* Angelicins)  *40*, 291 (1986)
Angelicin plus ultraviolet radiation (*see also* Angelicin and some  *Suppl. 7*, 57 (1987)
   synthetic derivatives)
Angelicins                                               *Suppl. 7*, 57 (1987)
Aniline                                                  *4*, 27 (1974) (*corr. 42*, 252); *27*, 39
                                                         (1982); *Suppl. 7*, 99 (1987)

*ortho*-Anisidine                                        *27*, 63 (1982); *Suppl. 7*, 57 (1987)

## B

| | |
|---|---|
| Benz[*a*]anthracene | *3*, 45 (1973); *32*, 135 (1983); *Suppl. 7*, 58 (1987) |
| Benzene | *7*, 203 (1974) (*corr. 42*, 254); *29*, 93, 391 (1982); *Suppl. 7*, 120 (1987) |
| Benzidine | *1*, 80 (1972); *29*, 149, 391 (1982); *Suppl. 7*, 123 (1987) |
| Benzidine–based dyes | *Suppl. 7*, 125 (1987) |
| Benzo[*b*]fluoranthene | *3*, 69 (1973); *32*, 147 (1983); *Suppl. 7*, 58 (1987) |
| Benzo[*j*]fluoranthene | *3*, 82 (1973); *32*, 155 (1983); *Suppl. 7*, 58 (1987) |
| Benzo[*k*]fluoranthene | *32*, 163 (1983); *Suppl. 7*, 58 (1987) |
| Benzo[*ghi*]fluoranthene | *32*, 171 (1983); *Suppl. 7*, 58 (1987) |
| Benzo[*a*]fluorene | *32*, 177 (1983); *Suppl. 7*, 58 (1987) |
| Benzo[*b*]fluorene | *32*, 183 (1983); *Suppl. 7*, 58 (1987) |
| Benzo[*c*]fluorene | *32*, 189 (1983); *Suppl. 7*, 58 (1987) |
| Benzo[*ghi*]perylene | *32*, 195 (1983); *Suppl. 7*, 58 (1987) |
| Benzo[*c*]phenanthrene | *32*, 205 (1983); *Suppl. 7*, 58 (1987) |
| Benzo[*a*]pyrene | *3*, 91 (1973); *32*, 211 (1983); *Suppl. 7*, 58 (1987) |
| Benzo[*e*]pyrene | *3*, 137 (1973); *32*, 225 (1983); *Suppl. 7*, 58 (1987) |
| *para*-Benzoquinone dioxime | *29*, 185 (1982); *Suppl. 7*, 58 (1987) |
| Benzotrichloride (*see also* α–Chlorinated toluenes) | *29*, 73 (1982); *Suppl. 7*, 148 (1987) |
| Benzoyl chloride | *29*, 83 (1982) (*corr. 42*, 261); *Suppl. 7*, 126 (1987) |
| Benzoyl peroxide | *36*, 267 (1985); *Suppl. 7*, 58 (1987) |
| Benzyl acetate | *40*, 109 (1986); *Suppl. 7*, 58 (1987) |
| Benzyl chloride (*see also* α–Chlorinated toluenes) | *11*, 217 (1976) (*corr. 42*, 256); *29*, 49 (1982); *Suppl. 7*, 148 (1987) |
| Benzyl violet 4B | *16*, 153 (1978); *Suppl. 7*, 58 (1987) |
| Bertrandite (*see* Beryllium and beryllium compounds) | |
| Beryllium and beryllium compounds | *1*, 17 (1972); *23*, 143 (1980) (*corr. 42*, 260); *Suppl. 7*, 127 (1987) |

Beryllium acetate (*see* Beryllium and beryllium compounds)
Beryllium acetate, basic (*see* Beryllium and beryllium compounds)
Beryllium–aluminium alloy (*see* Beryllium and beryllium compounds)
Beryllium carbonate (*see* Beryllium and beryllium compounds)
Beryllium chloride (*see* Beryllium and beryllium compounds)
Beryllium–copper alloy (*see* Beryllium and beryllium compounds)
Beryllium–copper–cobalt alloy (*see* Beryllium and beryllium compounds)
Beryllium fluoride (*see* Beryllium and beryllium compounds)
Beryllium hydroxide (*see* Beryllium and beryllium compounds)
Beryllium–nickel alloy (*see* Beryllium and beryllium compounds)

# C

Cadmium chloride (*see* Cadmium and cadmium compounds)
Cadmium oxide (*see* Cadmium and cadmium compounds)
Cadmium sulphate (*see* Cadmium and cadmium compounds)
Cadmium sulphide (*see* Cadmium and cadmium compounds)
Calcium arsenate (*see* Arsenic and arsenic compounds)
Calcium chromate (*see* Chromium and chromium compounds)
Calcium cyclamate (*see* Cyclamates)
Calcium saccharin (*see* Saccharin)

| | |
|---|---|
| Cantharidin | *10*, 79 (1976); *Suppl. 7*, 59 (1987) |
| Caprolactam | *19*, 115 (1979) *(corr. 42*, 258); *39*, 247 (1986) *(corr. 42*, 264); *Suppl. 7*, 390 (1987) |
| Captan | *30*, 295 (1983); *Suppl. 7*, 59 (1987) |
| Carbaryl | *12*, 37 (1976); *Suppl. 7*, 59 (1987) |
| Carbazole | *32*, 239 (1983); *Suppl. 7*, 59 (1987) |
| 3–Carbethoxypsoralen | *40*, 317 (1986); *Suppl. 7*, 59 (1987) |
| Carbon blacks | *3*, 22 (1973); *33*, 35 (1984); *Suppl. 7*, 142 (1987) |
| Carbon tetrachloride | *1*, 53 (1972); *20*, 371 (1979); *Suppl. 7*, 143 (1987) |
| Carmoisine | *8*, 83 (1975); *Suppl. 7*, 59 (1987) |
| Carpentry and joinery | *25*, 139 (1981); *Suppl. 7*, 378 (1987) |
| Carrageenan | *10*, 181 (1976) *(corr. 42*, 255); *31*, 79 (1983); *Suppl. 7*, 59 (1987) |
| Catechol | *15*, 155 (1977); *Suppl. 7*, 59 (1987) |

CCNU (*see* 1–(2–Chloroethyl)–3–cyclohexyl–1–nitrosourea)
Ceramic fibres (*see* Man–made mineral fibres)
Chemotherapy, combined, including alkylating agents
    (*see* MOPP and other combined chemotherapy including
    alkylating agents)

| | |
|---|---|
| Chlorambucil | *9*, 125 (1975); *26*, 115 (1981); *Suppl. 7*, 144 (1987) |
| Chloramphenicol | *10*, 85 (1976); *Suppl. 7*, 145 (1987) |
| Chlorendic acid | *48*, 45 (1990) |
| Chlordane (*see also* Chlordane/Heptachlor) | *20*, 45 (1979) *(corr. 42*, 258) |
| Chlordane/Heptachlor | *Suppl. 7*, 146 (1987) |
| Chlordecone | *20*, 67 (1979); *Suppl. 7*, 59 (1987) |
| Chlordimeform | *30*, 61 (1983); *Suppl. 7*, 59 (1987) |
| Chlorinated dibenzodioxins (other than TCDD) | *15*, 41 (1977); *Suppl. 7*, 59 (1987) |
| Chlorinated paraffins | *48*, 55 (1990) |
| α–Chlorinated toluenes | *Suppl. 7*, 148 (1987) |
| Chlormadinone acetate (*see also* Progestins; Combined oral contraceptives) | *6*, 149 (1974); *21*, 365 (1979) |

Chlornaphazine (*see* N,N–Bis(2–chloroethyl)–2–naphthylamine)

| | |
|---|---|
| Chlorobenzilate | *5*, 75 (1974); *30*, 73 (1983); |

# D

| | |
|---|---|
| Dibenzo[*a,i*]pyrene | *3*, 215 (1973); *32*, 337 (1983); *Suppl. 7*, 62 (1987) |
| Dibenzo[*a,l*]pyrene | *3*, 224 (1973); *32*, 343 (1983); *Suppl. 7*, 62 (1987) |
| 1,2–Dibromo–3–chloropropane | *15*, 139 (1977); *20*, 83 (1979); *Suppl. 7*, 191 (1987) |
| Dichloroacetylene | *39*, 369 (1986); *Suppl. 7*, 62 (1987) |
| *ortho*–Dichlorobenzene | *7*, 231 (1974); *29*, 213 (1982); *Suppl. 7*, 192 (1987) |
| *para*–Dichlorobenzene | *7*, 231 (1974); *29*, 215 (1982); *Suppl. 7*, 192 (1987) |
| 3,3′–Dichlorobenzidine | *4*, 49 (1974); *29*, 239 (1982); *Suppl. 7*, 193 (1987) |
| *trans*–1,4–Dichlorobutene | *15*, 149 (1977); *Suppl. 7*, 62 (1987) |
| 3,3′–Dichloro–4,4′–diaminodiphenyl ether | *16*, 309 (1978); *Suppl. 7*, 62 (1987) |
| 1,2–Dichloroethane | *20*, 429 (1979); *Suppl. 7*, 62 (1987) |
| Dichloromethane | *20*, 449 (1979); *41*, 43 (1986); *Suppl. 7*, 194 (1987) |
| 2,4–Dichlorophenol (*see* Chlorophenols; Chlorophenols, occupational exposures to) | |
| (2,4–Dichlorophenoxy)acetic acid (*see* 2,4–D) | |
| 2,6–Dichloro–*para*–phenylenediamine | *39*, 325 (1986); *Suppl. 7*, 62 (1987) |
| 1,2–Dichloropropane | *41*, 131 (1986); *Suppl. 7*, 62 (1987) |
| 1,3–Dichloropropene (technical–grade) | *41*, 113 (1986); *Suppl. 7*, 195 (1987) |
| Dichlorvos | *20*, 97 (1979); *Suppl. 7*, 62 (1987) |
| Dicofol | *30*, 87 (1983); *Suppl. 7*, 62 (1987) |
| Dicyclohexylamine (*see* Cyclamates) | |
| Dieldrin | *5*, 125 (1974); *Suppl. 7*, 196 (1987) |
| Dienoestrol (*see also* Nonsteroidal oestrogens) | *21*, 161 (1979) |
| Diepoxybutane | *11*, 115 (1976) (*corr. 42*, 255); *Suppl. 7*, 62 (1987) |
| Diesel and gasoline engine exhausts | *46*, 41 (1989) |
| Diesel fuels | *45*, 219 (1989) (*corr. 47*, 505) |
| Diethyl ether (*see* Anaesthetics, volatile) | |
| Di(2–ethylhexyl)adipate | *29*, 257 (1982); *Suppl. 7*, 62 (1987) |
| Di(2–ethylhexyl)phthalate | *29*, 269 (1982) (*corr. 42*, 261); *Suppl. 7*, 62 (1987) |
| 1,2–Diethylhydrazine | *4*, 153 (1974); *Suppl. 7*, 62 (1987) |
| Diethylstilboestrol | *6*, 55 (1974); *21*, 173 (1979) (*corr. 42*, 259); *Suppl. 7*, 273 (1987) |
| Diethylstilboestrol dipropionate (*see* Diethylstilboestrol) | |
| Diethyl sulphate | *4*, 277 (1974); *Suppl. 7*, 198 (1987) |
| Diglycidyl resorcinol ether | *11*, 125 (1976); *36*, 181 (1985); *Suppl. 7*, 62 (1987) |

Dulcin                                              *12*, 97 (1976); *Suppl. 7*, 63 (1987)


# E

Endrin                                              *5*, 157 (1974); *Suppl. 7*, 63 (1987)
Enflurane (*see* Anaesthetics, volatile)
Eosin                                               *15*, 183 (1977); *Suppl. 7*, 63 (1987)
Epichlorohydrin                                     *11*, 131 (1976) (*corr. 42*, 256);
                                                    *Suppl. 7*, 202 (1987)
1,2-Epoxybutane                                     *47*, 217 (1989)
1-Epoxyethyl-3,4-epoxycyclohexane                   *11*, 141 (1976); *Suppl. 7*, 63 (1987)
3,4-Epoxy-6-methylcyclohexylmethyl-3,4-epoxy-6-methyl-   *11*, 147 (1976); *Suppl. 7*, 63 (1987)
  cyclohexane carboxylate
*cis*-9,10-Epoxystearic acid                        *11*, 153 (1976); *Suppl. 7*, 63 (1987)
Erionite                                            *42*, 225 (1987); *Suppl. 7*, 203 (1987)
Ethinyloestradiol (*see also* Steroidal oestrogens)  *6*, 77 (1974); *21*, 233 (1979)
Ethionamide                                         *13*, 83 (1977); *Suppl. 7*, 63 (1987)
Ethyl acrylate                                      *19*, 57 (1979); *39*, 81 (1986);
                                                    *Suppl. 7*, 63 (1987)
Ethylene                                            *19*, 157 (1979); *Suppl. 7*, 63 (1987)
Ethylene dibromide                                  *15*, 195 (1977); *Suppl. 7*, 204 (1987)
Ethylene oxide                                      *11*, 157 (1976); *36*, 189 (1985)
                                                    (*corr. 42*, 263); *Suppl. 7*, 205 (1987)
Ethylene sulphide                                   *11*, 257 (1976); *Suppl. 7*, 63 (1987)
Ethylene thiourea                                   *7*, 45 (1974); *Suppl. 7*, 207 (1987)
Ethyl methanesulphonate                             *7*, 245 (1974); *Suppl. 7*, 63 (1987)
*N*-Ethyl-*N*-nitrosourea                           *1*, 135 (1972); *17*, 191 (1978);
                                                    *Suppl. 7*, 63 (1987)
Ethyl selenac (*see also* Selenium and selenium compounds)  *12*, 107 (1976); *Suppl. 7*, 63 (1987)
Ethyl tellurac                                      *12*, 115 (1976); *Suppl. 7*, 63 (1987)
Ethynodiol diacetate (*see also* Progestins; Combined oral   *6*, 173 (1974); *21*, 387 (1979)
  contraceptives)
Eugenol                                             *36*, 75 (1985); *Suppl. 7*, 63 (1987)
Evans blue                                          *8*, 151 (1975); *Suppl. 7*, 63 (1987)


# F

Fast Green FCF                                      *16*, 187 (1978); *Suppl. 7*, 63 (1987)
Ferbam                                              *12*, 121 (1976) (*corr. 42*, 256);
                                                    *Suppl. 7*, 63 (1987)
Ferric oxide                                        *1*, 29 (1972); *Suppl. 7*, 216 (1987)
Ferrochromium (*see* Chromium and chromium compounds)
Fluometuron                                         *30*, 245 (1983); *Suppl. 7*, 63 (1987)
Fluoranthene                                        *32*, 355 (1983); *Suppl. 7*, 63 (1987)

# G

# H

γ-HCH (*see* Hexachlorocyclohexanes)
Heating oils (*see* Fuel oils)
Heptachlor (*see also* Chlordane/Heptachlor)          *5*, 173 (1974); *20*, 129 (1979)
Hexachlorobenzene                                     *20*, 155 (1979); *Suppl. 7*, 219 (1987)
Hexachlorobutadiene                                   *20*, 179 (1979); *Suppl. 7*, 64 (1987)
Hexachlorocyclohexanes                                *5*, 47 (1974); *20*, 195 (1979)
                                                      (*corr. 42*, 258); *Suppl. 7*, 220 (1987)

Hexachlorocyclohexane, technical-grade (*see* Hexachloro-
    cyclohexanes)
Hexachloroethane                                      *20*, 467 (1979); *Suppl. 7*, 64 (1987)
Hexachlorophene                                       *20*, 241 (1979); *Suppl. 7*, 64 (1987)
Hexamethylphosphoramide                               *15*, 211 (1977); *Suppl. 7*, 64 (1987)
Hexoestrol (*see* Nonsteroidal oestrogens)
Hycanthone mesylate                                   *13*, 91 (1977); *Suppl. 7*, 64 (1987)
Hydralazine                                           *24*, 85 (1980); *Suppl. 7*, 222 (1987)
Hydrazine                                             *4*, 127 (1974); *Suppl. 7*, 223 (1987)
Hydrogen peroxide                                     *36*, 285 (1985); *Suppl. 7*, 64 (1987)
Hydroquinone                                          *15*, 155 (1977); *Suppl. 7*, 64 (1987)
4-Hydroxyazobenzene                                   *8*, 157 (1975); *Suppl. 7*, 64 (1987)
17α-Hydroxyprogesterone caproate (*see also* Progestins)   *21*, 399 (1979) (*corr. 42*, 259)
8-Hydroxyquinoline                                    *13*, 101 (1977); *Suppl. 7*, 64 (1987)
8-Hydroxysenkirkine                                   *10*, 265 (1976); *Suppl. 7*, 64 (1987)

# I

Indeno[1,2,3-*cd*]pyrene                              *3*, 229 (1973); *32*, 373 (1983);
                                                      *Suppl. 7*, 64 (1987)

IQ                                                    *40*, 261 (1986); *Suppl. 7*, 64 (1987)
Iron and steel founding                               *34*, 133 (1984); *Suppl. 7*, 224 (1987)
Iron–dextran complex                                  *2*, 161 (1973); *Suppl. 7*, 226 (1987)
Iron–dextrin complex                                  *2*, 161 (1973) (*corr. 42*, 252);
                                                      *Suppl. 7*, 64 (1987)

Iron oxide (*see* Ferric oxide)
Iron oxide, saccharated  (*see* Saccharated iron oxide)
Iron sorbitol–citric acid complex                     *2*, 161 (1973); *Suppl. 7*, 64 (1987)
Isatidine                                             *10*, 269 (1976); *Suppl. 7*, 65 (1987)
Isoflurane (*see* Anaesthetics, volatile)
Isoniazid (*see* Isonicotinic acid hydrazide)
Isonicotinic acid hydrazide                           *4*, 159 (1974); *Suppl. 7*, 227 (1987)
Isophosphamide                                        *26*, 237 (1981); *Suppl. 7*, 65 (1987)
Isopropyl alcohol                                     *15*, 223 (1977); *Suppl. 7*, 229 (1987)
Isopropyl alcohol manufacture (strong–acid process)   *Suppl. 7*, 229 (1987)
    (*see also* Isopropyl alcohol)
Isopropyl oils                                        *15*, 223 (1977); *Suppl. 7*, 229 (1987)
Isosafrole                                            *1*, 169 (1972); *10*, 232 (1976);
                                                      *Suppl. 7*, 65 (1987)

# J

| | |
|---|---|
| Jacobine | *10*, 275 (1976); *Suppl. 7*, 65 (1987) |
| Jet fuel | *45*, 203 (1989) |
| Joinery (*see* Carpentry and joinery) | |

# K

| | |
|---|---|
| Kaempferol | 31, 171 (1983); *Suppl. 7*, 65 (1987) |
| Kepone (*see* Chlordecone) | |

# L

| | |
|---|---|
| Lasiocarpine | *10*, 281 (1976); *Suppl. 7*, 65 (1987) |
| Lauroyl peroxide | *36*, 315 (1985); Suppl. 7, 65 (1987) |
| Lead acetate (*see* Lead and lead compounds) | |
| Lead and lead compounds | *1*, 40 (1972) (*corr. 42*, 251); *2*, 52, 150 (1973); *12*, 131 (1976); *23*, 40, 208, 209, 325 (1980); *Suppl. 7*, 230 (1987) |
| | |
| Lead arsenate (*see* Arsenic and arsenic compounds) | |
| Lead carbonate (*see* Lead and lead compounds) | |
| Lead chloride (*see* Lead and lead compounds) | |
| Lead chromate (*see* Chromium and chromium compounds) | |
| Lead chromate oxide (*see* Chromium and chromium compounds) | |
| Lead naphthenate (*see* Lead and lead compounds) | |
| Lead nitrate (*see* Lead and lead compounds) | |
| Lead oxide (*see* Lead and lead compounds) | |
| Lead phosphate (*see* Lead and lead compounds) | |
| Lead subacetate (*see* Lead and lead compounds) | |
| Lead tetroxide (*see* Lead and lead compounds) | |
| Leather goods manufacture | *25*, 279 (1981); *Suppl. 7*, 235 (1987) |
| Leather industries | *25*, 199 (1981); *Suppl. 7*, 232 (1987) |
| Leather tanning and processing | *25*, 201 (1981); *Suppl. 7*, 236 (1987) |
| Ledate (*see also* Lead and lead compounds) | *12*, 131 (1976) |
| Light Green SF | *16*, 209 (1978); *Suppl. 7*, 65 (1987) |
| Lindane (*see* Hexachlorocyclohexanes) | |
| The lumber and sawmill industries (including logging) | *25*, 49 (1981); *Suppl. 7*, 383 (1987) |
| Luteoskyrin | *10*, 163 (1976); *Suppl. 7*, 65 (1987) |
| Lynoestrenol (*see also* Progestins; Combined oral contraceptives) | *21*, 407 (1979) |

# M

| | |
|---|---|
| Magenta | *4*, 57 (1974) (*corr. 42*, 252); *Suppl. 7*, 238 (1987) |

Magenta, manufacture of (*see also* Magenta)                    *Suppl. 7*, 238 (1987)
Malathion                                                       *30*, 103 (1983); *Suppl. 7*, 65 (1987)
Maleic hydrazide                                                *4*, 173 (1974) (*corr. 42*, 253);
                                                                *Suppl. 7*, 65 (1987)
Malonaldehyde                                                   *36*, 163 (1985); *Suppl. 7*, 65 (1987)
Maneb                                                           *12*, 137 (1976); *Suppl. 7*, 65 (1987)
Man–made mineral fibres                                         *43*, 39 (1988)
Mannomustine                                                    *9*, 157 (1975); *Suppl. 7*, 65 (1987)
MCPA (*see also* Chlorophenoxy herbicides; Chlorophenoxy        *30*, 255 (1983)
    herbicides, occupational exposures to)
MeA–α–C                                                         *40*, 253 (1986); *Suppl. 7*, 65 (1987)
Medphalan                                                       *9*, 168 (1975); *Suppl. 7*, 65 (1987)
Medroxyprogesterone acetate                                    *6*, 157 (1974); *21*, 417 (1979)
                                                                (*corr. 42*, 259); *Suppl. 7*, 289 (1987)
Megestrol acetate (*see* also Progestins; Combined oral
    contraceptives)
MeIQ                                                            *40*, 275 (1986); *Suppl. 7*, 65 (1987)
MeIQx                                                           *40*, 283 (1986); *Suppl. 7*, 65 (1987)
Melamine                                                        *39*, 333 (1986); *Suppl. 7*, 65 (1987)
Melphalan                                                       *9*, 167 (1975); *Suppl. 7*, 239 (1987)
6–Mercaptopurine                                                *26*, 249 (1981); *Suppl. 7*, 240 (1987)
Merphalan                                                       *9*, 169 (1975); *Suppl. 7*, 65 (1987)
Mestranol (*see also* Steroidal oestrogens)                    *6*, 87 (1974); *21*, 257 (1979)
                                                                (*corr. 42*, 259)
Methanearsonic acid, disodium salt (*see* Arsenic and arsenic
    compounds)
Methanearsonic acid, monosodium salt (*see* Arsenic and arsenic
    compounds
Methotrexate                                                    *26*, 267 (1981); *Suppl. 7*, 241 (1987)
Methoxsalen (*see* 8–Methoxypsoralen)
Methoxychlor                                                    *5*, 193 (1974); *20*, 259 (1979);
                                                                *Suppl. 7*, 66 (1987)
Methoxyflurane (*see* Anaesthetics, volatile)
5–Methoxypsoralen                                               *40*, 327 (1986); *Suppl. 7*, 242 (1987)
8–Methoxypsoralen (*see also* 8–Methoxypsoralen plus ultraviolet  *24*, 101 (1980)
    radiation)
8–Methoxypsoralen plus ultraviolet radiation                    *Suppl. 7*, 243 (1987)
Methyl acrylate                                                 *19*, 52 (1979); *39*, 99 (1986);
                                                                *Suppl. 7*, 66 (1987)
5–Methylangelicin plus ultraviolet radiation (*see also* Angelicin
    and some synthetic derivatives)                             *Suppl. 7*, 57 (1987)
2–Methylaziridine                                               *9*, 61 (1975); *Suppl. 7*, 66 (1987)
Methylazoxymethanol acetate                                    *1*, 164 (1972); *10*, 131 (1976);
                                                                *Suppl. 7*, 66 (1987)

| | |
|---|---|
| Mirex | 5, 203 (1974); 20, 283 (1979) (corr. 42, 258); Suppl. 7, 66 (1987) |
| Mitomycin C | 10, 171 (1976); Suppl. 7, 67 (1987) |
| MNNG (see N-Methyl-N'-nitro-N-nitrosoguanidine) | |
| MOCA (see 4,4'-Methylene bis(2-chloroaniline)) | |
| Modacrylic fibres | 19, 86 (1979); Suppl. 7, 67 (1987) |
| Monocrotaline | 10, 291 (1976); Suppl. 7, 67 (1987) |
| Monuron | 12, 167 (1976); Suppl. 7, 67 (1987) |
| MOPP and other combined chemotherapy including alkylating agents | Suppl. 7, 254 (1987) |
| Morpholine | 47, 199 (1989) |
| 5-(Morpholinomethyl)-3-[(5-nitrofurfurylidene)amino]-2-oxazolidinone | 7, 161 (1974); Suppl. 7, 67 (1987) |
| Mustard gas | 9, 181 (1975) (corr. 42, 254); Suppl. 7, 259 (1987) |
| Myleran (see 1,4-Butanediol dimethanesulphonate) | |

# N

| | |
|---|---|
| Nafenopin | 24, 125 (1980); Suppl. 7, 67 (1987) |
| 1,5-Naphthalenediamine | 27, 127 (1982); Suppl. 7, 67 (1987) |
| 1,5-Naphthalene diisocyanate | 19, 311 (1979); Suppl. 7, 67 (1987) |
| 1-Naphthylamine | 4, 87 (1974) (corr. 42, 253); Suppl. 7, 260 (1987) |
| 2-Naphthylamine | 4, 97 (1974); Suppl. 7, 261 (1987) |
| 1-Naphthylthiourea | 30, 347 (1983); Suppl. 7, 263 (1987) |
| Nickel acetate (see Nickel and nickel compounds) | |
| Nickel ammonium sulphate (see Nickel and nickel compounds) | |
| Nickel and nickel compounds | 2, 126 (1973) (corr. 42, 252); 11, 75 (1976); Suppl. 7, 264 (1987) (corr. 45, 283); 49, 257 (1990) |
| Nickel carbonate (see Nickel and nickel compounds) | |
| Nickel carbonyl (see Nickel and nickel compounds) | |
| Nickel chloride (see Nickel and nickel compounds) | |
| Nickel-gallium alloy (see Nickel and nickel compounds) | |
| Nickel hydroxide (see Nickel and nickel compounds) | |
| Nickelocene (see Nickel and nickel compounds) | |
| Nickel oxide (see Nickel and nickel compounds) | |
| Nickel subsulphide (see Nickel and nickel compounds) | |
| Nickel sulphate (see Nickel and nickel compounds) | |
| Niridazole | 13, 123 (1977); Suppl. 7, 67 (1987) |
| Nithiazide | 31, 179 (1983); Suppl. 7, 67 (1987) |
| Nitrilotriacetic acid and its salts | 48, 181 (1990) |
| 5-Nitroacenaphthene | 16, 319 (1978); Suppl. 7, 67 (1987) |
| 5-Nitro-ortho-anisidine | 27, 133 (1982); Suppl. 7, 67 (1987) |

3-(*N*-Nitrosomethylamino)propionaldehyde                    *37*, 263 (1985); *Suppl. 7*, 68 (1987)
3-(*N*-Nitrosomethylamino)propionitrile                      *37*, 263 (1985); *Suppl. 7*, 68 (1987)
4-(*N*-Nitrosomethylamino)-4-(3-pyridyl)-1-butanal           *37*, 205 (1985); *Suppl. 7*, 68 (1987)
4-(*N*-Nitrosomethylamino)-1-(3-pyridyl)-1-butanone          *37*, 209 (1985); *Suppl. 7*, 68 (1987)
*N*-Nitrosomethylethylamine                                  *17*, 221 (1978); *Suppl. 7*, 68 (1987)
*N*-Nitroso-*N*-methylurea (*see N*-Methyl-*N*-nitrosourea)
*N*-Nitroso-*N*-methylurethane (*see N*-Methyl-*N*-methylurethane)
*N*-Nitrosomethylvinylamine                                  *17*, 257 (1978); *Suppl. 7*, 68 (1987)
*N*-Nitrosomorpholine                                        *17*, 263 (1978); *Suppl. 7*, 68 (1987)
*N'*-Nitrosonornicotine                                      *17*, 281 (1978); *37*, 241 (1985);
                                                             *Suppl. 7*, 68 (1987)
*N*-Nitrosopiperidine                                        *17*, 287 (1978); *Suppl. 7*, 68 (1987)
*N*-Nitrosoproline                                           *17*, 303 (1978); *Suppl. 7*, 68 (1987)
*N*-Nitrosopyrrolidine                                       *17*, 313 (1978); *Suppl. 7*, 68 (1987)
*N*-Nitrososarcosine                                         *17*, 327 (1978); *Suppl. 7*, 68 (1987)
Nitrosoureas, chloroethyl (*see* Chloroethyl nitrosoureas)
5-Nitro-*ortho*-toluidine                                    *48*, 169 (1990)
Nitrous oxide (*see* Anaesthetics, volatile)
Nitrovin                                                     *31*, 185 (1983); *Suppl. 7*, 68 (1987)
NNA (*see* 4-(*N*-Nitrosomethylamino)-4-(3-pyridyl)-1-butanal)
NNK (*see* 4-(*N*-Nitrosomethylamino)-1-(3-pyridyl)-1-butanone)
Nonsteroidal oestrogens (*see also* Oestrogens, progestins and      *Suppl. 7*, 272 (1987)
   combinations)
Norethisterone (*see also* Progestins; Combined oral                *6*, 179 (1974); *21*, 461 (1979)
   contraceptives)
Norethynodrel (*see also* Progestins; Combined oral                 *6*, 191 (1974); *21*, 461 (1979) (*corr.*
   contraceptives                                                  *42*, 259)
Norgestrel (*see also* Progestins, Combined oral contraceptives)    *6*, 201 (1974); *21*, 479 (1979)
Nylon 6                                                             *19*, 120 (1979); *Suppl. 7*, 68 (1987)

# O

Ochratoxin A                                                 *10*, 191 (1976); *31*, 191 (1983) (*corr.*
                                                             *42*, 262); *Suppl. 7*, 271 (1987)
Oestradiol-17β (*see also* Steroidal oestrogens)             *6*, 99 (1974); *21*, 279 (1979)
Oestradiol 3-benzoate (*see* Oestradiol-17β)
Oestradiol dipropionate (*see* Oestradiol-17β)
Oestradiol mustard                                           *9*, 217 (1975)
Oestradiol-17β-valerate (*see* Oestradiol-17β)
Oestriol (*see also* Steroidal oestrogens)                   *6*, 117 (1974); *21*, 327 (1979)
Oestrogen-progestin combinations (*see* Oestrogens, progestins
   and combinations)
Oestrogen-progestin replacement therapy (*see also* Oestrogens,     *Suppl. 7*, 308 (1987)
   progestins and combinations)

Oestrogen replacement therapy (*see also* Oestrogens, progestins and combinations) — *Suppl. 7*, 280 (1987)

Oestrogens (*see* Oestrogens, progestins and combinations)

Oestrogens, conjugated (*see* Conjugated oestrogens)

Oestrogens, nonsteroidal (*see* Nonsteroidal oestrogens)

Oestrogens, progestins and combinations — *6* (1974); *21* (1979); *Suppl. 7*, 272 (1987)

Oestrogens, steroidal (*see* Steroidal oestrogens)

Oestrone (*see also* Steroidal oestrogens) — *6*, 123 (1974); *21*, 343 (1979) (*corr. 42*, 259)

Oestrone benzoate (*see* Oestrone)

Oil Orange SS — *8*, 165 (1975); *Suppl. 7*, 69 (1987)

Oral contraceptives, combined (*see* Combined oral contraceptives)

Oral contraceptives, investigational (*see* Combined oral contraceptives)

Oral contraceptives, sequential (*see* Sequential oral contraceptives)

Orange I — *8*, 173 (1975); *Suppl. 7*, 69 (1987)

Orange G — *8*, 181 (1975); *Suppl. 7*, 69 (1987)

Organolead compounds (*see also* Lead and lead compounds) — *Suppl. 7*, 230 (1987)

Oxazepam — *13*, 58 (1977); *Suppl. 7*, 69 (1987)

Oxymetholone (*see also* Androgenic (anabolic) steroids) — *13*, 131 (1977)

Oxyphenbutazone — *13*, 185 (1977); *Suppl. 7*, 69 (1987)

# P

Paint manufacture and painting (occupational exposures in) — *47*, 329 (1989)

Panfuran S (*see also* Dihydroxymethylfuratrizine) — *24*, 77 (1980); *Suppl. 7*, 69 (1987)

Paper manufacture (*see* Pulp and paper manufacture)

Parasorbic acid — *10*, 199 (1976) (*corr. 42*, 255); *Suppl. 7*, 69 (1987)

Parathion — *30*, 153 (1983); *Suppl. 7*, 69 (1987)

Patulin — *10*, 205 (1976); *40*, 83 (1986); *Suppl. 7*, 69 (1987)

Penicillic acid — *10*, 211 (1976); *Suppl. 7*, 69 (1987)

Pentachloroethane — *41*, 99 (1986); *Suppl. 7*, 69 (1987)

Pentachloronitrobenzene (*see* Quintozene)

Pentachlorophenol (*see also* Chlorophenols; Chlorophenols, occupational exposures to) — *20*, 303 (1979)

Perylene — *32*, 411 (1983); *Suppl. 7*, 69 (1987)

Petasitenine — *31*, 207 (1983); *Suppl. 7*, 69 (1987)

*Petasites japonicus* (*see* Pyrrolizidine alkaloids)

Petroleum refining (occupational exposures in) — *45*, 39 (1989)

Some petroleum solvents — *47*, 43 (1989)

Phenacetin — *13*, 141 (1977); *24*, 135 (1980); *Suppl. 7*, 310 (1987)

Phenanthrene                                         *32*, 419 (1983); *Suppl. 7*, 69 (1987)
Phenazopyridine hydrochloride                        *8*, 117 (1975); *24*, 163 (1980) (*corr.*
                                                     *42*, 260); *Suppl. 7*, 312 (1987)
Phenelzine sulphate                                  *24*, 175 (1980); *Suppl. 7*, 312 (1987)
Phenicarbazide                                       *12*, 177 (1976); *Suppl. 7*, 70 (1987)
Phenobarbital                                        *13*, 157 (1977); *Suppl. 7*, 313 (1987)
Phenol                                               *47*, 263 (1989)
Phenoxyacetic acid herbicides (*see* Chlorophenoxy herbicides)
Phenoxybenzamine hydrochloride                       *9*, 223 (1975); *24*, 185 (1980);
                                                     *Suppl. 7*, 70 (1987)
Phenylbutazone                                       *13*, 183 (1977); *Suppl. 7*, 316 (1987)
*meta*-Phenylenediamine                              *16*, 111 (1978); *Suppl. 7*, 70 (1987)
*para*-Phenylenediamine                              *16*, 125 (1978); *Suppl. 7*, 70 (1987)
*N*-Phenyl-2-naphthylamine                           *16*, 325 (1978) (*corr. 42*, 257);
                                                     *Suppl. 7*, 318 (1987)
*ortho*-Phenylphenol                                 *30*, 329 (1983); *Suppl. 7*, 70 (1987)
Phenytoin                                            *13*, 201 (1977); *Suppl. 7*, 319 (1987)
Piperazine oestrone sulphate (*see* Conjugated oestrogens)
Piperonyl butoxide                                   *30*, 183 (1983); *Suppl. 7*, 70 (1987)
Pitches, coal-tar (*see* Coal-tar pitches)
Polyacrylic acid                                     *19*, 62 (1979); *Suppl. 7*, 70 (1987)
Polybrominated biphenyls                             *18*, 107 (1978); *41*, 261 (1986);
                                                     *Suppl. 7*, 321 (1987)
Polychlorinated biphenyls                            *7*, 261 (1974); *18*, 43 (1978) (*corr.*
                                                     *42*, 258);
                                                     *Suppl. 7*, 322 (1987)
Polychlorinated camphenes (*see* Toxaphene)
Polychloroprene                                      *19*, 141 (1979); *Suppl. 7*, 70 (1987)
Polyethylene                                         *19*, 164 (1979); *Suppl. 7*, 70 (1987)
Polymethylene polyphenyl isocyanate                  *19*, 314 (1979); *Suppl. 7*, 70 (1987)
Polymethyl methacrylate                              *19*, 195 (1979); *Suppl. 7*, 70 (1987)
Polyoestradiol phosphate (*see* Oestradiol-17β)
Polypropylene                                        *19*, 218 (1979); *Suppl. 7*, 70 (1987)
Polystyrene                                          *19*, 245 (1979); *Suppl. 7*, 70 (1987)
Polytetrafluoroethylene                              *19*, 288 (1979); *Suppl. 7*, 70 (1987)
Polyurethane foams                                   *19*, 320 (1979); *Suppl. 7*, 70 (1987)
Polyvinyl acetate                                    *19*, 346 (1979); *Suppl. 7*, 70 (1987)
Polyvinyl alcohol                                    *19*, 351 (1979); *Suppl. 7*, 70 (1987)
Polyvinyl chloride                                   *7*, 306 (1974); *19*, 402 (1979);
                                                     *Suppl. 7*, 70 (1987)
Polyvinyl pyrrolidone                                *19*, 463 (1979); *Suppl. 7*, 70 (1987)
Ponceau MX                                           *8*, 189 (1975); *Suppl. 7*, 70 (1987)
Ponceau 3R                                           *8*, 199 (1975); *Suppl. 7*, 70 (1987)
Ponceau SX                                           *8*, 207 (1975); *Suppl. 7*, 70 (1987)
Potassium arsenate (*see* Arsenic and arsenic compounds)

# Q

# R

# T

# U

# V

# W

# X

# Y